Comprehensive Exam Review *for* the Pharmacy Technician

Comprehensive Exam Review for the Pharmacy Technician

Jahangir Moini, MD, MPH

Director of Pharmacy Technician Programs
Florida Metropolitan University
Melbourne, Florida

DELMAR
CENGAGE Learning™

Australia Canada Mexico Singapore Spain United Kingdom United States

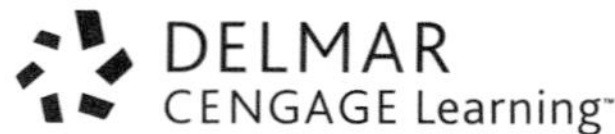

Comprehensive Exam Review for the Pharmacy Technician
Jahangir Moini

Vice President, Health Care Business Unit:
William Brottmiller

Editorial Director:
Cathy L. Esperti

Acquisitions Editors:
Maureen Rosener

Senior Developmental Editor:
Darcy M. Scelsi

Editorial Assistant:
Elizabeth Howe

Marketing Director:
Jennifer McAvey

Channel Manager:
Lisa Stover

Art and Design Specialist:
Alex Vasilakos

Production Coordinator:
Jessica McNavich

Project Editor:
Daniel Branagh

Technology Project Manager:
Sherry Conners

Library of Congress Control Number: 2004058810
ISBN-13: 978-1-4018-4131-7

ISBN-10: 1-4018-4131-7

Delmar Cengage Learning
5 Maxwell Drive
Clifton Park, NY 12065-2919
USA

Cengage Learning products are represented in Canada by Nelson Education, Ltd.

For your lifelong learning solutions, visit **delmar.cengage.com**

Visit our corporate website at **www.cengage.com**

Notice to the Reader
Publisher does not warrant or guarantee any of the products described herein or perform any independent analysis in connection with any of the product information contained herein. Publisher does not assume, and expressly disclaims, any obligation to obtain and include information other than that provided to it by the manufacturer. The reader is expressly warned to consider and adopt all safety precautions that might be indicated by the activities described herein and to avoid all potential hazards. By following the instructions contained herein, the reader willingly assumes all risks in connection with such instructions. The publisher makes no representations or warranties of any kind, including but not limited to, the warranties of fitness for particular purpose or merchantability, nor are any such representations implied with respect to the material set forth herein, and the publisher takes no responsibility with respect to such material. The publisher shall not be liable for any special, consequential, or exemplary damages resulting, in whole or part, from the readers' use of, or reliance upon, this material.

Printed in the United States of America
10 11 12 13 12 11 10 09 08

Contents

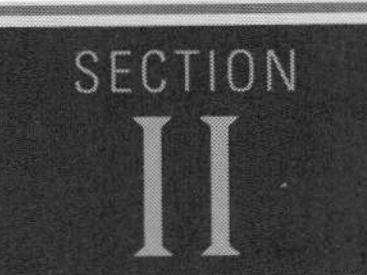

SECTION II THE SCIENCE OF PHARMACOLOGY ▪ 33

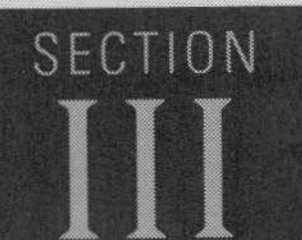

SECTION III HOSPITAL AND RETAIL PHARMACY ▪ 47

15 Computer Applications in Drug-Use Control ▪ 111

16 Communications ▪ 116

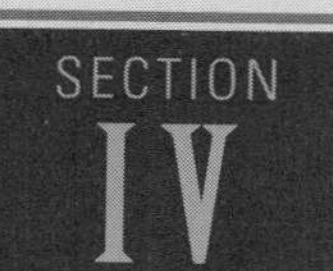

SECTION IV DRUG CLASSIFICATIONS ▪ 123

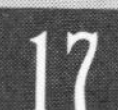

17 Biopharmaceutics ▪ 124

Dedication

This book is dedicated to:
My lovely wife, Hengameh,
and to my daughters, Mahkameh and Morvarid
who have sacrificed much time away from me
while I was writing this book.

Preface

The rapid and substantial progress made in the field of pharmacy within the past two decades has created a necessity for changing the role and responsibility of pharmacists. Therefore, pharmacy services in the hospital and organized delivery systems have changed dramatically. Modifications in pharmacy practice reflect the transformation that has occurred in health care delivery. This evolution encompasses a renewed emphasis on outpatient care and an increased focus on patient care outcomes and treatment costs. Because pharmacists traditionally have provided services in both the ambulatory and inpatient environments, the pharmacy profession has adapted well to the movement of care delivery to the outpatient setting.

Biotechnology has grown rapidly as a means to identify disease pathology and to develop effective drugs to treat a specific disease process. Pharmacies and pharmacists have made adjustments to secure biotechnology drug therapies and to deliver them in a timely and cost-effective manner.

The pharmacy profession has changed to meet the new demands of society. Pharmacists have accepted direct patient care responsibilities, supported by information systems, automation, robotics, and enhanced roles for pharmacy technicians.

Today, many of the drug preparation and distribution tasks of pharmacists have been delegated to trained pharmacy technicians. Pharmacy technicians work under the direct supervision of a pharmacist. All pharmacy technicians have completed high school and most have completed one or two years of college.

Pharmacy technicians are trained and educated to work in a variety of care delivery areas, including inpatient care, home care, and ambulatory care. Most states register or license pharmacy technicians and require applicants to pass an examination and complete continuing education to maintain registration. A growing number of pharmacy technicians seek certification on a national level to document skills and knowledge to serve in this profession.

Certified technicians are able to provide valuable support for the pharmacist and pharmacy services. Since I became Director of the Pharmacy program at Florida Metropolitan University, I have become increasingly aware of the valuable role of pharmacy technicians in supporting pharmacists to serve patients more effectively. The requirements for pharmacy technicians to pass difficult certification examinations prompted me to write these books, *Comprehensive Exam Review for the Pharmacy Technician,* and *Pharmacy Technician: A Comprehensive Approach.*

The *Comprehensive Exam Review for the Pharmacy Technician* contains 36 chapters and a practice CD. Throughout the preparation of this text, making the content as clear and understandable as possible for today's pharmacy technicians and students has been of great importance. Each chapter contains 15 to 20 multiple-choice questions. At the end of the book, Appendix A contains 150 questions similar to those on the Pharmacy Technician Certification Board exam, and Appendix B contains 30 case study questions. The CD-ROM that accompanies this book contains 600 multiple-choice questions. The goals of this book have been to focus on only the essential information that the technician needs to know for preparation for the national certification exam. Emphasis has been placed on federal law, calculation of medications, medical terminology, the role of pharmacy technicians in different areas of the pharmacy (including hospital, retail, and ambulatory pharmacy settings), and pharmacology.

Jahangir Moini, MD, MPH

Contributors and Reviewers

Contributors

Maggie Carpenter, PharmD
Adjunct Professor
Florida Metropolitan University
Director of Pharmacy Department
Sea Pines Hospital
Melbourne, FL

Joseph Infantino, MD
Retired Gynecologist
Adjunct Professor
Florida Metropolitan University
Melbourne, FL

Patricia A. Lawton, RN
Retired Nurse
Adjunct Professor
Florida Metropolitan University
Melbourne, FL

Mahkameh Moini
Nova-Southeastern University
School of Dental Medicine
Fort Lauderdale, FL

Stephanie K. Mullen, RN, MSN, CPNP
Pediatric Nurse Practioner
Medical College of Wisconsin
Children's Hospital of Wisconsin
Milwaukee, WI

Susan Neil, MBA, RNP, LMIF
Chief Operating Officer
Alternate Family Care, Inc.
West Palm Beach, FL

Nicole Ostroff-Bologna, CMA, BS
Academic Advisor
Adjunct Professor
Florida Metropolitan University
Melbourne, FL

Jeanette Pham, ARNP, BC
Adjunct Professor
Florida Metropolitan University
Melbourne, FL

Vincent E. Trunzo, RPh, MSM
Adjunct Professor
Florida Metropolitan University
Director of Pharmacy, Health First Inc.
Holmes Regional Medical Center
Melbourne, FL

Greg Vadimsky, Pharm Tech
Pharmacy Technician in Training
Florida Metropolitan University
Melbourne, FL

Reviewers

Renee Acosta, RPh, MS
Pharmacy Technician Department Chair
Austin Community College
Austin, TX

Jeanie Barkett, BS, RPh
Professor
Clark College
Vancouver, WA

Nora Chan, Pharm D
Pharmacy Technician Program Coordinator
San Francisco Community College
San Francisco, CA

Christopher Miller, Pharm D, BCPP
Director of Pharmacy Services
Circles of Care, Inc.
Melbourne, FL

James Mizner, RPh, MBA
Pharmacy Technician Program Coordinator
Applied Career Training
Rosslyn, VA

Stephanie K. Mullen, RN, MSN, CPNP
Pediatric Nurse Practitioner
Medical College of Wisconsin
Children's Hospital of Wisconsin
Milwaukee, WI

Agnes Pucillo, BSN, ACHI, RHE
Educational Supervisor for Allied Health
The Cittone Institute
Edison, NJ

Karen Snipe, CPhT, AS, BA, MAEd
Pharmacy Technician Program Coordinator
Trident Technical College
Charleston, SC

About the Author

Dr. Moini is a/an:
Husband
Father
Author
Physician
Professor
Director
Chairman
Chief Proctor
Biological Scientist III
Epidemiologist
Health Educator Consultant
Physician Liaison of the Florida Society of Medical Assistants

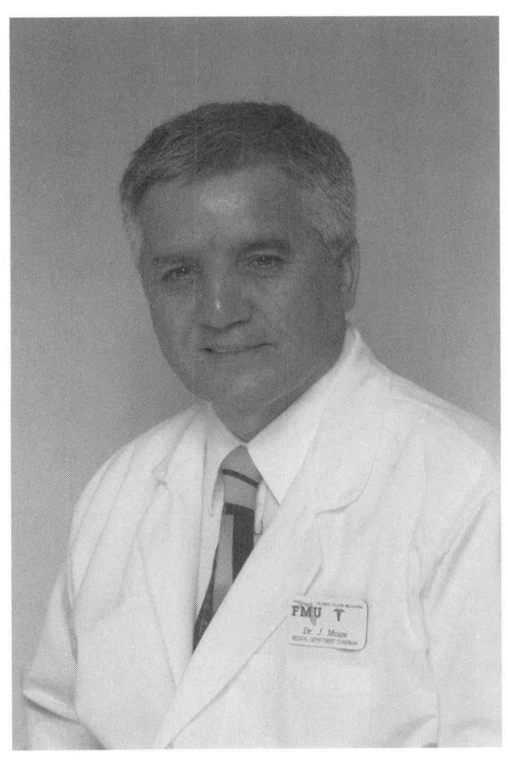

SECTION I

Introduction

1 The Foundation of Pharmaceutical Care

OUTLINE

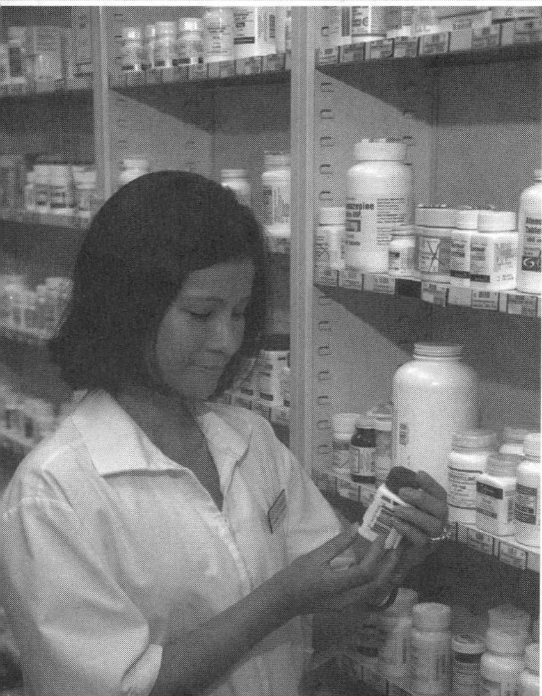

GLOSSARY

pharmaceutical care The role of the pharmacist is to be responsible for providing drug therapy for the purpose of achieving the improvement of a patient's quality of life.

pharmacist An individual who is educated and licensed to dispense drugs and to provide drug information.

pharmacy The art and science of dispensing and preparing medication and providing drug-related information to the public.

pharmacy technician An individual who helps licensed pharmacists provide medication and other health care products to patients.

Pharmacy Technician Certification Board A national organization that provides certification to pharmacy technicians based on a national examination and continuing education.

PHARMACEUTICAL CARE

The current philosophy or approach to professional practice in pharmacy is referred to as **pharmaceutical care**. This concept holds that the important role of the pharmacist is to ensure "the responsible provision of drug therapy for the purpose of achieving definite outcomes that improve a patient's quality of life." A **Pharmacist** then, is one who is educated and licensed to dispense drugs and provide drug information. Pharmacists are experts on medications. They are the most accessible member of today's health care team. Increased drug knowledge, medical progress, commerce, technology, and professional development have come together to produce modern pharmacy and pharmaceutical care throughout the world.

The Profession of Pharmacy

The profession of pharmacy involves a specialized body of knowledge. Practitioners perform a highly useful social and health care–related function. All lawful occupations provide some positive benefit to society and are based on specialized knowledge. Working in the field of pharmacy is typically considered a more socially useful profession than many other occupations, but social utility alone does not make an occupation a profession. Pharmacists are not considered professionals because they have good typing skills—it is their relevant professional knowledge about medications and patient care and interactions that set them apart. Pharmacists advise patients and prescribers concerning drug therapy, are alert for potential drug interactions, select appropriate product sources, and exercise professional judgment. Exercising proper judgment is an essential skill. In addition to these characteristics, specific attitudes also influence professional behavior. Professionals are concerned with matters that are vital to the health or well-being of their patients.

Pharmacy Practice

Pharmacy is the art and science of dispensing and preparing medication and providing drug-related information to the public. It involves interpreting prescription orders; compounding, labeling, and dispensing drugs and devices; selecting drug products and conducting drug utilization reviews; monitoring patients and intervening as necessary; and providing cognitive services related to use of medications and devices. Today, pharmaceutical care is a necessary element of total health care. There are currently two professional degrees in pharmacy: the baccalaureate (BS Pharm) and the doctorate (PharmD). The curriculum of the BS in pharmacy usually requires 5 academic years of study. The PharmD curriculum usually requires 6 academic years to complete the degree requirements.

Pharmaceutical Testing, Analysis, and Control

Developing methods for standardizing and controlling medicines is vital. (Control is a method used to eliminate or reduce the potential harm of the drug distributed. Drug control provides knowledge, understanding, judgments, procedures, skills, controls, and ethics that ensure optimal safety in distribution and use of medication.) In manufacturing laboratories, pharmacists often perform physical and chemical analyses either in the course of developing dosage forms of new products or in the control of standard products. In small laboratories, the responsibility for performing analyses may be delegated entirely to pharmacy staff members. However, even if pharmacists are not conducting analyses, they should at a minimum understand the basic principles involved in the standardization and control of the medicinal agents dispensed. The use of an analytical method is justified only after it has been proved to be valid, accurate, and selective. Drug control is the most important goal for medications that may be taken by patients.

PHARMACY TECHNICIANS

To keep up with the increasing demand for pharmaceutical products and services, pharmacy technicians can play a vital role in supporting pharmaceutical care. A **pharmacy technician** helps licensed pharmacists provide medication and other health care products to patients. Technicians usually perform routine tasks, such as counting tablets and labeling bottles, to help prepare prescribed medication for patients. Technicians refer any questions regarding prescription, drug information, or health matters to a pharmacist.

Two-thirds of all pharmacy technician jobs in the United States are in retail pharmacies, and one-third in hospitals. Pharmacy technicians who work in retail pharmacies have varying responsibilities, depending on the rules and regulations of the state in which they are working. In hospitals, pharmacy technicians have additional responsibilities. They read patient charts and prepare and deliver the medicine to patients. The pharmacist must check the order before it is dispensed to the patient. Pharmacy technicians also may assemble a 24-hour supply of medicine for patients within an institutional setting.

The National Certification Exam

Certification (via the national exam) is a valuable component of the pharmacy technician's career. This certification exam is performed by the **Pharmacy Technician Certification Board** (PTCB). This test is a standardized national exam that tests knowledge and competency in basic functions of the pharmacy and its activities. Skills are measured in three general areas:

1. Assisting the pharmacist in serving patients
2. Maintaining medication and inventory control systems

3. Participating in the administration and management of the pharmacy

The exam, which lasts for 3 hours, contains 140 multiple-choice questions, 15 of which are not actually scored (these are pretest questions that serve only to gather statistics for future exams). The questions are not presented in distinct sections relating to the three general areas being tested; rather, they are presented randomly throughout the exam. A score of at least 650 (of a possible 300 to 900) is required to pass.

Assisting the Pharmacist in Serving Patients

The exam questions that address assisting pharmacists in serving patients make up 64% of the exam. This portion includes approximately 60 to 70 questions and covers both retail and hospital settings. Technicians must prepare themselves for questions about how to interpret the prescription order; the structure and use of the patient profile; and the dispensing, labeling, storage, and delivery of medications. Questions related to this area also include drug calculations.

Maintaining Medication and Inventory Control Systems

The exam questions that address maintaining medications and inventory control systems include questions about the storage of medications in the pharmacy, the ordering and inventory process, prepackaging and unit dose distribution, labeling, and record keeping. These questions account for 25% of the exam (40 to 50 questions).

Participating in the Administration and Management of the Pharmacy

The questions that test knowledge about participating in the administration and management of the pharmacy deal with topics such as safety, cleanliness, infection control, pharmacy law, communications, and computers. These questions make up 11% of the exam.

Continuing Education

Certification for the pharmacy technician is good for 2 years and must then be renewed. To become eligible for recertification every 2 years, certified pharmacy technicians (CPhTs) must meet requirements of 20 contact hours of pharmacy-related continuing education. At least 1 contact hour must be in pharmacy law. This can be accomplished through various means, such as educational meetings, seminars, workshops, and conventions. Up to 10 contact hours can be earned when the technician is employed under the direct supervision and instruction of a pharmacist. The annual American Association of Pharmacy Technicians (AAPT) or National Pharmacy Technician Association (NPTA) convention provides an excellent forum for attaining knowledge through its educational offerings and for networking with other pharmacy technicians. Continuing education is a lifelong process.

PROFESSIONAL ORGANIZATIONS

Professional people in the pharmacy, like other businesses, have created organizations or associations to advance the purposes of their professions. The most important organizations in the pharmacy profession are discussed in the following sections.

American Association of Colleges of Pharmacy

The American Association of Colleges of Pharmacy (AACP), established in 1900, represents all 79 pharmacy colleges and schools in the United States and is the national organization representing the interests of pharmaceutical education and educators. The AACP publishes the journal *American Journal of Pharmaceutical Education,* a monthly newsletter, as well as some other publications.

American Association of Pharmaceutical Scientists

The American Association of Pharmaceutical Scientists (AAPS), formerly an academy of the American Pharmacists Association, represents pharmaceutical scientists employed in academia, industry, government, and other research institutions. The AAPS publishes the journals *Pharmaceutical Research, Pharmaceutical Development and Technology,* and *Journal of Pharmaceutical Marketing and Management* and its newsletter.

American Association of Pharmacy Technicians

The American Association of Pharmacy Technicians (AAPT), formerly called the APT, was founded in 1979. It is a national organization and has chapters in many states. It represents pharmacy technicians and promotes certification of technicians. The association has established a Code of Ethics for Pharmacy Technicians.

American College of Clinical Pharmacy

The American College of Clinical Pharmacy (ACCP) is a professional and scientific society that provides leadership, education, advocacy, and resources for clinical pharmacists.

American Council on Pharmaceutical Education

The American Council on Pharmaceutical Education (ACPE), founded in 1932, is the national accrediting agency for pharmacy education programs recognized by the Secretary of Education.

American Pharmacists Association

The largest of the national pharmacy organizations, the American Pharmacists Association (APhA), consists of three academies: the Academy of Pharmacy Practice and Management (APhA-APPM), the Academy of Pharmaceutical Research and Science (APhA-APRS), and the Academy of Students of Pharmacy (APhA-APS). The APhA publishes the bimonthly *Journal of the American Pharmacists Association,* the monthly *Pharmacy Today Newsletter,* and the monthly *Journal of Pharmaceutical Sciences*. The APhA also operates a political action committee, or PAC. According to the APhA, its mission is "to advocate the interests of pharmacists; influence the profession, government, and others in addressing essential pharmaceutical care issues; promote the highest professional and ethical standards; and foster science and research in support of the practice of pharmacy."

American Society of Health-System Pharmacists

The American Society of Health-System Pharmacists (ASHP) is a large organization that represents pharmacists who practice in hospitals, health maintenance organizations (HMOs), long-term care facilities, home care agencies, and other institutions. The ASHP is a national accrediting organization for pharmacy residency and pharmacy technician training programs. The ASHP publishes the *American Journal of Health-System Pharmacy*.

United States Drug Enforcement Administration

The U.S. Drug Enforcement Administration (DEA) enforces federal laws and regulations related to controlled substances.

United States Food and Drug Administration

The U.S. Food and Drug Administration (FDA) is the federal government agency charged with primary responsibility for creating regulations governing the safety of foods, drugs, and cosmetics. The FDA enforces the Food, Drug, and Cosmetic Act of 1938 and its subsequent amendments, oversees new drug development, approves or disapproves applications to market new drugs, monitors reports of adverse reactions, and has the authority to recall drugs deemed dangerous.

Pharmacy Technician Certification Board

The Pharmacy Technician Certification Board (PTCB) administers the Pharmacy Technician Certification Examination (PTCE). The PTCE is taken voluntarily by anyone who wishes to be certified in the United States. This organization also oversees a recertification program for technicians.

Pharmacy Technician Educators Council

The Pharmacy Technician Educators Council (PTEC) is an association of educators who prepare people for careers as pharmacy technicians. Its official publication is the *Journal of Pharmacy Technology*.

United States Pharmacopeia

The U.S. Pharmacopoeia (USP) is a nonprofit organization that sets standards for the identity, strength, quality, purity, packaging, and labeling of drug products. The USP provides drug information online.

JOB OUTLOOK

Excellent job opportunities are expected for full-time and part-time work, especially for pharmacy technicians with formal training or previous experience. Job openings for pharmacy technicians will result from the expansion of retail pharmacies and other employment settings and from the need to replace workers who leave the field. Employment of pharmacy technicians is expected to grow much faster than the average for all occupations through 2010 as a result of the increased pharmaceutical needs of a larger and older population. The increased number of middle-aged and elderly people, who, on average, use more prescription drugs than do younger people, will spur demand for pharmacy technicians in all practice settings. With advances in science, newer medications are becoming available to treat more conditions. Cost-conscious insurers, pharmacies, and health systems will continue to emphasize the role of pharmacy technicians. As a result, pharmacy technicians will assume responsibility for more routine tasks previously performed by pharmacists. Pharmacy technicians also will need to learn and master new pharmacy technology as it surfaces. For example, robotic machines are used to dispense medicine into containers, and pharmacy technicians must oversee the machines, stock the bins, and label the containers. Thus, although automation is increasingly incorporated into the job, it will not necessarily reduce the need for pharmacy technicians.

WEB SITES OF INTEREST

American Association of Colleges of Pharmacy:
http://www.aacp.org
American Association of Pharmaceutical Scientists:
http://www.aaps.org
American Association of Pharmacy Technicians:
http://www.pharmacytechnician.com
American College of Clinical Pharmacology: http://www.accp1.org
Accreditation Council for Pharmacy Education:
http://www.acpe-accredit.org
American Pharmacists Association: http://www.aphanet.org
American Society of Health-System Pharmacists:
http://www.ashp.org

Pharmacy Technician Certification Board: http://www.ptcb.org
Pharmacy Technician Educators Council: http://www.rxptec.org
U.S. Drug Enforcement Administration: http://www.usdoj.gov/dea
U.S. Food and Drug Administration: http://www.fda.gov
U.S. Pharmacopeia: http://www.usp.org

REVIEW QUESTIONS

1. The national testing of a pharmacy technician is administered by the
A. Illinois Council of Health-System Pharmacists.
B. American Society of Health-System Pharmacists.
C. Pharmacy Technician Certification Board.
D. National American Pharmacy Technicians.

2. Recertification of a pharmacy technician occurs when the individual has completed
A. 10 hours of credit every 2 years in pharmacy-related study.
B. 10 contact hours of credit in pharmacy law.
C. 20 hours of credit every 2 years in pharmacy-related study.
D. 40 hours of credit; it is not required for recertification.

3. Pharmacists are those who are educated and licensed to
A. dispense drugs and provide drug information.
B. dispense information but not drugs.
C. dispense alternative remedies rather than the drugs prescribed.
D. test pharmacy technicians and provide their certification.

4. The key elements of professionals in the pharmacy include all of the following, except
A. using proper judgment.
B. having good typing skills.
C. having specific attitudes that influence professional behavior.
D. possessing relevant professional knowledge about drugs.

5. Pharmacy is
A. the art of drug therapy.
B. only about drug product selection.
C. exclusively about interpreting prescriptions from doctors' handwriting.
D. the art and science of dispensing and preparing medication and providing drug-related information to the public.

6. The most important goal for patients' medication is
A. that it be inexpensive.
B. drug control.
C. that it be easy to open.
D. drug therapy.

7. Pharmacy technicians perform some routine tasks, such as
A. prescribing medications.
B. counting tablets and labeling bottles.
C. referring questions to medical assistants.
D. counting patients and giving out free samples.

8. Of the questions on the National Certification Exam, 64% concern
A. medication distribution and inventory control.
B. the Pharmacy Technician Certification Board.
C. pharmacy operations.
D. assisting the pharmacist in serving patients.

9. *AAPT* stands for
A. American Association of Pharmaceutical Terminology.
B. Automatic Accreditation of Pharmacy Technicians.
C. American Association of Pharmacy Technicians.
D. American Association of Pharmaceutical Torts.

10. Which government bureau enforces federal laws and regulations related to controlled substances?
A. DEA
B. FDA
C. DDA
D. LSD

Pharmacy Law and Ethics for Technicians 2

OUTLINE

Law and Ethics in Pharmacy
Governing Bodies
Types of Law
- Constitutional Law
- Statutory Law
- Administrative Law
- Common Law
- International Law

State and Federal Pharmacy Laws, Regulations, and Agencies
- The Pure Food and Drug Act of 1906
- The Food, Drug, and Cosmetic Act of 1938
- The Durham-Humphrey Amendment of 1951
- The Kefauver-Harris Amendment of 1962
- The Comprehensive Drug Abuse Prevention and Control Act of 1970
- The Poison Prevention Act of 1970
- The Drug Listing Act of 1972
- The Drug Regulation Reform Act of 1978
- The Orphan Drug Act of 1983
- The Drug Price Competition and Patent-Term Restoration Act of 1984
- The Prescription Drug Marketing Act of 1987
- The Omnibus Budget Reconciliation Act of 1990
- The Occupational Health and Safety Administration
- Health Insurance Portability and Accountability Act of 1996
- Centers for Disease Control and Prevention

Drug Standards
The Ethical Foundation of Pharmacy

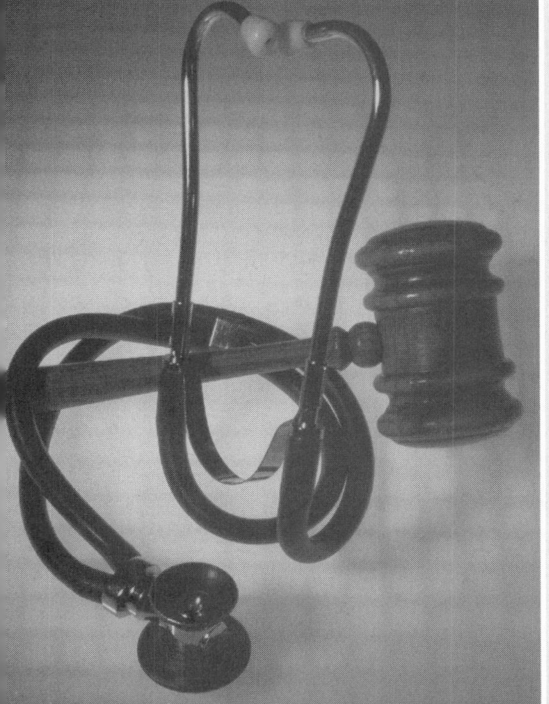

GLOSSARY

administrative law Regulations set forth by governmental agencies, such as the Internal Revenue Service (IRS) and the Social Security Administration (SSA).
bioethics A discipline dealing with the ethical and moral implications of biological research and applications.
case law Law established by judicial decision in legal cases and used as legal precedent.
common law Derives authority from ancient usages and customs affirmed by court judgments and decrees.
constitutional law Deals with interpretation and implementation of the United States Constitution.
ethics The branch of philosophy that deals with the distinction between right and wrong and with the moral consequences of human actions.
international law Law based on treaties and other agreements between two or more countries.
law A principle or rule that is advisable or obligatory to observe.
National Drug Code (NDC) A unique and permanent product code assigned to each new drug as it becomes available in the marketplace; it identifies the manufacturer or distributor, the drug formulation, and the size and type of its packaging.
National Formulary (NF) A database of officially recognized drug names.
regulatory law Regulations set forth by governmental agencies. It is also called administrative law.
standards Established by authority, custom, or general consent as a model or example; something set up and established by authority as a rule for the measure of quantity, weight, extent, value, or quality.
statutory law The body of laws enacted by a legislative body with the power to make law.
U.S. Pharmacopeia (USP) A database of drugs and their preparation that serves as the standard for drugs used in the United States.

LAW AND ETHICS IN PHARMACY

Laws, standards, and ethics can exercise controls on pharmacy and drugs. A **law** is a rule or regulation established by a governing body. Laws are enacted both to protect society as a whole and to maintain order and standards of living. **Ethics** is the study of values or principles governing personal relationships. These values and principles are used to determine whether actions are right or wrong. Ethics are based on morals, a particular behavior or rule of conduct that is formed through the influences of family, culture, and society. **Standards** are guidelines for practice established by professional organizations. Professionals in a particular area of practice share a common philosophy (a basic viewpoint or shared beliefs, concepts, attitudes, and values). This common philosophy dictates the etiquette, or standards of behavior, considered appropriate for that profession. The philosophy and etiquette established within a profession drive the standards that are established for the profession. Pharmacists and pharmacy technicians are responsible for upholding legal and ethical standards in their profession.

GOVERNING BODIES

Laws are created and upheld by federal, state, and local government. In the United States, the federal government is divided into three branches:

1. The legislative branch consists of the Congress (that is, the House of Representatives and the Senate). This branch is responsible for creating laws.
2. The executive branch consists of the president, vice president, cabinets, and various smaller organizations. This branch of government enforces law.
3. The judicial branch consists of the Supreme Court and lower federal courts. This branch interprets laws.

The federal government creates, issues, and interprets laws for the general population. State and local governments are responsible for determining the specifics of certain laws within their jurisdictions.

Regulatory agencies are government-based departments that create specific rules about what is and is not legal within a specific field or area of expertise. The regulatory agency for the field of pharmacy is the U.S. Food and Drug Administration (FDA), which is a branch of the Department of Health and Human Services. Among other things, the FDA regulates all drugs with the exception of illegal drugs. All legislation pertaining to drug administration is initiated, implemented, and enforced by the FDA. The FDA is responsible for the approval of drugs, over-the-counter (OTC) and prescription drug labeling, and standards for drug manufacturing.

TYPES OF LAW

As society grows and changes, the laws change to conform to current realities and to try to govern future realities. The main types of law are constitutional, statutory, administrative, common, and international.

Constitutional Law

In the broadest sense, **constitutional law** deals with the interpretation and implementation of the U.S. Constitution. This type of law deals with the fundamental relationships within our society, such as relationships among states, relationships among states and the federal government, and the rights of the individual in relation to state and federal government.

Statutory Law

Statutory law is the body of laws enacted by a legislative body with the power to make law. In the federal government, this legislative body is Congress.

Administrative Law

Administrative law is the rules and regulations established by agencies of the federal government. This law is also called the **regulatory law.** Administrative law agencies are given authority by Congress to write these rules.

Common Law

Common law, also known as **case law**, describes law created by judges based on previous court decisions. Areas of common law include contracts, property law, domestic law, and torts.

International Law

International law is based on treaties and other agreements between two or more countries. International law defines the rules and principles governing the relations between nations, specifically the rights between several countries or between countries and the citizens of other countries.

STATE AND FEDERAL PHARMACY LAWS, REGULATIONS, AND AGENCIES

Pharmacy practice is regulated by a series of rules, regulations, and laws that are enforced by local, state, and federal governments. In 1906, the U.S. Congress passed the first laws to regulate the development, compounding, distribution, storage, and dispensing of drugs.

The Pure Food and Drug Act of 1906

The purpose of the Pure Food and Drug Act of 1906 was to forbid the interstate distribution or sale of adulterated and misbranded food and drugs. The act did not require that drugs be labeled, only that the label not contain false information about the strength or purity of the drug. Therefore, the act, after amended, proved unenforceable, and new legislation was required. In 1937, the need for new legislation was tragically demonstrated by 107 deaths caused by the sale of a sulfa drug product that contained diethylene glycol, used today as an antifreeze for automobile radiators.

The Food, Drug, and Cosmetic Act of 1938

The Food, Drug, and Cosmetic Act (FDCA) of 1938 created the FDA and required pharmaceutical manufacturers to file a New Drug Application with the FDA. Under this act, manufacturers must maintain the purity, strength, effectiveness, safety, and packaging of drugs. Food and cosmetics are also regulated under this act. This act empowers the FDA to approve or deny new drug applications and to conduct inspections to ensure compliance. The FDA approves the investigational use of drugs on humans and ensures that all approved drugs are safe and effective. Any adverse reaction to a drug should be reported to the FDA.

The Durham-Humphrey Amendment of 1951

The Durham-Humphrey Amendment of 1951 states that drug containers do not have to include "adequate directions for use" as long as they bear the legend "Caution: Federal law prohibits dispensing without a prescription." The dispensing of the drug by a pharmacist with a label giving directions from the practitioner meets the law's requirements. Therefore, this amendment established the difference between legend, or prescription, drugs and OTC, or nonprescription, drugs. This amendment also authorized the acceptance of verbal prescriptions and the refilling of prescriptions.

The Kefauver-Harris Amendment of 1962

The Kefauver-Harris Amendment of 1962 was passed in response to the birth of newborn infants with severe anatomical abnormalities to mothers who had taken the tranquilizer thalidomide. It extended the FDCA to require that drug products, both prescription and nonprescription, be shown to be effective and safe. At this time, provisions were added to the act concerning factory inspections and investigational drugs, and the responsibility for regulating prescription drug advertising was shifted from the Federal Trade Commission (FTC) to the FDA.

The Comprehensive Drug Abuse Prevention and Control Act of 1970

The Comprehensive Drug Abuse Prevention and Control Act of 1970, referred to as the Controlled Substance Act (CSA), controls the manufacture, importation, sale, and distribution of drugs that have the potential for addiction and abuse. Drugs with a strong potential for abuse are identified, and their manufacture and distribution are monitored closely. Under this act, drugs are classified with potential for abuse into five types, or schedules (see Table 2-1).

The Drug Enforcement Administration (DEA), an arm of the Department of Justice, is primarily charged with enforcing laws and regulations related to the abuse of controlled substances, both legal and illegal. The DEA manages most of its funds and personnel toward the illegal trafficking of Schedule

TABLE 2-1. Drug Schedules

SCHEDULE	ABUSE POTENTIAL	PRESCRIPTION REQUIREMENT	EXAMPLES
I	High abuse potential; no accepted medical use	No prescription permitted	Heroin, LSD, marijuana, mescaline, peyote, PCP, hashish, and amphetamine variants
II	High abuse potential; accepted medical use	Prescription required; no refills permitted without a new written prescription	Cocaine, codeine, amphetamine salts (Adderall), Desoxyn, methadone hydrochloride, morphine, opium, codeine, methylphenidate (Ritalin), meperidine (Demerol), and secobarbital (Seconal)
III	Moderate abuse potential; accepted medical use	Prescription required; 5 refills permitted in 6 months	Certain drugs compounded with small quantities of narcotics, other drugs with high potential for abuse (Tylenol or Empirin with codeine tablets), and certain barbiturates such as butabarbital (Butisol)
IV	Low abuse potential; accepted medical use	Prescription required; 5 refills permitted in 6 months	Barbital, chloral hydrate (Noctec), diazepam (Valium), chlordiazepoxide (Librium), pentazocine hydrochloride (Talwin), and propoxyphene (Darvon)
V	Low abuse potential; accepted medical use	No prescription required for individuals 18 or older	Cough syrups with codeine, diphenoxylate hydrochloride with atropine sulfate (Lomotil), and kaolin/pectin/opium (Parepectolin)

I drugs. This agency also has responsibilities regarding the legal use of narcotics and other controlled substances. The DEA issues practitioners and pharmacies a license (number) that enables them to write prescriptions for scheduled drugs and, in the case of a pharmacy, order scheduled drugs from wholesalers. A special form—the DEA Form 222 (see Figure 2-1)—must be used when ordering Schedule II narcotics.

The Poison Prevention Act of 1970

The Poison Prevention Act of 1970 required that the majority of OTC and legend drugs be packaged in child-resistant containers. These containers cannot be opened by 80% of children younger than age 5 but can be opened by 90% of adults. The Consumer Product Safety Commission enforces this act.

The Drug Listing Act of 1972

Under the Drug Listing Act of 1972, each new drug is assigned a unique and permanent product code, known as a **National Drug Code (NDC)** that identifies the manufacturer or distributor, the drug formulation, and the size and type of its packaging. Using this code, the FDA is able to maintain a database of drugs by use, manufacturer, and active ingredients and of newly marketed, discontinued, and remarketed drugs. The NDC for one product may not be used for another. If any changes occur in product characteristic, a new NDC number must be assigned to the new product version.

The Drug Regulation Reform Act of 1978

The Drug Regulation Reform Act of 1978 was enacted to permit a shorter period for the investigation of new drugs. This law was developed in response to public pressure to allow for quicker consumer access.

The Orphan Drug Act of 1983

The Orphan Drug Act of 1983 offers federal financial incentives to commercial and nonprofit organizations to develop and market drugs previously unavailable in the United States. The orphan drug can be used to treat a disease that affects fewer than 200,000 people in the United States. This law offers tax breaks and a 7-year monopoly on drug sales to induce companies to undertake the development and manufacturing of such drugs. Since the 1983 act went into effect, more than 100 orphan drugs have been approved, including those for the treatment of conditions such as acquired immunodeficiency syndrome (AIDS), cystic fibrosis, blepharospasm (uncontrolled rapid blinking), and snake bites.

The Drug Price Competition and Patent-Term Restoration Act of 1984

The Drug Price Competition and Patent-Term Restoration Act of 1984 encouraged the creation of both generic drugs (those not protected by trademark) and innovative new drugs by streamlining the process for generic drug approval and extending patent license as a function of the time required for the drug application approval process.

The Prescription Drug Marketing Act of 1987

The Prescription Drug Marketing Act of 1987 deals with safety and competition issues raised by secondary markets for drugs and prohibits the reimportation of a drug into the United States by anyone except the manufacturer. This act also prohibits the sale or trading of drug samples, the distribution of samples to persons other than those licensed to prescribe them, and the distribution of samples except by mail or by common carrier.

The Omnibus Budget Reconciliation Act of 1990

The Omnibus Budget Reconciliation Act of 1990 (OBRA-90) requires the pharmacist to offer to discuss information about new and refill prescriptions with each patient. Matters discussed in counseling should include the following information:

- Name and description of medication
- Dosage form, dosage, route of administration, and duration of drug therapy
- Common severe side effects or adverse effects
- Interactions (with other drug or food) and therapeutic contraindications
- Self-monitoring of the medication therapy
- Proper storage
- Action in the event of a missed dose
- Special directions and precautions to be taken by the patient

The Occupational Safety and Health Administration

The Occupational Safety and Health Administration (OSHA) was established in 1970 to set standards and protocols for occupational health and safety. OSHA is a part of the Department of Labor. The involvement of OSHA with medical practices accelerated during the 1980s, partly because of the risk of exposure to the hepatitis B virus and later because of the spread of AIDS. As a result of the increasing danger of bloodborne pathogens, regulations were introduced in 1991. Enforcement of this standard, which is mandated by federal law, is meant to minimize, if not eliminate, occupational exposure to bloodborne pathogens. The health care facility is subject to an OSHA compliance inspection at any time during regular office hours. To comply with the OSHA standard, employers must have a written exposure control plan. The plan must be reviewed and updated at least annually to document review and implementation of safer medical devices. Nonmanagerial employees with risk of exposure must be involved in the identification, review, and selection of engineering and work practice, and their participation in the procedure must be documented.

See Reverse of PURCHASER'S Copy for Instructions

No order form may be issued for Schedule I and II substances unless a completed application form has been received, (21 CFR 1305.04).

OMB APPROVAL No. 1117-0010

TO: *(Name of Supplier)* STREET ADDRESS

CITY and STATE DATE

TO BE FILLED IN BY SUPPLIER

SUPPLIERS DEA REGISTRATION No.

	TO BE FILLED IN BY PURCHASER			**TO BE FILLED IN BY SUPPLIER**		
LINE No.	No. of Packages	Size of Package	Name of Item	National Drug Code	Packages Shipped	Date Shipped
1						
2						
3						
4						
5						
6						
7						
8						
9						
10						

◀ **LAST LINE COMPLETED** ***(MUST BE 10 OR LESS)*** SIGNATURE OF PURCHASER OR ATTORNEY OR AGENT

Date Issued | DEA Registration No. | Name and Address of Registrant

Schedules

Registered as a | No. of this Order Form

DEA Form -222
(Oct. 1992)

U.S. OFFICIAL ORDER FORMS - SCHEDULES I & II
DRUG ENFORCEMENT ADMINISTRATION
SUPPLIER'S Copy 1

92527420

Figure 2-1. DEA Form 222.

Health Insurance Portability and Accountability Act of 1996

The Health Insurance Portability and Accountability Act (HIPAA) of 1996 was signed into law on August 21, 1996, and required all health care providers to be in compliance by April 14, 2003. HIPAA was designed with many goals in mind; limiting administrative costs of health care and privacy issues and preventing fraud and abuse are of primary importance.

It was thought that the use of electronic transmissions would lower the administrative costs of providing health care, but this has led to problems related to privacy of health information. Therefore, the law also had to provide security and confidentiality guarantees for each individual patient. Extensive privacy rules, including the use of unique identifiers, have shaped the law.

The final regulations regarding the privacy legislation sections of HIPAA were published in December 2000, after the Centers for Medicare & Medicaid Services (CMS) reviewed more than 50,000 comments and concerns on this important subject. All health care organizations that transmit any health information electronically must comply with HIPAA; fines and prison terms can be imposed on those who do not comply with the regulations.

Centers for Disease Control and Prevention

The Centers for Disease Control and Prevention (CDC) is a federal agency of the U.S. government that provides facilities and services for the investigation, identification, prevention, and control of disease, injury, and disability. It provides statistics and information to health professionals about the treatment of common and rare diseases worldwide. Its primary function is to issue regulations for infection control. It was established in 1946 as the Communicable Disease Center and became the Centers for Disease Control in 1970; "and Prevention" was added in 1992, but Congress requested that "CDC" remain the agency's initials. This agency has also been deeply involved in the war against human immunodeficiency virus (HIV) infection and AIDS.

DRUG STANDARDS

Drug standards are the set of requirements for the formulation of drug substances, ingredients, and dosage forms. Drugs stocked in the pharmacy must be compendia drugs, and a drug formulary, or list of drugs stocked by the pharmacy, must be maintained. The pharmaceutical services must be under the general supervision of a licensed pharmacist. The pharmacist must schedule regular visits to the facility to supervise the drug handling and administration procedures. At least monthly, he or she must review the drug regimen of each patient and report any discrepancies or irregularities to the administrator and the medical director. This is a significant requirement in terms of patient safety and professional integrity. These drug standards are contained in the **U.S. Pharmacopeia (USP)** and the **National Formulary (NF),** published by the U.S. Pharmacopeia.

THE ETHICAL FOUNDATION OF PHARMACY

Ethics concerns the thoughts, judgments, and actions on issues that have the greater implications of moral right and wrong. Providing information about the risks and side effects of drug regimens is an ethical responsibility of physicians, pharmacists, and nurses. It is grounded in the principle of respect for the distinctive capacity of humans to make their own choices about their own lives. Patients must be aware of the benefits and risks of drugs that they may be taking.

Bioethics, relating to the sciences that underlie medicine, is a discipline dealing with the ethical and moral implications of biological research and applications, especially as they relate to life and death. These include pharmacology, anatomy, physiology, microbiology, pathology, and biochemistry. This is a new area of ethics resulting from genetic research in the current era.

WEB SITES OF INTEREST

American Society for Pharmacy Law: http://www.aspl.org
Centers for Disease Control and Prevention: http://www.cdc.gov
Occupational Safety and Health Association: http://www.osha.gov
U.S. Drug Enforcement Administration: http://www.usdoj.gov/dea
U.S. Department of Health and Human Services: http://www.hhs.gov
U.S. Food and Drug Administration: http://www.fda.gov
U.S. Pharmacopeia: http://www.usp.org

REVIEW QUESTIONS

1. Which of the following types of law is derived from previous court decisions?
   A. Constructional
   B. Common
   C. Administrative
   D. Statutory

2. Which of the following acts requires pharmaceutical manufacturers to file a New Drug Application with the FDA?
   A. The Pure Food and Drug Act of 1906
   B. The Comprehensive Drug Abuse Prevention and Control Act of 1970
   C. The Drug Listing Act of 1972
   D. The Food, Drug, and Cosmetic Act of 1938

3. Which of the following drugs are examples of Schedule IV drugs?
   A. Cocaine, morphine, and opium
   B. Valium, barbital, and chloral
   C. Lomotil and Parepectolin
   D. Tylenol with codeine

4. Which of the following laws permit a shorter period for the investigation of new drugs?
   A. The Orphan Drug Act of 1983
   B. The Drug Regulation Reform Act of 1978
   C. The Prescription Drug Marketing Act of 1987
   D. Controlled Substance Act

5. The Drug Enforcement Administration is a branch of the
   A. U.S. Department of Health and Human Services.
   B. U.S. Department of Justice.
   C. U.S. Department of Labor.
   D. Centers for Disease Control and Prevention.

6. Which of the following agencies has been deeply involved in the war against AIDS?
   A. U.S. Department of Labor
   B. American Red Cross
   C. U.S. Department of Health and Human Services
   D. Centers for Disease Control and Prevention

7. Which of the following is encompassed by the Food, Drug, and Cosmetic Act of 1938?
   A. Labeling requirements for safe consumer use of OTC drugs
   B. Collection of adverse drug reaction reports
   C. Protection of public health
   D. A and C

8. The Durham-Humphrey Amendment of 1951 established the difference between
   A. the pharmacist and technician.
   B. prescription and nonprescription drugs.
   C. legend and OTC drugs.
   D. B and C.

9. All health care providers were required to comply with HIPAA by what year?
   A. 1906
   B. 1970
   C. 2003
   D. 2000

10. Which federal law was enacted in 1970 to regulate the use and distribution of substances with high abuse potential?
    A. FDA
    B. DEA
    C. EPA
    D. CSA

11. Which of the following is the goal of OSHA?
    A. To ensure safe and effective drug therapy
    B. To ensure a safe and healthful workplace
    C. To ensure that all drugs are labeled
    D. To control outdated drugs

12. Any adverse reaction of drug should be reported to the
    A. FDA.
    B. DEA.
    C. FAA.
    D. CSA.

13. All health care organizations that transmit any health information electronically must comply with the
    A. CDC.
    B. FDA.
    C. DEA.
    D. HIPAA.

14. Basic viewpoints, general beliefs, and attitudes are known as
    A. morals.
    B. ethics.
    C. etiquette.
    D. philosophy.

15. Which of the following agencies is primarily charged with enforcing laws and regulations related to the abuse of controlled substances?
    A. FBI
    B. DEA
    C. NIH
    D. CDC

16. The drug standards are contained in which of the following?
    A. U.S. Pharmacopeia
    B. Federal and state statutes
    C. National formulary
    D. A and C

Continues

17. Which of the following agencies was established as a result of the first act to regulate the development, compounding, storage, and dispensing of drugs?
A. DEA
B. FDA
C. EPA
D. CDC

18. Which federal organization controls and oversees the safety of health facilities?
A. CDC
B. DEA
C. OSHA
D. WHO

19. The term that refers to the rules and principles of conduct that are required of citizens by legislative enactments is
A. *philosophy.*
B. *morals.*
C. *ethics.*
D. *laws.*

20. Which of the following schedules of drug is ordered by using a Federal Triplicate Order Form (DEA Form 222) that is obtained from the Drug Enforcement Administration (DEA)?
A. I
B. II
C. III
D. IV

21. Which of the following laws requires that a pharmacist counsel patients?
A. Patient Counseling Act
B. The Orphan Drug Act of 1983
C. The Omnibus Budget Reconciliation Act of 1990
D. Occupational and Safety Act

3 Pharmaceutical Terminology and Abbreviations

OUTLINE

- Word Building
  - Root
  - Prefix
  - Suffix
- Abbreviations
- Brand or Trade Names and Generic Names
- Commonly Used Apothecary Symbols

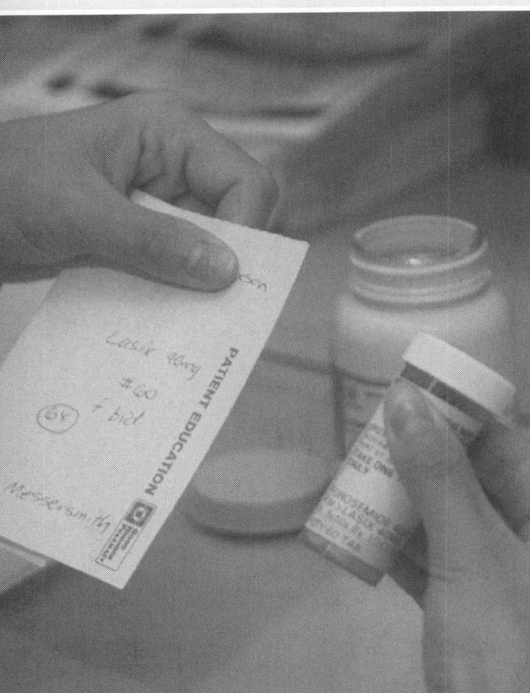

GLOSSARY

abbreviations Shortened forms of words.

root The main part of a word that gives the word its central meaning.

prefix A part of a word structure that occurs before or in front of the word and modifies the meaning of the root.

suffix A word ending that modifies the meaning of the root.

WORD BUILDING

Pharmacy technicians must have appropriate knowledge and understanding of specialized words, phrases, abbreviations, and symbols used in pharmacy and medicine to communicate precisely with other health care professionals. They must learn and utilize terminology, words, and phrases to explain the particular elements of their field. Medical terminology is derived from word parts that are placed together to form specific words and phrases in the medical fields. This is called word building. Word building is accomplished through the use of roots, prefixes, and suffixes.

Root

The main part of a word that gives the word its central meaning is its **root.** Word parts can be added to the root to offer more specific meanings to words. For example, *brady* is a prefix meaning "slow" and *cardi* is a root meaning "heart." If the two word parts are placed together to form the word *bradycardia,* the meaning is "slowness of the heart." Some examples of roots are shown in Table 3-1.

Prefix

A structure at the beginning of a word that modifies the meaning of the root is a **prefix.** Not all medical words have a prefix, but every medical word has a root and ending, which is either a suffix or another root, that is itself a word. *Hyperglycemia* is an example of a word containing a prefix. *Hyper* is the prefix, *glyc* is the root, and *emia* is the suffix. For a list of common prefixes, see Table 3-2.

Suffix

A word ending that modifies the meaning of the root is called a **suffix.** The root to which a suffix is attached may or

TABLE 3-1. Commonly Used General Roots

ROOT	MEANING	EXAMPLE	ROOT	MEANING	EXAMPLE
Acu	Abrupt, sudden	Acute	Mal	Bad	Malpractice
Adeno	Gland	Adenoid	Mast, mamm	Breast	Mastectomy
Adipo	Fat	Adipose	Melano	Black	Melanoma
Aero	Air	Aerosol	Meter	Measure	Thermometer
Alb	White	Albumin	My	Muscle	Myalgia
Ambulo	Walk	Ambulatory	Nas	Nose	Nasal
Andro	Male	Androgen	Necro	Dead	Necrosis
Angio	Vessel	Angiogram	Nephr	Kidney	Nephrosis
Arthr	Joint	Arthritis	Ocul	Eye	Ocular
Bucc	Inside of cheek	Buccal	Odont	Shaped like a tooth	Orthodontist
Canc	Crab	Cancer	Onc	Tumor	Oncology
Carcin	Crab, cancer	Carcinogen	Ophthalm	Eye	Ophthalmoscope
Cardi	Heart	Cardiology	Optic	Eye	Optician
Cereb	Brain	Cerebrum	Oste	Bone	Osteoarthritis
Chemo	Chemistry	Chemotherapy	Ot	Ear	Otalgia
Chol	Bile	Cholangiogram	Patho	Disease	Pathology
Cyst	Urinary bladder	Cystoscopy	Phleb, ven	Vein	Phlebotomy, venipuncture
Cyt	Cell	Cytology			
Dactyl	Finger	Syndactylism	Procto	Rectum	Proctologist
Dermat	Skin	Dermatology	Psych	Mind	Psychology
Encephal	Brain	Electroencphalogram	Ren	Kidney	Renal
Erythro	Red	Erythrocyte	Rhino	Nose	Rhinovirus
Gastr	Stomach	Gastric acid	Spir	Breathing	Spirometer
Gluco	Sugar	Glucose	Thrombo	Blood clot	Thrombolysis
Hemo	Blood	Hematoma	Tom, tome	Cut	Phlebotomy
Hepat	Liver	Hepatoma	Tox, toxo	Poisonous	Toxic, toxicology
Hydro	Water	Hydrocephalus	Uro	Urine	Urology
Lachry	Tear	Lachrymal fluid	Uter/o, hyster	Uterus	Intrauterine, hysterectomy
Lacto	Milk	Lactose			
Lapar	Abdomen	Laparoscope	Vaso	Blood vessel	Vasoconstriction
Laryng	Larynx (voice box)	Laryngitis	Xantho	Yellow	Xanthin
Leuko	White	Leukemia	Xero	Dry	Xeroderma
Lingua	Tongue	Sublingual	Zyme	Ferment	Enzyme

may not need a combining vowel. Not all words have a suffix. An example of a word with a suffix is *pharmacology*. *Pharmaco* is the root and *logy* is the suffix. For a list of common suffixes, see Table 3-3.

ABBREVIATIONS

Abbreviations are shortened forms of words. Health care professionals are required to know many abbreviations. The common abbreviations used in medical offices or hospitals are presented in Table 3-4. The most common abbreviations associated with measurements are shown in Table 3-5, and the abbreviations used for writing prescriptions are listed in Table 3-6. Tables 3-7 through 3-16 list common abbreviations related to each body system.

BRAND OR TRADE NAMES AND GENERIC NAMES

Pharmacy technicians must know all names for a given drug. Pharmaceutical literature usually has three different names listed for each medication:

1. Generic or nonproprietary
2. Trade or brand
3. Chemical

The most commonly used name is the generic name. This is the name the manufacturer uses for a drug, and it is the same in any country. The trade name is capitalized and followed by the symbol®, which indicates that the name is registered to a specific manufacturer or owner and no one else can use it. The chemical name is derived from the chemical composition of the drug. This name is usually hyphenated and may be long. Table 3-17 shows the brand and trade names and the corresponding generic names of some commonly used medications.

COMMONLY USED APOTHECARY SYMBOLS

The definitions of all apothecary symbols are not absolute; many of them have more than one meaning when used in different contexts. The symbols used most commonly in medicine are shown in Table 3-18.

TABLE 3-2. Commonly Used General Prefixes

PREFIX	MEANING	EXAMPLE	PREFIX	MEANING	EXAMPLE
A-	Without	Aphonia	Iso-	Equal	Isometric
Ab-	From, away from	Abduct	Juxta-	Near, beside	Juxtaarticular
Ad-	Toward	Adduct	Macro-	Large	Macrocytic
Ambi-	Both	Ambidextrous	Mal-	Bad	Malnutrition
Ana-	Up to-toward	Anaphylactic	Mega-	Large	Megacephaly
Ante-	Before	Antecubital	Meso-	Middle	Mesoderm
Auto-	Self	Autoimmune	Meta-	Change, after	Metastasis
Bi-	Two, double	Biceps, bilateral	Micro-	Small	Microscope
Bio-	Life	Biopsy, biology	Milli-	One-thousandth	Milliliter
Brady-	Slow	Bradycardia	Neo-	New	Neonatal
Cata-	Down	Cataleptic	Non-	Not	Noninvasive
Circum-	Around	Circumcision	Para-	Near, beside, beyond	Paramedic
Con-	Together	Congestion	Per-	Through	Percutaneous
Contra-	Against	Contraceptive	Peri-	Around	Perianal
De-	From, away from, down	Decalcify	Poly-	Many	Polyarthritis
Deca-	Ten	Dekaliter	Post-	Behind, after	Postpartum
Dia-	Through, complete	Diagnosis	Pre-	Before	Premature
Dis-	Separate	Dislocation	Re-	Again, back	Reactivate
Dys-	Bad, abnormal, painful	Dyspepsia, dysuria	Retro-	Backward, behind	Retrograde
Ec-	Out, away	Ectopic	Semi-	Half	Semiconscious
Ecto-	Outside	Ectoplasm	Sub-	Under, beneath, below	Sublingual
Em-	In	Embolism	Super-	Above, over	Superficial
En-	In	Endemic	Supra-	Above, excessive	Suprarenal
Endo-	Into, within	Endoscope, endometriosis	Syn-	Together, with	Synthetic
			Tri-	Three	Triceps
Epi-	Upon, high	Epidermis	Uni-	One	Unicellular
Eu-	Well, good	Eupnea	Ultra-	Beyond, excessive	Ultrasound
Intra-	Within, inside	Intravenous			

TABLE 3-3. Commonly Used General Suffixes

SUFFIX	MEANING	EXAMPLE	SUFFIX	MEANING	EXAMPLE
-ar	Pertaining to	Lumbar	-lysis	Breaking down	Hemolysis
-clasis	Break	Osteoclasis	-megaly	Enlargement	Hepatomegaly
-desis	Binding	Arthrodesis	-ol	Alcohol	Ethanol
-dipsia	Thirst	Polydipsia	-oma	Tumor	Melanoma
-ectomy	Cut out, remove	Appendectomy	-opia	Vision	Hyperopia
-emesis	Vomit	Hematemesis	-ose	Carbohydrate	Glucose
-form	Resembling, like	Vermiform	-pathy	Disease	Homeopathy
-genic	Originating, producing	Toxigenic	-penia	Abnormal reduction	Leukocytopenia
-gram	Record	Electrocardiogram	-pepsia	Digestion	Dyspepsia
-graph	Device for recording	Electrocardiograph	-philia	Attraction	Hydrophilia
-iasis	Condition	Nephrolithiasis	-phobia	Abnormal fear	Photophobia
-iatry	Treatment	Podiatry	-plasty	Surgical repair	Rhinoplasty
-ic	Pertaining to	Thoracic	-rrhea	Discharge, flow	Diarrhea
-ical	Pertaining to	Neurological	-sis	Process	Diagnosis
-ism	Condition	Alcoholism	-stasis	Control, stoppage	Hemostasis
-ist	Specialist	Cardiologist	-stomy	Surgical opening	Colostomy
-itis	Inflammation	Nephritis	-tomy	Cut, incision	Nephrotomy
-logist	Specialist in the study of	Microbiologist	-tropia	Turning	Hypertropia
-logy	Study of	Etiology			

TABLE 3-4. Abbreviations Used in Medical Care Facilities

ABBREVIATION	MEANING	ABBREVIATION	MEANING
CCU	Coronary care unit	IP	Inpatient
CDS	Controlled drug substance	OP	Outpatient
CICU	Coronary intensive care unit	OR	Operating room
COPD	Chronic obstructive pulmonary disease	PAR	Postanesthetic recovery
CP	Chest pain	Peds	Pediatrics
CXR	Chest x-ray	Post-op	After surgery
Dx	Diagnosis	Pre-op	Preoperative
ECU	Emergency care unit	pt.	Patient
ER	Emergency room	R/O	Rule out
Fx	Fracture	RR	Recovery room
F(X)	Function	RTC	Return to clinic
GU	Genitourinary	RTO	Return to office
Hg	Mercury	Tx	Treatment
H.O.	House officer	U	Unit
H.T.	Hypodermic tablet	VO	Verbal order
Hx	History	VS	Vital sign
ICU	Intensive care unit		

TABLE 3-5. Abbreviations Commonly Used for Measurements

ABBREVIATION	MEANING	ABBREVIATION	MEANING
C or °C	Celsius	gt	Drop
cc	Cubic Centimeter (1cc = 1 mL)	gtt	Drops
cm	Centimeter (2.5 cm = 1 inch)	ht	Height
°F	Fahrenheit	lb	Pound
g or gm	Gram	kg	Kilogram (kg = 1000 gm = 2.2 pounds)
Gr	Grain	L or l	Liter = 100 ml (1 gallon = 4 quarts=8 pints)

Continues

TABLE 3-5. Abbreviations Commonly Used for Measurements—cont'd

ABBREVIATION	MEANING	ABBREVIATION	MEANING
m^2	Square meter	Ss	One-half
mcg, µg	Microgram	T	Temperature
mEq	Milliequivalent	tbs or tbsp	Tablespoon
mg	Milligram	tsp	Teaspoon
mg/kg	Milligram of drug per kilogram of body weight	U	Unit
ml, mL	Millilitermm Millimeter	wt	Weight
no or NO	Number	w/v	Weight-to-volume ratio

TABLE 3-6. Abbreviations Commonly Used in Prescriptions

ABBREVIATION	MEANING	ABBREVIATION	MEANING
$\bar{a}$	Before	P	After
$\bar{a}\bar{a}$, aa	Of each	p.c.	After meals
a.c.	Before meals	Per.	By, through
ad	To, up to	PM, p.m.	After noon
AD	Right ear	PO, p.o.	By mouth, orally
Ad lib.	As desired	PR, p.r.	Through the rectum
AL	Left ear	PRN, p.r.n.	As needed
AM, a.m.	Morning	PV, vag.	Through the vagina
Amt	Amount	Pulv.	A powder
aq.	Water	q	Every
AS	Left ear	q AM	Every morning
a.u.	Each ear	q.d., QD	Every day
b.i.d.	Twice a day	q h	Every hour
BAA	Body surface area	q2h	Every two hours
Buc.	Buccal	q.i.d.	Four times a day
$\bar{c}$	With	q.o.d.	Every other day
Cap.	Capsule	q.v.	As much as you wish
Comp.	Compound	®	Right; registered trademark
d	Day	Rχ	Prescription, take
dil	Dilute	$\bar{s}$	Without
Disp.	Dispense	Sat.	Saturated
el., elix.	Elixir	Sig.	Instruction to patient
Fl, fld	Fluid	SL	Sublingual
h, hr	Hour	Sol., Soln.	Solution
h.s.	At bedtime, at the hour of sleep	SP	Spirits
IM	Intramuscular	SS, ss	One half
IV	Intravenous	S.O.S.	There is a need
Liq	Liquid	Stat	Immediately
M.	Mix	Supp., Suppos.	Suppository
Mixt., mist.	A mixture	Syr.	Syrup
No.	Number	T	Topical
Noc., N., n	Night	Tab	Tablet
Non. Rep.	Do not repeat, no refills	t.i.d., TID	Three times a day
NPO	Nothing by mouth	Tiw	Three times a week
OD	Right eye	tr., tinct.	Tincture
Oint. Ung.	Ointment	w.a.	While awake
OS	Left eye	WK	Week
OU	Each eye or both eyes	X	Times, for

TABLE 3-7. Abbreviations Related to the Integumentary System

ABBREVIATION	MEANING
Bx	Biopsy
Derm	Dermatology
SC, sub-Q, SQ, sub CU, Subq.	Subcutaneous

TABLE 3-8. Abbreviations Related to the Musculoskeletal System

ABBREVIATION	MEANING
C1, C2, ...C7	Individual cervical vertebrae
Ca	Calcium
CTS	Carpal tunnel syndrome
EMG	Electromyography
Fx	Fracture
Ortho	Orthopedics
ROM	Range of motion
SLE	Systemic lupus erythematosus

TABLE 3-9. Abbreviations Related to the Eye

ABBREVIATION	MEANING
Ast	Astigmatism
IOP	Intraocular pressure
OD	Right eye
OS	Left eye
OU	Both eyes
REM	Rapid eye movement
VA	Visual acuity
VF	Visual field

TABLE 3-10. Abbreviations Related to the Nervous System

ABBREVIATION	MEANING
AD	Alzheimer's disease
ALS	Amyotrophic lateral sclerosis
CAT	Computed axial tomography
CNS	Central nervous system
CP	Cerebral palsy
CSF	Cerebrospinal fluid
CT	Computed tomography
CVA	Cerebrovascular accident
EEG	Electroencephalogram
LP	Lumbar puncture
MRI	Magnetic resonance imaging
MS	Multiple sclerosis
TIA	Transient ischemic attack

TABLE 3-11. Abbreviations Related to the Ear

ABBREVIATION	MEANING
AD	Right ear
AS	Left ear
AU	Each ear
EENT	Eyes, ears, nose, and throat
Oto	Otology

TABLE 3-12. Abbreviations Related to the Endocrine System

ABBREVIATION	MEANING
ACTH	Adrenocorticotropic hormone
BMR	Basal metabolic rate
DI	Diabetes insipidus
DM	Diabetes mellitus
FBS	Fasting blood sugar
FSH	Follicle-stimulating hormone
GH	Growth hormone
GTT	Glucose tolerance test
IDDM	Insulin-dependent diabetes mellitus
K	Potassium
Na	Sodium
PRL	Prolactin
TFT	Thyroid function test

TABLE 3-13. Abbreviations Related to the Cardiovascular System

ABBREVIATION	MEANING
AF	Atrial fibrillation
AS	Aortic stenosis
ASD	Atrial septal defect
BP	Blood pressure
CAD	Coronary artery disease
CHD	Coronary heart disease
CHF	Congestive heart failure
ECG, EKG	Electrocardiogram
ECHO	Echocardiography
MI	Myocardial infarction
MVP	Mitral valve prolapse
PDA	Patent ductus arteriosus
PVC	Premature ventricular contraction
VT	Ventricular tachycardia

TABLE 3-14. Abbreviations Related to the Digestive System

ABBREVIATION	MEANING
BE	Barium enema
EUS	Endoscopic ultrasound
GERD	Gastroesophageal reflex disease
GI	Gastrointestinal
IBS	Irritable bowel syndrome

TABLE 3-15. Abbreviations Related to the Urinary System

ABBREVIATION	MEANING
ADH	Antidiuretic hormone; vasopressin
ARF	Acute renal failure
BUN	Blood urea nitrogen
Cath	Catheter
CRF	Chronic renal failure
HD	Hemodialysis
IVP	Intravenous pyelogram
KUB	Kidney, ureter, and bladder
PKU	Phenylketonuria
UA	Urinalysis
UTI	Urinary tract infection

TABLE 3-16. Abbreviations Related to the Reproductive System

ABBREVIATION	MEANING
AB	Abortion
AIDS	Acquired immunodeficiency syndrome
BPH	Benign prostatic hyperplasia
CS, C-section	Cesarean section
CX	Cervix
D & C	Dilation and curettage
ECC	Endocervical curettage
EMB	Endometrial biopsy
FHT	Fetal heart tones
FSH	Follicle-stimulating hormone
GYN	Gynecology
HCG	Human chorionic gonadotropin
HIV	Human immunodeficiency virus
HSV	Herpes simplex virus
LH	Luteinizing hormone
Multip	Multipara
Pap Smear	Papanicolaou Smear (test for cervical of vaginal cancer)
PMS	Premenstrual Syndrome
PSA	Prostate-Specific Antigen
STD	Sexually Transmitted Disease

TABLE 3-17. Brand/Trade Names and Generic Names of Commonly Used Drugs

BRAND	GENERIC	BRAND	GENERIC
Achromycin	tetracycline	Biomox	amoxicillin trihydrate
Activase	alteplase, recombinant	Bufferin	aspirin
Adalat	nifedipine	BuSpar	buspirone
Advil	ibuprofen	Capoten	captopril
Airet	albuterol sulfate	Carafate	sucralfate
Aldomet	methyldopa	Cardizem	diltiazem
Amerge	naratriptan	Catapres	clonidine
Amoxil	amoxicillin	Ceclor	cefaclor
Amphojel	aluminum hydroxide	Celexa	citalopram
Ancef	cefazolin	Cipro	ciprofloxacin
Anzemet	dolasetron	Claritin	loratadine
Apresoline	hydralazine	Cleocin	clindamycin
Atarax	hydroxyzine	Compazine	prochlorperazine
Ativan	lorazepam	Corgard	nadolol
Axid	nizatidine	Corlopam	fenoldopam
Bactrim	sulfamethoxazole	Coumadin	warfarin
Benadryl	diphenhydramine	Crystodigin	digitoxin
Bentyl	dicyclomine	Cytotec	misoprostol
Brethine	terbutaline	Decadron	dexamethasone
Biaxin	clarithromycin	Deltasone	prednisone

Continues

TABLE 3-17. Brand/Trade Names and Generic Names of Commonly Used Drugs—cont'd

BRAND	GENERIC	BRAND	GENERIC
Demerol	meperidine	Pepcid	famotidine
Depakene	valproic acid	Phenergan	promethazine
DiaBeta	glyburide	Prilosec	omeprazole
Diabinese	chlorpropamide	Prinivil	lisinopril
Diamox	acetazolamide	Procardia	nifedipine
Dilantin	phenytoin	Pronestyl	procainamide
Dramamine	dimenhydrinate	Prozac	fluoxetine
Dulcolax	bisacodyl	Proventil	albuterol
Dyazide	hydrochlorothiazide	Retrovir	zidovudine
Effexor	venlafaxine	Robitussin	guaifenesin
Elavil	amitriptyline	Rocephin	ceftriaxone
Ery-Tab	erythromycin base	Rufen	ibuprofen
Flagyl	metronidazole	Septra	trimethoprim
Floxin	ofloxacin	Stadol	butorphanol
Folvite	folic acid	Synthroid	levothyroxine
Fungizone	amphotericin B	Tagamet HB	cimetidine
Garamycin	gentamicin	Talwin	pentazocine
Genprin	aspirin	Tamoxifen	tamoxifen citrate
Glucotrol	glipizide	Tapazole	methimazole
Haldol	haloperidol	Tavist	clemastine fumarate
Hexadrol	dexamethasone	Teargen	artificial tears solution
Hycort	hydrocortisone, topical	Tebamide	trimethobenzamide HCl
Hytrin	terazosin	Tebrazid	pyrazinamide
Ilosone	erythromycin estolate	Tega-cort	hydrocortisone, topical
Ilotycin	erythromycin base	Tegopen	cloxacillin sodium
Impril	imipramine HCl	Tegretol	carbamazepine
Inderal	propranolol	Terramycin	oxytetracycline HCl
Indocin	indomethacin	Tobrex	tobramycin
Integrilin	eptifibatide	Tofranil	imipramine
Isoptin	verapamil	Totacillin	ampicillin, oral
Kantrex	kanamycin sulfate	Trilafon	perphenazine
Keflex	cephalexin	Tums	calcium carbonate
Kefzol	cefazolin	Tylenol	acetaminophen
Kenalog	triamcinolone	Tyzine	tetrahydrozoline HCl, nasal
Klonopin	clonazepam	Ultiva	remifentanil HCl
Lanoxin	digoxin	Ultralente	insulin
Lasix	furosemide	Ultram	tramadol
Levate	amitriptyline HCl	Uritrol	furosemide
Lipitor	atorvastatin	Urobak	sulfamethoxazole
Lopid	gemfibrozil	Vasotec	enalapril
Lopressor	metoprolol	Valisone	betamethasone valerate
Maxalt	rizatriptan	Valium	diazepam
Mefoxin	cefoxitin	V-Cillin K	penicillin V potassium
Mellaril	thioridazine	Ventolin	albuterol
Micronase	glyburide	Vibramycin	doxycycline
Minipress	prazosin	Virilon	methyltestosterone
Motrin	ibuprofen	Vivarin	caffeine
Mycostatin	nystatin	Vivol	diazepam
Mylicon	simethicone	Volmax	albuterol sulfate
Naprosyn	naproxen sodium	Wellferon	interferon alfa-N1
Nebcin	tobramycin	Wycillin	penicillin G procaine
Nizoral	ketoconazole	Xalatan	latanoprost
Oretic	hydrochlorothiazide	Xanax	alprazolam

Continues

TABLE 3-17. Brand/Trade Names and Generic Names of Commonly Used Drugs—cont'd

BRAND	GENERIC	BRAND	GENERIC
Xylocaine	lidocaine HCl, local	Zithromax	azithromycin
YF-Vax	yellow fever vaccine	Zocor	simvastatin
Yocon	yohimbine HCl	Zonalon	doxepin, topical
Zantac	ranitidine	Zovirax	acyclovir
Zestril	lisinopril	Zyloprim	allopurinol
Zetar	coal tar	Zyrtec	cetirizine HCl
Zincate	zinc sulfate		

TABLE 3-18. Symbols Commonly Used in Medicine

SYMBOL	MEANING	SYMBOL	MEANING
□	Left	″	Seconds
®	Right	°	Hours
>	Greater than	1°	Primary
<	Less than	2°	Secondary
=	Equal to	ʒ	Teaspoonful, 5ml (dram)
↑	Increase	♍	Minim
↓	Decrease	#	Pound
∅	None	×	Times (as in two times a week)
Δ	Change	♂	Male
′	Minutes	♀	Female

REVIEW QUESTIONS

1. Which of the following abbreviations means "centimeter"?
A. ct
B. cr
C. cn
D. cm

2. Which of the following abbreviations means "four times a day"?
A. q4h
B. q.o.d.
C. q.i.d.
D. b.i.d.

3. The suffix "-itis" means
A. pain.
B. swelling.
C. softening.
D. inflammation.

4. Which of the following prefixes means "surrounding tissue"?
A. Pre
B. Peri
C. Post
D. Para

5. The abbreviation that means "right eye" is
A. OC.
B. OD.
C. OS.
D. OU.

6. Which of the following is the symbol for "female"?
A. ∅
B. X
C. ♀
D. ♂

Continues

7. The abbreviation that means "every other day" is
   A. q.i.d.
   B. q.o.d.
   C. q.o.h.
   D. q.d.

8. Which of the following terms means "death of tissue"?
   A. *Necrosis*
   B. *Nephrosis*
   C. *Stenesis*
   D. *Sclerosis*

9. Which of the following abbreviations means "diagnosis"?
   A. CXR
   B. CDS
   C. Dx
   D. BX

10. The abbreviation that means "drops" is
    A. g.
    B. gr.
    C. gt.
    D. gtt.

11. Which of the following means "before meals"?
    A. a
    B. aa
    C. a.c.
    D. ad

12. Which of the following terms means distribution of a drug in labeled containers to a patient?
    A. *Prescription*
    B. *Administration*
    C. *Prepackaging*
    D. *Dispense*

13. Which of the following symbols means "none"?
    A. >
    B. Δ
    C. ∅
    D. <

14. The brand name is also called the
    A. generic name.
    B. chemical name.
    C. trade name.
    D. physical name.

15. Which of the following is the brand name of ibuprofen?
    A. Dulcolax
    B. Axid
    C. Ativan
    D. Advil

16. Pentazocine is the generic name of
    A. Talwin.
    B. Tylenol.
    C. Tums.
    D. Tegopen.

17. The abbreviation "OU" indicates
    A. right ear.
    B. right eye.
    C. left eye.
    D. both eyes.

18. Which of the following symbols means "sodium"?
    A. Cl
    B. Ca
    C. Na
    D. K

19. EKG is also called
    A. EEG.
    B. EEM.
    C. ECHO.
    D. ECG.

20. The trade name of diphenhydramine is
    A. bentyl.
    B. amerge.
    C. benadryl.
    D. capoten.

21. Which of the following roots means "cut"?
    A. Thrombo
    B. Tox
    C. Tom
    D. Vaso

22. Which of the following is the generic name for Zocor?
    A. simvastatin
    B. ranitidine
    C. zidovidine
    D. prozosin

23. Which of the following is a trade name for nifedipine?
    A. Prolosec
    B. Pronestyl
    C. Prozac
    D. Procardia

24. Which of the following roots means "bone"?
    A. Oste
    B. Onc
    C. Ot
    D. Zo

Medication and Dosage Forms 4

OUTLINE

Medical Uses of Drugs
- Therapeutic Agents
- Diagnostic Agents
- Replacement Agents
- Anesthetic Agents
- Prophylactic or Preventative Agents
- Destructive Agents

Drug Classification

Dosage Forms
- Solid Drugs
- Semisolid Drugs
- Liquid Drugs

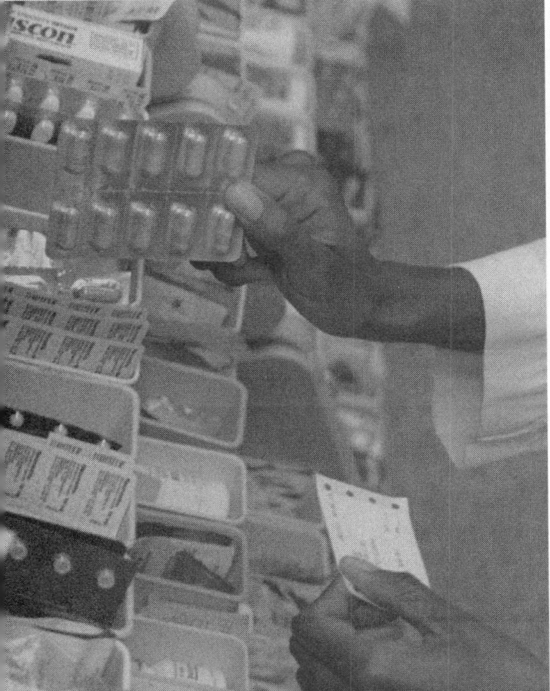

GLOSSARY

aerosol A liquid or fine powder that is sprayed in a fine mist.

caplet A tablet shaped like a capsule.

capsule A solid dosage form in which the drug is enclosed in either a hard or soft shell of soluble material.

cream A semisolid emulsion of either the oil-in-water or the water-in-oil type, ordinarily intended for topical use.

elixir A clear, sweetened, hydroalcoholic liquid intended for oral use.

emulsion A system containing two liquids that cannot be mixed together in which one is dispersed, in the form of very small globules, throughout the other.

fluidextract A pharmacopeial liquid preparation of vegetable drugs, made by filtration, containing alcohol as a solvent or as a preservative or both.

gel A jelly or the solid or semisolid phase of a colloidal solution.

gelcap An oil-based medication that is enclosed in a soft gelatin capsule.

granule A very small pill, usually gelatin- or sugar-coated, containing a drug to be given in a small dose.

implants or pellets Implants or pellets are dosage forms that are placed intradermally, or under the skin, by means of minor surgery or special injections.

liniment A liquid preparation for external use, usually applied by friction to the skin.

lozenge A small, disk-shaped tablet composed of solidifying paste containing an astringent, an antiseptic, or an oil-based drug used for local treatment of the mouth or throat. It is held in the mouth until dissolved. Also known as a troche.

medication A substance used in the treatment or maintenance of an illness.
mixture A mutual incorporation of two or more substances, without chemical union, in which the physical characteristics of each of the components are retained.
ointment A semisolid preparation that usually contains medicinal substances and is intended for external application.
parenteral Administration by some means other than through the gastrointestinal tract; referring particularly to introduction of substances into an organism by intravenous, subcutaneous, intramuscular, or intramedullary injection.
pill A small, globular mass of soluble material containing a medicinal substance to be swallowed.
plaster A solid preparation that can be spread when heated and that becomes adhesive at the temperature of the body.
powder A dry mass of minute separate particles of any substance.
solution The incorporation of a solid, a liquid, or a gas into a liquid.
spirits An alcoholic or hydroalcoholic solution of volatile substances.
suppository A small, solid body shaped for ready introduction into one of the orifices of the body other than the oral cavity (e.g., rectum, urethra, or vagina), made of a substance, usually medicated, that is solid at ordinary temperature but melts at body temperature.
suspension A class of pharmacopeial preparations of finely divided, undissolved drugs dispersed in liquid vehicles for oral or parenteral use.
syrup A liquid preparation in a concentrated aqueous solution of a sugar used for medicinal purposes or to add flavor to a substance.
tablet A solid dosage form containing medicinal substances with or without suitable diluents.
tincture An alcoholic solution prepared from vegetable materials or from chemical substances.
troche A small, disk-shaped tablet composed of solidifying paste containing an astringent, antiseptic, or oil-based drug used for local treatment of the mouth or throat. It is held in the mouth until dissolved. Also known as a lozenge.
water A mixture of distilled water with an aromatic volatile water.

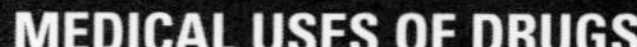

MEDICAL USES OF DRUGS

A **medication** is a drug or other substance that is legally used to treat an illness or disease state. There are six medical uses of drugs: therapeutic, diagnostic, replacement, anesthetic, prophylactic or preventive, and destructive.

Therapeutic Agents

The therapeutic use of a drug is intended to relieve signs and symptoms of a disease or for curative purposes to combat and remove the agent causing the disease. Therapeutic agents include prescription or over-the-counter medications. For example, antibiotics are able to kill or destroy microorganisms. Cough medicines may relieve coughing, and painkillers are used to relieve pain.

Diagnostic Agents

Diagnostic drugs are used to determine the location of a disease by specific radiologic procedures and other diagnostic imaging techniques. Examples of diagnostic agents include the radiopharmaceutical thallium chloride for computed tomographic scans and barium meals or enemas to facilitate X-ray observation of the gastrointestinal tract.

Replacement Agents

The purpose of replacement drugs is to restore substances normally found in the body. Examples are vitamins, minerals, and hormones.

Anesthetic Agents

Anesthetics are used in a procedure in which an altered state of consciousness is induced to a depth adequate to permit comfortable performance of moderately painful diagnostic procedures of short duration. These agents may also be used for local or general surgical procedures. Examples are lidocaine for local procedures and nitrous oxide (laughing gas), ether, and chloroform for general surgery.

Prophylactic or Preventative Agents

Drugs used as prophylactic or preventive agents are intended to prevent a disease or disorder from occurring. Examples are vaccines and gamma globulin.

Destructive Agents

Destructive agents are able to destroy bacteria or cancer cells. Specific types are antiseptics and antineoplastics.

Chemotherapy with these drugs is used to destroy malignant tumors. An example is radioiodine, which is used to destroy thyroid cancer.

DRUG CLASSIFICATION

Drugs are classified according to clinical indication or action on a particular body system. Drugs may have a principal action on the body or can act on specific body systems or organs. Drugs may also be classified by the preparation such as liquid, suppository, or solid. Table 4-1 lists common drug classifications by clinical indication.

DOSAGE FORMS

Drug preparation consists of three basic types: solid, semisolid, and liquid. Certain drugs are soluble in water, some in alcohol, and others in a mixture of several solvents. The route for administering a medication depends on its form, its properties, and the effects desired.

Solid Drugs

Solid drugs include tablets, pills, plasters, capsules, caplets, gelcaps, powders, granules, troches, or lozenges (see Figure 4-1).

TABLE 4-1. Common Classifications of Drugs and Their Actions

CLASSIFICATION	ACTION
Analgesic	A drug that relieves pain without loss of consciousness
Anesthetic	A drug that causes a lack of feeling
Antacid	A drug that neutralizes stomach acid
Antianemic	A drug that replaces iron
Antiarrhythmic	A drug that corrects and controls cardiac arrhythmias
Anticoagulant	A drug that prevents or reduces blood clotting
Anticonvulsant	A drug that relieves or prevents convulsions
Antidepressant	A drug that reduces feelings of depression
Antidiarrheal	A drug that relieves or prevents diarrhea
Antidote	A drug that counteracts poisons and their effects
Antiemetic	A drug used to treat vomiting
Antiepileptic	A drug used to treat or prevent epileptic seizures
Antiflatulent	A drug intended to reduce intestinal gas
Antifungal	A drug that kills or inhibits reproduction of fungi
Antihistamine	A drug that prevents histamine from interacting with its receptors
Antihypertensive	An agent that reduces high blood pressure
Anti-inflammatory	A drug that reduces inflammation
Antimalarial	A drug that kills or inhibits the reproduction of malaria parasites
Antimanics	A drug used for the treatment of the manic episode of manic-depressive disorder
Antineoplastic	A drug that kills or inhibits reproduction of cancer cells
Antiparasitic	A drug or chemical that kills or inhibits reproduction of parasites
Antiparkinsonian	A drug that helps to control symptoms of Parkinson's disease
Antipruritic	A drug or other material that reduces itching
Antipsychotic	A drug that relieves symptoms of schizophrenia and chronic brain syndrome
Antipyretic	A drug that reduces fever
Antitoxin	An antibody that forms in response to a toxin produced by an infecting microorganism (examples are antitoxins against diphtheria and tetanus toxins)
Antitussive	A drug that reduces coughing
Antiulcer	A drug that relieves and heals ulcers
Antiviral	A drug that kills or inhibits reproduction of a virus
Bronchodilator	A drug that dilates the bronchi
Contraceptive	An agent, a device, or a method, that prevents pregnancy
Decongestant	An agent that relieves nasal congestion due to infection or allergy and inflammation in the eyes
Diuretic	A drug that promotes urine formation and excretion of excess interstitial fluid
Expectorant	A medication that facilitates removal of mucus secretion in the lungs
Hemostatic	A medication that controls or stops bleeding
Hypnotic	A drug that causes sleep; it is also called a sleeping pill or sedative
Hypoglycemic	A drug that lowers blood glucose level
Laxative	A drug that promotes bowel movements
Muscle relaxant	A drug that reduces the contraction of muscles
Sedative	Any agent that produces calm or sleep
Tranquilizer	A drug that acts on the central nervous system to reduce anxiety or emotional stress
Vasodilator	An agent that causes blood vessels to relax and lowers blood pressure
Vasopressor	A drug that causes vasoconstriction and raises blood pressure
Virucide	An agent that kills viruses either in a living organism or inanimate surfaces

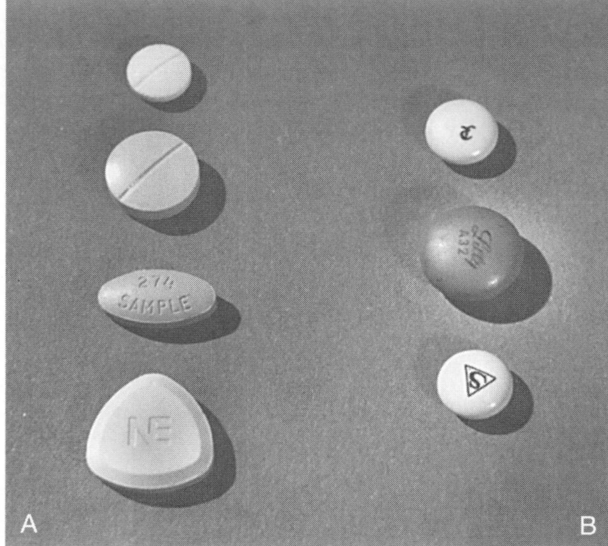

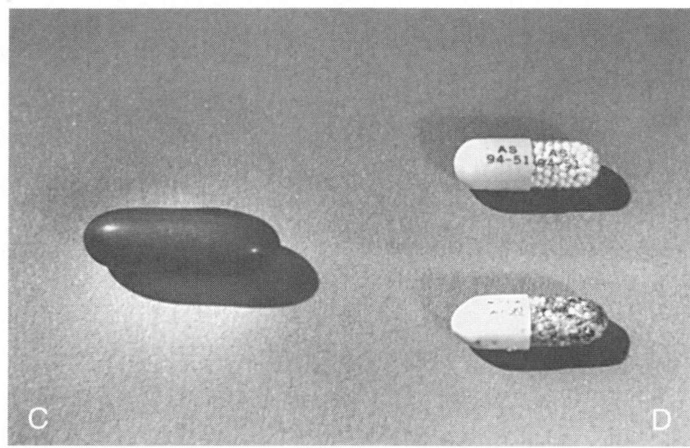

Figure 4-1. Solid forms of drugs include tablets and capsules and are generally administered orally. (A) Tablets, scored and unscored, (B) enteric-coated tablets, (C) gelatin capsules, and (D) timed-release capsules.

The most common route of administration for solid drugs is the oral route. This will be discussed further in Chapter 5.

Tablets

A **tablet** is a pharmaceutical preparation made by compressing the powdered form of a drug and bulk filling material under high pressure. Special forms of tablets include sublingual tablets (to be dissolved under the tongue) and enteric-coated tablets (to which a special outside layer has been applied to certain tablets or capsules to ensure that they are passed through the stomach into the small intestine, where their special coating will dissolve). Most tablets are intended to be swallowed whole for dissolution and absorption in the gastrointestinal tract. Some are intended to be dissolved in the mouth or dissolved in water. Many times tablets are mistakenly called pills. Tablets come in various sizes, shapes, colors, and compositions. Examples of various forms of tablets include enteric-coated, chewable, sublingual, buccal, and buffered.

Pills

A **pill** is a medicine initially compounded or manufactured as a putty. Measured portions of the putty are rolled into spheres that may or may not be coated. Pills are intended for oral administration. Tablets are produced by an entirely different process and are often mistakenly referred to as pills. Birth control pills, for example, are actually tablets. The terms *tablet* and *capsule* have replaced the term *pill* and this term should not be used in medicine today.

Plasters

Any composition of a liquid and a powder that hardens when it dries is a **plaster**. Plasters may be solid or semisolid. An example is the salicylic acid plaster used to remove corns.

Capsules

A medication dosage form in which the drug is contained in an external shell is a **capsule**. Capsule shells are usually made of hard gelatin and enclose or encapsulate powder, granules, liquids, or some combinations of these. Liquids may be placed in soft gelatin capsules. Examples include vitamin E capsules, Benadryl capsules, and cod liver oil capsules.

Caplets

A **caplet** is shaped like a capsule but has the consistency of a tablet. It is a coated, solid preparation for oral administration. An example is a Tylenol caplet.

Gelcaps

A **gelcap** is an oil-based medication that is enclosed in a soft gelatin capsule. An example is a vitamin A gelcap.

Powders

A drug dried and ground into fine particles is a **powder**. An example is potassium chloride powder (Kato powder).

Granules

A **granule** is a small pill, usually accompanied by many others, encased within a gelatin capsule. In most cases, granules within capsules are specially coated to gradually release medication over a period of up to 12 hours. An example of a granule is Metamucil, which is a popular bulk-forming laxative. Metamucil also comes in powder and water forms.

Troches or Lozenges

A hard or semisolid dosage form containing a medication intended for local application in the mouth or throat is called a **troche** or **lozenge**. Typically, a troche is placed on the tongue or between the cheek and gum and left in place until it dissolves. The medications most commonly administered by means of troches include cough suppressants and medications used for relief of a sore throat. Many other drugs, such as nystatin or clotrimazole, are available in lozenge form.

Semisolid Drugs

Semisolid drugs are often used as topical applications (applied to the surface of the body). Topical drug administration is addressed in greater detail in Chapter 5. Semisolid drugs include suppositories, ointments, creams, and gels (see Figure 4-2). These types of drugs can be used topically to treat burns, insect bites, and itching.

Suppositories

A bullet-shaped dosage form intended to be inserted into a body orifice is called a **suppository**. Suppositories contain medication usually intended for a local effect at the site of insertion. They are semisolid dosage forms designed for insertion into bodily orifices. Suppositories maintain their shape at room temperature but melt or dissolve when inserted. The most common sites of administration for suppositories are the rectum and vagina and a less common site is the urethra. Rectal suppositories are often used for systemic administration of drugs because of the large number of blood vessels in the rectum. Suppositories are available in a variety of forms, including cocoa butter, glycerinated gelatin, and hydrogenated vegetable oils.

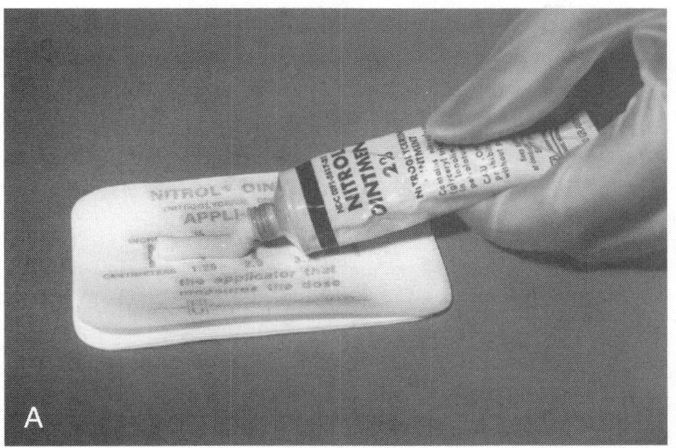

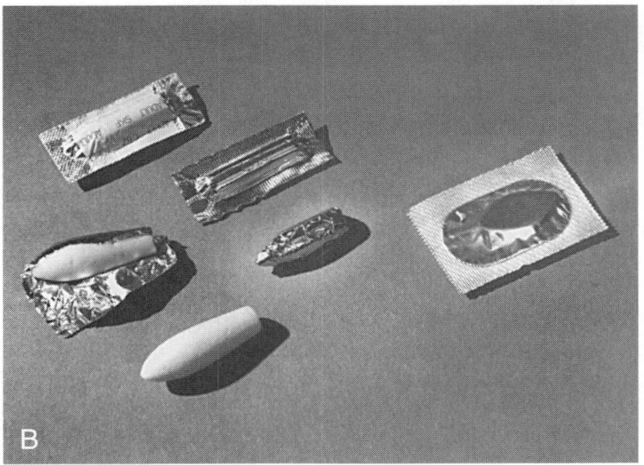

Figure 4-2. Semisolid forms of drugs include creams and suppositories and are generally administered topically. (A) Cream to be applied dermally and (B) suppositories to be applied rectally or vaginally.

Ointments

An **ointment** is a semisolid, oil-based medication intended for external application, usually by rubbing. Medications that may be administered in ointment form include anti-inflammatory drugs, topical anesthetics, and antibiotics. Examples are zinc oxide ointment and Ben-Gay ointment.

Creams

A **cream** is a pharmaceutical preparation that combines an oil with water. Creams are usually used topically and may or may not contain medication. Creams are usually dispensed in a tube or jar. Creams differ from lotions in that lotions contain more water and are more fluid.

Gels

A jelly-like substance that may be used for topical medication is a **gel**. Some gels have a high alcohol content and can cause stinging if applied to broken skin.

Implants or Pellets

Implants or **pellets** are dosage forms that are placed intradermally, or under the skin, by means of minor surgery or special injections. This form of drug is used for the long-term, controlled release of medications, especially hormones. Radioactive isotopes, used in the treatment of cancer, may also be administered in the form of implants.

Liquid Drugs

Liquid preparations include drugs that have been dissolved or suspended. Examples of liquid drugs are syrups, spirits, elixirs, tinctures, fluidextracts, liniments, emulsions, solutions, mixtures, suspensions, waters, sprays, and aerosols (see Figure 4-3). They are also classified by site or route of administration such as local (topical) on or through the skin, through the mouth, through the eye (ophthalmic), through the ear (otic), or through the rectum, urethra, or vagina. Liquid drugs may also be administered systemically by mouth or by injection (throughout the body).

Syrups

A **syrup** is a drug dosage form that consists of a high concentration of a sugar in water. A syrup may contain addi-

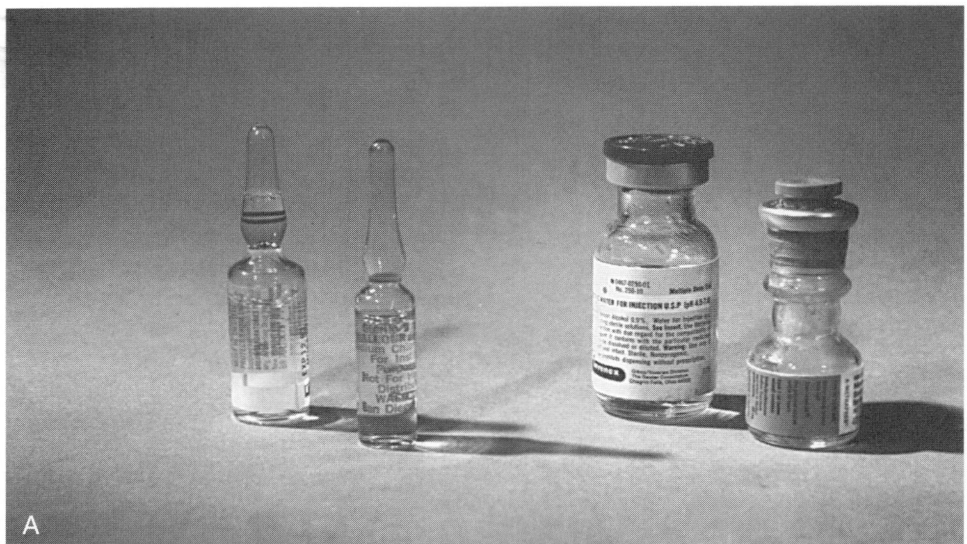

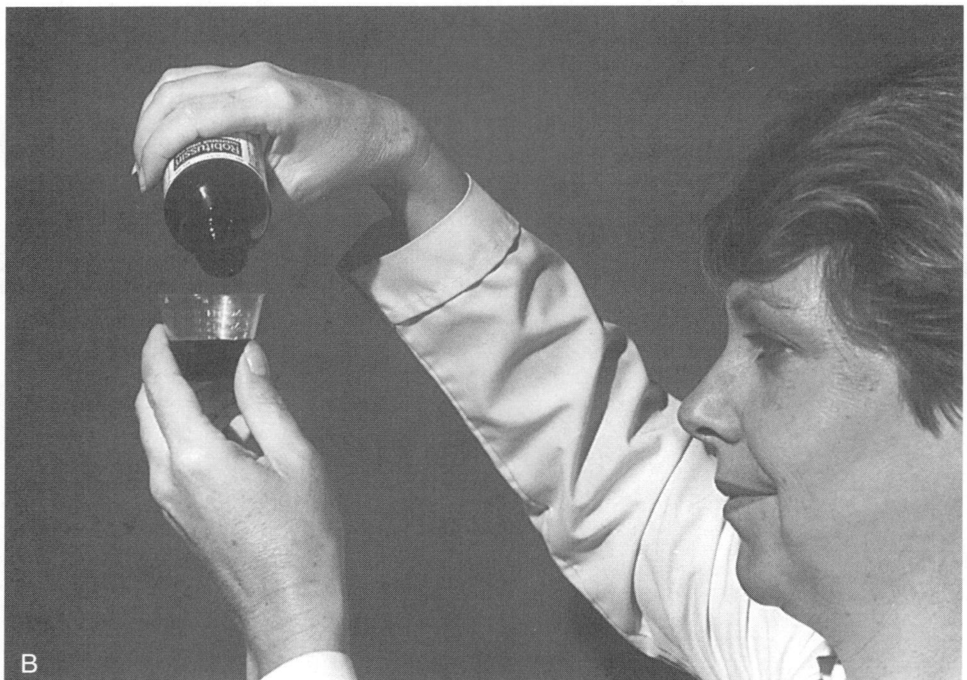

Figure 4-3. Liquid drug forms include syrups and mixtures and can be administered via many different routes depending on the preparation. (A) Mixtures administered intravenously and (B) syrup administered orally.

tional flavorings, colors, or aromatic agents. Syrups come in two varieties. One type is medicated syrup that contains active ingredients such as simple syrup, lithium citrate syrup, or ipecac syrup. Another type is nonmedicated syrup, such as cherry syrup or cocoa syrup, used as a vehicle because it does not contain alcohol.

Solutions

A **solution** is a drug or drugs dissolved in an appropriate solvent. An example of a solution is normal saline.

Spirits

Spirits are alcohol-containing liquids that may be used pharmaceutically as solvent vehicles for medication or as flavoring agents. Spirits are also known as essences (e.g., essence of peppermint, aromatic ammonia spirits, and camphor spirit).

Elixirs

An **elixir** is a drug vehicle that consists of water, alcohol, and sugar. It may or may not be aromatic and may or may not have active medicine. Their alcohol content makes elixirs convenient liquid dosage forms for many drugs that are only slightly soluble in water. In these cases, the drug is first dissolved in alcohol, and the other elixir components are added. All elixirs contain alcohol (e.g., terpin hydrate elixir and phenobarbital elixir).

Tinctures

An alcoholic solution of a drug is called a **tincture**. In some cases, the solution may also contain water (e.g., iodine tincture and digitalis tincture).

Fluidextracts

A concentrated solution of a drug removed from a plant source by mixing ground parts of the plant with a suitable solvent, usually alcohol, and then separating the plant residue from the solvent is called a **fluidextract**. Typically, 1 ml (1 cc) contains 1 g of the drug. Fluidextracts are not intended to be administered directly to a patient. Instead, they are used to provide a source of drug in the manufacture of final dosage forms. Only vegetable drugs are used (e.g., glycyrrhiza fluidextract and ergot fluidextract).

Liniments

A **liniment** is a mixture of drugs with oil, soap, water, or alcohol, intended for external application with rubbing. Most liniments are counterirritants intended to treat muscle or joint pain. They produce a feeling of heat in the area (e.g., camphor liniment and chloroform liniment).

Emulsions

An **emulsion** is a pharmaceutical preparation in which two agents that cannot ordinarily be combined are mixed. In the typical emulsion, oil is dispersed inside water. Most creams and lotions are emulsions (e.g., Haley's MO and Petrogalar).

Mixtures and Suspensions

In a **mixture** or a **suspension** an agent is mixed with a liquid, but not dissolved. These preparations must be shaken before being taken by the patient. An example is milk of magnesia.

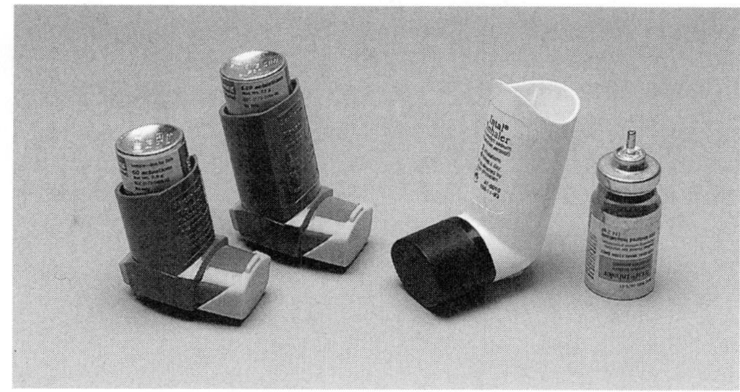

Figure 4-4. Metered-dose inhalers allow aerosolization of a liquid medication for inhalation.

Waters

In pharmacy, a mixture of distilled water with an aromatic volatile oil is called a **water**. Waters may be used for medicinal purposes (e.g., peppermint water and camphor water).

Aerosolized Drugs

An **aerosol** is a liquid or fine powder that is sprayed in a fine mist. The most commonly used aerosols are respiratory treatments for asthma and skin sprays. Although most aerosolized medicines are liquids, some are powders whose particles are small enough to pass through the spray apparatus. An example is the inhaler in a metered-dose aerosol unit used in the treatment of asthma (see Figure 4-4).

Parenteral Medication Forms

Parenteral refers to the injection of a liquid substance into the body by using a sterile needle and a sterile syringe. This form of medication can be selected when a rapid response time to a medication is desired or the patient is not able to take the medication orally. Injectable drug forms may be available as a solution or powder. A solution is a mixture of one or more substances dissolved in another substance. A solution is usually a fluid to form a homogeneous mixture. Powder is dry particles of medications. The powder itself cannot be injected. It must be reconstituted to a liquid for injection. A diluent such as sterile water is added to the powder and mixed well. Parenteral medications can be administered via different routes such as intravenous, intramuscular, subcutaneous, and intradermal, which will be discussed in Chapter 5.

REVIEW QUESTIONS

1. A troche is also called a
   A. tincture.
   B. lozenge.
   C. gel.
   D. liniment.

2. All of the following are examples of liquid drugs, except
   A. fluidextract.
   B. emulsion.
   C. tincture.
   D. gel.

3. Which of the following is an example of a drug used to remove corns?
   A. Decongestant
   B. Salicylic acid plaster
   C. Kato powder
   D. Cod liver oil

4. All of the following drugs are classified as a semisolid, except
   A. gel.
   B. tincture.
   C. suppository.
   D. ointment.

5. Implants or pellets are dosage forms that are placed
   A. intramuscularly.
   B. intravenously.
   C. intradermally.
   D. all of the above.

6. An example of a plaster is
   A. cough suppressant.
   B. zinc oxide.
   C. salicylic acid.
   D. Ben-Gay.

7. Which of the following medications is semisolid and oil-based for external use by rubbing?
   A. Gel
   B. Tincture
   C. Suppository
   D. Ointment

8. Milk of magnesia is an example of
   A. a water.
   B. a suspension.
   C. an emulsion.
   D. a fluidextract.

9. Which of the following forms of medications may be applied directly to the skin?
   A. Gels
   B. Liniments
   C. Lotions
   D. All of the above

10. Which of the following medications can be spread by heating and becomes adhesive at body temperature?
    A. Pill
    B. Mixture
    C. Plaster
    D. Troche

11. Creams differ from lotions in that lotions contain
    A. more alcohol.
    B. less alcohol.
    C. less water.
    D. more water.

12. An elixir is a drug vehicle that consists of
    A. sugar.
    B. water.
    C. alcohol.
    D. all of the above.

13. If a tablet is dissolved in the intestines and not in the stomach, it is called
    A. layered.
    B. scored.
    C. sublingual.
    D. enteric-coated.

14. Which of the following drug and dosage forms is a mixture of drugs with water, alcohol, soap, or oil?
    A. Liniment
    B. Fluidextract
    C. Tincture
    D. Elixir

15. What type of agent is used to determine the location of a disease by a specific procedure?
    A. Diagnostic
    B. Preventative
    C. Therapeutic
    D. Replacement

SECTION II

The Science of Pharmacology

Administration of Medication 5

OUTLINE

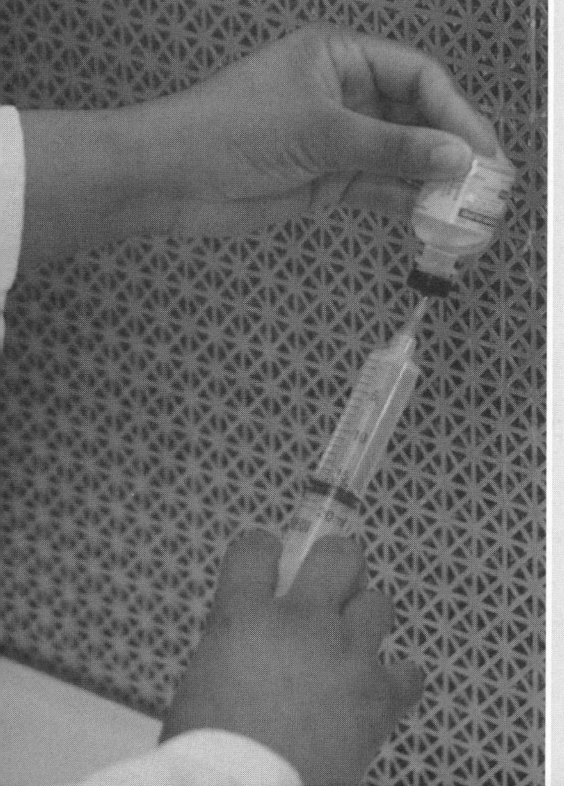

GLOSSARY

ampule A sealed glass container that usually contains a single dose of medicine. The top of the ampule must be broken off to open the container.

buccal Pertaining to the inside of the cheek.

implant An insert or a graft.

intradermal injection Between the layers of the skin. A dose of an agent administered between the layers of the skin.

intramuscular injection Inside a muscle. Normally used in the context of an injection given into a muscle.

intravenous injection Into a vein. Most commonly used in the context of an injection given directly into a vein.

oral Pertaining to the mouth. Medication given by mouth.

parenteral Administered by some means other than through the gastrointestinal tract; referring particularly to introduction of substances into an organism by intravenous, subcutaneous, intramuscular, or intramedullary injection.

subcutaneous injection The administration of medication by means of a needle and syringe into the layer of fat and blood vessels beneath the skin.

sublingual Pertaining to the area under the tongue.

topical Pertaining to a drug that is applied to the surface of the body.

transdermal drug delivery (TDD) Pertaining to a passage through the skin. Dosage forms that release minute amounts of drug at a consistent rate.

vial A small glass or plastic bottle intended to hold medicine.

wheal An intensely itchy skin eruption larger than a hive.

Z-track method A method of intramuscular injection of medication in which the skin must be pulled to one side before the tissue is grasped for the injection of such medication. It is used when a drug is highly irritating to subcutaneous tissues or has the ability to permanently stain the skin.

PRINCIPLES OF DRUG ADMINISTRATION

When any medication is administered, the seven rights of drug administration—right patient, right drug, right dose, right time, right route, right technique, and right documentation—should always be followed (see Figure 5-1).

Right Patient

Always verify that you have the right patient. Ask the patient to tell you his or her name. Check the patient's identification band if available, especially if the patient's mental status is decreased. You should also check the patient's middle initial in the event that more than one patient with the same first and last name is in the facility.

Right Drug

Verify that you are using the correct drug before you administer the drug. The label should be checked three times: when the medication is taken from the drawer or cabinet, when the medication is removed from the bottle, and when the medication is returned to storage. Make sure generic names and pharmaceutical names are for the same medication.

Right Dose

It is vital that patients receive the right dose of a medication. Giving less medication may be ineffective; giving too much may result in harm to the patient.

Right Time

Giving medications to the patient at the proper time is essential. Ensure that directions, such as before or after meals, with milk, etc., are adhered to.

Right Route

The medication must be administered following the manufacturer's order or the physician's order to clarify the route of administration, whether it is oral or parenteral, to have the desired effect. The effectiveness of the drug depends on the correct route of administration. The various routes of administration will be addressed later in this chapter.

Right Technique

A pharmacy technician, like other health care workers, must be familiar with proper techniques for all routes of administration.

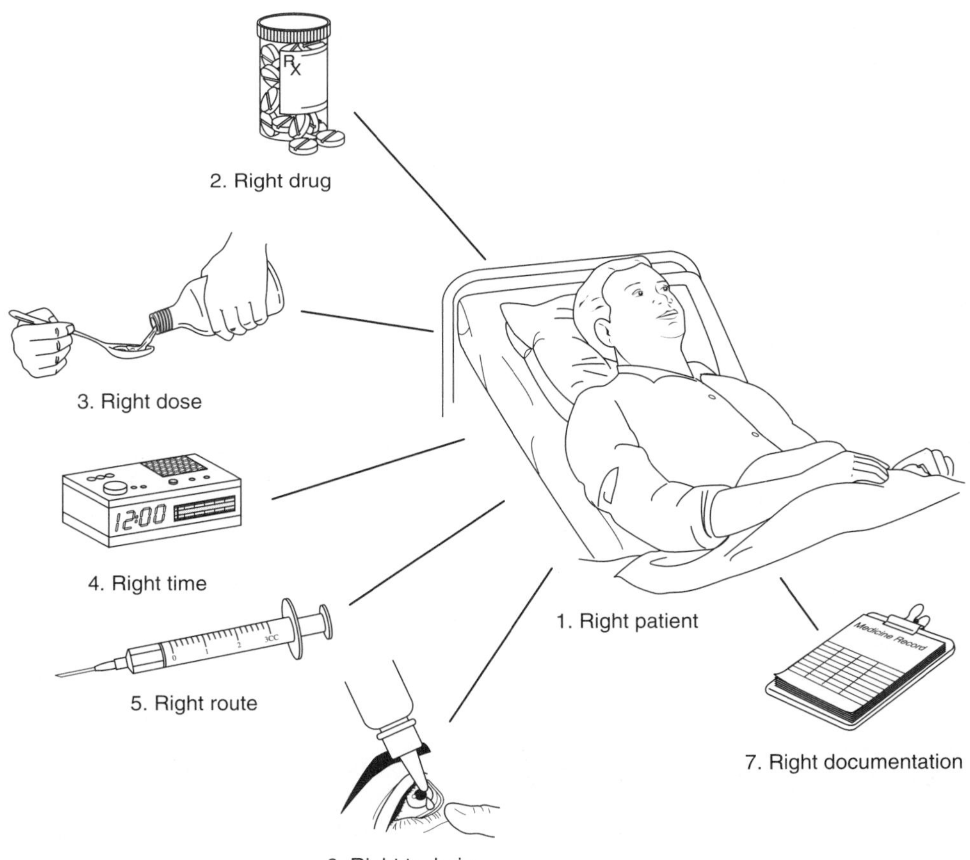

Figure 5-1. The seven rights of medication administration.

If there are any doubts about your ability to administer a particular drug, you should always ask for help.

Right Documentation

After a medication is given, it should be documented immediately in the patient's medical record. The following information must be included: date, time given, name of the medication, administration route, dosage of medication, and patient reaction. The signature of the person who gave the medication must accompany the documentation.

All documentation for administering drugs must be carefully recorded in the patient's file in the medication administration record (MAR). The record must be accurate and precise. Any medication errors have to appear in the patient's record.

MEDICATION ERRORS

Any incorrect or wrongful administration of a medication may result in serious untoward effects for the patient. Mistakes may be made in prescribing, administering, or dispensing a medication. Causes of medication errors may include difficulty in reading handwritten orders, confusion about different drugs with similar names, differences between pharmaceutical and generic names, or lack of information about a patient's drug allergies or sensitivities.

When a medication error occurs, it is very important that the error be reported as soon as it is noticed and that the patient be monitored to see if any adverse reaction to the medication develops. Medication errors must be documented in the medical record with the signature of the person who made the error. Pharmacists should consider reporting of errors as one of their professional duties. The U.S. Pharmacopeia (USP) and the Institute for Safe Medication Practices (ISMP) have developed a standardized form and method for reporting medication errors. Information about preventing medication errors can be obtained by calling 1-800-23-ERROR or by accessing the Web site for the USP (http://www.usp.org) or the ISMP (http://www.ismp.org). If you follow the seven rights of proper drug administration and dispensing guidelines, medication errors should not happen, but unfortunately, errors may be made periodically. When the pharmacy technician or the nurse has doubts, administration of a drug should be delayed until confirmation is made by a physician.

METHODS OF ADMINISTERING MEDICATIONS

The route of a drug refers to how it is administered to the patient. Certain medications can be administered by more than one route, whereas others must be administered via a specific route. The route of administration is determined by a number of factors:

- The action of medication on the body
- The physical and emotional state of the patient
- The characteristics of the drug

Other factors, such as age (pediatric and geriatric), the disease being treated, and the absorption, distribution, metabolism, and elimination of drugs, are important. There are generally three methods of administration: oral, topical, and parenteral.

Oral Route

The **oral** route is the safest and most convenient route chosen for most medications. Medication taken by mouth is solid (tablet) or liquid (syrup). The presence or lack of food in the stomach affects absorption of many oral medications. Some drugs taken with food may have a slow absorption rate. Oral drugs may be swallowed or may be taken by the buccal or sublingual route.

Sublingual Route

To administer a drug by the **sublingual** route, the drug is placed under the patient's tongue until it is completely dissolved. This method is used when rapid action is desired; for example, ergotamine tartrate (Ergostat) for migraines and nitroglycerin for angina pectoris can be administered by the sublingual route (see Figure 5-2).

Buccal Route

To administer a medication via the **buccal** route, the medication is placed between the gum and the mucous membranes of the cheek and left there until it is dissolved (see Figure 5-3). Drugs administered buccally are given for a local rather than a systemic effect. They are absorbed slowly

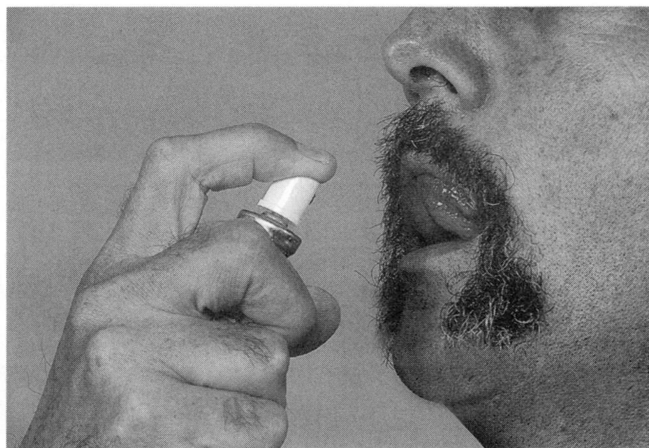

Figure 5-2. Nitroglycerin is a medication administered via the sublingual route.

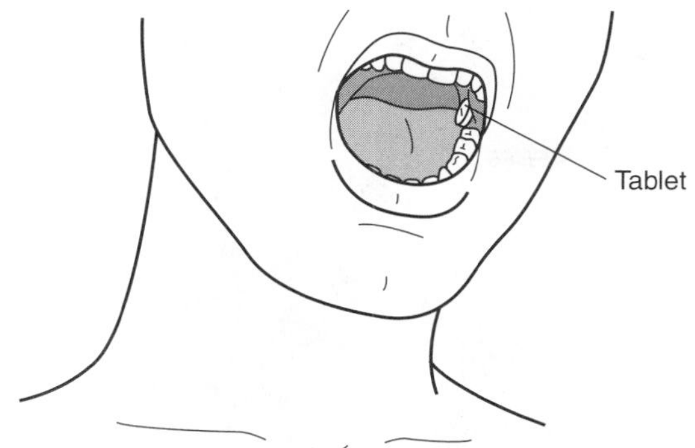

Figure 5-3. The medication is placed between the cheek and gum for administration via the buccal route.

from the mucous membranes of the mouth. Drugs given buccally may be given as a tablet.

Topical Route

Medications administered via the **topical** route are applied directly to the surface of the body. For instance, topical anesthesia is the application to the skin of a drug that temporarily deadens nerve sensations. Topical anesthetics are most commonly administered in aerosol, cream, or lotion form and may be used for conditions that include burns, insect bites, and itching. Other topical routes are transdermal absorption via mucous membranes, such as ophthalmic, otic, nasal, rectal, vaginal, and urethral membranes, for local or systemic effects.

Transdermal Drug Delivery

In **transdermal drug delivery (TTD)**, medication passes through unbroken skin. For example, transdermal patches are dosage forms that release minute amounts of medication at a consistent rate (see Figure 5-4). The drug is released from the patch and absorbed into the skin and bloodstream. Examples of drugs administered transdermally include nicotine, nitroglycerin, estrogen, testosterone, and scopolamine.

Inhalation Administration

The act of drawing breath, vapor, or gas into the lungs is called inhalation. Inhalation therapy may involve the administration of medicines, water vapor, and gases such as oxygen, carbon dioxide, and helium. The medication is inhaled to achieve local effects within the respiratory tract through an aerosol, nebulizer, Spinhaler, or metered-dose inhaler (see Figure 5-5). Medications that are administered via an inhaler include bronchodilators, mucolytic agents, and steroids.

Oxygen therapy is also administered via the inhalation route. When oxygen is administered, the dosage is based on individual needs. Oxygen is a drug; it is prescribed according to the flow rate, concentration, method of delivery, and length of time for administration. The dosage of oxygen is ordered as liters per minute (LPM) and as percentage of oxygen concentration (%). There are several ways to use oxygen. Methods prescribed most often include the use of nasal cannulas and masks (see Figure 5-6).

Oxygen toxicity may develop when 100% oxygen is breathed for a prolonged period. A high concentration of inhaled oxygen causes alveolar collapse, intra-alveolar hemorrhage, hyaline membrane formation, and disturbance of the central nervous system and retrolental fibroplasias in newborns.

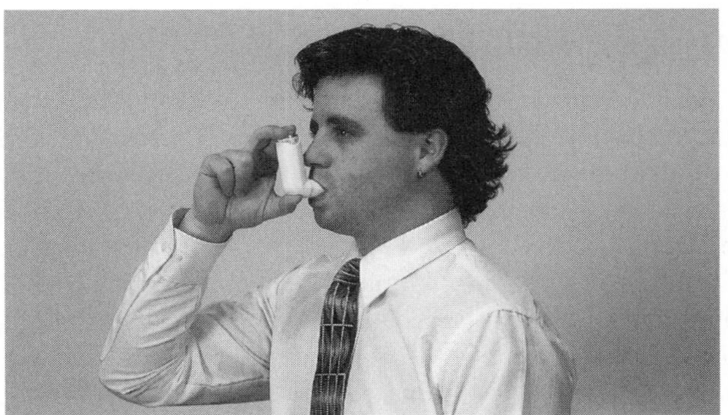

Figure 5-5. A metered-dose inhaler delivers medications topically through inhalation.

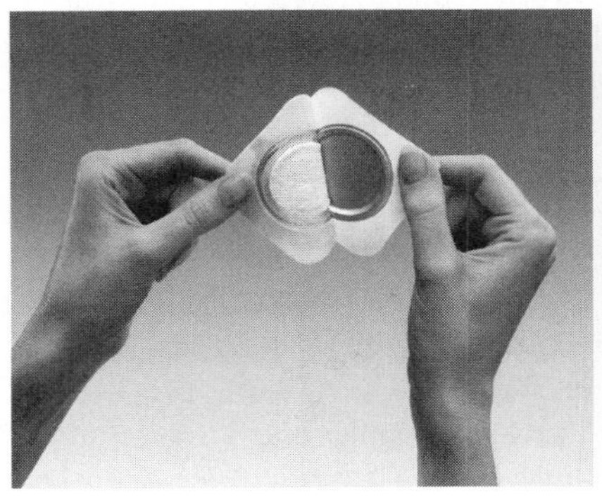

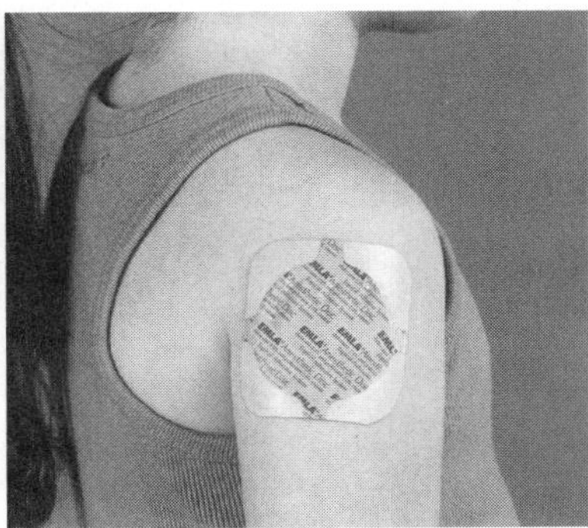

Figure 5-4. Transdermal patches deliver medication directly through the skin. (Courtesy of AstraZeneca, LP, Wayne, PA.)

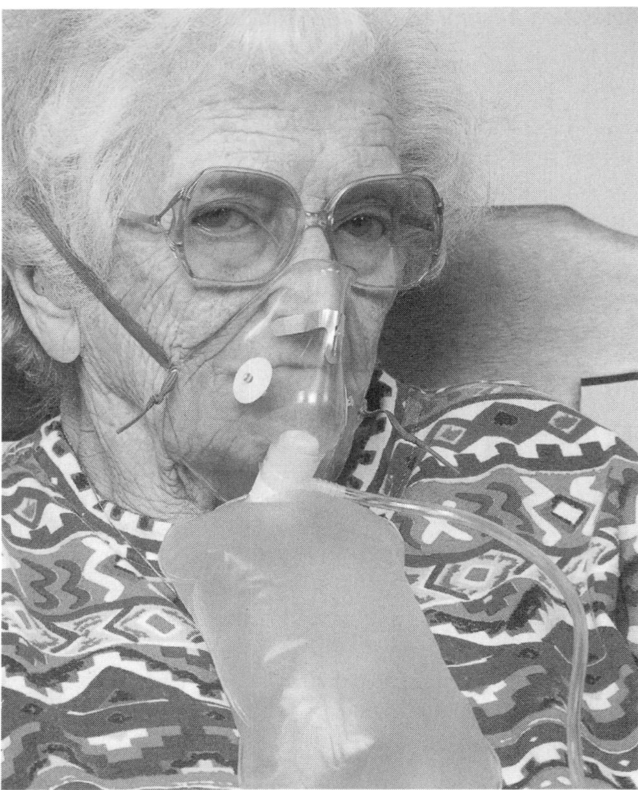

Figure 5-6. Oxygen is delivered topically in a gaseous form via a mask.

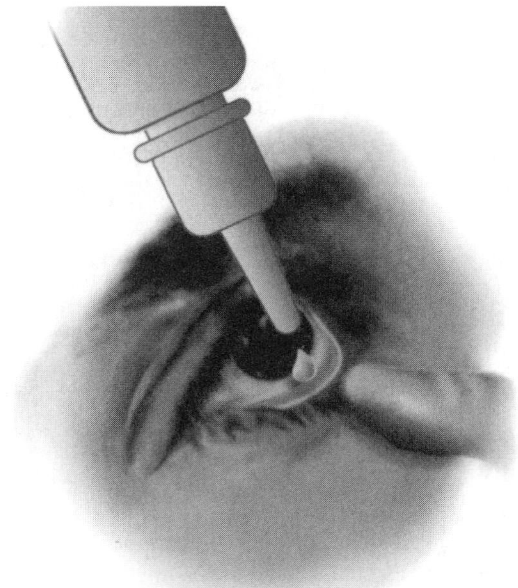

Figure 5-7. Eyedrops are administered between the eyeball and lower lid.

Ophthalmic Administration

Drops and ointments instilled into the eye are generally absorbed slowly and affect only the area in contact. The medications are placed between the eyeball and the lower lid (see Figure 5-7). Ophthalmic preparations must be sterile to prevent eye infections and should be isotonic to minimize burning. Medications in ophthalmic preparations include antibiotics, antivirals, decongestants, artificial tears, and topical anesthetics.

Otic Route

Localized infection or inflammation of the ear is treated by dropping a small amount of a sterile medicated solution into the ear. Very low dosages of medication are required, and the manufacturer must indicate that the medication is meant for otic usage. In children younger than 3 years of age, gently pull the earlobe down and back; in adults, gently pull the earlobe up and out (see Figure 5-8). The patient must remain on that side for 5 minutes to allow the medication to coat the surface of the inner ear canal. The use of eardrops is usually contraindicated if the patient has a perforated eardrum.

Nasal Route

Nasal solutions act locally to treat minor congestion or infection. The medication should be drawn up in the dropper and held just over one nostril, and then the required number of nose drops should be administered (see Figure 5-9). If a nasal spray is used, the patient sits upright; one nostril is blocked, and the tip of the nasal spray is inserted into the nostril. As the patient takes a deep breath, a puff of spray is squeezed into the nostril.

Rectal Route

Rectal medications are useful if the patient is nauseated, vomiting, or unconscious. Manufacturers supply rectal medications in the form of gelatin- or cocoa butter-based suppositories, which melt in the warmth of the rectum and release the medication (see Figure 5-10). Rectal medications also come in the form of enemas as a solution. Rectal medications may be used to soften the stool or stimulate evacuation of the bowel.

The best time to administer a rectal drug intended to produce a systemic effect is after a bowel movement or enema. An enema is the means of delivering a solution or medication into the rectum and colon. An enema is also used to cleanse the lower bowel in preparation for radiography, proctoscopy, sigmoidoscopy, and surgery.

Fleet Ready-To-Use Enema promotes bowel evacuation by softening the feces and stimulating peristalsis. Fleet Ready-To-Use Enema does not cause burning, irritation, or dehydration and does not interfere with the absorption of vitamins or the actions of drugs.

Vaginal Route

Vaginal suppositories, tablets, creams, and fluid solutions are used to treat local infections. Medications are deposited

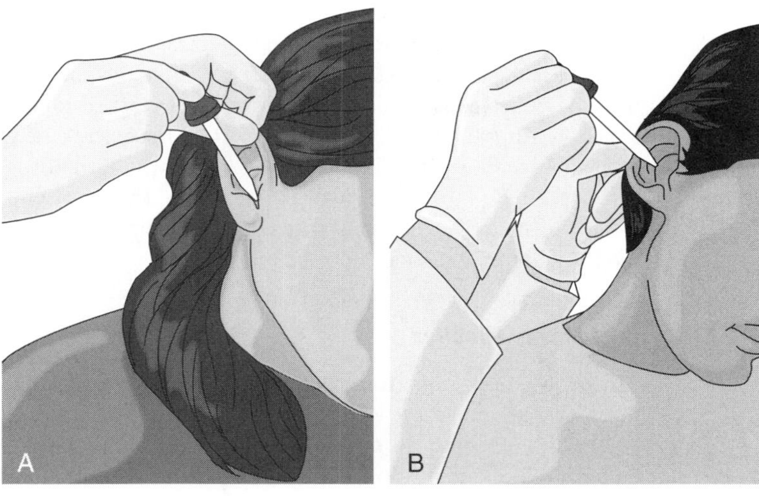

Figure 5-8. Eardrops are administered in the adult by pulling the ear up and outward (A); in the pediatric patient they are administered by pulling the ear down and back (B).

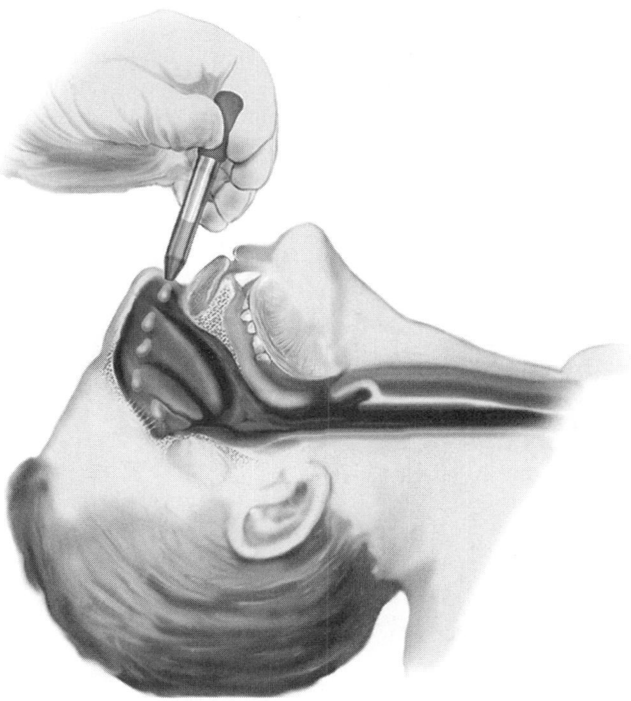

Figure 5-9. Nose drops are instilled while the patient is lying down.

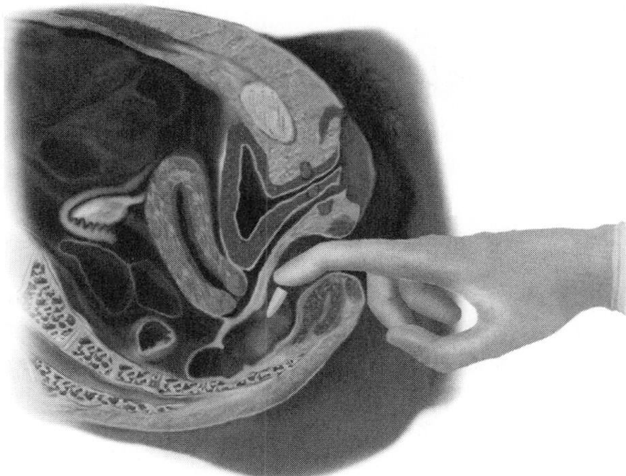

Figure 5-10. Rectal suppositories can be administered to the patient who is nauseous, vomiting, or unconscious.

into the vagina. Douches may be used as anti-infectives. Creams and foams are available for use as local contraceptives. Vaginal instillation is most effective if the patient is lying down. Creams are instilled with applicators.

Urethral Route

When a medication is administered via the urethral route, a solution is instilled into the urinary bladder using a catheter, or specially formulated suppositories may be administered.

Parenteral Route

Parenteral administration is the injection of medications into the tissues of the body with a syringe and a needle for rapid effects and absorption. There are four main categories for parenteral administration according to the site of the injection. Drugs may be injected into muscles, veins, skin (intradermal or subcutaneous), and the spinal column.

Intradermal Injection

Intradermal injections are given within the skin. If drugs are injected correctly, a small **wheal** (bump) occurs on the skin. The angle of insertion is 15 degrees, almost parallel to the skin surface. The common site of injection is the center of the forearm. Other sites that may be used are the upper chest and back areas (see Figure 5-11). Skin tests for allergies and tuberculin tests are the most common uses for intradermal injections.

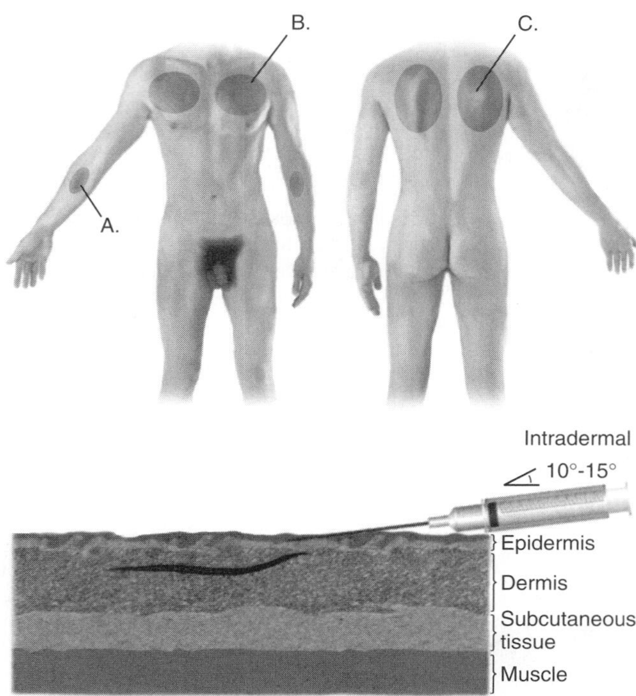

Figure 5-11. Intradermal injection sites and proper angle of injection.

Subcutaneous Injections

Subcutaneous injections are given just below the skin and the layer of fatty tissue called adipose tissue. The most common sites for subcutaneous injections are the deltoid area, anterior thigh, abdomen, and upper back (see Figure 5-12). The angle of insertion is 45 degrees for local anesthetics, allergy treatments, and epinephrine; however, insulin and heparin are usually injected at a 90-degree angle. The amount of drug administered through the subcutaneous route should not be more than 2 ml.

Intramuscular Injection

An **intramuscular injection** is given into a large muscle. The preferred sites are the gluteus, deltoid, and vastus lateralis muscles in adults (see Figure 5-13). The vastus lateralis is part of the quadriceps muscle in the thigh and is also considered the safest site of administration for infants. The deltoid site is acceptable for adults and older children. Muscles can absorb a greater amount of fluid than is usually given by subcutaneous administration. Dosage may vary from 0.5 to 5 ml. The needle should be 1 to 3 inches in length or may sometimes be longer. The gauge of the needle ranges from 18 to 23.

Drugs are injected into a muscle for the following reasons:

- The drug being given irritates skin tissues.
- A more rapid absorption is desired.
- The volume of the medication to be injected is large.

There are some intramuscular drugs that are irritating to skin tissue. For these the **Z-track method** of intramuscular injection is used. To administer a drug by this method, the skin must be pulled to one side before the tissue is grasped for the injection. After the needle is withdrawn, the tissue is released, with the needle tract to one side of the site where the drug was deposited in the muscle (see Figure 5-14). The sites of injection of many medications that require administration by the Z-track method should not be massaged after injection.

Intravenous Injection

An **intravenous injection** is used during emergency situations, when immediate effects are required, or when drugs or fluids are being administered by infusion. Sometimes large doses of medication must be given, either every few hours or over a long period of time. The rate of absorption and the onset of action by intravenous medication are faster. Intravenous injections are generally inserted into the smallest veins and as close to the hands as possible. The metacarpal, dorsal, basilic, and cephalic veins are commonly used in adults. Veins commonly used in infants and children include the scalp vein in the temporal area and veins in the dorsum of the foot and the back of the hand. Peripheral veins used in adults include the back of the hand, arm and forearm, and dorsal plexus of the foot.

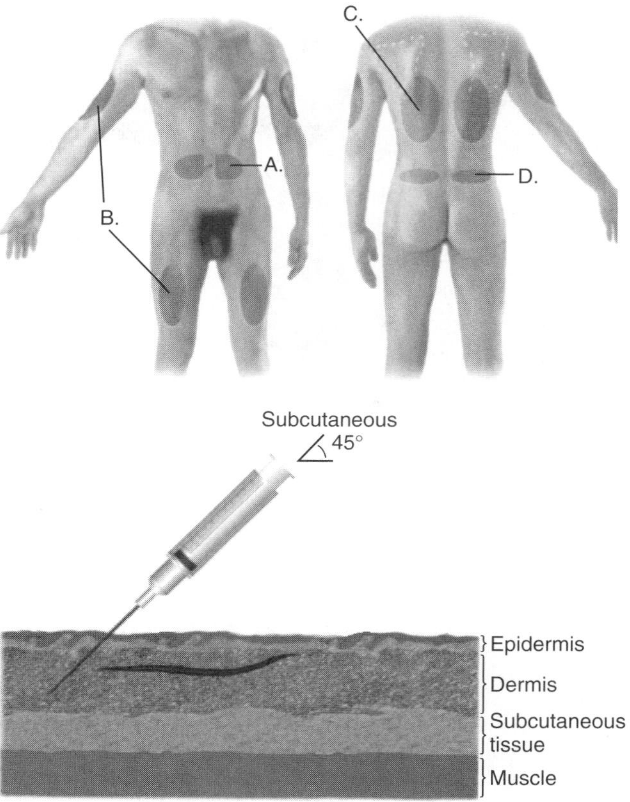

Figure 5-12. Subcutaneous injection sites and proper angle of injection.

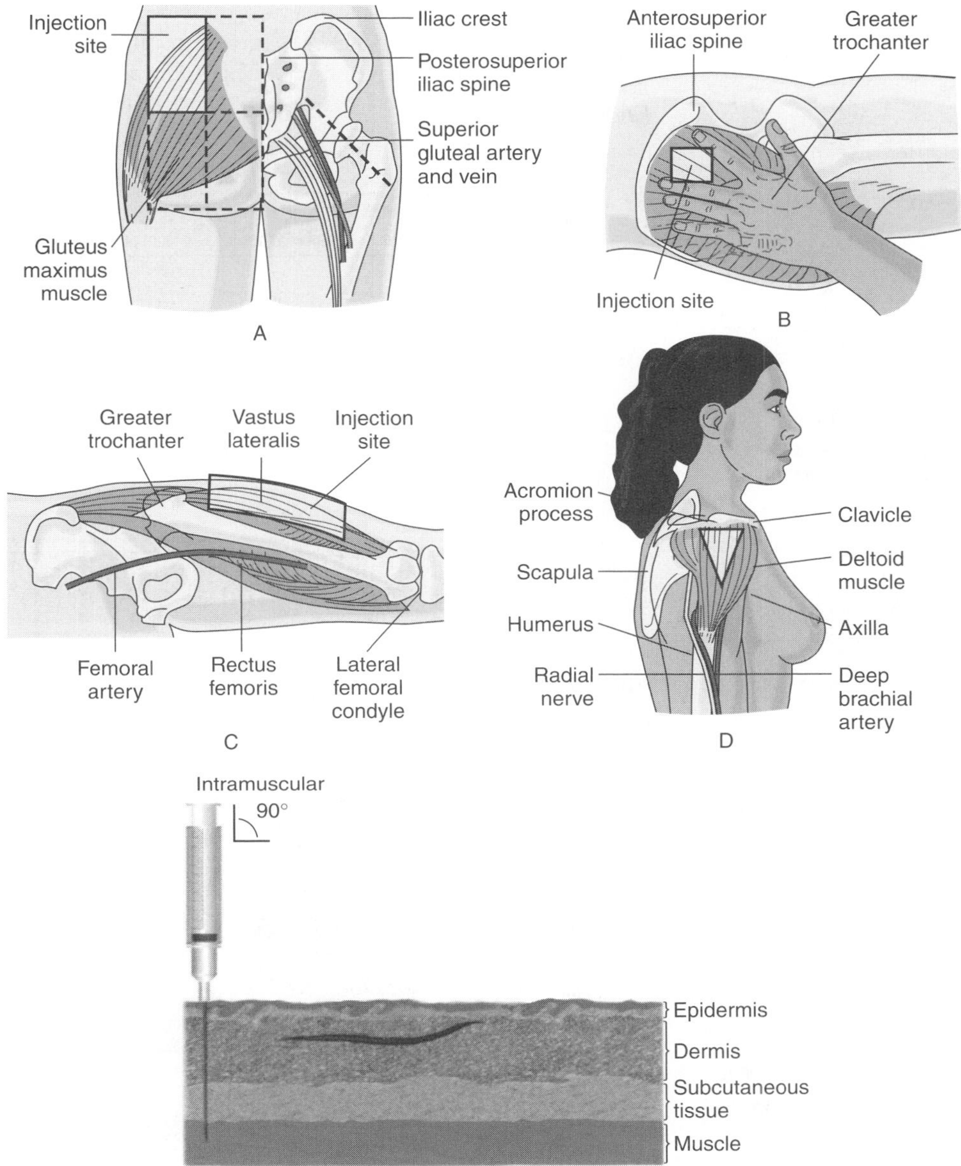

Figure 5-13. Intramuscular injection sites and proper angle of injection.

Implants

An **implant** is a device inserted surgically under the skin for the delivery of medications. Female contraception involves surgically inserting hormone-containing rods (e.g., Norplant) beneath the skin of the forearm. Once the device is implanted, the medication slowly and consistently secretes enough hormones to prevent conception. The rods may be removed if the woman wants to reestablish fertility. If left in place, the implants are effective for up to 5 years.

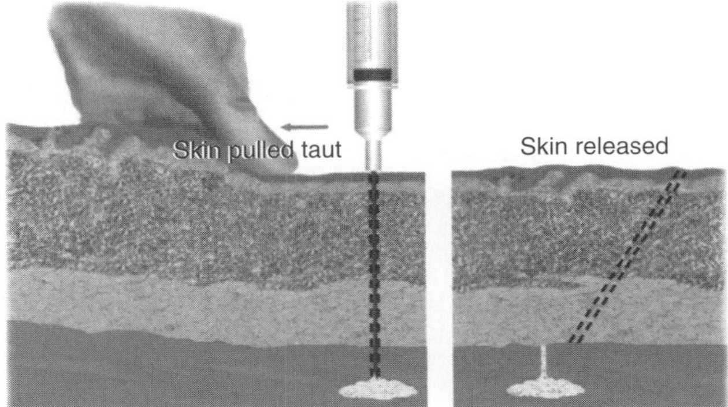

Figure 5-14. *Z*-track injection method.

Pumps

Medication can be administered via a pump to provide continuous flow into the system. Pumps are electronic devices

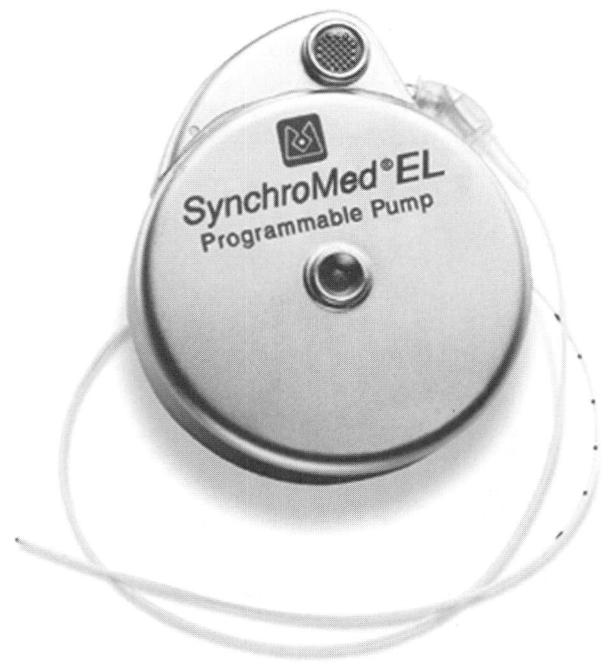

Figure 5-15. Implantable medication pump. (Courtesy of Medtronic, Minneapolis, MN.)

that force a precisely measured amount of intravenous fluid into a patient's vein over a predetermined amount of time (see Figure 5-15). The pump is a very popular way of administering a constant dose of insulin to a diabetic patient.

EQUIPMENT USED FOR ORAL ADMINISTRATION

There are three measuring devices used in the administration of oral medications: the medicine cup, the medicine dropper, and the calibrated spoon (see Figure 5-16). The medicine cup may be calibrated in fluid ounces, fluidrams, cubic centimeters (cc), milliliter (ml), teaspoons, or tablespoons. The medicine dropper may be calibrated in milliliter, minims, or drops.

EQUIPMENT USED FOR PARENTERAL ADMINISTRATION

Various types of equipment are used to administer medication via a parenteral route. Needles, syringes, intravenous

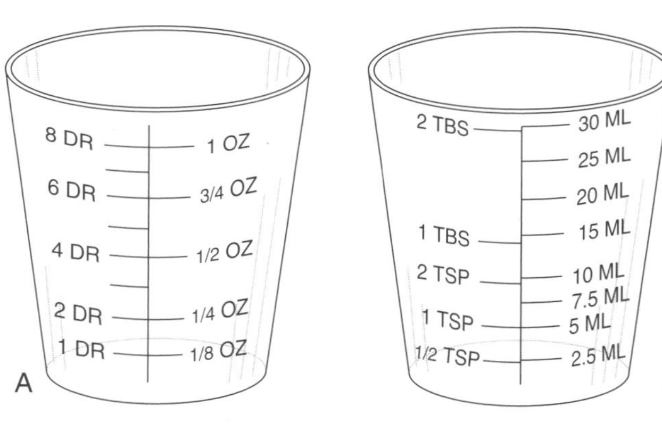

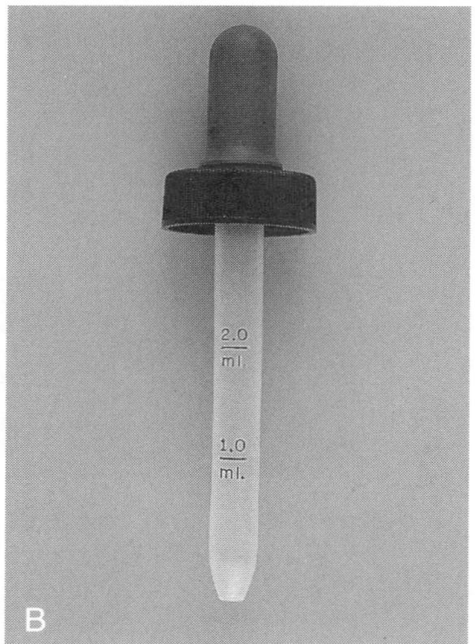

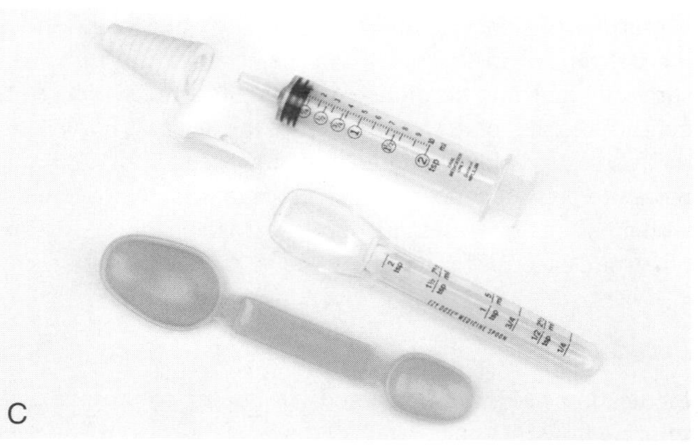

Figure 5-16. (A) Medicine cup, (B) calibrated dropper, and (C) calibrated spoon.

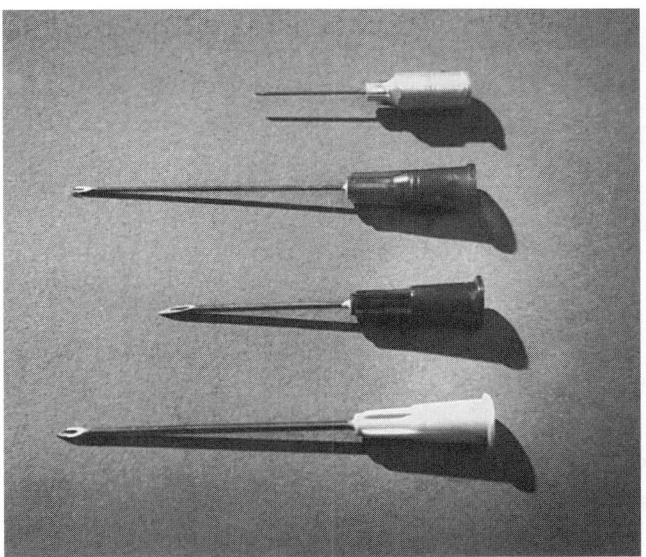

Figure 5-17. Needles come in various size gauges and lengths.

devices, and unit- and multiple-dose forms of injections are some of the equipment you should be familiar with.

Needles

There are two types of needles available for parenteral medication administration: disposable and nondisposable. Disposable needles are the most commonly used.

The gauge (G) of a needle is determined by the diameter of the lumen or opening at its beveled tip. Needle gauges range from 16 to 30 G and needle lengths vary from ⅜ inch to 2 inches. The larger the needle gauge is, the smaller the diameter of its lumen. Various sizes and types of needles are shown in Figure 5-17. Needles consist of five parts: the point, the lumen, the shaft, the hub, and the hilt.

Syringes

Both disposable and nondisposable syringes are available. Disposable syringes are sterilized, prepackaged, nontoxic, nonpyrogenic, and ready for use. The size of the syringes varies from ½ to 50 cc. The 1-, 3-, and 5-cc syringes are the ones most commonly used (see Figure 5-18).

A disposable syringe and needle unit consists of a syringe with an attached needle. Syringes are named according to their sizes and uses. In general there are two types of syringes: hypodermic and prefilled.

Hypodermic syringes are available in sizes of 3, 5, 10, 20, and 50 cc. These typically are used for intramuscular or subcutaneous injections. They are also used for venipuncture, medical or surgical treatment, aspiration, irrigations, and gavage (tube-to-stomach) feedings. There are several types of hypodermic syringes, which include needleless, insulin, and tuberculin.

Retractable needle syringes are used for prevention of needle sticks, as required by Occupational Health and Safety Administration (OSHA) standards. These syringes come with retractable needle covers to prevent needle sticks from contaminated syringes (see Figure 5-19).

Another type of syringe called an injector pen is used most commonly for insulin administration. The insulin syringe is calibrated in units (U) specifically for use by diabetic patients. The sizes of syringes are U-100 (0.5 cc) and U-100 (1 cc).

The tuberculin syringe is used for small quantities of drugs, because it holds only up to 1.0 ml of injectable material. Tuberculin syringes inject minute amounts intradermally and are used in allergy testing and allergy injections.

A prefilled syringe is a sterile disposable syringe and needle unit packaged by the manufacturer with a single dose of medication inside and ready to administer (see Figure 5-20). These syringes are meant for one-time use only and should by properly disposed of after medication administration.

Proper Needle and Syringe Disposal

All needles and syringes must be disposed of in proper containers. These containers are called sharps containers and are made of hard plastic to prevent needles from poking through them. Proper disposal of needles will reduce the risk of needle stick injuries.

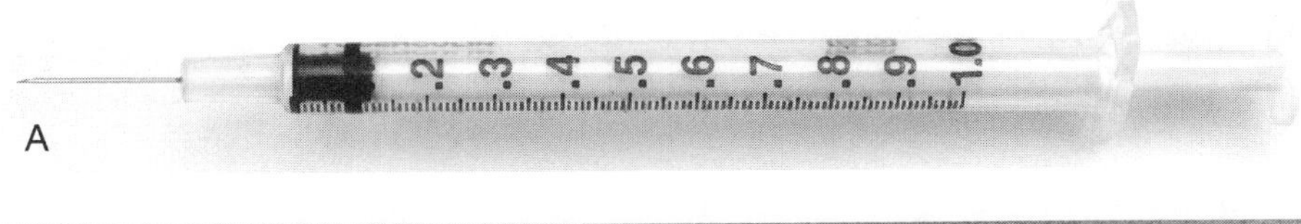

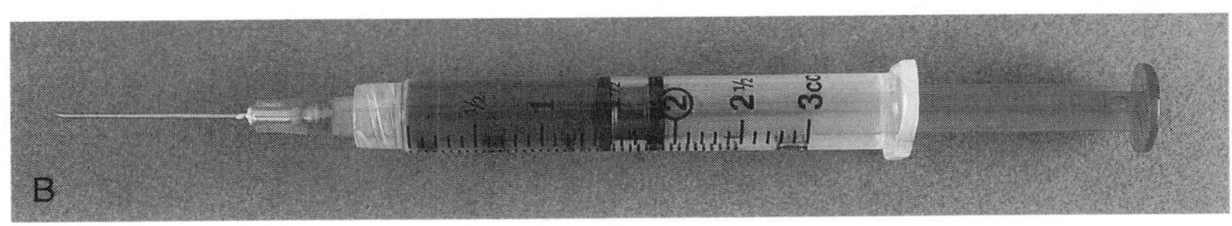

Figure 5-18. (A) 1-cc syringe and (B) 3-cc syringe.

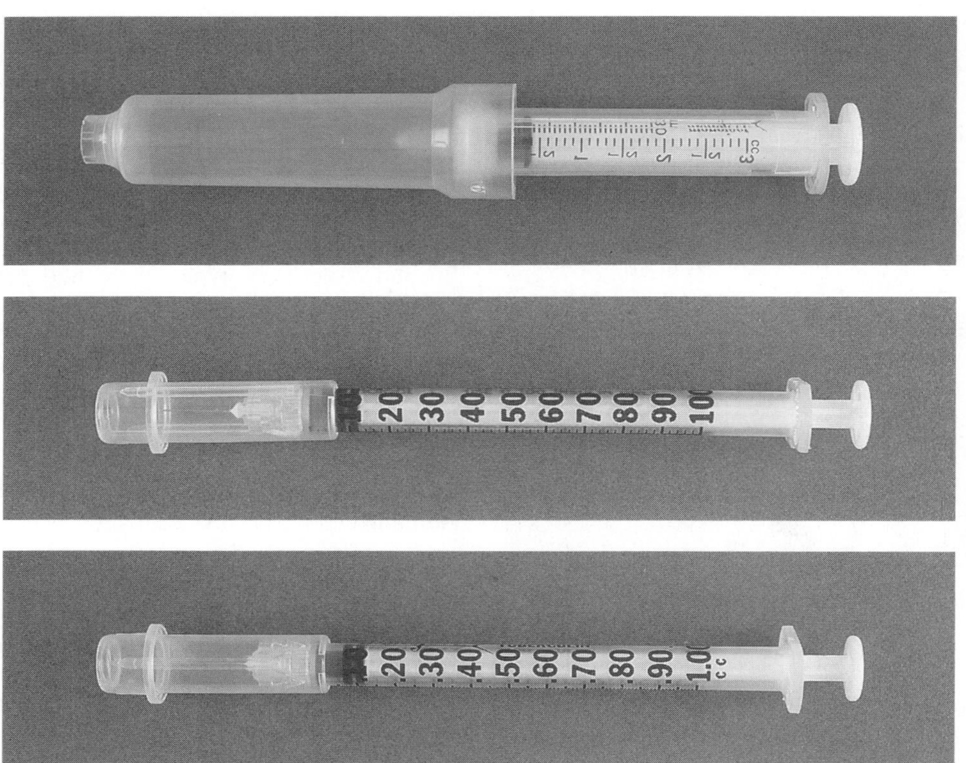

Figure 5-19. Syringes that have a safety device to slide over the needle or retractable needles are now preferred.

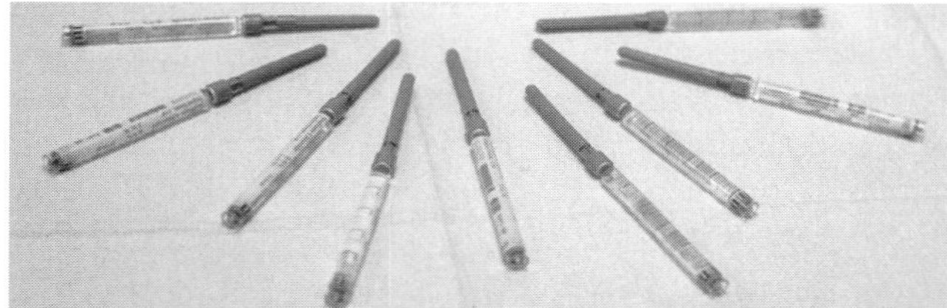

Figure 5-20. Prefilled, single-dose syringe.

Unit- and Multiple-Dose Forms

Medications prescribed by injection are available in different forms such as ampules, vials, and sterile cartridges with premeasured doses of medication. The **ampule** is a small, hermetically sealed glass container that holds a single dose of medication. The **vial** is a small bottle with a rubber stopper through which you insert a sterile needle to withdraw a single dose of medication. There are two types of vials: single and multiple dose. A multiple-dose vial may contain a varying number of doses of a drug. Vials vary in size from 2 to 100 ml or more doses (see Figure 5-21). A disposable sterile cartridge, containing a premeasured amount of medication, is available in single-dose forms.

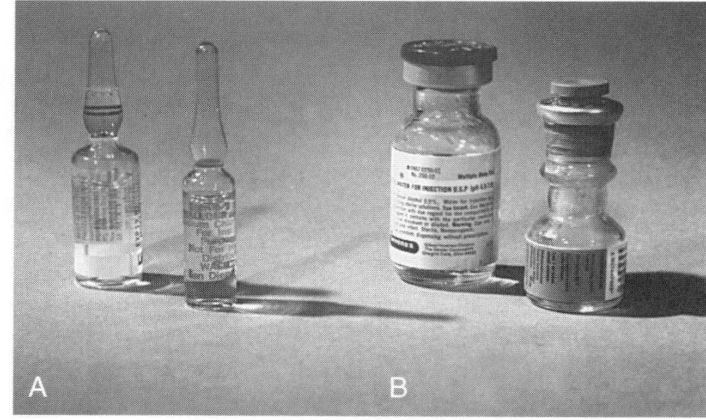

Figure 5-21. (A) Ampules and (B) vials.

WEB SITES OF INTEREST

Institute for Safe Medication Practices: http://www.ismp.org
U.S. Pharmacopeia: http://www.usp.org

REVIEW QUESTIONS

1. Oxygen is prescribed according to all of the following factors except
A. flow rate.
B. age of patient.
C. method of delivery.
D. length of time of administration.

2. The best time to administer a rectal drug intended for a systemic effect is
A. before bedtime.
B. before eating breakfast.
C. after a bowel movement.
D. at any time.

3. Which of the following would require an injection of medication at an angle of insertion of 15 degrees, almost parallel to the skin surface?
A. Tuberculin test
B. Allergy treatments
C. Allergy tests
D. A and C

4. Implants (surgically inserting hormone-containing rods to prevent conception) are effective for up to
A. 1 year.
B. 3 years.
C. 5 years.
D. 10 years.

5. Needle gauge is determined by the diameter of the lumen. Needle gauges range from
A. 13 to 20.
B. 16 to 20.
C. 16 to 30.
D. 20 to 35.

6. Which of the following syringes are calibrated in units?
A. Insulin syringes
B. Needleless syringes
C. Tuberculin syringes
D. Disposable syringes

7. All of the following are examples of drugs administered transdermally, except
A. ergotamine tartrate.
B. nicotine.
C. scopolamine.
D. nitroglycerin.

8. Which of the following injection methods should be used for medications that are irritating or may cause discoloration of the skin?
A. Intravenous
B. Intradermal
C. Subcutaneous
D. Z-track

9. Which of the following types of injections is inserted just below the surface of the skin and forms a wheal?
A. Subcutaneous
B. Intradermal
C. Intramuscular
D. Z-track

10. To perform irrigation of the ear in adult patients, the ear canal should be straightened by gently pulling the ear lobe in which of the following directions?
A. Up and back
B. Up and out
C. Down and out
D. Down and back

11. Which of the following is the route of administration of a drug that is placed between the gums and the cheek?
A. Transdermal
B. Sublingual
C. Buccal
D. Topical

12. Which of the following is the most appropriate site for intramuscular injections in infants and children?
A. Gluteus maximus
B. Deltoid
C. Ventrogluteal
D. Vastus lateralis

13. Which of the following is the most common route of drug administration?
A. Intravenous
B. Parenteral
C. Oral
D. Transdermal

14. Suppositories may be used for all of the following except
A. vaginal.
B. rectal.
C. buccal.
D. urethral.

15. OSHA standards require which of the following devices for the prevention of needle sticks?
A. Retractable needle syringes
B. Injector pen
C. Tuberculin syringe
D. None of the above

16. The angle of insertion for subcutaneous injections is
A. 15 degrees.
B. 25 degrees.
C. 45 degrees.
D. 90 degrees.

Continues

17. The advantages of Fleet Ready-To-Use Enemas include that it
A. does not cause burning or irritation.
B. does not interfere with bowel evacuation.
C. does not interfere with the absorption of vitamins or the action of the drug.
D. A and C.

18. All of the following are examples of sublingual administration of drugs, except
A. oxytocin.
B. ergotamine tartrate.
C. nitroglycerin.
D. B and C.

SECTION III

Hospital and Retail Pharmacy

The Policy and Procedure Manual 6

OUTLINE

The Policy and Procedure Manual
- The Need for Policies and Procedures
- Benefits of a Policy and Procedure Manual

Developing the Policy and Procedure Manual
- Writing Policies and Procedures

Review and Revision of the Policy and Procedure Manual

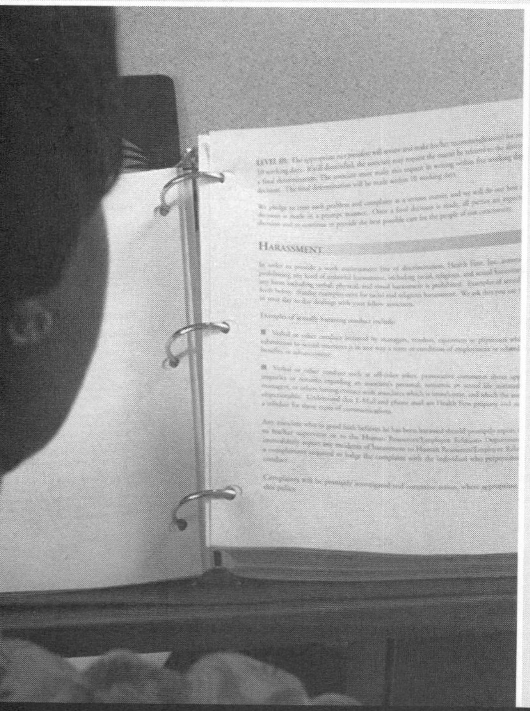

GLOSSARY

Centers for Medicare & Medicaid Services (CMS) The federal organization that administers Medicare and Medicaid. Its official Web site offers information about programs, statistical highlights, and the full text of laws and regulations affecting the agency. Formerly known as the Health Care Financing Administration (HCFA).

Department of Public Health (DPH) An organization in which sciences, skills, and beliefs that are directed to the maintenance and improvement of the health of all the people are combined.

Joint Commission on Accreditation of Healthcare Organizations (JCAHO) Not-for-profit organization that sets standards to ensure effective quality services (e.g., optimal standards for the operation of hospitals).

policy and procedure manual A set of standard procedural statements or documents that aid an organization in operating effectively and efficiently and support the overall goals of the organization.

The State Board of Pharmacy The organization responsible for the registration of pharmacists, pharmacy interns, and pharmacy technicians.

THE POLICY AND PROCEDURE MANUAL

Hospitals today are very complex organizations. In addition, the hospital may be a member of an integrated health care delivery system. This complexity dictates that the hospital and all its departments must have a set of standard procedural statements to operate effectively and efficiently. The regulatory and quasi-legal organizations that oversee hospitals require a manual to fulfill this need. In support of the hospital and the health care delivery system, the pharmacy department must develop a guideline for operations. This document is formally called the **policy and procedure manual**. The policy and procedure manual contains statements of the definite course or method of action selected to support the goals of the overall organization (policies) and statements of a series of steps to implement the policies of the department within the organization (procedures). This document provides a standard direction for operation and function within an organization and its specific departments.

The policy and procedure statements in the manual should answer the following questions:

- What action must be undertaken?
- What is its purpose (why must it be done)?
- When should it be done?
- Where should it be done?
- Who should do it?
- How should it be done?

A policy and procedure manual should be created and implemented in all pharmacy departments. All pharmacy personnel should use it as a guide for daily operations. However, it should not be used as a substitute for good judgment. A policy and procedure manual will never cover every situation that may arise. For these situations personnel must use their problem-solving skills and draw on their education and knowledge to formulate a course of action. There is no substitute for human judgment.

The Need for Policies and Procedures

The primary reason for developing policies and procedures is that regulatory agencies such as the Food and Drug Administration (FDA) and state boards of pharmacy, governing the delivery of pharmaceutical services, require that certain policies and procedures be developed and many times prescribe the content of the document. The Joint Commission on Healthcare Accreditation (JCAHO) and the American Society of Health-System Pharmacists (ASHP) are quasi-legal organizations that have defined a standard of practice for pharmacy departments which includes certain policies and procedures with a defined content. Table 6-1 lists organizations requiring polices and procedures.

Regulatory Agencies Overseeing the Hospital Pharmacy

The agencies that oversee all aspects of hospital operations, including the pharmacy department, are as follows:

- **Joint Commission on Accreditation of Healthcare Organizations (JCAHO):** This organization surveys and accredits health care services. All health care organizations must undergo this accreditation process every 3 years. JCAHO identifies specific guidelines for every department within the hospital.
- **The State Board of Pharmacy (BOP):** This agency registers pharmacists, pharmacy interns, and pharmacy technicians.
- **Centers for Medicare & Medicaid Services (CMS):** The CMS inspects and approves hospitals to provide care for Medicaid patients. Approval by this organization is required to receive reimbursement for any patients covered by Medicaid.
- **Department of Public Health (DPH):** This organization oversees hospitals including the pharmacy department. Hospitals undergo inspections by the DPH to ensure compliance with laws concerning hospital practice.

TABLE 6-1. Organizations Requiring the Use of a Policy and Procedure Manual

ORGANIZATION	POLICIES AND PROCEDURES REQUIRED
Food and Drug Administration (FDA)	■ Investigation of drug policies and procedures in hospital pharmacies ■ Policies and procedures for drug recall
Drug Enforcement Agency (DEA)	■ Policies and procedures showing proper handling of controlled substances
Occupational Safety and Health Administration (OSHA)	■ Policies and procedures that ensure the health and safety of people in the workplace
Joint Commission on Accreditation of Healthcare Organizations (JCAHO)	■ Policies and procedures that guide the pharmacy department in providing safe, effective, and cost-effective drug therapy
American Society of Health System Pharmacists (ASHSP)	■ Policies and procedures showing implementation of its guidelines and standards of practice

Benefits of a Policy and Procedure Manual

The primary benefit of having a policy and procedure manual is to document compliance with the rules of accrediting, certifying, and regulatory bodies. The second most beneficial effect of having a policy and procedure manual is to create a more effective departmental management program. Other benefits include the following:

- Establishing standards of practice for delivering pharmaceutical services
- Coordinating use of resources
- Improving intradepartmental relationships
- Providing consistency in orientation and training of personnel
- Providing a reference guide to all personnel in the performance of daily activities
- Creating a positive work environment, increased job satisfaction, and productivity

A department with a functioning policy and procedure manual will operate more efficiently and effectively.

DEVELOPING THE POLICY AND PROCEDURE MANUAL

The pharmacy director is responsible for initiating and developing the policies and procedures for the pharmacy department. This is done in cooperation with and with the approval of the hospital director, chief executive officer or president, and the pharmacy and therapeutics committee. The policy and procedure manual should be continually revised to reflect changes in procedures and organization. All pharmacy personnel should be familiar with the contents of the manual. The minimum standards for pharmacies in the hospital include the following:

1. Preparation of a comprehensive operations manual
2. Clearly defined lines of authority and areas of responsibility
3. Written job descriptions that are developed and revised as needed
4. Manual revisions that include continuing changes
5. Familiarization of all personnel with the contents of the manual
6. Input from other disciplines

Policies and procedures should relate to the selection, distribution, and safe and effective use of drugs in the facility. These should be established by the combined efforts of the director of pharmaceutical services, the medical staff, the nursing service, and the administration.

Policies and procedures will be either administrative or professional. The administrative policies and procedures are related to the control of resources (human resources, financial resources, supplies and equipment, job descriptions, and the physical plant) and relationships with other departments and administration. Professional policies and procedures pertain either directly or indirectly to patient care services. This section should represent the major portion of the manual. It should include all dispensing and clinical functions. A list of the topics contained in a policy and procedure manual is found in Table 6-2.

Writing Policies and Procedures

The pharmacy director must undertake the creation and writing of policies and procedures. Either the hospital administration or the pharmacy and therapeutics committee should approve all pharmacy policies and procedures. The information should be clear, direct, and simple. Creative writing techniques should not be used in writing policies and procedures. The policies and procedures should be developed with the input of all affected parties and the staff of other departments. The content, format, and design of each policy and procedure manual will vary with each organization. There is general information that should be included in each policy and procedure manual. A system of indexing each policy and procedure must be created. It is also imperative that a method of tracking origination date, reviews, and revisions of the policy or procedure be established. Because the practices of medicine and pharmacy are ever-changing, the policy and procedure manual should always be in a state of development. Thus, it would be beneficial to have a dedicated staff member who is skilled in the process of creating and managing a policy and procedure manual. The person(s) writing policies and procedures should be able to think analytically. The policy and procedure manual should inform and guide but not suppress professional judgment, personal initiative, or creativity.

A copy of the policy and procedure manual needs to be located in each area of the pharmacy department so that it is available to any department employee. The document should start with a policy title followed by a policy statement. The next section of the document should contain the step-by-step procedure for placing the policy into operation. A section should be devoted to references to source material used in the creation of the policies and procedures. Signatures indicating proper approvals should be obtained after the policies and procedures have been defined.

REVIEW AND REVISION OF THE POLICY AND PROCEDURE MANUAL

The information in the policy and procedure manual must be current and reliable. It must be flexible and change accordingly; thus, the manual must be readily revisable. The entire contents should be reviewed or revised at least annually. Reasons for this are to ensure currency and conformity with new laws, rules, and regulations of government agencies and to ensure compliance with the standards of the Joint

TABLE 6-2. Hospital Pharmacy—Policy and Procedure Manual

SECTION 1: INTRODUCTION	SECTION 2: ORGANIZATIONAL STRUCTURE	SECTION 3: ADMINISTRATION	SECTION 4: CLINICAL PHARMACY	SECTION 5: DISPENSING	SECTION 6: DRUG DISTRIBUTION SYSTEMS	SECTION 7: SAFE USE OF MEDICATIONS	SECTION 8: PHARMACY COMMUNICATIONS	SECTION 9
Purpose	Hospital	Develops budget	Patient care	Inpatients	Floor stock			Index
Hospital	Pharmacy	Purchasing and inventory control	Research	Outpatients	Unit doses			
Mission/vision statement		Medical service representative and pharmacy relations	Teaching	Ancillary supplies	Automation			
Pharmacy		Drug charges	Pharmacy and therapeutic committee	Controlled substances	Mixed systems			
Mission/vision statement		Pharmacy policy and procedure manual	Formulary	After hours				
Scope of practice		Accreditation—JCAHO	Drug research studies	Intravenous admixtures				
		Physical plant and facilities	Drug utilization and evaluation	Pharmacist and radioisotopes				
		Professional practices and relations	Pharmacy library—drug information center	Prepackaging				
		Preparation of annual report		Manufacturing—bulk and sterile				
		Human resources						
		Job descriptions						
		Performance evaluations						
		Quality improvement						

Commission of Accreditation of Healthcare Organizations. Policies and procedures that clearly identify the method for handling revisions in the manual should be established. These should address who can initiate change, how change is accomplished, who reviews and comments on change, and how to process revision of material no longer in effect.

WEB SITES OF INTEREST

Centers for Medicare & Medicaid Services: http://cms.hhs.gov

Joint Commission on Accreditation of Healthcare Organizations (JCAHO): http://www.jcaho.org

State department of public health: Each state has its own department of public health. Search for the department in your state.

REVIEW QUESTIONS

1. A statement of a series of steps to implement the policies of the pharmacy department is called
A. organization.
B. regulation.
C. benefits of a policy.
D. procedures.

2. All of the following are the primary benefits of having a policy and procedure manual, except
A. good judgment.
B. certifying.
C. regulatory bodies.
D. accrediting.

3. The Centers for Medicare & Medicaid Services (CMS) inspects and approves hospitals to provide care for
A. elderly patients.
B. Medicaid patients.
C. only inpatients.
D. only pregnant patients.

4. The information in the policy and procedure manual must be all of the following except
A. flexible and change accordingly.
B. readily revisable.
C. accessible to patients.
D. current and reliable.

5. Providing a policy and procedure manual is a responsibility of the
A. pharmacy technician.
B. pharmacy director.
C. director of the hospital.
D. director of human resources.

6. Who should approve all pharmacy policies and procedures?
A. Pharmacy and therapeutics committee
B. State government
C. Hospital administration
D. A and C

7. The entire contents of the policy and procedure manual should be reviewed or revised at least
A. daily.
B. weekly.
C. monthly.
D. annually.

8. Which of the following organizations accredits health care services?
A. CMS
B. JCAHO
C. DPH
D. BOP

9. Which of the following agencies or organizations registers pharmacists and pharmacy technicians?
A. BOP
B. DPH
C. JCAHO
D. CMS

10. The primary reason for developing policies and procedures is that all of the following regulatory agencies require certain policies and procedures, except
A. the Food and Drug Administration (FDA).
B. State Boards of Pharmacy.
C. the Centers for Disease Control and Prevention (CDC).
D. A and B.

7 Hospital Pharmacy

OUTLINE

The History of Pharmacy Practice
Hospital Pharmacy
Organization of the Hospital
    Organization of the Hospital Pharmacy
Medication Orders
    Medication Dispensing Systems
Sterile Products
Inventory Control
Automation
The Future of the Hospital Pharmacy

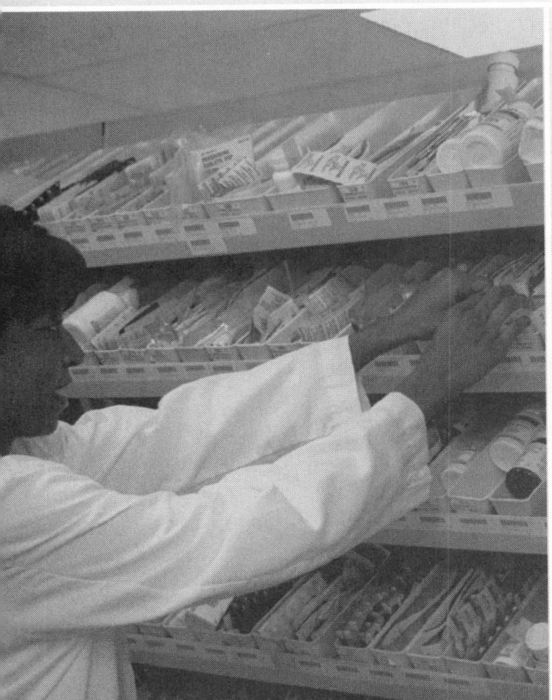

GLOSSARY

computerized physician order entry system (CPOE) A process in which the physician enters medication orders directly into a computerized system to eliminate the need for interpretation and thus reduce the risk for medication error.

floor stock system A system of drug distribution in which the pharmacy buys medications in bulk and distributes bulk orders to patient care units, where they are stored in medication rooms. Nurses are then responsible for preparing individual doses of medications.

patient prescription system A system of drug distributions in which the nurse transcribes a physician's medication order on an order form for the pharmacy and the pharmacy provides a 3-day supply of the medication for the nurse to prepare upon use.

sterile product One that contains no living organisms.

unit-dose drug distribution system A system of drug distributions in which a copy of the physician's order is sent to the pharmacy, the pharmacist prepares individual doses of medication, and a 24-hour supply of medication is delivered to the patient care floor.

THE HISTORY OF PHARMACY PRACTICE

The practice of pharmacy is as old as man. Early mankind, living alone, had to survive injuries and diseases with little help. A handful of mud, astringent leaves, and cool water was probably the first medicine used by ancient man to soothe his wounds. From such simple beginnings came the profession of pharmacy. As man became socialized and communities developed, houses of refuge for the sick and infirm evolved to provide more sophisticated health care. These houses were the earliest forms of what we know today as hospitals. With the evolution of Christianity and other religions a mission to care for this group of people was identified. The houses of refuge then moved into monasteries. The religious influence helped to foster the scientific directions of caring for the sick and infirm, because the monasteries were also centers of learning and science. Wars and conflict also influenced the need for health care. With the vast number of injuries sustained by soldiers during wars, a need for more sophisticated methods of treating injuries developed, and the hospital developed into the place where this care would be provided. The need for hospitals was also confirmed by the occurrence of catastrophic illnesses, such as the plague, cholera, and small pox. Patients with psychiatric illnesses were secluded from society in confined quarters, which eventually led to the development of psychiatric hospitals.

In early times the physician was both the doctor and pharmacist. As the practice of medicine became more sophisticated and demand for treatment increased, some physicians began to specialize in the art and science of preparing materials from natural sources to care for the sick, injured, and infirm; this was the advent of the profession of pharmacy. Many descriptions of early hospitals mention the apothecary and the herb garden. The concept of the hospital was brought to the Americas when the first hospital was opened in 1752. It was funded by a grant obtained by Benjamin Franklin and was known as the Pennsylvania Hospital. Jonathan Roberts was hired as the first American hospital pharmacist. The term *pharmacy* may refer to the practice of the profession of pharmacy or it may refer to a place where the profession of pharmacy is practiced. Some examples of these places are a retail pharmacy (called an *apothecary* in earlier times), a clinic, a medical center, a hospital, or any place where a pharmacist practices pharmacy. This chapter will focus on the practice of pharmacy in the hospital.

HOSPITAL PHARMACY

What is the definition of *hospital pharmacy* in today's setting? Simply stated, it is the practice of pharmacy in the hospital setting or the provision of pharmaceutical care in the institutional setting. The practice of pharmacy in the institution is comprised of the following:

- Support services—ordering and properly storing medications and maintaining an inventory of pharmaceuticals and associated medical supplies, billing for services, and installing and maintaining computer systems
- Product services—dispensing, preparing, and processing medication orders for inpatients and maintaining required patient records and drug control records
- Clinical services—managing the formulary system, evaluating drug use, and reviewing drug orders for appropriateness
- Educational services—providing education about medications to pharmacy staff, other health care professionals, the public, and patients and their caregivers

Hospital pharmacy practice has come to encompass all aspects of drug therapy through the total continuum of medical care.

ORGANIZATION OF THE HOSPITAL

The structure of a hospital or a health care system varies greatly from organization to organization. The basic structure includes a board of directors, who are responsible for the overall governance of the organization. Answering to the board are several layers of management. The primary leadership position is chief executive officer (CEO). This position may also be called hospital director or hospital president. Depending upon the size of the hospital, a senior vice president or chief operating officer (COO) who answers to the CEO may be present. The CEO usually works with the medical staff leadership and the COO with the operating staff leadership, which both consist of vice presidents, functional department heads, assistant department heads, and supervisors. At the vice president level, there may be positions such as chief financial officer (CFO), director of nursing (many times this position is called vice president of patient care services), vice president of professional or clinical services, and chief information officer (CIO). The functional directors are the directors of departments with a specific function or specialty. These are usually departments such as radiology, respiratory care, dietary services, pharmacy, environmental services, plant operations, medical records, finance and accounting, and many more.

In the preceding description, there is no mention of the medical staff, who are ultimately responsible for the diagnosis and treatment of the patients of the hospital. The medical staff members have a unique relationship with the hospital in that they are not employees of the hospital. They function as independent medical practitioners in private practice. Their income is derived not from the hospital but from their independent practice. Often they perform procedures in the hospital, but their income is derived through their office practices. The medical staff has a unique structure that links it to the hospital's organization. There is a chief of staff or a medical director who is elected by the medical staff of the hospital. This person acts as the liaison with the hospital director or CEO. A medical staff executive committee is elected to govern the medical staff. This committee is composed of functional medical department (e.g., medicine, surgery, cardiology, and pediatrics) chairpersons or chiefs of services and the medical director or chief of staff. This committee is responsible for overseeing the activities of the medical staff. It recommends the granting of clinical privileges to medical staff members and conducts quality assurance processes to ensure that the medical staff is providing appropriate medical care. The committee functions are performed through the formation of specific committees to oversee credentialing, pharmacy, therapeutics, and quality assurance. There is also a joint conference committee composed of representatives from the board of directors, the hospital executive staff, and the medical staff. Meetings of this committee are generally convened when there are issues to be addressed between the medical staff and the hospital administration and the board of directors. Figure 7-1 presents a sample organizational chart for the hospital setting.

Organization of the Hospital Pharmacy

The pharmacy department is responsible for all aspects of drug use. These include both product-related services and clinical services. The personnel in a hospital pharmacy are classified into three categories:

- Professional—comprises all pharmacists and management
- Technical—comprises the pharmacy technicians involved in drug-related processes
- Support—comprises nonlicensed personnel involved in providing services that support the drug-related processes and/or management functions

All hospital pharmacies have a leadership position in the department, usually titled director of pharmacy. This individual is responsible for all the pharmacy services provided in or by the organization. The rest of the department's structure depends on the size of the organization. Smaller hospitals may have a small staff, consisting of a pharmacy director and a staff pharmacist. As the size of the institution grows, additional pharmacists may be added along with pharmacy technicians. Larger hospital systems will have many different positions categorized by functions:

1. Management—almost always pharmacists
   a. Director
   b. Manager

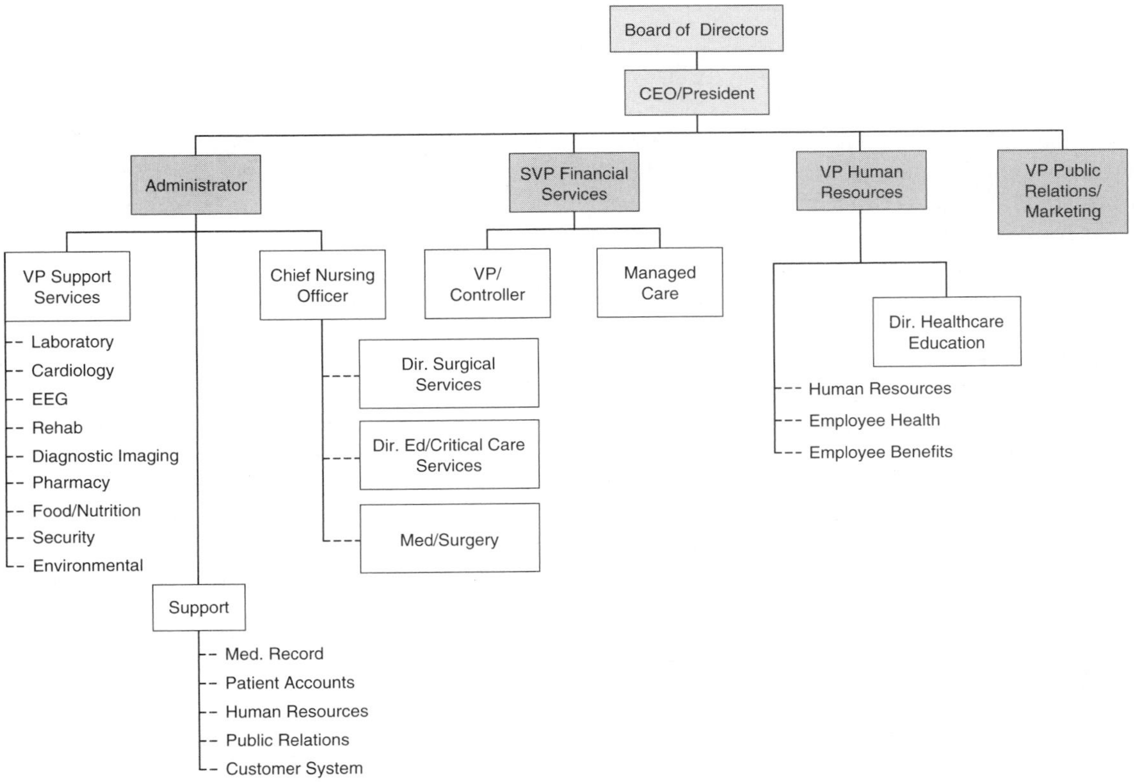

Figure 7-1. Hospital organizational chart.

   c. Supervisor—may have a technician supervisor supervising technicians
2. Dispensing and preparation
   a. Pharmacist—unit dose, satellite
   b. Technician—unit dose, cart fill, medication and supply delivery
   c. Central intravenous (IV) admixture and sterile processing
   d. Controlled drug storage and distribution
3. Support—generally nonpharmacists
   a. Department secretary
   b. Buyer
   c. Biller
   d. Systems analyst
4. Clinical
   a. Clinical coordinator
   b. Clinical pharmacist
   c. Clinical specialist
5. Education and research
   a. Drug information specialist
   b. Research coordinator

As the pharmacy department becomes more involved in the provision of direct patient care, many departments are beginning to redesign their organizational structure to support the practices of the future.

MEDICATION ORDERS

The practice of hospital pharmacy begins with the medication order generated by the physician. In the hospital pharmacy the medication order is the equivalent to the prescription in the retail pharmacy. All medications, including prescription medications and over-the-counter (OTC), ordered in a hospital require a medication order. The medication process begins in the pharmacy department when a copy of the original medication order is received in the department. Pharmacists and technicians must be able to distinguish between the various types of orders that are written on this document because there may be orders on this document that do not pertain to pharmacy. Diet, laboratory, radiology, and physical activity orders are a few examples of nonmedication orders. A variety of types of medication orders may also be encountered (see Figure 7-2). The types of orders are the following:

- Scheduled medication orders—medications that are given on a continuous schedule according to the medication order
- Scheduled IV/total parenteral nutrition (TPN) solution orders—medications that are given by the injectable route and must be prepared in a controlled environment
- PRN (as needed) medication orders—medications that may be given in response to a given parameter or condition defined in the medication order. If the defined situation does not occur, the medication is not given.
- Controlled substances medication orders—narcotics that require controlled documentation of procurement, dispensing, and administration. Storage is usually in a secured environment.
- Demand/stat medication orders—medications that are needed for a rapid response to a given medical condition
- Emergency medication orders—medications that are needed in response to a medical emergency, e.g., cardiac arrest
- Investigational medication orders—medications that are given under the direction of research protocols. Strict documentation of the procurement, dispensing, and administration of the medication is required.

Medication Dispensing Systems

The role of the pharmacist has changed from being a product dispenser to having expanding responsibility for the entire medication process. Because the pharmacist now is responsible for the complete medication process, medication dispensing systems have changed to support this increased responsibility. In the past, medications were stored in the pharmacy in bulk quantities. The medications were then dispensed in bulk quantities and multidose containers to "mini" pharmacies located on the patient care units. Nurses prepared doses for administration to patients. This system has evolved into sophisticated processes for unit doses and automated dispensing to allow pharmacists and their support personnel to concentrate on the final preparation of the medications for administration to the patient and the monitoring of the proper use of medications.

Floor Stock

In the **floor stock system**, the role of the pharmacy in the medication process is product related only. Drugs are purchased in bulk and multidose dosage forms. The drugs are then issued to patient care units via a bulk drug order form and are stored in medication rooms. Once placed in the medication room, drugs for administration to the patient are prepared by a nurse. A medication could be used for more than one patient. In this system the nurse is responsible for most of the steps in the medication process.

The disadvantages of this system are the following:

- Potential for medication errors
- Potential for drug diversion and misappropriation resulting in economic loss
- Increased inventory needs
- Inadequate space for medication storage on the patient care unit

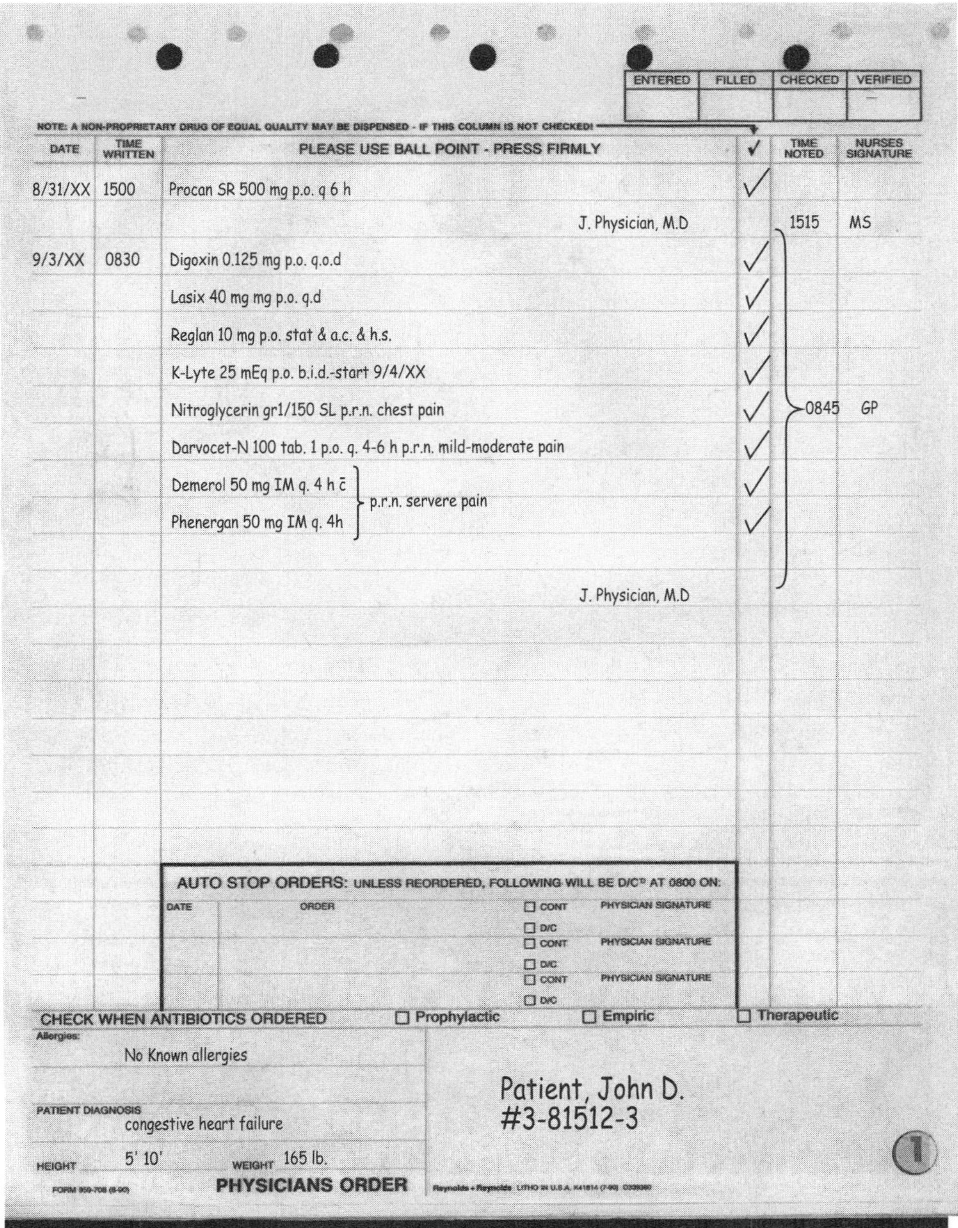

ENTERED	FILLED	CHECKED	VERIFIED

NOTE: A NON-PROPRIETARY DRUG OF EQUAL QUALITY MAY BE DISPENSED - IF THIS COLUMN IS NOT CHECKED!

DATE	TIME WRITTEN	PLEASE USE BALL POINT - PRESS FIRMLY	✓	TIME NOTED	NURSES SIGNATURE
8/31/XX	1500	Procan SR 500 mg p.o. q 6 h	✓		
		J. Physician, M.D		1515	MS
9/3/XX	0830	Digoxin 0.125 mg p.o. q.o.d	✓		
		Lasix 40 mg mg p.o. q.d	✓		
		Reglan 10 mg p.o. stat & a.c. & h.s.	✓		
		K-Lyte 25 mEq p.o. b.i.d.-start 9/4/XX	✓		
		Nitroglycerin gr1/150 SL p.r.n. chest pain	✓	0845	GP
		Darvocet-N 100 tab. 1 p.o. q. 4-6 h p.r.n. mild-moderate pain	✓		
		Demerol 50 mg IM q. 4 h c̄ } p.r.n. servere pain	✓		
		Phenergan 50 mg IM q. 4h	✓		
		J. Physician, M.D			

AUTO STOP ORDERS: UNLESS REORDERED, FOLLOWING WILL BE D/C'D AT 0800 ON:

DATE	ORDER		
		☐ CONT ☐ D/C	PHYSICIAN SIGNATURE
		☐ CONT ☐ D/C	PHYSICIAN SIGNATURE
		☐ CONT ☐ D/C	PHYSICIAN SIGNATURE

CHECK WHEN ANTIBIOTICS ORDERED ☐ Prophylactic ☐ Empiric ☐ Therapeutic

Allergies: No Known allergies

PATIENT DIAGNOSIS congestive heart failure

HEIGHT 5' 10' WEIGHT 165 lb.

Patient, John D.
#3-81512-3

PHYSICIANS ORDER

Figure 7-2. Physician's medication order.

Patient Prescription System

In an attempt to improve on the floor stock system, the **patient prescription system** was developed. In this system the nurse orders medications on a specific patient form. The nurse transcribes information from the medication order prepared by the physician to this specific patient form. The pharmacy then dispenses a 3-day supply of medication. The nurse still prepares the medications for administration to the patient. In this system, the pharmacy still has little patient information and cannot properly monitor medication utilization. The system is an improvement over the floor stock system but is an inefficient method of drug distribution.

Unit-Dose System

In response to the increasing number of new and more complex medications available, pharmacists have been expected to play an expanded role in the medication process. The system that evolved is the **unit-dose drug distribution system**. It is considered to be the safest, most efficient, most effective medication system for distributing medications. The features of the unit-dose system are the following:

- A copy of the original physician's order is received by the pharmacy and used as the dispensing document.
- Medications, including liquid and injectable medications, are prepared in ready-to-use forms and are dispensed per individual patient.
- Individual doses of medications are labeled.
- The pharmacy receives more patient information, including drug allergies, weight, and possibly a medication history.
- No more than a 24-hour supply of medication is dispensed.

The advantages of using the unit-dose system are the following:

- Reduction in medication errors
- Improved medication control
- Decreased overall cost of medication distribution
- More precise medication billing
- Reduction in medication credits (medications returned unused)
- Reduced drug inventories

STERILE PRODUCTS

The term **sterile product** is usually associated with drugs that are administered by injection. A sterile product contains no living microorganisms. The need for sterility is based on the fact that by injection the major body defense mechanisms are bypassed. The greatest protection against infection is the intact skin.

Even products that are administered to porous, membranous tissues must be sterile. An example of this is ophthalmic preparations, including ointments and solutions and suspensions. Because of improvements in manufacturing processes and technology, most products requiring sterility are prepared commercially. When a product of this nature that is not available commercially is required, the responsibility for preparing the medication resides in the pharmacy department. The pharmacy department will do the following:

- Ensure that the person preparing these products is properly and carefully trained in the use of aseptic technique.
- Prepare the product in an environment (clean room or laminar flow hood) that will prevent contamination.
- Prepare the product using aseptic technique to prevent contamination.
- Ensure that all contents of the preparation are chemically, physically, and therapeutically compatible.
- Ensure that the product is stable over the time it is to be used.
- Ensure that the prepared product is stored under proper conditions.
- Ensure that the product is labeled properly.
- Keep records of preparation.
- Use proper quality control processes to ensure that a proper preparation has been produced.

Handwashing is a very important procedure for preventing contamination. In preparing sterile products, the primary concern must be safety and accuracy.

INVENTORY CONTROL

The director of pharmacy is responsible for maintaining an adequate medication inventory and establishing specifications for the procurement of all drugs, chemicals, and biological agents related to the practice of pharmacy. This duty is usually delegated to a pharmacy buyer or pharmacy technician. The expectation of the customers of pharmacy services is that drugs are quickly available, cost effectively purchased, of high quality, and stored properly. In the hospital pharmacy the pharmacy and therapeutics committee determines which medications will be purchased and maintained in stock. The hospital must then decide on the system of purchasing the medications. The two types of systems are the following:

1. Independent purchasing: The director of pharmacy or pharmacy buyer will contract directly with pharmaceutical manufacturers to negotiate prices and other conditions affecting purchases from that manufacturer. Larger institutions are more likely to use independent purchasing because they can offer larger committed volumes independent of other institutions. Smaller hospitals will form coalitions to achieve the larger committed volumes needed to obtain competitive prices.
2. Group purchasing (group purchasing organization [GPO]): This type of purchasing involves the collaboration of several hospitals in negotiations with pharmaceutical manufacturers to achieve advantageous pricing and other benefits. The main advantage of this process is the promise of high, committed volumes to the manufacturer. This will allow the manufacturer to offer more competitive pricing.

The next consideration is to determine the method of acquisition of the pharmaceuticals. There are three modes of purchasing:

1. Direct purchasing from the pharmaceutical manufacturer
2. Purchase from a wholesaler
3. Purchase from a prime vendor

Direct purchasing eliminates the middle man and handling fees but requires a significant commitment of time, larger inventories, and more storage space. Purchases must be made from many vendors. Purchasing from a wholesaler means many items are bought from one source. The wholesaler is usually located closer to the institution, can provide next day delivery, and will maintain the larger portion of the inventory. This enables the hospital to reduce inventory costs. Wholesaler purchasing also reduces the need for a large commitment of personnel to support the purchasing process. The primary disadvantage is the higher acquisition costs of the pharmaceuticals. The prime vendor system of purchasing is a relationship established between the hospital and a single wholesaler. A contract is established, which stipulates a committed volume of purchases. In return the vendor will charge a highly competitive service fee and provide a guaranteed service level, a guaranteed delivery schedule, and a guarantee that individual or group contract prices will be the base price. A contract with a prime vendor may be an independent agreement with the hospital or an agreement made through the GPO. Generally the GPO is better able to negotiate a competitive contract. The prime vendor system has the advantages of both direct and wholesaler processes without the disadvantages. To reduce inventory costs, most pharmacy departments will attempt to have a just-in-time (JIT) inventory system. In this system sufficient inventory is maintained for the pharmacy to function until the next reorder period. With the prime vendor system this reorder period could be as little as 24 hours.

The pharmacy department must select a method of inventory management. Types of inventory management are the following:

1. Order book system
2. Inventory record card system
3. ABC inventory system
4. Economic order quantity (EOQ)/economic order value (EOV) systems
5. Computerized inventory system
8. Minimum/maximum (min/max) level system

In general, most of these systems require a large commitment of personnel. The EOQ/EOV systems are mathematical equations with parameters that are not easily obtained, rendering them unusable in the normal hospital. The inventory record card system, minimum/maximum level system, and ABC inventory system are laborious manual record-keeping processes. Most hospital pharmacies use the order book system or the computerized inventory system. The computerized inventory system can also be laborious, but this problem is being addressed by the use of bar coding and wireless technology (personal digital assistants [PDAs]).

Many pharmacy departments use the inventory turnover rate to determine the effectiveness of their inventory control system. This is a mathematical calculation of the number of times the average inventory is replaced over a period of time, usually annually. The target figure is 10 to 12 times per year. This generally means that the entire inventory value is turned over once a month.

Inventory turnover rate = Purchases for period/ Average inventory for period

Average inventory = (Beginning inventory for period + Ending inventory for period)/2

AUTOMATION

One of the disadvantages of the increased involvement of the pharmacy in the medication process is the need for massive amounts of information and the need to process many transactions quickly. The advent of automation (pharmacy information systems) has greatly enhanced the ability of the pharmacy to achieve these requirements. Automation provides the ability to rapidly process large volumes of medication orders accurately and quickly. From the automated processing of medication orders, patient profiles are generated, medication labels are produced, medication fill lists are produced, medication administration records are produced, and medication charges are processed.

Clinical screening can occur to check for drug interactions, drug allergies, and dosage ranges. Reports can also be generated to produce data to monitor appropriate drug utilization. Utilization and usage data from the pharmacy information system can be used to order and maintain medication inventory. One of the problems identified with this process is the medication order. It is a document handwritten by the physician that is very prone to error because the handwriting may be illegible. For this reason, a suggestion for the future is that the physician rather than the pharmacy be responsible for entering medication orders into the hospital information system. This type of system is generically called a **computerized physician order entry system (CPOE)**.

Many unit-dose systems use the 24-hour medication cart exchange process. This cart contains a 24-hour supply of medication for each patient on a patient care unit. The cart is usually filled by pharmacy technicians and checked by a pharmacist. A robotic device interfaced with the pharmacy information system will fill each patient medication tray in the cart. This robotic device is also capable of returning credited medication to proper stock locations.

Automation is also used to create point-of-service storage cabinets that are interfaced with the pharmacy information system. Use of these cabinets eliminates the medication cart filling process. An example of this type of automation is the automated dispensing cabinet. Many fear that the use of automation will decrease the need for pharmacy personnel. However, these devices require human intervention for appropriate use. The pharmacy technician of the future will be controlling these machines and providing proper maintenance, repair, and quality assurance processes. If mechanical failure occurs, manual backup processes must be in place, and human intervention will be needed to repair the failed mechanical systems. Human intervention can never be replaced.

THE FUTURE OF THE HOSPITAL PHARMACY

With the aging population and the increasing number of medications being produced by research and used by practitioners, there will be an increasing need for pharmacy services in all settings. Trends for the future include the following:

1. Increasing expansion of the responsibilities of pharmacy technicians to allow pharmacists to concentrate on direct patient care activities
2. Increasing need for education of both pharmacists and pharmacy technicians
3. Increasing need for pharmacists and pharmacy technicians to obtain the skills necessary to work directly with patients
4. Increasing multiprofessional approach to providing patient care, thus requiring better communication skills
5. Increasing use of automation to perform routine tasks and to handle the massive amount of information and documentation that must occur as a result of providing patient care. Automation will also be used to make patient information available in the many settings in which patient care will be delivered.

The future is bright for those who choose pharmacy as a profession. It is the responsibility of those in the field to prepare for the requirements of the future directions of pharmacy.

REVIEW QUESTIONS

1. The pharmacy practice in the hospital comprises all of the following, except
   A. educational services.
   B. product services.
   C. engineering services.
   D. clinical services.

2. The basis for the practice of hospital pharmacy begins with the
   A. providing pharmacy technician.
   B. medication order.
   C. emergency department.
   D. administration of medication.

3. The unit dose is considered to have all of the following characteristics, except
   A. it is safest.
   B. it is the most efficient.
   C. it is the cheapest.
   D. it is the most effective.

4. In preparing sterile products, the primary concern must be
   A. safety and accuracy.
   B. saving time and moving quickly.
   C. availability and productivity.
   D. cost.

5. All of the following are among the three modes of purchasing, except
   A. purchase from wholesaler.
   B. purchase from a second vendor.
   C. purchase from a prime vendor.
   D. purchase from the pharmaceutical manufacturer.

6. Which of the following personnel will be running the automation machines?
   A. The pharmacy technician
   B. The secretarial department
   C. The pharmacist
   D. The supervisor

7. The disadvantages of the floor stock system include all of the following, except
   A. potential for drug diversion and misappropriation resulting in economic loss.
   B. increased inventory needs.
   C. inadequate space for medication storage on the patient care unit.
   D. potential for scheduling errors.

8. The inventory turnover rate equals
   A. purchases for period plus average inventory for period.
   B. purchases for previous year divided by average inventory of this year.
   C. purchases for period divided by average inventory for period.
   D. beginning inventory for period plus ending inventory for period.

9. CPOE means
   A. certified physician-ordered examination.
   B. computerized physician order entry.
   C. computerized physical order entry.
   D. certified physician order entry.

Continues

10. In the hospital pharmacy, the medications that are purchased and stocked are determined by
A. the pharmacy buyer and the pharmacy technician.
B. the pharmacy supervisors.
C. the pharmacists on staff.
D. the pharmacy and therapeutics committee.

11. The term *sterile product* means
A. one that contains fluid.
B. one that produces enzymes.
C. one that contains no living organism.
D. all of the above.

12. The provision of pharmaceutical care in the institutional setting is known as
A. nuclear pharmacy.
B. hospital pharmacy.
C. retail pharmacy.
D. mail-order pharmacy.

13. The main advantage of group purchasing is
A. the manufacturer can offer competitive pricing.
B. the buyer can order low volumes from the manufacturer.
C. the manufacturer can offer less volume of its product.
D. the buyer can offer more competitive pricing.

14. One of the advantages of a computerized physician order entry system is to prevent
A. conflict with patients.
B. side effects of the drugs.
C. infectious diseases.
D. errors.

15. The unit-dose drug distribution system is considered to be the
A. safest system.
B. cheapest system.
C. most effective system.
D. A and C.

Community (Retail) Pharmacy 8

OUTLINE

Community Pharmacy
The Prescription
- Processing Prescriptions—Dispensing

Floor Plan of the Retail Pharmacy
- Drop-Off Window
- Input Terminals
- Prescription Counter
- Drive-Through
- Consultation Area
- Customer Service Area
- Refrigerator
- Prescription Shelves
- Cash Register Area

Pharmacy Computer System
Compounding

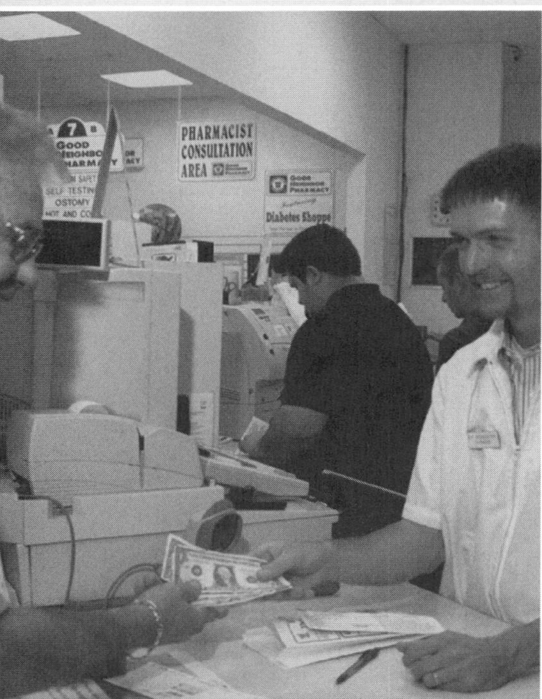

GLOSSARY

drive-through An external site at a pharmacy that can be accessed by driving up in a car.

legend drug A medication that may be dispensed only with a prescription; also known as prescription drug.

over-the-counter (OTC) A medication that may be purchased without a prescription directly from the pharmacy.

pharmacy compounding The preparation, mixing, assembling, packaging, or labeling of a drug or device.

COMMUNITY PHARMACY

There are more than 60,000 community pharmacies across the United States. They are the primary providers of pharmaceuticals and pharmaceutical care services to patients. Community pharmacies are found in a variety of locations such as shopping centers, grocery stores, department stores, and medical office buildings. These are classified into two main categories: independent pharmacies or chain pharmacies. Independent pharmacies are owned by local individuals. On the contrary, chain pharmacies are usually regionally or nationally based, such as CVS, Walgreens, and Eckerd. Giant regional or national mass merchandisers such as Wal-Mart or Kmart also have pharmacies inside most of their stores. Pharmacists in the community pharmacy provide several important functions:

1. They provide distribution of prescribed drug products.
2. They are caretakers of the nation's drug supply.
3. They compound prescriptions to meet the specific needs of individual patients.
4. They educate the public to maximize the intended benefits of drug therapy while minimizing unintended side effects and adverse reactions.

THE PRESCRIPTION

An order for medication issued by a physician, dentist, or other licensed medical practitioner is called a prescription. In certain states, nurse practitioners and even pharmacists can issue prescriptions with certain restrictions. The prescription order is a part of the professional relationship among the prescriber, the pharmacist, and the patient. It is the pharmacist's responsibility in this relationship to provide quality pharmaceutical care that meets the medication needs of the patient. The pharmacist or pharmacy technicians not only must be precise in the manual aspects of filling the prescription order but also must provide the patient with the necessary information and guidance to ensure the patient's compliance in taking the medication properly. There are two broad legal classifications of medications: those that can be obtained only by prescription and those that may be purchased without a prescription. The latter are termed *nonprescription drugs* or **over-the-counter (OTC)** drugs. Medications that may be dispensed legally only on prescription are referred to as prescription drugs or **legend drugs.** Prescriptions may be written by the prescriber and given to the patient for presentation at the pharmacy, telephoned or sent directly to the pharmacist by means of a fax machine, or sent electronically from a physician's computer to a pharmacist's computer. The component parts of a prescription include the following:

- Information on prescriber's office
- Information on patient
- Date
- Medication prescribed (inscription), which states the name and quantities of ingredients.
- Rx symbol (superscription), which gives directions to the pharmacist.
- Dispensing directions to pharmacist (subscription)
- Directions for patient (Signa)
- Refill and special labeling
- Prescriber's signature and license or Drug Enforcement Administration (DEA) number

An example of a physician's prescription is shown in Figure 8-1.

Processing Prescriptions—Dispensing

Proper procedures and correct steps for processing prescriptions and dispensing drugs include receiving, reading and checking, numbering and dating, labeling, preparing, packaging, rechecking, delivering and patient counseling, recording and filing, pricing, and refilling.

Receiving

The pharmacy technician receives the prescription order directly from the patient. This is a good opportunity to enhance the pharmacist- or the technician-patient relationship and to facilitate the gathering of essential information from the patient, such as a history of diseases and other drugs

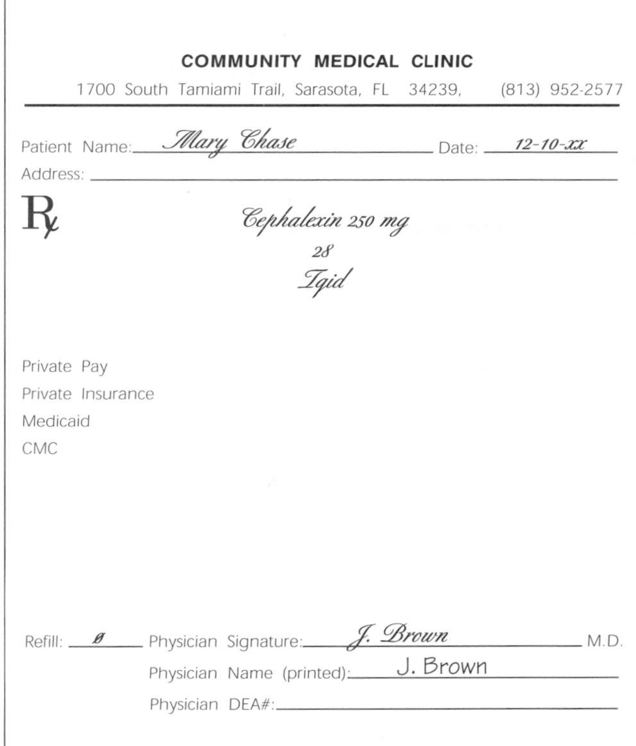

COMMUNITY MEDICAL CLINIC
1700 South Tamiami Trail, Sarasota, FL 34239, (813) 952-2577

Patient Name: Mary Chase Date: 12-10-xx
Address:

℞ Cephalexin 250 mg
28
Tqid

Private Pay
Private Insurance
Medicaid
CMC

Refill: ø Physician Signature: J. Brown M.D.
Physician Name (printed): J. Brown
Physician DEA#:

Figure 8-1. Prescription.

being taken. This information is critical for the provision of quality pharmaceutical care. The technician can also obtain the patient's correct name, address, and other necessary information and determine whether the patient's medications are provided through insurance coverage. Pharmacy technicians should ask the patient whether he or she wishes to wait, call back, or have the medication delivered. Many pharmacists try to price prescriptions before dispensing, especially for unusually expensive medication, to avoid subsequent questions concerning the charge.

Reading and Checking

Pharmacy technicians should read the prescription completely and carefully to be sure the ingredients or quantities prescribed are clear. The pharmacy technician should take the time to update the patient's profile. From the computer, the technician should determine the compatibility of the newly prescribed medication with other drugs being taken by the patient. The technician should determine whether any drug-food or drug-disease interactions are possible. If some part of the information is illegible or if it appears that an error has been made, the technician should notify the pharmacist. Then the pharmacist should consult another pharmacist or the prescriber. Unfamiliar or unclear abbreviations represent a source of errors in interpreting and filling prescriptions. The pharmacist must take great care and use his or her broad knowledge of drug products to prevent dispensing errors. The amount and frequency of a dose must be noted carefully and checked. In determining the safety of the dose of a medicinal agent, the age, weight, and condition of the patient, dosage form prescribed, possible influence of other drugs being taken, and the frequency of administration all must be considered.

Numbering and Dating

It is a legal requirement that the prescription order be numbered and that the same number be placed on the label. This numbering helps to identify the bottle or package. Consecutive numbers are assigned by prescription computers or manually by use of numbering machines. Including the date the prescription is filled on the label is also a legal requirement. This information is important in determining the appropriate refill frequency and patient compliance and can be used as an alternate means of locating the prescription order if the prescription number is lost by the patient.

Labeling

The prescription label may be typewritten or prepared by computer, using the information entered by the pharmacist or pharmacy technician. Figure 8-2 shows a computer-prepared prescription, including the label.

A prescription should have a professional-appearing label. The size of the label used should be appropriate to the size of the prescription container. The name, address, and

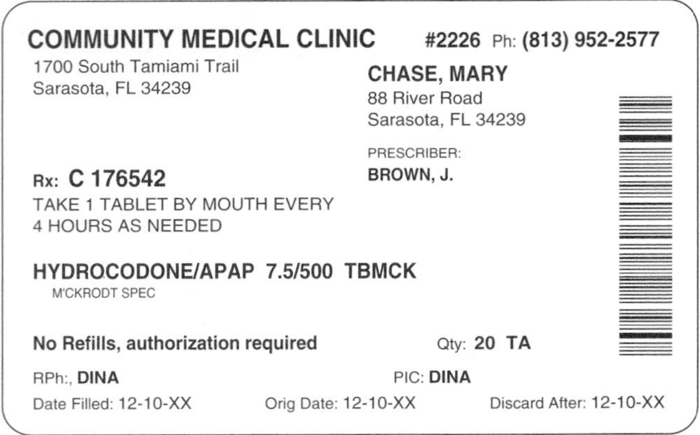
COMMUNITY MEDICAL CLINIC #2226 Ph: (813) 952-2577
1700 South Tamiami Trail
Sarasota, FL 34239
CHASE, MARY
88 River Road
Sarasota, FL 34239
PRESCRIBER:
BROWN, J.
Rx: C 176542
TAKE 1 TABLET BY MOUTH EVERY
4 HOURS AS NEEDED
HYDROCODONE/APAP 7.5/500 TBMCK
M'CKRODT SPEC
No Refills, authorization required Qty: 20 TA
RPh:, DINA PIC: DINA
Date Filled: 12-10-XX Orig Date: 12-10-XX Discard After: 12-10-XX

Figure 8-2. Computer-prepared prescription and label.

telephone number of the pharmacy are all legally required to appear on the label. The prescription number, prescriber's name, patient's name, directions for use, and date of dispensing also are legally required. The patient's name and address and strength of the medication are also commonly included. Some state laws require that the name or initials of the pharmacist dispensing the medication appear on the label. Auxiliary labels are used to emphasize important aspects of the dispensed medication, including its proper use, handling, storage, refill status, and necessary warnings or precautions. Auxiliary labels are available in various colors to give them special prominence. Figure 8-3 shows some examples of pharmacy auxiliary labels.

Preparing

Most prescriptions call for dispensing of medications already prefabricated into dosage forms by pharmaceutical manufacturers. In filling prescriptions with prefabricated products, the pharmacist should compare the manufacturer's label with the prescription to be certain it is the correct medication. Medications that show signs of poor

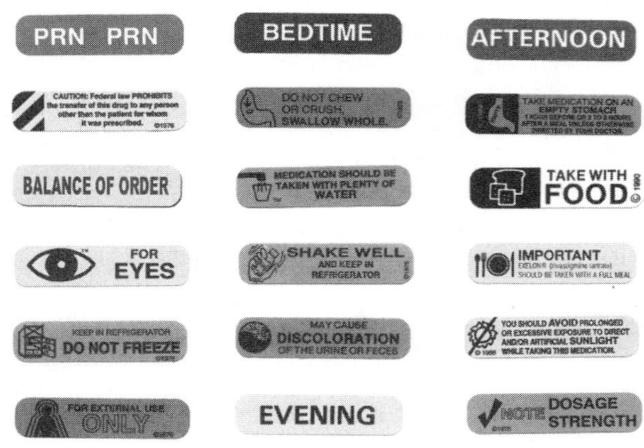

Figure 8-3. Auxiliary labels.

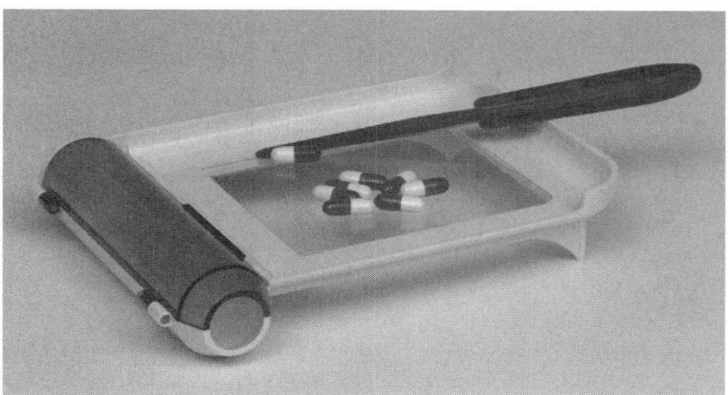

Figure 8-4. Counting tray.

manufacture or deterioration or for which the stated expiration date on the label has passed should never be dispensed.

Tablets, capsules, and some other solid, prefabricated dosage forms usually are counted in the pharmacy using a device called the counting tray, which is shown in Figure 8-4. This device facilitates the rapid and sanitary counting and transferring of medication from the stock packages to the prescription container. To prevent contamination of capsules and tablets, the counting tray should be wiped clean with a dry cloth after each use, because powder, especially from uncoated tablets, tends to remain on the tray.

Some prescriptions may require compounding, but these represent only a small percentage of the total. The pharmacist must have the knowledge and skills needed to prepare them accurately. **Pharmacy compounding** is defined as the preparation, mixing, assembling, packaging, or labeling of a drug or device. Extemporaneous compounding is essential in the course of professional practice to prepare drug formulations in dosage forms or strengths that are not otherwise commercially available.

Packaging

When the pharmacy technician is in the process of filling a prescription, he or she may select a container from among various types with different shapes, sizes, mouth openings, colors, and compositions. Selection is based primarily on the type and quantity of medication to be dispensed and the method of its use. Figure 8-5 shows some types of medication containers.

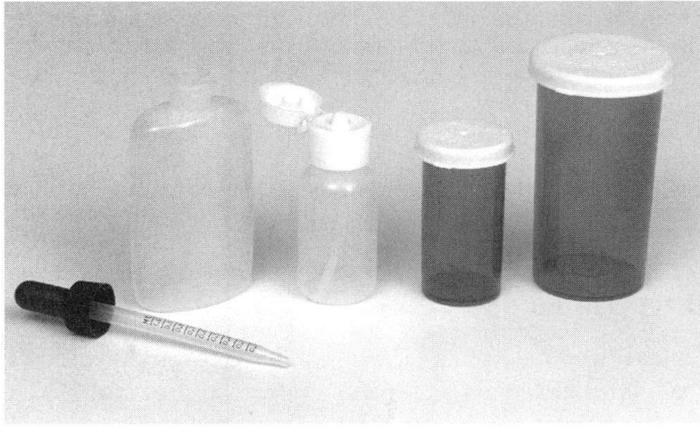

Figure 8-5. Various types of medication containers.

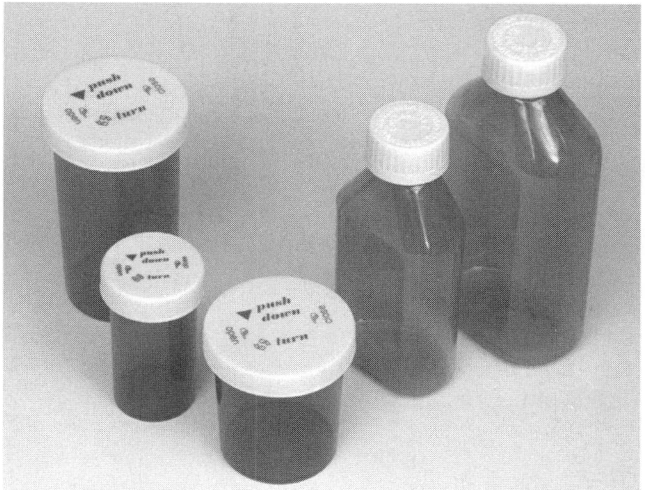

Figure 8-6. Various child-resistant caps.

All legend drugs intended for oral use must be dispensed by the pharmacist or pharmacy technician to the patient in containers having child-resistant safety closures, unless the prescriber or the patient specifically requests otherwise. Drugs that are used by or given to patients in hospitals, nursing homes, and extended-care facilities need not be dispensed in containers with safety closures unless they are intended for patients who are leaving the confines of the institution. Examples of child-resistant containers are shown in Figure 8-6.

Rechecking

The pharmacist must recheck every prescription that has been dispensed for verification. All details of the label should be rechecked against the prescription order to verify directions, patient's name, prescription number, date, and prescriber's name. Rechecking is especially important for those drug products available in multiple strengths.

Delivering and Patient Counseling

The pharmacist should personally present the prescription medication to the patient or his or her family member unless it is to be delivered to the patient's home or workplace. There has been increased awareness that labeling instructions are often inadequate to ensure the patient's understanding of his or her medication. The prescriber and the pharmacist share the responsibility for ensuring that the patient receives specific instructions, precautions, and warnings for safe and effective use of the prescribed drugs.

Recording and Filing

A record of the prescriptions dispensed is maintained in the pharmacy through the use of computers and hard copy prescription files. Many chain drug stores have central computers today, which allows pharmacists from any place in the system to access a patient's record and refill a prescription previously dispensed at another store. There are various types of units available to keep original prescription orders. Metal or cardboard units, which conveniently store approximately 1000 prescriptions, are commonly used. Partitioned drawers often may be used for filing (Figure 8-7). The least common method of filing is microfilming of prescriptions.

Pricing

The pharmacy is a business practice. The pharmacy technician must assist in the financial aspects of this practice so that the pharmacy is maintained and makes a fair profit. A method of pricing prescriptions should be established to ensure the profitable operation of the prescription section. The charge applied to a prescription should cover the costs of the ingredients, which include the container and label, the time of the pharmacist or pharmacy technician and auxiliary personnel involved, the cost of inventory maintenance, and operational costs of the pharmacy. It is obvious that pricing the prescription must provide a reasonable margin of profit on investment.

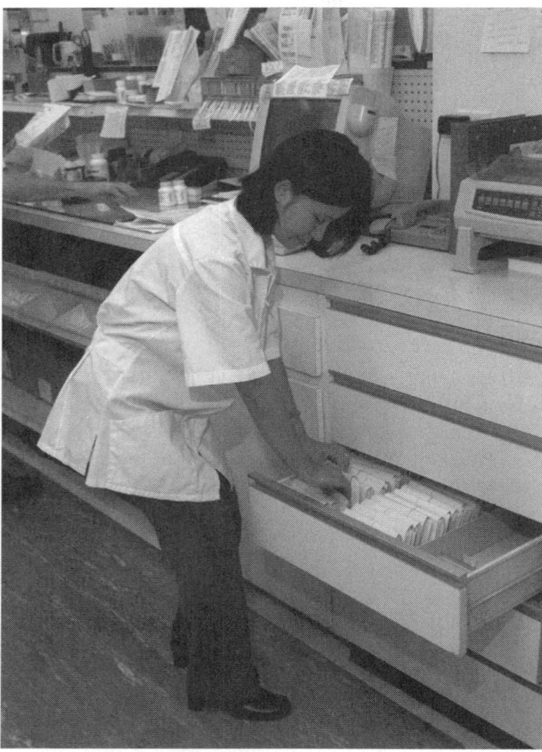

Figure 8-7. Partitioned drawers may be used for filing.

Refilling

The prescriber must provide instructions for refilling a prescription by indicating on the original prescription the number of appropriate refills. The number of refills of prescriptions for noncontrolled medications is not limited by federal law. State laws may impose such limits. On the other hand, the refilling of prescriptions for controlled agents is strictly regulated. No prescription should be renewed indefinitely without the patient being reevaluated by the prescriber to ensure that the medication as originally prescribed remains the drug of choice. The maintenance of accurate records of refilling is important not only for complying with federal and state laws, but also for providing information on the patient's medication history.

FLOOR PLAN OF THE RETAIL PHARMACY

Almost all community pharmacies have similar floor plans and are generally organized into two areas: the front area and the prescription processing area. OTC drugs, cosmetics, and other merchandise items are located in the front area. Dispensing of legend drugs, which are regulated under federal law, always requires a prescription because these drugs are off limits to customers. Only authorized individuals are able to enter the prescription processing areas. By state regulations, a description of the space and equipment is required. Figures 8-8 and 8-9 show the front and prescription dispensing areas of community pharmacies.

Drop-Off Window

The customer drops off the prescription, new hard copy (or Rx) or refill, or verbally asks for a refill. The technician will obtain all personal information that is required for a hard copy prescription.

Input Terminals

The technician must put the information in the computer before starting the order. When the information for the prescription has been entered, the order goes to be filled.

Prescription Counter

The prescription counter is an area that a pharmacist or a technician can use to prepare prescriptions.

Drive-Through

Some community pharmacies have **drive-through** windows that allow customers or patients to drop off prescriptions or purchase their medications (Figure 8-10). Pharmacy technicians need to make sure that the correct person is receiving

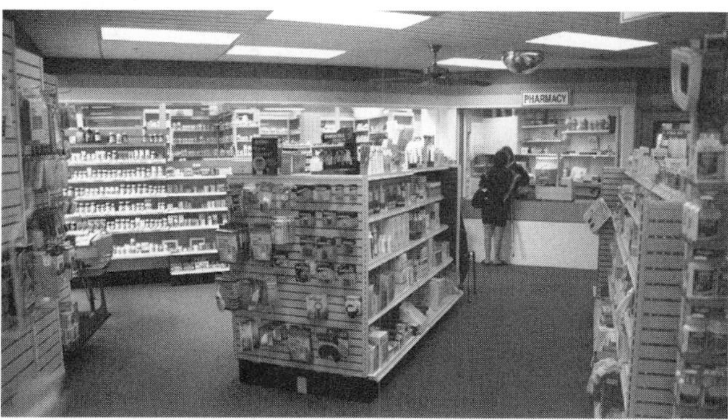

Figure 8-8. The front area of the retail pharmacy.

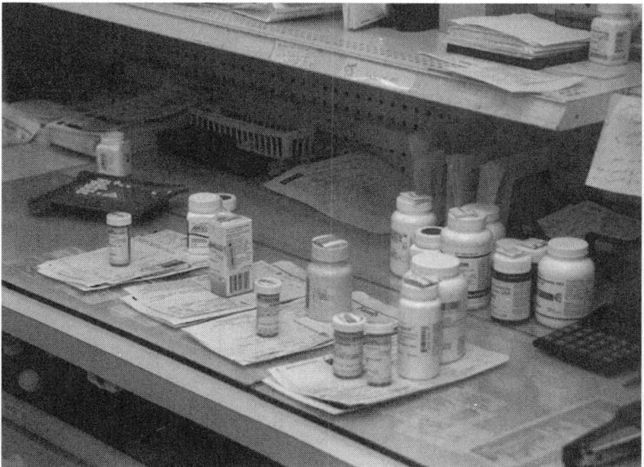

Figure 8-9. The dispensing area of the retail pharmacy.

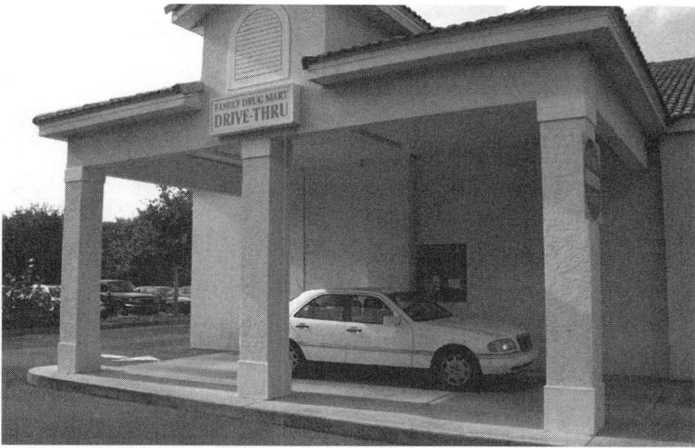

Figure 8-10. Drive-through windows allow patients to drop off prescriptions or purchase their medications.

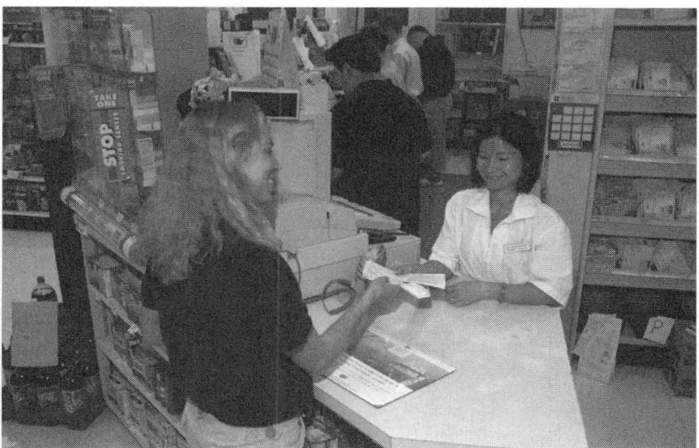

Figure 8-11. Technicians in the community pharmacy interact with patients as customers.

his or her order and not another person's order. The technician must ask if the patient has any questions for the pharmacist about the prescription. The pharmacist should be available for consultation.

Consultation Area

The consultation area is strictly for the pharmacist to counsel patients privately. The technician must always remember that he or she is not legally permitted to counsel patients about medications. This is the role and responsibility of the pharmacist.

Customer Service Area

The community pharmacy is different from the hospital pharmacy. Technicians in the community pharmacy interact with patients as customers (Figure 8-11). Therefore, customer service is one of the most important aspects of the community pharmacy, and technicians must have strong interpersonal skills. Customers can also pick up their prescription in this area.

Refrigerator

Each pharmacy must have a refrigerator to store drugs that are required to be kept at temperatures between 2 and 8°C. It must be used exclusively for medications. No food or beverages are permitted to be stored in any refrigerator in which medication is stored.

Prescription Shelves

When prescriptions are completed and customers do not pick them up right away, they should be placed in a specific area or on shelves (Figure 8-12). For storage, prescriptions should be alphabetized by the name of the patient.

Cash Register Area

The technician may ring up prescriptions and other items such as OTC products into the cash register and accept payment for their purchase. Cash register machines are connected into the pharmacy's computer and can provide prices automatically by using barcode scanners. The pharmacy

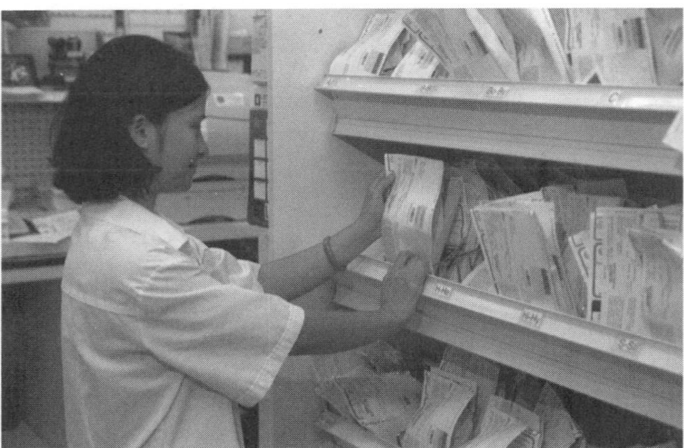

Figure 8-12. Shelves for storing completed prescriptions that customers are not going to pick up right away.

technician must handle payments properly. For cash payments, he or she must count the payment in the presence of the customer, confirming the amount verbally.

PHARMACY COMPUTER SYSTEM

The use of computers is now standard in pharmacy practice because of the expanded informational needs of the pharmacist. Another factor is the increased amount of paperwork required in practice. Computer systems are essential for promoting efficiency by offering improving technology and expanding databases that provide needed support. Most chain pharmacies are linked together by dedicated telephone lines or satellites, thus facilitating the sharing of information between pharmacies.

There are three areas in the pharmacy in which computerized systems can be used:

1. Prescription dispensing and associated record maintenance
2. Clinical support and accounting
3. Business management

Many insurance and prescription plans now require online verification and authorization before the dispensing of any medication. Pharmacists and pharmacy technicians can now use the Internet to obtain and download information about disease states and drug therapy for their patients.

COMPOUNDING

The vast majority of prescriptions dispensed are for dosage forms that are produced by manufacturers approved by the Food and Drug Administration (FDA). These standardized dosages meet the needs for most patients. Many patients, however, need custom-made dosages to treat specific problems. Many community pharmacists offer specialized compounding services. Extremely small doses for pediatric or geriatric use may be needed. Compounding has always been a skill unique to pharmacists, and it continues to be a part of contemporary pharmacy practice.

WEB SITES OF INTEREST

CVS/Pharmacy: http://www.cvs.com
Eckerd Corporation: http://www.eckerd.com
Walgreens: http://www.walgreens.com

REVIEW QUESTIONS

1. Prescribed medication is also called
   A. superscription.
   B. subscription.
   C. inscription.
   D. legend drug.

2. Auxiliary labels are used to emphasize
   A. important aspects of aseptic technique.
   B. important characteristics of the dispensed medication.
   C. that technicians complete the dispensed medication.
   D. that technicians satisfy the customers.

3. Child-resistant containers are used in which of the following situations?
   A. Dispensed medications for patients in the hospital
   B. Dispensed medications for patients in nursing homes
   C. The dispensing of all legend drugs
   D. Dispensed drugs for extended-care facilities

4. Which of the following areas in the community pharmacy is the most important?
   A. Customer service area
   B. Consultation area
   C. Drive-through area
   D. All of the above

Continues

5. The pharmacy technician may do which of the following?
   A. Count or pour medications
   B. Empty returned medications to stock containers
   C. Take prescriptions over the phone
   D. Counsel a patient

6. Refills for a prescription may be completed when the
   A. prescription is lost.
   B. refill blank is filled in.
   C. refill blank is left blank.
   D. pharmacist tells the technician to refill the prescription.

7. Which of the following is correct in regard to a prescription?
   A. It must include the full first and last name of the patient.
   B. It must include the patient's social security number.
   C. It must include the pharmacy technician's signature.
   D. It must include the pharmacist's signature.

8. Why do some pharmacists try to price prescriptions before dispensing?
   A. The medication is close to being expired.
   B. The medication is manufactured in another country.
   C. Some medications are unusually expensive.
   D. To keep a good relationship with the patients.

9. The size of the prescription label should be appropriate for the
   A. amount of medication prescribed.
   B. size of the prescription container.
   C. age of the patient.
   D. patient's wishes.

10. To prevent contamination of capsules and tablets, the counting tray should be wiped clean after each use with which of the following?
    A. Cold water
    B. Alcohol
    C. Bleach
    D. Dry cloth

11. Original prescription orders are most commonly stored using
    A. computers.
    B. microfilm.
    C. partitioned drawers.
    D. metal or cardboard units.

Advanced Pharmacy

9

OUTLINE

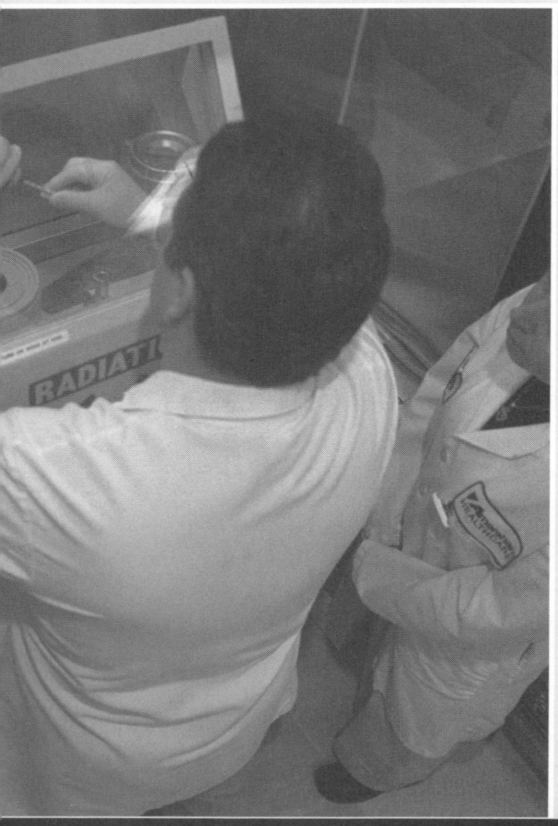

GLOSSARY

ambulatory care Medical care that is given on an outpatient basis. Patients are able to come and go to an office or clinic for diagnostic tests or treatments.

enteral nutrition Feedings given into the gastrointestinal system. Although normal eating qualifies as enteral nutrition, the term is usually applied to specially prepared liquid feedings.

hospice Originally a facility, usually within a hospital, intended to care for the terminally ill, in particular, by providing physical comfort to the patient and emotional support and counseling to the patient and the family.

long-term care A wide range of health and health-related support services.

long-term care pharmacy organization An organization involving a licensed professional pharmacy or practice that provides medications and clinical services to long-term care facilities and their residents.

mail-order pharmacy A licensed pharmacy that uses the mail or other carriers (e.g., overnight carriers or parcel services) to deliver prescriptions to patients.

nuclear pharmacy A pharmacy that is specially licensed to work with radioactive materials. Previously called radiopharmacy.

parenteral nutrition A combination of amino acids, dextrose, fats, vitamins, minerals, electrolytes, and water administered intravenously. Parenteral nutrition is capable of providing all the nutrients needed to sustain life.

radiopharmaceutical A drug that is or has been made to be radioactive. Although a few radiopharmaceuticals are used to treat diseases (e.g., radioactive iodine), most are used as diagnostic agents.

starter kit A group of medicines provided to a hospice patient to treat urgent problems that develop in the last days of life.

total parenteral nutrition (TPN) An intravenous feeding that supplies all of the nutrients necessary for life.

THE EXPANDING ROLE OF THE PHARMACIST

Today the role of the pharmacist is expanding. This evolution has guided the differentiation of pharmacy practice in various subspecialties. The rapid development of new drugs and drug delivery systems, changes in the health care delivery system, an increase in the acuity of illness of institutionalized patients, and increased emphasis on patient outcomes and quality of health care are very important factors in this matter. The primary goal of changes in the heath care system is to reduce health care costs and increase the overall quality of life for the patient. Pharmacy technicians can be very effective in assisting pharmacists in the advancement of pharmacy practice. They must be trained, skillful, and knowledgeable in these areas.

Long-Term Care Pharmacy Services

Long-term care is defined as a wide range of health and health-related support services. The recipients may be people of any age, ranging from children with congenital anomalies to young adults with lengthy recovery periods from trauma to frail elderly persons with chronic diseases and the multifaceted changes associated with aging (mental or physical impairment). The goal of long-term care is to enable a person to maintain the maximum possible level of functional independence.

Because of limited resources, most long-term care facilities will contract out dispensing and clinical pharmacy services. This means that they will pay another company to take care of the majority of patient medications. The licensed professional pharmacy or practice that provides medications and clinical services to long-term care facilities and their residents is called a **long-term pharmacy organization.** A pharmacist or pharmacy technician does not have to physically be present at the facility during all hours; however, pharmacy services must be made available 24 hours a day.

Pharmacists perform two types of functions for long-term care: distributive and consultant. The distributive pharmacist is responsible for making sure patients are receiving the correct medicines that were ordered. This job is mainly done outside of the long-term care facility itself. The impact and cost savings of the use of consultant pharmacist services in long-term care have been documented. The role of the consultant pharmacist has been shown to decrease overall medication costs, the occurrence of medication errors and adverse drug reactions and interactions, the length of hospitalization, and mortality rates of long-term care patients. The consultant pharmacist in long-term care is, in many ways, like a hospital pharmacy director in that he or she must supervise all aspects of the comprehensive pharmaceutical services delivered to patients. The consultant pharmacist interacts with doctors, nurses, and other health professionals. The consultant pharmacist is responsible for several different nursing homes or other facilities and may only visit each at certain weekly or monthly intervals.

Home Health Care Pharmacy

Home health care service is one of the fastest growing parts of the health care market. Today, the majority of serious medical conditions and problems are treated outside of the hospital setting, many times at home. Home health care is an important part of the continuum of care. The growth of this system is related to several factors, such as the increase in the number of elderly persons, patient preference, lower costs, improvement of technology, managed care, and physician acceptance. There are several types of home health care services that may be available. These include the following:

- Pharmaceutical services
- Nursing services
- Personal care services
- Rehabilitation services
- Home medical supply services

The use of home care is a viable alternative that is safe and cost effective. It is also mutually satisfying to the patient and caregiver. The major sources of payment for home care are Medicare and Medicaid (see Table 9-1).

There are many home health care products and services provided by pharmacies today. These services include providing durable medical supplies, orthopedic supplies, oxygen therapy, wound care, artificial limbs, medical devices, prescription medications, and infusion therapy (intravenous [IV] and nutritional therapy). The patient may have multiple conditions that require monitoring of treatment beyond high-tech therapy for which other home care providers and the patient's regular physician continue to be involved. The most common high-tech therapies include the following:

- IV antibiotic therapy
- Chemotherapy
- Pain medication
- Total parenteral nutrition (TPN)
- Enteral nutrition
- Renal dialysis
- Respiratory and ventilation therapy

TABLE 9-1. Sources of Payment for Home Care

PAYMENT SOURCE	PERCENT
Medicare	39.0
Medicaid	27.2
Private insurance	12.0
Out-of-pocket	20.5
Other and unknown	1.3
Total	100.0

High-tech home care requires close collaboration of the physician, the pharmacist, the registered nurse, and, depending on the type of therapy, the medical supply company.

Home Infusion Pharmacy

Home infusion pharmacy practice is a unique area for pharmacists and pharmacy technicians. In this type of pharmacy practice infusion therapies are prepared and dispensed to patients in the home. Home infusion pharmacy includes IV solutions, other injectable drugs, and enteral nutrition therapy. This type of service involves safe compounding of an IV solution and its delivery to the patient. Equipment and supplies needed to infuse the solution are also provided. Home infusion pharmacies may be established in different areas, such as community pharmacies, long-term care pharmacies, and hospital pharmacies. There are several types of infusion therapies prescribed for home infusion that depends upon the condition of patients. These therapies include antibiotic therapy, pain management therapy, hydration therapy, nutrition therapy, and chemotherapy.

There is a wide variety of equipment used in the home infusion pharmacy such as automated compounding and dispensing devices, horizontal and vertical laminar flow hoods, a refrigerator with a locked compartment for storage of drugs, computer hardware, and printers. Supplies found in the home infusion pharmacy include syringes, needles, dispensing pins, IV solution containers, filters, transfer sets, IV tubing, alcohol preparation pads, gloves, masks, gowns, beard and shoe covers, and others. One of the main duties of the pharmacy technician in the home infusion pharmacy is the processing of equipment and supply orders. The pharmacy technician must be familiar with vascular access and vascular access devices, infusion devices, and other IV delivery systems. The pharmacy technician performs the compounding of sterile products (Figure 9-1) and handling of home infusion equipment and supplies. He or she must have knowledge and skills specific to home infusion therapies and nutritional products, sterile compounding, aseptic technique, pharmaceutical calculations, and computer skills and understanding of the laws and regulations pertaining to home infusion pharmacy. The pharmacy technician may be responsible for compounding, equipment and supplies, and computer functions in the home infusion pharmacy.

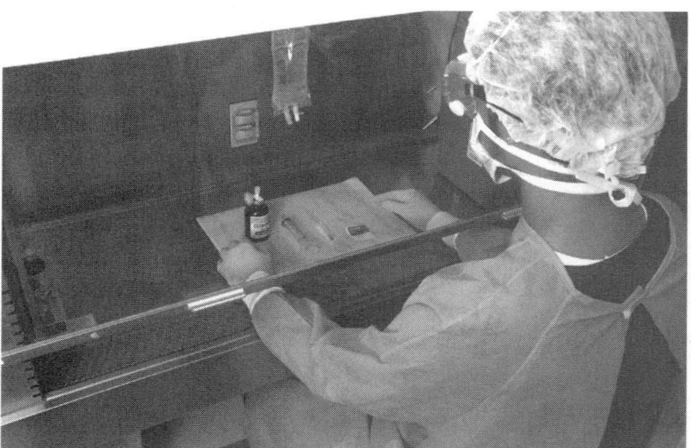

Figure 9-1. The technician is ready to perform the compounding of sterile products.

Pharmacy technicians must be familiar with nutrition therapy. There are two types of nutritional therapy provided by a home infusion pharmacy: parenteral and enteral nutrition therapy.

In **parenteral nutrition** therapy, nutrients are delivered directly into the bloodstream. **Total parenteral nutrition (TPN)** consists of amino acid (protein), dextrose (carbohydrate), fats, electrolytes, vitamins, trace elements, and medication (insulin and heparin). TPN formulations are highly complex, and proper mixing is important (Figure 9-2). A safe and effective order of mixing ingredients should be followed. TPN formulations for home infusion are usually prepared several days before they are administered.

In **enteral nutrition** therapy, foods and nutrients are delivered into the gastrointestinal (GI) tract through a tube. This process is called tube feeding and is the most common home infusion nutritional therapy (Figure 9-3). Enteral nutrition can be used to supplement oral or parenteral nutrition, or it can be used to meet the patient's entire nutritional needs. Patients with swallowing problems resulting from conditions such as stroke, dementia, trauma, cancer, or

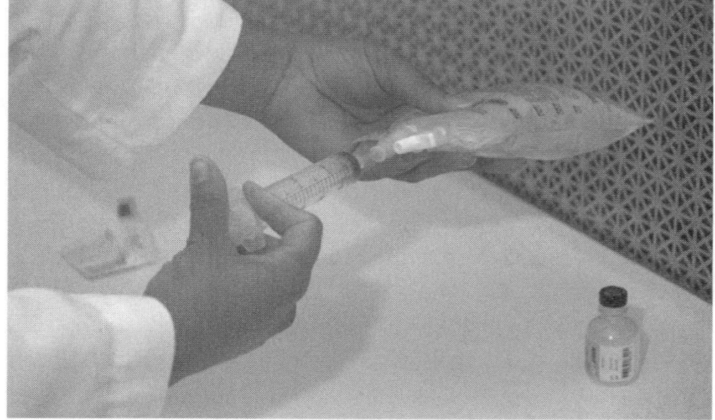

Figure 9-2. The technician is mixing total parenteral nutrition (TPN).

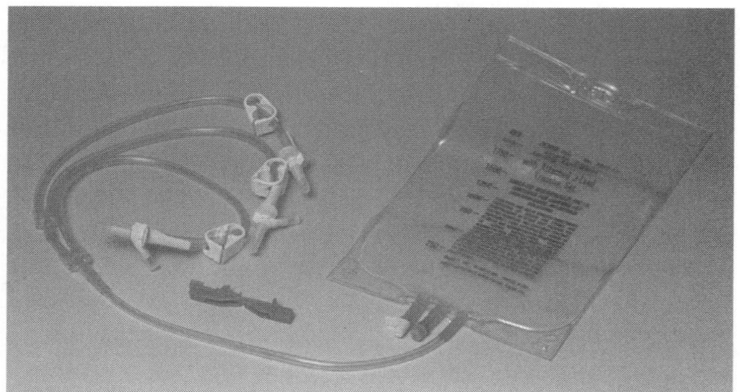

Figure 9-3. The patient's entire nutritional needs.

acquired immunodeficiency syndrome (AIDS) are candidates for home enteral nutrition. Feeding tubes placed into the stomach through the nose are used for short-term therapy of up to 3 to 4 weeks. Feeding tubes placed into the stomach or small intestine through the skin are used for long-term enteral therapy.

Hospice Pharmacy

Hospice is an organized program of services to meet the physical, emotional, spiritual, and social needs of a patient who is terminally ill. Hospice care focuses on the patient's comfort rather than on a cure for the disease. Hospice care allows the patient to live the remainder of his or her life as free from pain and other symptoms as possible. Hospice serves all types and ages of patients and is provided in a variety of settings. The preferred setting is in the patient's home. An inpatient hospice facility may provide a safe and comfortable alternative. Funding for hospice programs comes from Medicare, Medicaid, and private insurance. For a patient to be eligible for hospice care under Medicare, a physician must certify that death is expected within 6 months.

Pharmacists have become involved in hospice by providing needed medications and pharmaceutical care services to patients who are terminally ill or nearing the end of life. A pharmacy must prepare and dispense medications, medication-related equipment and supplies, and pharmaceutical care services to hospice patients at home or in a facility. A hospice pharmacy can be part of a traditional community pharmacy, in which hospice is a part of its business, or it can be a pharmacy that services only hospice patients. Hospice pharmacy services can be divided into two areas: clinical services and dispensing services. Clinical services include pain management, symptom management, medication monitoring, drug regimen review, drug information services, and formulary development and management. Dispensing services include medications and related equipment and supplies, sterile IV infusion compounding (pain, hydration, and chemotherapy), starter kits, and 24-hour on-call coverage. A **starter kit** is a group of medications that is given to a hospice patient by the hospice pharmacy to provide a "start" in treatment for the majority of urgent problems that can develop during the last days or weeks of life. Patients may suffer from pain, fever, nausea, vomiting, anxiety, agitation, increased secretions, and constipation.

Ambulatory Care Pharmacy

One of the most significant trends in health care has been the emphasis on shorter hospital stays and on outpatient care. Ambulatory care has become the standard for health care delivery. The term **ambulatory care** includes a wide range of services such as outpatient pharmacies, emergency departments, primary care clinics, specialty clinics, ambulatory care centers, and family practice groups.

The increase in ambulatory care services has greatly expanded the opportunities for ambulatory care pharmacy practitioners. Many outpatient pharmacies provide only traditional pharmaceutical services. Ambulatory care pharmacy practitioners, more commonly referred to as clinical pharmacists, practice in a wide variety of primary care clinics. The clinical pharmacist improves drug therapy documentation, improves patient compliance, decreases duplicate prescriptions, and prevents the risk of overdosage. The pharmacy clinic provides refills to drop-in patients. Patients are referred by physicians to the clinical pharmacists, who provide physical assessment, order laboratory tests, alter dosages, and change medications. One of the most successful pharmacist-managed ambulatory clinics has been the anticoagulation clinic. The value of clinical pharmacists in the chronic management of patients with hypertension, diabetes, or allergies and patients receiving anticoagulation therapy is obvious. One of the most important aspects of ambulatory care practice is the involvement of the clinical pharmacist in drug therapy decisions. This requires the pharmacist to be available and accessible when the patient is being seen. It is clear that successful ambulatory care pharmacy services must be comprehensive and continual. Clinical pharmacy services must be provided 80% to 90% of the time.

Mail-Order Pharmacy

Mail-order pharmacy is defined as a pharmacy that dispenses maintenance medications to patients through mail delivery. It is one of the fastest growing areas in pharmacy practice. It is offered by the majority of health plans today as an option to the traditional retail pharmacy for obtaining prescriptions. The medications are sent to patients through mail or delivery services. Mail-order pharmacy is a unique practice setting for pharmacists and pharmacy technicians. The staff members consist of licensed pharmacists, registered nurses, and technicians. Mail-order pharmacies can provide services to all 50 states. Therefore, they can operate at a high volume, which results in discounts, and will be more economical for patients. Mail-order pharmacies can serve more patients, particularly those who have chronic illnesses such as diabetes, high blood pressure, depression, heart disease, arthritis, or gastrointestinal disorders. The need for medication can be predicted and the supply can be easily maintained by mail delivery. This type of medication, which is required on a continuous basis for the treatment of a chronic condition, is called a maintenance medication. In most cases, mail-order pharmacies contract with health insurers and fill prescriptions at discounted rates for members of those plans.

Nuclear Pharmacy

Nuclear pharmacy is a branch of the pharmacy profession that deals with the provision of services related to radiopharmaceuticals. A **radiopharmaceutical** is a radioactive drug that is used in the diagnosis and treatment of disease. The radioactive drugs contain radioactive elements. There are three types of radiation that can be released by a radionuclide: alpha, beta, and gamma radiation. Gamma radiation is the most penetrating type of radiation. Nuclear medicine uses very small quantities of radionuclides for the diagnosis and treatment of disease. Radiopharmaceuticals are used as tracers for assessing the structure, function, secretion, excretion, and volume of a particular organ or tissue. They are also used to analyze biological specimens; to treat specific diseases such as hyperthyroidism, thyroid cancer, and polycythemia vera; and to alleviate bone pain. Most radiopharmaceuticals are prepared as sterile, pyrogen-free intravenous solutions or suspensions to be administered directly to the patient. An important component of nuclear medicine is imaging, which involves administering radiopharmaceuticals to a patient orally, intravenously, or by inhalation to localize a specific organ or system and its structure and function. Nuclear pharmacy is essentially a sterile compounding practice. The most commonly used radionuclides are iodine and technetium compounds. Technetium-99m (^{99m}Tc) is used in about 80% of radioactive drugs. Most technetium compounds are used for diagnosis. Iodine-131 (^{131}I) is used for treatment of hyperthyroidism or, more recently, for ovarian and prostate cancer. There are numerous other radionuclides used in medicine. These include xenon (a gas used to image the lungs), thallium, gallium, cobalt, chromium, indium, and strontium. Nuclear pharmacy practice involves the procuring, storage, compounding, dispensing, and provision of information about radiopharmaceuticals and is one possible area of specialization for both pharmacists and pharmacy technicians (Figure 9-4).

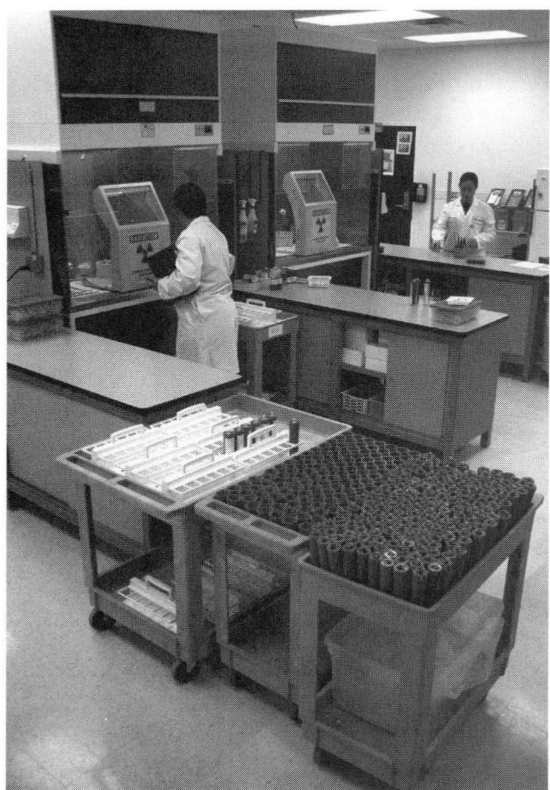

Figure 9-4. The pharmacist and the technician are working in the nuclear pharmacy dealing with radiopharmaceuticals.

REVIEW QUESTIONS

1. Which of the following types of radiation released by radionuclides is the most penetrating type?
   A. Beta
   B. Gamma
   C. Alpha
   D. Xenon

2. Which of the following radionuclides is the most commonly used in nuclear pharmacy practice?
   A. ^{99m}Tc
   B. ^{133}Xe
   C. ^{123}I
   D. ^{67}Ga

3. Radiopharmaceutical agents can be administered
   A. intravenously.
   B. orally.
   C. by inhalation.
   D. all of the above.

4. One of the fastest growing areas in pharmacy is
   A. mail-order pharmacy.
   B. ambulatory care pharmacy.
   C. nuclear pharmacy.
   D. home infusion therapy.

5. The major source of payment for home care is
   A. Medicaid.
   B. private insurance.
   C. Medicare.
   D. A and C.

6. The most common high-tech therapies include all of the following, except
   A. chemotherapy.
   B. rectal drug therapy.
   C. pain medication.
   D. IV antibiotic therapy.

Continues

7. All of the following equipment can be found in home infusion pharmacy practice except
A. horizontal laminar flow hoods.
B. refrigerators with locked compartments.
C. automated compounding.
D. rehabilitation equipment.

8. Total parenteral nutrition (TPN) formulations for home infusion are usually prepared how long before they are administered?
A. Less than 1 hour
B. Several hours
C. Several days
D. Several years

9. The goal of long-term care is to enable a person to
A. stay in the hospital longer.
B. maintain the maximum possible level of functional independence.
C. be sent home as soon as possible.
D. afford to pay the minimum for home care.

10. The role of the pharmacist in long-term care includes all of the following, except
A. decreasing overall medication costs.
B. decreasing medication errors.
C. increasing mortality rates.
D. consulting with doctors and nurses.

11. A starter kit is defined as
A. medications from an organization who is responsible for day-care services.
B. a group of medications provided for a hospice patient by the hospice pharmacy to provide treatment for a majority of urgent problems.
C. medications for a hospital patient who is discharged right away.
D. medications for a hospice patient who is discharged.

12. Home infusion pharmacies include all of the following, except
A. IV solutions.
B. radiation therapy.
C. other injectable drugs.
D. enteral nutrition therapy.

13. There are several types of infusion therapies prescribed for home infusion, which include all of the following, except
A. nutrition therapy.
B. enteral nutrition therapy.
C. pain management.
D. chemotherapy.

14. The increase in ambulatory care services has greatly expanded the opportunities for
A. physicians who seek to be retained.
B. pharmacy technicians to get a license.
C. hospital pharmacy technicians.
D. ambulatory pharmacy practitioners.

15. Which of the following is one of the fastest growing parts of the health care market?
A. Home nuclear pharmacy
B. Home health care services
C. Home mental care services
D. All of the above

The Role and Duties of Technicians at Retail Pharmacies

10

OUTLINE

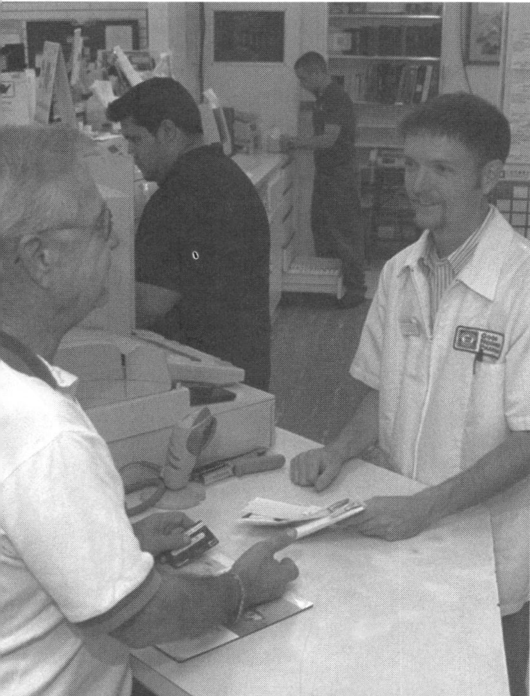

GLOSSARY

auxiliary labeling Supplementary or secondary labeling.

professionalism The conduct or qualities characterized by or conforming to the technical or ethical standards of a profession; exhibiting a courteous, conscientious, and generally businesslike manner in the workplace.

THE ROLE OF THE PHARMACY TECHNICIAN

As the practice of pharmacy develops, so does the role of the pharmacy technician. The number of prescriptions dispensed in the United States has rapidly increased, as has the number of settings in which pharmacists practice. To keep up with the rising demand for pharmaceutical products and services, pharmacy technicians will play a greater role in support of pharmaceutical care in their communities.

Job Responsibilities

Recent studies indicate that pharmacy technicians are now involved in more areas of pharmacy practice. Studies show that in addition to assisting with outpatient prescription dispensing, many community pharmacy technicians participate in purchasing, inventory control, billing, and repackaging products.

Receiving and Reviewing Prescriptions

Prescriptions come to the pharmacy in three main ways: by a person, via fax, or by telephone. In the community setting, the prescription is typically written by the prescriber and delivered to the pharmacy by the patient. There are rules that govern special prescriptions such as those for controlled substances or narcotics and those that need special compounding. Many states require that prescriptions be phoned in by a licensed professional. Another requirement is that telephone prescriptions must be received by a pharmacist. Technicians should consult the pharmacy's policy and procedure manual. The technician should screen prescriptions for anything that looks unusual, such as a dispense quantity in excess of normal quantities or an unrecognizable signature. Any suspicious prescription should be presented to the pharmacist for more evaluation. The technician must recognize the legitimate Drug Enforcement Administration (DEA) number of the practitioner.

The pharmacy technician must enter the following information into the computer for dispensing a prescription:

- The patient information
- The patient profile
- Correct drug and dosage
- Correct physician's name
- DEA number of physician for controlled substances
- Directions for use
- Quantity of medication
- Refill number
- Brand name or a generic product
- Patient counseling provided
- The dispensing pharmacist's initials

One of the major duties of the pharmacy technician is processing new and refill prescriptions. This process may differ depending on the community pharmacy. Most pharmacies are using computers. It is important that technicians process the prescription accurately and efficiently on the computer system.

Most pharmacy computers allow pharmacists or technicians to look up a refill through the patient profile for the medication. Technicians must be sure that a refill is available. When no refill is available, the technician should notify the pharmacist that he or she should contact the patient's physician for a new prescription.

Prescription Dispensing

The last step in the prescription-processing function is dispensing. To prepare medication for the patient, a prescription label will be printed from the computer with all the patient and prescription information that the technician entered into the system. When the label is ready, the technician should prepare the medication. A large and important component of the dispensing function is patient counseling, which must be performed by the pharmacist.

Labeling the Prescription

In addition to the name of the patient, the pharmacy, and the prescriber, the prescription label should accurately identify the medication and provide directions for its use. The label for a prescription order for a controlled substance must contain the following information (see Figure 10-1):

1. Name and address of the pharmacy
2. Serial number assigned to the prescription by the pharmacy
3. Date of the initial filling
4. Name of the patient
5. Name of the prescriber
6. Directions for use
7. Cautionary statements as required by law
8. Refill information

The patient needs to be informed of some specific properties of the medication. For example, the medication may

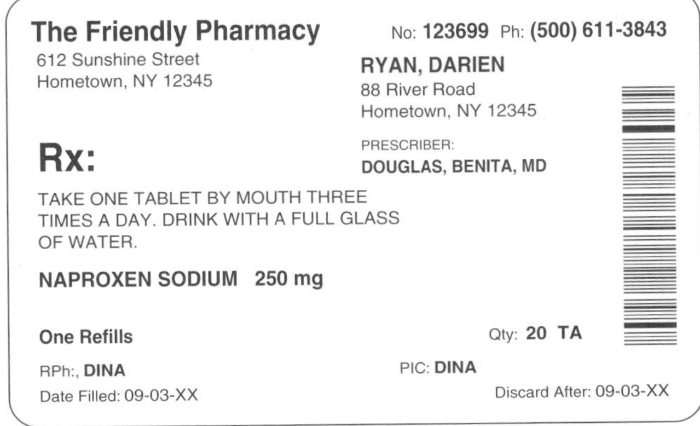

Figure 10-1. The prescription label.

BEDTIME
AFTERNOON
DO NOT CHEW OR CRUSH, SWALLOW WHOLE.
TAKE MEDICATION ON AN EMPTY STOMACH 1 HOUR BEFORE OR 2 TO 3 HOURS AFTER A MEAL UNLESS OTHERWISE DIRECTED BY YOUR DOCTOR.
MEDICATION SHOULD BE TAKEN WITH PLENTY OF WATER
TAKE WITH FOOD
PRN PRN
IMPORTANT EXELON® (rivastigmine tartrate) SHOULD BE TAKEN WITH A FULL MEAL
CAUTION: Federal law PROHIBITS the transfer of this drug to any person other than the patient for whom it was prescribed.
YOU SHOULD AVOID PROLONGED OR EXCESSIVE EXPOSURE TO DIRECT AND/OR ARTIFICIAL SUNLIGHT WHILE TAKING THIS MEDICATION.
BALANCE OF ORDER
NOTE DOSAGE STRENGTH
FOR EYES
SHAKE WELL AND KEEP IN REFRIGERATOR
KEEP IN REFRIGERATOR DO NOT FREEZE
MAY CAUSE DISCOLORATION OF THE URINE OR FECES
FOR EXTERNAL USE ONLY
EVENING

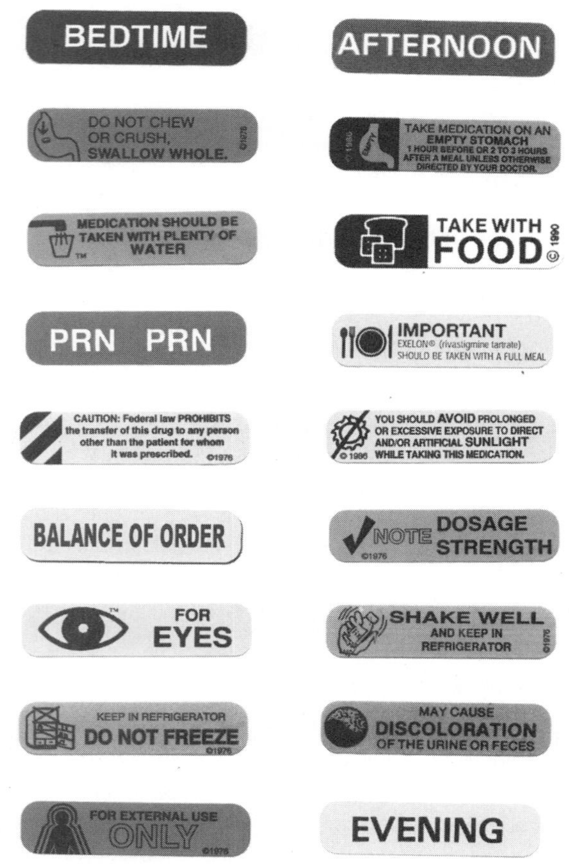

Figure 10-2. Auxiliary labels.

make the patient sensitive to sunlight; a drug may change the color of urine or must be taken with food. **Auxiliary labeling**, also referred to as strip labels, must be applied to the container to warn the patient of these properties (see Figure 10-2).

Record Keeping

A medication order or prescription becomes part of the patients' medical record (see Figure 10-3). The information must be kept in the computer record of the patient. It is also important in the current environment because third-party payers such as insurance companies rely on the correct patient-identifying information to properly process and pay submitted claims for drugs.

Pricing

A pharmacy, as any other business, must deal with expense and receipts. The pharmacy must make a profit. Thus, another responsibility of the pharmacy technician is to help ensure that the receipts are greater than the expenses so that the pharmacy can continue to operate. He or she often takes care of pricing in the pharmacy by marking products up a certain percentage over the cost, or the average wholesale price, and by marking products down by a percentage discount at other times. Insurance companies often use either a percentage-based payment for prescription products or a capitation fee. Pharmacy technicians also have responsibility for monitoring and correcting insurance billing for prescription products.

Patient Profiles and Billing Records

Patient profiles include all the patient's prescription information such as original date, refill dates, and prescribing physician. Patient medication profiles are usually organized by medication type or by order of input. Active medication orders should be listed first, and they should be separated from the discontinued medications. Discontinued medications should be available only for review upon entering of an appropriate command at the end of the profile. In the patient profiles, third-party payer information such as medical insurance information, including any co-payment amount, is included. When the prescription has been filled and the label prepared, billing can be done. Many pharmacy customers have prescription drug insurance, and a third party must be billed. A prescription card contains information such as the name of the insured person, the insurance carrier, a group number, a cardholder identification number, information on dependents covered, an expiration date, and the amount of the co-payment (see Figure 10-4). The technician must enter all of the information into the computer system.

Answering Telephone Calls

The pharmacy technician should field phone calls for the pharmacist. Patients, customers, or health care professionals may contact pharmacies by telephone. This task is one of the major responsibilities of the technician. He or she must answer the phone in a pleasant and courteous manner. Any questions from patients that the technician cannot answer should be handled by the pharmacist (e.g., when a call requires the pharmacist's judgment or questions are about medication or general health).

Operating the Pharmacy Cash Register

Another duty of the pharmacy technician is handling the pharmacy cash register. Operating a cash register successfully requires taking care of payments properly. The cash register is connected to the pharmacy's computer so that prices for any product can be automatically entered by using bar code scanners.

Purchasing

The pharmacy technician often orders products for use or sale. He or she may work alone with a purchasing agent and deal directly with pharmaceutical or medical supply companies on matters such as price. The technician must complete a purchase order that includes the product name, amount, and price. The order is then transmitted directly to manufacturers or wholesalers. Although selection of drugs must al-

COMMUNITY MEDICAL CLINIC
1700 South Tamiami Trail, Sarasota, FL 34239, (813) 952-2577

Patient Name: *Mary Chase* Date: *12-10-xx*
Address:

℞ *Cephalexin 250 mg*
28
Tqid

Private Pay
Private Insurance
Medicaid
CMC

Refill: *0* Physician Signature: *J. Brown* M.D.
Physician Name (printed): J. Brown
Physician DEA#:

A

ENTERED	FILLED	CHECKED	VERIFIED

NOTE: A NON-PROPRIETARY DRUG OF EQUAL QUALITY MAY BE DISPENSED - IF THIS COLUMN IS NOT CHECKED!

DATE	TIME WRITTEN	PLEASE USE BALL POINT - PRESS FIRMLY	✓	TIME NOTED	NURSES SIGNATURE
11/3/XX	0815	Keflex 250 mg p.o. q.6h	✓	0830	G. Pickar, R.N.
		Human NPH Insulin 40 U SC a breakfast	✓		
		Demerol 75 mg IM q. 3–4 h p.r.n severe pain	✓		
		Codeine 30 mg p.o. q. 4h p.r.n. mild–mod pain	✓		
		Tyenol 650 mg p.o. q. 4h p.r.n., fever > 101 degrees F	✓		
		Lasix 40 mg p.o. q.d.	✓		
		Slow-K 8 mEq p.o. b.i.d.	✓		
		J. Physician, M.D			
11/3/XX	2200	Lasix 80 mg IV stat			
		J. Physician, M.D	✓	2210	M. Smith, R.N.

AUTO STOP ORDERS: UNLESS REORDERED, FOLLOWING WILL BE D/C'D AT 0800 ON:

CHECK WHEN ANTIBIOTICS ORDERED ☐ Prophylactic ☐ Empiric ☐ Therapeutic

Allergies: None Known
PATIENT DIAGNOSIS: Diabetes
HEIGHT 5' 15' WEIGHT 130 lb.
PHYSICIANS ORDER

Patient, Mary Q.
#3-11316-7

1

B

Figure 10-3. (A) The prescription form in the retail setting. (B) The physician's order in the institutional setting.

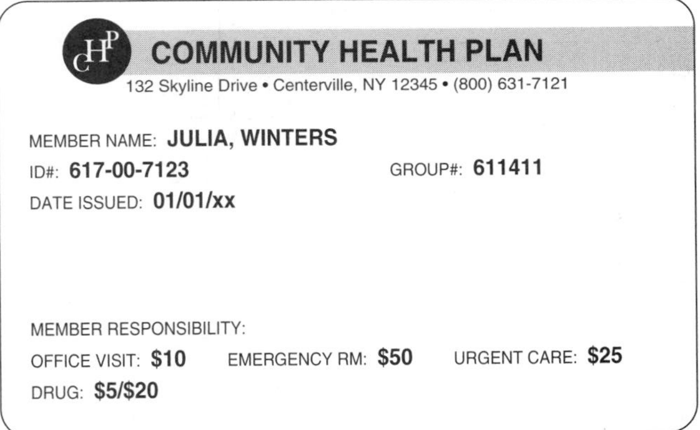

COMMUNITY HEALTH PLAN
132 Skyline Drive • Centerville, NY 12345 • (800) 631-7121

MEMBER NAME: **JULIA, WINTERS**
ID#: **617-00-7123** GROUP#: **611411**
DATE ISSUED: **01/01/xx**

MEMBER RESPONSIBILITY:
OFFICE VISIT: **$10** EMERGENCY RM: **$50** URGENT CARE: **$25**
DRUG: **$5/$20**

Figure 10-4. Patient insurance card.

ways be the responsibility of the pharmacist, purchase orders may be prepared by a pharmacy technician (see Figure 10-5).

Receiving and Inventory Control

When pharmaceutical products are received, the technician must carefully check the product against the purchase order. Damaged products must be reported without delay and returned to the manufacturer or wholesaler. The pharmacy technician must check all products for expiration dates.

Computer Applications in Control of Drug Use

After the telephone, the computer is probably the most frequently used and possibly the most important piece of equipment in the modern pharmacy. The pharmacy technician must be familiar with the computer equipment used in the pharmacy and with all different programs that he or she will be asked to use. All patient information for pharmacy record keeping such as insurance carriers and diagnostic codes can be computerized. Other information entered into the computer may include payroll and bills paid by the pharmacy.

ACCOUNTABILITY

Pharmacy technicians must understand the boundaries of what they can and cannot do legally. They must be accountable for their performance and also their mistakes. An error, even a small one, can have disastrous consequences for a patient, a customer, or the pharmacy itself. The pharmacy technician must develop work habits to ensure accuracy and expect to be held responsible for what he or she does on the job. The technician must always double-check everything to avoid mistakes.

INVOICE

DAY	DIV	RTE	STP
THU	035	105	230

5342 GATOR WAY
ORLANDO FL 12347
405 929-8999 DEA# RA0289492

PLEASE REMIT TO:

P.O. BOX 774
ATLANTA GA 74312

56 SUNSHINE DR
ROCKLEDGE FL 71342

* * * ORIGINAL * * *
SHIP DATE 09/04/xx

INVOICE NO.	INV DATE	PAGE
035–322713	09/04/xx	1
ACCOUNT NO.	**CUST DEA#**	**OF**
035–033100	AL 4994679	1

ST LIC#: PH1982

QTY	DESCRIPTION	CL	CD	ITEM NO	AWP	CUST RTL	G/P PCT	UNIT PRICE	EXTENSION
	THE ORLANDO – B DISTRIBUTION CENTER WILL BE CLOSED ON MONDAY, 09/01/xx.								
	PURCHASE ORDER NO. – 1								
	* * * PICKING NUMBER – 193957 * * *								
1CS	BL FIT BRIEF XLG BRF 4X14	MS	RP	398–750	43.56	13.99	29.87	39.24	39.24
1CS	OWENS OVL GLS AMBCRC1OZ 72	GM		481–994	49.87	74.79	50.48	37.03	37.03
1CS	OWENS OVL PET AMBPL CAP 25X16OZ	GM		476–705	32.29	48.45	50.50	23.98	23.98
2CS	OWENS P/PK CV S/LAM VL 300X13DR	GM		055–285	38.67	57.99	50.49	28.71	57.42
5	TOTAL NUMBER OF PIECES FOR THIS INVOICE	***							

TOTAL	RETAIL	COST	G/P %
OTC	295.18	157.67	46.58

CL } BC - BEHIND THE COUNTER; C2 - CONTROLLED SUBSTANCE - CLASS 2; C3 - CONTROLLED SUBSTANCE - CLASS 3; C4 - CONTROLLED SUBSTANCE - CLASS 4; C5 - CONTROLLED SUBSTANCE - CLASS 5; GM - GENERAL MERCHANDISE; HB - HEALTH AND BEAUTY AIDS; MS - MEDICAL SUPPLIES; OT - OVER THE COUNTER MEDICATION; RX - PRESCRIPTION DRUGS

CL } B - BEST PRICE; C - CONTRACT PRICE CHNG - LAST 30 DAYS; E - FREE GOODS; F - TAX FREE TO CONSUMER; N - NET ITEM; P - PRICE CHANGE; Q - CONTRACT ITEM; R - PROGRAM PRICE; S - SPECIAL PRICE; T - RETAIL TAX; W - WHOLESALE TAX; Z - SUPERNET ITEM

5 *** C14

PURCHASES 1ST THRU 15TH DUE BY 25TH OF SAME MONTH:
16TH THRU EOM DUE BY 10TH OF FOLLOWING MONTH.

157.67
DUE 09/25/xx

ABC-18 (3/02)

TERMS OF SALE AND CLAIMS ON REVERSE SIDE

Figure 10-5. Purchase order.

ETHICAL STANDARDS AND PROFESSIONAL BEHAVIOR

Ethics is the study of moral values or principles, and a professional is an individual qualified to perform the activities of a specific occupation. **Professionalism** goes beyond the knowledge, skills, and abilities required to perform those activities. The pharmacy technician as a professional represents the profession of pharmacy. He or she must always be courteous and listen with focus. The technician must respect the privacy of patients and keep all information confidential. He or she is accountable for the new laws and regulations dictated by the Health Insurance Portability and Accountability Act of 1996 (HIPAA). The most important character traits of a good pharmacy technician are honesty, organization, reliability, and dependability. The pharmacist must be able to count on the technician to maintain confidentiality and privacy of patients and behave ethically, even when not under direct supervision, because of the higher level of trust needed to provide excellent patient care. The HIPAA privacy rule became effective on April 14, 2001. *Compliance was required by April 14, 2003.* This rule sets national standards for the protection of health information of patients. To be in compliance, the covered entities must implement standards to protect individually identifiable health information and guard against the misuse of that information. The privacy rule does not replace federal, state, or other laws that grant individuals even greater privacy protection. Therefore, pharmacy technicians must always keep in mind that they must maintain confidentiality and privacy of patients.

Communication Skills

One of the fundamental skills that the pharmacy technician must acquire to function effectively in the pharmacy is effective verbal communication. Verbal communication is either oral (spoken) or written. Written communication has traditionally been thought of as being more formal than oral conversation. Today, however, with the increasing use of e-mail, written communication is often as informal as oral communication.

Nonverbal communication is easy to understand and one needs only to pay attention to the other party to interpret what is being conveyed. Facial expression, eye contact, and body position are all methods of communicating without using words. Listening to the words and the tone of voice is important. The pharmacy technician must always use a nonjudgmental expression and tone of voice. Communication skills are covered in more depth in Chapter 16.

Teamwork

A pharmacy technician needs to be genuinely interested in helping people and be warm and caring. He or she should be able to put the needs of others first. An effective health care team working together does not just happen. To be effective, team members work together to provide appropriate care for each patient. Each member of the team must be committed to problem solving, focusing on the patient, and communicating. A team approach to patient care ensures comprehensive service without expensive duplication of effort. Teamwork is also necessary for the smooth operation of the entire pharmacy. Technicians work closely with others to perform their duties.

Ability to Handle a Fast Pace and Stress

A pharmacy technician's ability to learn new ideas, modify his or her thinking, adapt to new situations, and handle stress in the pharmacy is an increasingly important skill in today's evolving and complex health care delivery system. Most difficult problems can be solved if one steps back and looks at the situation from the other person's point of view. Team members should try to see what obstacles are present and then work together to move past the problem. A team member in the pharmacy should expect to deal with a high stress environment. The pharmacy technician must handle any workload and other specific situations in a professional manner.

REVIEW QUESTIONS

1. Any suspicious prescription should be presented to the __________ by the pharmacy technician.
   A. physician
   B. pharmaceutical representative
   C. pharmacist
   D. co-worker

2. Patient medication profiles are usually organized by
   A. medication type.
   B. discontinued medications.
   C. physician's specialty.
   D. condition of the patient.

3. Which of the following is the most important thing that pharmacy technicians must understand?
   A. Computer
   B. Supervisor
   C. Performance
   D. Accountability

4. Which of the following is the last step in the prescription processing function?
   A. Putting all the patient information into the computer system
   B. Counseling with the pharmacist
   C. Dispensing
   D. Purchasing supplies

Continues

5. The label for a prescription order for a controlled substance must contain all of the following information, except
   A. the serial number assigned to the prescription by the pharmacy.
   B. the social security number of the patient.
   C. name of the prescriber.
   D. name and address of the pharmacy.

6. All of the following are job responsibilities of pharmacy technicians, except
   A. prescription dispensing.
   B. purchasing.
   C. advising and counseling the patient.
   D. repackaging.

7. Prescriptions come to the retail pharmacies in all of the following ways, except
   A. via fax.
   B. by mail.
   C. by a person.
   D. by telephone.

8. When there is no refill available, the technician should
   A. contact the patient's physician.
   B. contact the insurance company.
   C. notify the patient to see his or her physician.
   D. notify the pharmacist.

9. Which of the following is the most important component of the dispensing function?
   A. Patient counseling
   B. Computer system
   C. Labeling
   D. Pricing

10. A purchase order must be completed by the technician to include all of the following information, except
    A. amount of product.
    B. price.
    C. invoice number.
    D. product name.

11. Which of the following is the most frequently used and possibly the most important piece of equipment in the modern pharmacy, after the telephone?
    A. Typewriter
    B. Autoclave
    C. Durable supply
    D. Computer

12. The HIPAA privacy rule, which is the rule that sets national standards for the protection of health information of patients, became effective in
    A. April 1991.
    B. April 1999.
    C. April 2001.
    D. April 2003.

13. One of the fundamental skills that the pharmacy technician must acquire to function effectively in the pharmacy is
    A. verbal communication.
    B. passing the certification exam.
    C. learning math.
    D. showing leadership.

14. Operating a cash register requires taking care of
    A. patients properly.
    B. pharmacists.
    C. invoices.
    D. payments properly.

15. The study of morals or principles is called
    A. professional.
    B. ethics.
    C. skills.
    D. law.

16. Damaged products must be reported without delay to
    A. the pharmacist.
    B. the wholesaler.
    C. the manager of the pharmacy.
    D. co-workers.

17. A strip label is applied to the container to warn the patient about the property of a medication. This is known as
    A. part of the prescription.
    B. labeling.
    C. safety procedure.
    D. auxiliary labeling.

18. When the pharmaceutical products are received, the technician must carefully check
    A. the serial numbers of the boxes.
    B. for damaged boxes.
    C. the expiration dates of products.
    D. all of the above.

19. To prevent any errors, the technician must
    A. always ask the pharmacist for confirmation.
    B. double-check everything.
    C. perform all calculations three times.
    D. call the physician to verify the order.

20. In patient profiles, active medication orders should be listed
    A. first.
    B. after medical insurance information.
    C. at the end of profiles.
    D. after reviewing the prescription.

11 The Role and Duties of Pharmacy Technicians in Hospitals

OUTLINE

The Role of the Pharmacy Technician in the Hospital
Maintenance of Medication Records
Setting Up Unit-Dose System
Compounding Medications
Packaging
Administration of Medication
Setting Up Outpatient Prescriptions
Computer Data Input
Refilling Drug Carts
Filling Prescriptions
Inspecting Nursing Unit Drug Stocks
Inventory Maintenance
Preparation of Labels
Sensitive Information
Communication Skills
Safety Procedures

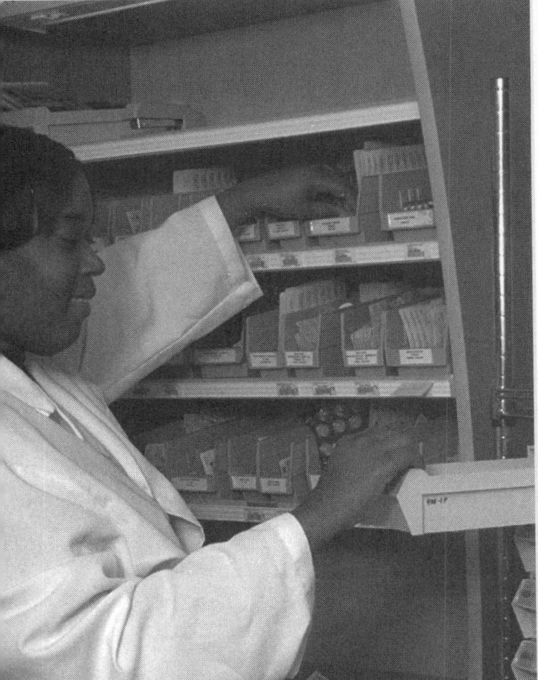

GLOSSARY

extemporaneous A medication that is made based upon a particular set of circumstances or criteria.
prn As needed.

THE ROLE OF THE PHARMACY TECHNICIAN IN THE HOSPITAL

The increasing complexity of health care in the modern hospital is creating ever-greater demands for the hospital pharmacy to broaden its scope of services. New health care legislation and rapid changes in health care technology are imposing new demands on hospital pharmacies, which result in a need for increased manpower. There is growing concern about the present shortage of hospital pharmacists and even greater concern about future shortages. The scope of pharmaceutical services being provided in most hospitals is limited largely by personnel shortages. The hospital pharmacist can be freed by delegating routine tasks to the pharmacy technician, as long as the pharmacist supervises the technician. Supportive hospital pharmacy personnel are used in most hospitals today. Therefore, it is essential to understand the roles and duties of the technician in the hospital setting, as outlined in this chapter.

MAINTENANCE OF MEDICATION RECORDS

Accurate and consistent documentation of medication is essential. The basis of the computerized control system is the medication database. The medication master file contains all of the information needed for ordering, inventory, pricing, and distributing. One of the most significant roles that the pharmacy technician plays involves the maintenance of medication records for usage reports, which indicate the utilization of drugs by individual services, cost centers, or individual physicians. Maintaining accurate medication records helps ensure that these records will be available when needed.

SETTING UP UNIT-DOSE SYSTEM

In hospital settings, the unit-dose system is commonly used. In unit-dose medication distribution systems, drugs are dispensed in single-unit packages. These types of packages contain a single dose that is ready to be administered to a patient. The unit-dose packages are delivered to patient care areas by pharmacy technicians. Hospital pharmacies may also employ automated distribution systems. These devices aid in the automatic storage and dispensing of and charges for medications. Therefore, another duty of the technician is to set up unit doses and deliver them to the appropriate floors.

COMPOUNDING MEDICATIONS

Compounded products may be produced in the hospital pharmacy. The technician should be able to handle this task. Compounded medications that may be produced in the pharmacy include oral liquids, topical preparations, or sterile products. Generally, compounded and repackaged products have short expiration dates, ranging from a few days to a few months. If expiration dates of compounded or repackaged medications have passed, they must be disposed of.

PACKAGING

One of the most rapidly expanding areas of modern hospital pharmacy dispensing has been unit-dose systems. The importance of the single-unit package as a central item has increased accordingly. Pharmaceutical manufacturers have not been able to supply all medication prescribed in single-unit packages. The first step in the design of a single-unit packaging program is to define a "standard inventory" for unit-dose use separate from those items to be packaged on an **extemporaneous** basis only. At the same time, anticipated usage should be determined. Packaging procedures vary from product to product, depending on factors such as moisture and light sensitivity. Other quality control concerns for solid packages are also important. The quality of the package seal depends on heat, pressure, wrinkles, and the thickness of the materials involved. Handling of the drugs in the packaging process should be minimized, and each package should be inspected individually. Also, temperature and humidity in the storage area should be monitored. Another major area of single-unit repackaging is liquid oral dosages. Most of the stability characteristics of liquid dosage forms will be considered in Chapter 7.

Another area of quality assurance important in dispensing of oral liquid doses is the handling procedure used. These dosage forms are generally not intended to be sterile, but cleanliness in the operation is mandatory. Doses should be sealed as soon as possible after filling. Another dosage form often packaged by hospitals is oral powders. These are generally placed into the single-unit vials or cups ordinarily used for liquid. The bioavailability of antibiotic stability after repackaging and problems of cross-contamination must be carefully considered before repackaging is attempted. Other powders generally present less risk. Filling is most accurately done by weight. The final dosage form prepared by the packaging area for unit-dose use is suppository packages. These usually are made up of the suppository, a packet of lubricant, and an examining glove, all packaged in a small plastic bag. The technicians maintain adequate stock of medications and supplies according to established policies and procedures. They should assist in ordering, receiving, unpacking, and storing pharmaceuticals and supplies in appropriate locations.

ADMINISTRATION OF MEDICATION

The total control of medications within the hospital is the responsibility of the pharmacy department. This responsibility extends to control over drug administration. However, the administration of medications to the hospitalized patient is the result of the thoughts and actions of every department within the institution. From environmental services staff (who prepare the patient's room) to the admitting department staff (who initially place the patient into the environment), the nursing staff (who care for the patient), the medical staff (who diagnose and prescribe), and finally, the pharmacy staff (who prepare the medication), all departments act to achieve the final result of the actual administration of the drug to the patient. The administration of medication also involves the clinical laboratories, pathology, radiology, and dietary departments. In today's environment, shifting the responsibility for the administration of medications to the pharmacy has far-reaching consequences. This shift requires that pharmacists be on the nursing unit and have a thorough knowledge of how to administer drugs. The function of medication administration, however, may be delegated to trained pharmacy technicians. For example, the Ohio State University Hospitals employ pharmacy technicians to administer all medications except those given intravenously. The pharmacy technician may also assist in preparation of intravenous solutions (Figure 11-1).

SETTING UP OUTPATIENT PRESCRIPTIONS

Sometimes technicians will be assigned to dispense prescriptions and deliver them to patients who are out of the hospital and may be located in other facilities, such as nursing homes, hospice, rehabilitation facilities, and others. The pharmacy technician here acts as an extension of the hospital pharmacy and also may be required to interface with the nursing staff in each of the delivery points to make sure that the correct dispensing of the prescriptions is both understood and followed.

COMPUTER DATA INPUT

Computer applications have been developed in each segment of the hospital pharmacy: clinical practice, administration, drug distribution, and ambulatory care. The greatest attention has been given to the administrative applications because they have the most impact on the financial health of the pharmacy. Drug distribution has been the focus of work because this has been seen as the primary problem area in hospital practice. From the time the use of a computer is considered until the system is implemented, everyone within the pharmacy, at every level of management from pharmacy technician to pharmacy administrator, must be involved. The primary aspects of computer system use and maintenance are input database administration, data entry, quality control, technical performance, and professional system implementation and maintenance. The technician should enter medication orders into a data processing system (Figure 11-2). Data entry may be accomplished through terminals located in the central pharmacy, in satellite pharmacies, or at each nursing station where pharmacists or technicians would go to review and enter orders.

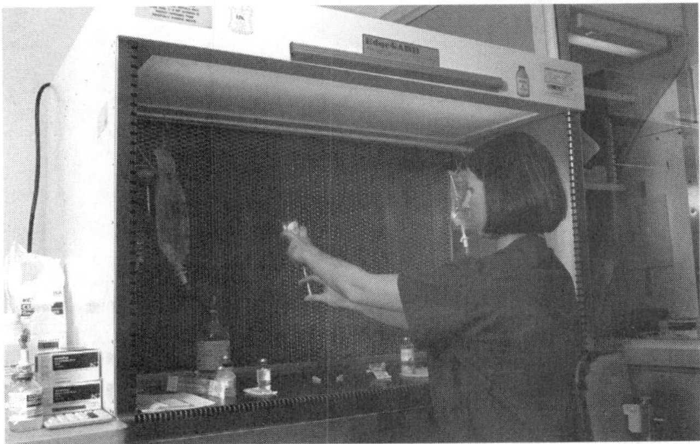

Figure 11-1. Pharmacy technicians will prepare intravenous solutions for use in the hospital setting.

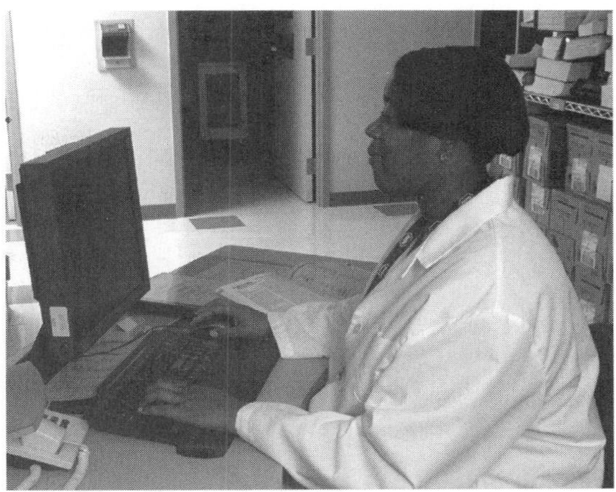

Figure 11-2. The pharmacy technician enters the prescription order into the hospital pharmacy computer system.

REFILLING DRUG CARTS

The pharmacy technicians may receive pharmacy refill requests and original medication containers via a dumbwaiter or courier. He or she should be able to determine the amount to be dispensed from the instructions on the prescription label or refill original container. If the original container is lost, the technician must treat the refill request as a new order (obtaining the original order by calling the nursing station and reviewing the patient's chart or information supplied on the refill request). When the refill order is dispensed, he or she must transmit the medication to the nursing station.

FILLING PRESCRIPTIONS

When the technician receives a copy of new orders for inpatients via a dumbwaiter, a courier, or the telephone, he or

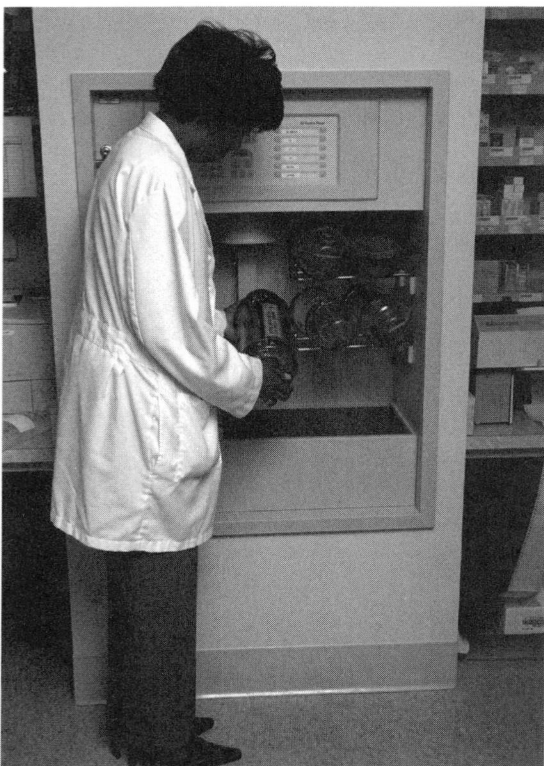

Figure 11-3. Orders may be received via a dumbwaiter in the pharmacy.

she must review and edit the order and then determine the quantity of medication to be supplied to the patient (Figure 11-3). For nonscheduled medications, a 5-day supply is usually dispensed unless the order states that a definite number of doses are required. The technician must select the proper medication and place the determined amount of medication into the proper container. Then, he or she should type the label, including the drug name, strength, patient's name, room number, the date filled, the instructions for administration, the prescribing physician, and the initials of the dispensing pharmacist. After these steps are taken, the technician must attach the label to the container and transmit the medication to the nursing station.

INSPECTING NURSING UNIT DRUG STOCKS

Specific space for storage or automated dispensing machines, both of which are used for stocking and keeping medications, are provided on each nursing unit. Floor drug stock contains those medications that are dispensed often on a **prn** (as needed) basis. Nursing unit drug stocks generally include emergency medications and items such as Tylenol® elixir or drops, antacids, cough syrup, inhalers, creams, ointments, pain relievers, and narcotics. The pharmacy technician is responsible for providing, maintaining, and inspecting nursing unit drug stocks. The inspection happens regularly to confirm proper storage and control of narcotics and to remove expired drugs and discontinued medications.

INVENTORY MAINTENANCE

When drugs arrive, they are stored and must be placed in inventory. Information about drugs such as the name, strength, and quantity must be put into the computer system. The pharmacy technician is involved with the process of inventory maintenance (Figure 11-4). He or she must answer the following questions: how much inventory should be maintained, when inventory levels should be adjusted, and where inventory should be stored. Too much inventory in stock may cause several problems, such as waste of product because of passed expiration dates, increased contamination, and the need for more storage space. As patient medication orders are filled, stock levels are automatically reduced in the inventory system. The technician must ensure that the transaction is recorded in the computer system. Medications in inventory must also be controlled based on their expiration dates. If drugs are close to expiring, they must be removed from inventory. When the pharmacy technician is adding new inventory, he or she should place the newest product toward the back of the storage area, and the older drugs, which are closer to expiring, toward the front (so that they may be dispensed first). Regular drugs can be stored on the pharmacy shelves with free access, and drugs under Schedules II to IV (particularly Schedule II drugs) must be kept in a locked cabinet (Figure 11-5 and Figure 11-6). The pharmacist usually retains the key. Expired drugs must be discarded with proper documentation but are often returned to the manufacturer for credit. Disposal of pharmaceutical products requires documentation for the Drug Enforcement Administration (DEA), which must be done by the pharmacist.

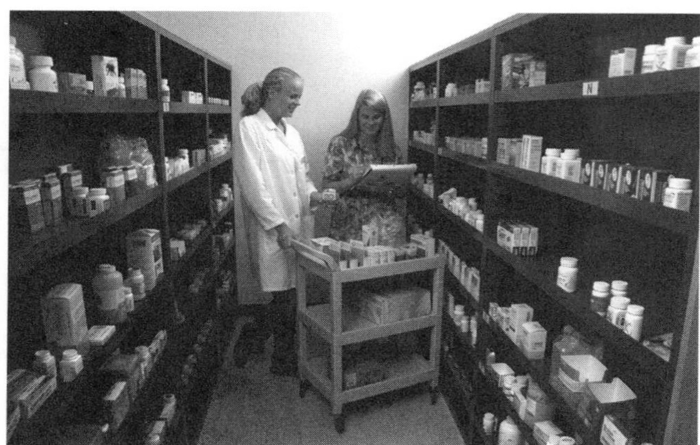

Figure 11-4. It is the pharmacy technician's responsibility to inspect and maintain inventory on nursing units.

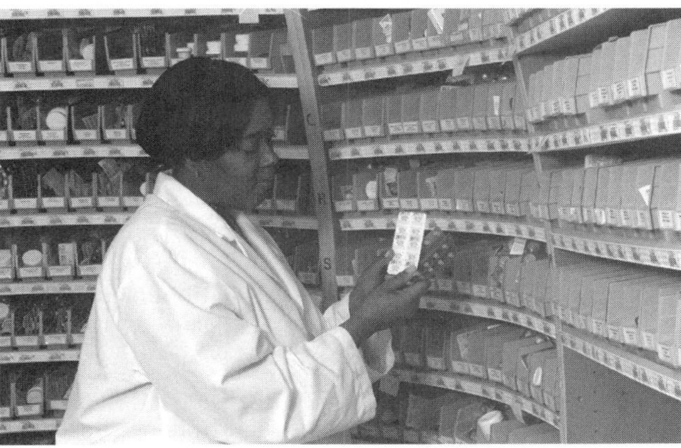

Figure 11-5. Free access is available to regular drugs.

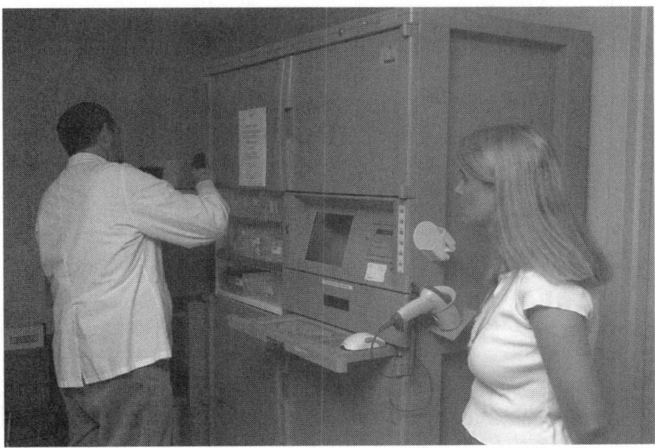

Figure 11-6. Schedule II drugs are kept under lock and key.

PREPARATION OF LABELS

A label includes all information provided with a drug by a manufacturer or pharmacist. When the drug is accurately measured, it should be placed into the proper container and labeled. A container label can be generated before or after the preparation of the order. The label may either be affixed directly to the container by the technician who generates the label, or it may be kept separate for review by the pharmacist before being affixed. The label usually is generated by computer, although sometimes labels are typed (Figure 11-7).

SENSITIVE INFORMATION

The pharmacy technician must preserve the dignity, privacy, and confidentiality of every person. He or she should maintain confidentiality of information and protect issues of patient privacy. The technician must not discuss internal policies, management, or operational issues in the presence of the customers. He or she must be 100% committed to providing the highest quality care for patients, their families, and customers. Technicians also must respect and honor the Patient's Bill of Rights. Patients have the right to know their diagnoses, the nature and purpose of their treatment, and to have enough information to be able to make an informed choice about their treatment protocol.

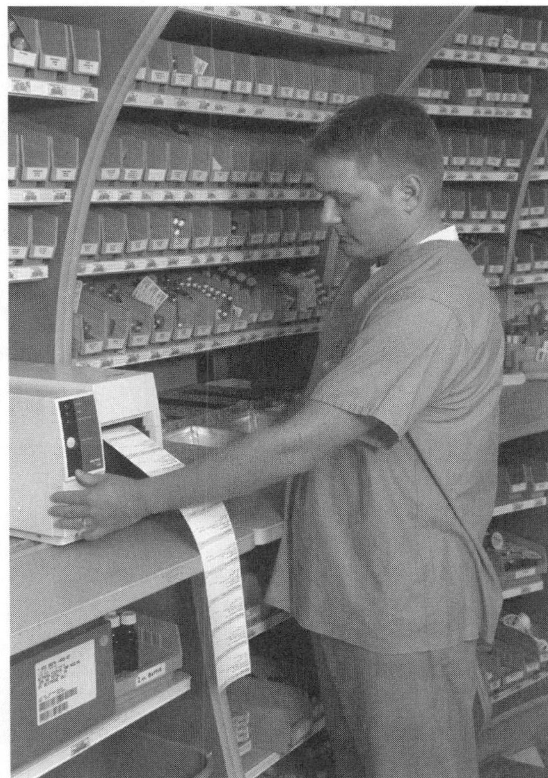

Figure 11-7. Prescription labels are generated by the computer.

COMMUNICATION SKILLS

Pharmacy technicians must be recognized by co-workers, patients, and customers as responsive, courteous, respectful, and cooperative. They should positively promote the mission, values, and goals of the organization. Technicians may answer the phone, demonstrating courteous, polite, friendly, and cooperative behavior toward others. They must actively communicate the mission of the organization, both on the premises and at outside functions or meetings where they represent the organization. Pharmacy technicians must consistently demonstrate a caring attitude and concern for everyone. They must volunteer for community outreach and hospital-sponsored events. The technician must demonstrate the ability to work with co-workers, setting aside personal differences to support the

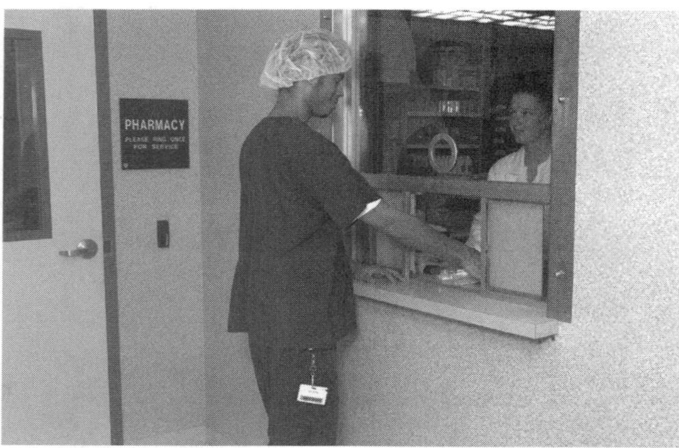

Figure 11-8. Teamwork is important in the hospital setting.

teamwork approach (Figure 11-8). He or she must use excellent interpersonal communication.

SAFETY PROCEDURES

One of the most important duties of the pharmacy technician is to protect himself or herself and others from biohazardous material during different procedures that are completed. The technician must be familiar with fire, disaster, and safety procedures. He or she must also know regulations that pertain to the work area. Handwashing must be a routine procedure, and cleanup of the assigned work area must occur each day, particularly when work is done with flow hoods. Cleaning the hood by washing down its surface with hood disinfectant, wiping from the back to the front, is essential. The pharmacy technician must keep pharmacy areas clean, neat, and well organized, and keep all pharmacy equipment clean.

REVIEW QUESTIONS

1. The basis of the computerized control system is the
A. computer station.
B. filing system.
C. medication database.
D. medication cabinet.

2. Unit dose medication distribution systems dispense drugs in
A. unit packages.
B. single-unit packages.
C. refill packages.
D. out-of-the-way locations.

3. Compounded medications that may be produced in the hospital pharmacy include
A. topical preparations.
B. oral liquids.
C. Schedule I drugs.
D. A and B.

4. Filling is most accurately done by
A. robots.
B. repackaging.
C. technicians.
D. weight.

5. The total control of medications within the hospital is the responsibility of
A. the chief surgeon.
B. the security department.
C. the pharmacy department.
D. the board of trustees.

6. If the original medication container is lost, the pharmacy technician must
A. treat the order as a new order and obtain the original order information.
B. find the original container at all costs.
C. treat the order as a reorder or refill.
D. none of the above.

7. Whose initials should be listed on the medication container's label?
A. The nurse on duty's initials
B. The pharmacy technician's initials
C. The prescribing doctor's initials
D. The dispensing pharmacist's initials

8. If drugs are close to expiration, which of the following must occur?
A. They must be dispensed quickly, at discounted prices to the patients.
B. They must be removed from inventory.
C. They must be tested to see if they are still potent.
D. They must be destroyed by the pharmacy technician.

9. Who usually retains the key(s) to the lockable drug cabinet?
A. The chief surgeon
B. The pharmacist
C. The pharmacologist
D. The pharmacy technician

Continues

10. The term *extemporaneous* refers to
A. destroying a single-unit package that is not immediately used.
B. destroying medication at the time of expiration.
C. preparing medication with materials on hand at the time it is required.
D. prepared labeling for all medications.

11. The quality of the package seal depends on which of the following?
A. Wrinkles
B. Heat
C. Thickness of the material involved
D. All of the above

12. Which of the following hospitals employ pharmacy technicians to administer all medications except those given intravenously?
A. The Ohio State University Hospital
B. The University of Miami Hospital
C. The University of Texas Hospital
D. None of the above

13. Which type of computer applications in the hospital pharmacy has been given the greatest attention?
A. Clinical
B. Administrative
C. Hospital security
D. Blood borne pathogens

14. The technician receives a copy of new orders for inpatients via which of the following?
A. Telephone
B. Dumbwaiter
C. Courier
D. All of the above

15. Floor drug stock in each nursing unit contains medications that are often dispensed on which of the following bases?
A. Abuse potential
B. As the nurse wishes
C. As needed
D. As the technician wishes

Management of Pharmacy Operations 12

OUTLINE

Managing the Pharmacy
Cost Analysis
Purchasing Procedures
  Ordering
  Invoice
Receiving
  Returning Products
Record Keeping
Inventory Control
  Computerized Inventory System
  Perpetual Inventory
  Drug Formulary
  Point of Sale
Repackaging
  Specific Guidelines for Repackaging

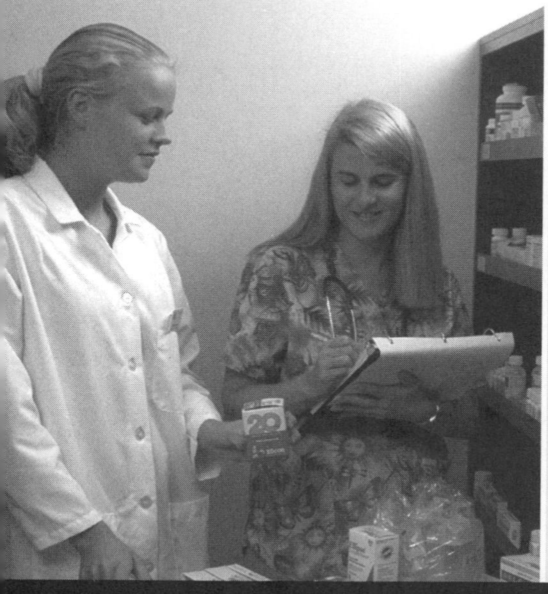

GLOSSARY

batch repackaging The reassembling of a specific dosage and dosage form of medication at a given time.

cost control The implementation of managerial efforts to achieve cost objectives.

group purchasing Procurement contracts are negotiated on behalf of the members of a group (e.g., hospitals, nursing home pharmacies, and home infusion pharmacies). The group purchasing organization uses the collective buying power of its members to negotiate discounts from manufacturers, wholesalers, and other suppliers.

independent purchasing The pharmacist or technician works alone and deals directly with pharmaceutical companies or wholesalers to negotiate price, quantity, and delivery.

inventory The stock of medications a pharmacy keeps immediately on hand.

invoice A form describing a purchase and the amount due.

purchase order The document created when an order is placed.

time purchase The time that the purchase order was made.

unit-of-use packaging The packaging from bulk containers into patient-specific containers.

want book A list of drugs and devices that routinely need to be reordered.

MANAGING THE PHARMACY

The concept of managerial effectiveness is extremely important for anyone involved in the management process. The effectiveness of an organization in providing a product or service that fits customers needs is critical if it is to survive. Management of pharmacy operations encompasses all of the experience, skills, judgment, abilities, knowledge, contacts, risk taking, and wisdom of the manager and other individuals associated with an organization. A complete understanding of strategic sources of competitive advantages must include an analysis of the internal strengths, opportunities, and weaknesses of an organization. The most important concerns of the pharmaceutical organization are productivity, quality, service, and price.

COST ANALYSIS

The pharmacist or manager is responsible and accountable for the finances of the pharmacy. The process of control in general involves the gathering of information and data, the establishment of standards based on this information, and the adjustment of operations to conform to the standards developed. Cost analysis involves all information of the disbursements of an activity, agency department, or program. **Cost control** can be considered to be the implementation of managerial efforts to achieve cost objectives. This process of monitoring and regulating the expenditure of funds by an agency or institution includes budget reports and cost-accounting procedures. These are performed to achieve cost control. There are several factors that should be considered when a cost analysis study is performed. These include cost finding, cost factors, and cost-benefit analysis. Generally, cost control studies are performed for one of two purposes:

1. To estimate the total cost of an operational or proposed system
2. To compare two or more methods or systems to determine which is more advantageous (profitable)

PURCHASING PROCEDURES

The pharmacy must order and buy the products for use or sale, which is usually carried out in one of two ways: independent purchasing or group purchasing. **Independent purchasing** means that the pharmacist or technician works alone and deals directly with representatives of pharmaceutical companies or wholesalers to negotiate price, quantity, and delivery. In **group purchasing**, a number of hospitals or pharmacies join together to obtain or negotiate discounts for high-volume purchases. A **purchase order** is the document created when an order is placed. It should contain complete information for each item that is ordered such as the name, brand, dosage form, size of the box or the package, strength, and quantity of product.

Ordering

Regular drugs, devices, and supplies may be ordered electronically by fax or telephone or online by computer. The order is normally made on a form known as a purchase order. The decision to order a drug or item depends on how well it sells in the pharmacy. Many pharmacies have a list of drugs and devices that routinely need to be reordered. This list is called the **want book**. Information to be specified when ordering includes the following:

- The item name and manufacturer. For a drug product, the generic or brand name must be specified.
- The strength and dosage form of the drug (or size, if ordering a device)
- The quantity of drug dosage forms per package (e.g., bottle of or boxes of 100, package of two or more)
- The type of packaging
- The number of bottles, packages, or devices being ordered

Invoice

An **invoice** is a paper describing a purchase and the amount due. When a **time purchase** is made, that is, when the item is not paid for at the time of purchase, the vendor usually includes a packing slip with delivery of the merchandise. A packing slip describes the item enclosed. The vendor may also enclose an invoice. Invoices should be placed in a special folder until paid. The pharmacy may be making more than one purchase from the same vendor during the month. Some vendors request that payment be made from the invoice: others send a statement later. A statement is a request for payment.

RECEIVING

Receiving is one of the most important parts of the pharmacy operation. When products that have been ordered arrive at the pharmacy, it is essential that a system for checking purchases and receiving is in place. Generally the individual who ordered the products should not do the receiving also. All items must be carefully checked against the purchase order. The following procedure should be followed when pharmaceuticals or medical supplies are received:

- They should be verified and compared against the purchase order for name of product, quantity of boxes, and package size, and examined for any gross damage of boxes.

- For drug products the name, brand, dosage form, size of the package, strength, quantity, and expiration date must be checked.
- After products are received and checked, they must be placed in an appropriate storage location. Products requiring refrigeration or freezing should be processed first.

Returning Products

For damaged or incorrect shipments or expired medications, the manufacturer should be notified immediately and a return merchandise authorization should be requested for the return of the rejected shipment.

RECORD KEEPING

A modern record-keeping system has three key components:

1. A symbol on the outside of the jacket or folder to indicate the active or inactive status of records
2. Safeguards to prevent misfiling
3. A filing technique that allows quick, accurate retrieval and proper refilling

Files may be kept as hard copy (on paper) or on the computer disk. Most medical facilities and pharmacies use a combination of computers and hard copy. The most popular system today is the use of color coding on open shelves. Some records are kept in card or tray files. Regardless of the type or style of filing system equipment, purchasing the best quality is always recommended. Some of the considerations in record keeping are size, type, and volume of records. It is also important to ensure confidentiality requirements and at the same time maximize retrieval speed. At the time of payment, the pharmacy technician should compare the statement with the invoice(s) to verify accuracy and fasten the statement and invoices together. Write the date and check number on the statement, and place it in the paid file.

Disbursements are recorded and distributed to specific expense accounts such as the following:

- Dues and meetings
- Equipment
- Insurance
- Medical supplies
- Pharmacy expenses
- Printing, postage, and stationery
- Rent and maintenance
- Salaries
- Taxes and licenses
- Travel
- Utilities
- Miscellaneous

All records for wholesale distributors need to be kept separate and distinct from the records for the rest of pharmacy operations. The wholesale records should not be filed by prescription number. The inventory and records of purchase from the wholesale transactions must be made available at the time of an inspection (e.g., FDA inspection), for which they should be centrally maintained. Wholesale records (purchase and sale) must be maintained for a minimum of 2 years from the date of disposition of the prescription drugs. Also, the pharmacy may have to keep required records for more than 2 years after the date of disposition of the prescription drug if notified that an investigation is underway.

INVENTORY CONTROL

Inventory is a list of articles in stock, with the description and quantity of each. In other words, inventory is the entire stock of products on hand at a given time in the pharmacy. Inventory control is closely associated with the function of purchasing. Inventory control is important to the pharmacist because it is the means by which he or she assures that all medications and products are accounted for and used legitimately, that adequate stocks are available when needed, and that the costs of too large an inventory are avoided (Figure 12-1). There are several important factors and issues with regard to inventory such as the following:

1. How much inventory should be maintained?
2. When should inventory levels be adjusted?
3. Where should inventory be stored?

In an ideal system, pharmaceutical products would arrive shortly before they are needed (just-in-time [JIT] system).

Computerized Inventory System

The traditional purchasing and inventory control system, which is still being used in a majority of pharmacies today, does not involve computers and is considered old-fashioned. It is more expensive and difficult to maintain all information accurately, in addition to being more time consuming. For

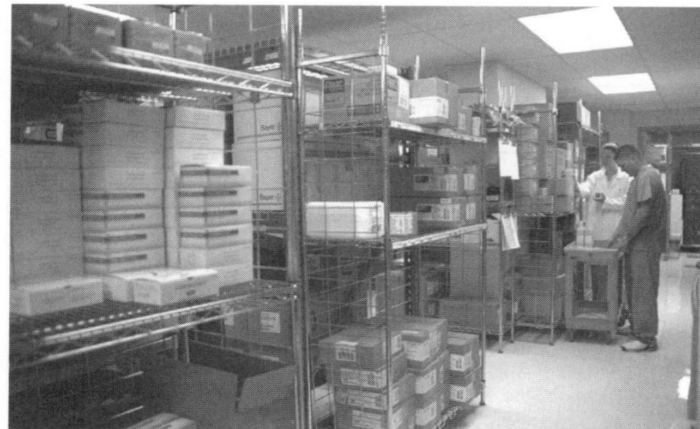

Figure 12-1. The pharmacy technician is responsible for maintaining inventory in the pharmacy.

these reasons, some pharmacists have attempted to implement more sophisticated purchasing and inventory control systems. Computers and computerized inventory systems increase accuracy, generate more data, and require less time compared with traditional systems. The basis of the computerized purchasing and control system is the medication database. The medication master file contains all of the information needed for ordering, inventory, pricing, and distribution of pharmaceuticals. Most computerized systems provide all of the information needed to write a purchase requisition and a few systems actually produce the final purchase order. The real advantage of computerized inventory control systems is the time savings for the pharmacy and the business office.

Perpetual Inventory

Perpetual inventory systems are being used today to show when it is time to reorder materials. These systems allow the pharmacist to review drug use monthly, allowing better monitoring of all information. The computer also enables the monitoring of the budget. Board regulations require that a pharmacist should keep a perpetual inventory of each controlled substance in Schedule II that has been received, dispensed, or disposed of, in accordance with the Controlled Substance Act of 1970, which is discussed in Chapter 2. This inventory must be reconciled at least every 10 days. The perpetual inventory is a written record of the amount of controlled substances in Schedule II that are physically contained with the pharmacy or pharmacy department. The technician must keep in mind that the computer system is only effective when all input information is accurate.

Drug Formulary

Drug formularies are lists or catalogs of drugs that are approved for use either within a hospital or for reimbursement by a third-party payer. The purpose of formularies is to eliminate therapeutic duplication and provide patients with the best drug at the lowest cost. In the early days of formularies, they were used by hospitals to control drug inventories and provide to prescribers a list of drugs of choice for various conditions. However, the absence of a drug from the formulary was not usually a great barrier to a prescriber's obtaining it for a patient. A special request could be made by the prescriber to a member of the pharmacy and therapeutic committee of the hospital, and usually the drug would be obtained. When managed-care organizations and pharmacy-benefit management companies began to use formularies, circumventing them became much more difficult. The restrictive use of formularies has led to a number of important ethical questions. For example, does the use of generic drugs for therapeutic substitution violate the autonomy of the patient and/or prescriber? Is the use of such substitution a violation of informed consent? Does the use of formularies violate the ethical principles of beneficence (doing good) and nonmaleficence (avoiding harm)?

Point of Sale

The point-of-sale (POS) master is the most suitable, flexible, and open-ended system on the market. The POS master can increase overall profitability, and it can be installed in all of the computers at the main pharmacy. POS systems can control stock in the pharmacy accurately. The system can handle a significant volume of customers and transactions and all the orders, credits, interstore transfers, and returns. A major benefit of the POS master is that it can cover every area that a user could conceivably be interested in and is driven by practical requests of the users themselves. The POS master can enhance every area of the pharmacy and is really easy to use; it is probably the best system and the best support team for the business.

REPACKAGING

As pharmaceutical manufacturers began to prepare, package, and distribute commonly prescribed medications, the role of pharmacist changed from formulator and packager to repackager of commercially prepared medication. Therefore, the pharmacist and technician repackage bulk containers of medication into patient-specific containers of medication. The amount of medication that is repackaged into the patient container is generally predicated on the course of therapy. This type of packaging from bulk containers into patient-specific containers is called **unit-of-use packaging.** Unit-of-use packaging, sometimes referred to as "repackaging," is a suitable concept for inpatient or outpatient dispensing. An advantage to this type of dispensing process is that it allows the pharmacist to prepare medications for administration before their use is anticipated. The unit-dose system of dispensing medication in organized health care settings has been the driving force behind repackaging programs as we know them today. Unit-dose distribution is the standard by which all other distribution systems are measured. The single-dose package always contains the dose of the drug for a given patient. A single-dose package may contain two tablets or two capsules in one package or container for a given patient if the dose calls for two tablets or two capsules. Single-unit packages will contain only one tablet or one capsule. One of the major advantages of unit-dose drug distribution systems is that they decrease the total cost of medication-related activities. Repackaging medications in advance of when they are needed allows the pharmacist to take advantage of periods of reduced staff activity to lessen the demands of peak activity. **Batch repackaging** is defined as the repackaging of a specific dosage and dosage form of medication at a given time.

Specific Guidelines for Repackaging

Drug packages must have four basic functions:

1. Protect their contents from deleterious environmental effects.

2. Protect their contents from deterioration resulting from handling.
3. Identify their contents completely and precisely.
4. Permit their contents to be used quickly, easily, and safely.

Manufacturers of repackaging materials and repackaging equipment describe their products based on the type of package that is achievable. There are four classes—A, B, C, and D—with class A being the best and class D the worst. The package types most often found in hospital pharmacy departments include those used for oral solids, oral liquids, injections, respiratory medications, and topical medications.

Compounded and repackaged products typically have short expiration dates, ranging from days to months. Expired compounded or repackaged pharmaceuticals cannot be returned and must be disposed of.

REVIEW QUESTIONS

1. The implementation of managerial efforts to achieve cost objectives is called
   A. purchasing procedures.
   B. cost control.
   C. ordering.
   D. record keeping.

2. After products ordered for the pharmacy are received, in the case of damage, incorrect shipment, or expired medications, the pharmacy technician should immediately notify the
   A. co-worker.
   B. purchasing department.
   C. manufacturer.
   D. logbook.

3. A list of articles in stock is called
   A. cost control.
   B. inventory control.
   C. record keeping.
   D. receiving.

4. One of the major advantages of unit-dose drug distribution systems is that they
   A. decrease the total cost of medication.
   B. decrease the total dosage for patients.
   C. increase the effectiveness of the medication.
   D. increase the absorption of the medication.

5. A list of drugs approved for use within a managed care or a health system such as a hospital is called
   A. drug inventory.
   B. drug formulary.
   C. drug prescription.
   D. open file.

6. When the pharmacist or technician works alone and deals directly with pharmaceutical companies' representatives to negotiate prices, quantities, and deliveries, it is called
   A. cost control.
   B. dependent purchasing.
   C. independent purchasing.
   D. inventory control.

7. All of the following are the most important concerns of the pharmaceutical organization, except
   A. operating hours.
   B. quality.
   C. price.
   D. productivity.

8. Many pharmacies have a list of drugs and devices that routinely need to be reordered. This list is called the
   A. red book.
   B. white book.
   C. want book.
   D. green book.

9. Which of the following is one of the most important parts of the pharmacy operation?
   A. Handwashing
   B. Receiving invoices
   C. Receiving products
   D. Returning products

10. Expired, compounded, or repackaged pharmaceuticals must be
    A. returned to the manufacturers.
    B. returned to the purchasing department.
    C. disposed of.
    D. used.

11. The repackaging of a specific dosage and dosage form of medication at a given time is called
    A. batch repackaging.
    B. unit-of-use repackaging.
    C. manufacturer repackaging.
    D. none of the above.

12. The basis of the computerized purchasing and control system is
    A. the repackaging database.
    B. the expired medications.
    C. the medication database.
    D. the manufacturers' database.

Continues

13. In a modern record-keeping system, there should be three key components, which include all of the following, except
   A. safeguards to prevent misfiling.
   B. a filing technique that shows a reminder sign.
   C. a filing technique that allows quick, accurate retrieval.
   D. a symbol on the outside of the jacket.

14. Specific guidelines for repackaging require that all of the following basic functions are fulfilled, except
   A. identifying the contents completely and precisely.
   B. protecting the contents from deleterious environmental effects.
   C. permitting the contents to be unstable or outdated.
   D. protecting the contents from deterioration resulting from handling.

15. The amount of medication that is repackaged into the patient container is predicated on which factor?
   A. The course of therapy
   B. The age of the patient
   C. The cost of medication
   D. All of the above

Financial Management and Health Insurance

13

OUTLINE

Financial Aspects of Pharmacy Practice
- Financial Issues
- Purchasing
- Accounting
- Pricing

Health Insurance
- Insurance Policy
- Health Insurance Terminology
- Types of Health Insurance

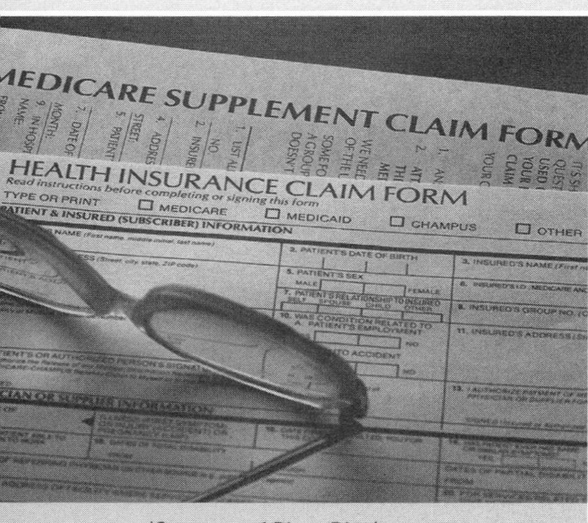

(Courtesy of PhotoDisc)

GLOSSARY

accounting A system of recording, classifying, and summarizing financial transactions for preparing a pharmacy budget.

amortize To spread the cost of services out over a period of several years.

assignment of benefits An authorization to an insurance company to make payment directly to the pharmacy or physician.

CHAMPVA Civilian Health and Medical Program of the Veterans Administration; a program to cover medical expenses of the dependent spouse and children of veterans with total, permanent service-connected disabilities.

coordination of benefits The prevention of duplicate payment for the same service.

co-payment Most policies have a coinsurance, or cost-sharing requirement, that is the responsibility of the insured.

deductible A specific amount of money that must be paid each year before the policy benefits begin (e.g., \$50, \$100, \$300, or \$500).

dependents The insured's spouse and children under the terms of the policy.

dispensing fee A pricing mechanism calculated by adding the operating expenses and profit margin and dividing by the total work units, either unit doses or inpatient prescriptions.

eligibility The specific terms of coverage under a policy.

health insurance A contract between a policyholder and an insurance carrier or government program to reimburse the policyholder for all or a portion of the cost of medical care rendered by health care professionals.
independent practice association (IPA) A type of health maintenance organization (HMO) in which the HMO contracts directly with physicians, who continue in their existing practices.
markup fee system A pricing mechanism in which the price charged to the patient is calculated by adding a percentage markup, in addition to a dispensing fee, to the acquisition cost of the drug.
Medicaid A federal/state medical assistance program to provide health insurance for specific populations.
Medicare A federal health insurance program created as part of the Social Security Act.
overpayment Payment by the insurer or by the patient of more than the amount due.
percentage markup system A system of establishing price that assumes that total operating expenses are directly related to the acquisition cost.
point of service Payment of services outside of an insurance plan at the time the service is rendered.
policy limitation Policies that exclude certain types of coverage.
policy terms and financial obligations Policy that becomes effective only after the company offers the policy and the person accepts it and pays the initial premium.
preauthorization The requirement of notification and permission to receive additional types of services before one obtains those services.
preferred provider organization (PPO) A managed care organization that contracts with a group of providers, who are called *preferred providers*, to offer services to the managed care organization's members.
premium The cost of the coverage that the insurance policy contains; this may vary greatly, depending on the age and health of the individual and the type of insurance protection.
subscriber The individual or organization protected in case of loss under the terms of an insurance policy.
third-party payer The fee for services provided is paid by an insurance company and not by the patient.
time limit The amount of time from the date of service to the date (deadline) the claim can be filed with the insurance company.
TRICARE A federally funded comprehensive health benefits program for dependents of personnel serving in the uniformed services.
waiting period The period of time that an individual must wait to become eligible for insurance coverage (e.g., 30 days) before coverage commences or for a specific benefit.

FINANCIAL ASPECTS OF PHARMACY PRACTICE

The practice of pharmacy is a business as well as a profession, and the details of conducting the business aspects of a pharmacy are often the responsibility of the pharmacy technician. Although service to the patient is the primary concern of the medical profession, a pharmacist must charge and collect a fee for such services to continue providing medical care. As a business, a pharmacy must charge competitive and fair prices for services and must receive payment for those services in cash or in a timely fashion. Even a patient or customer with medical insurance should be fully informed about the practice's fees and payment policies. He or she is ultimately responsible for the bill if the insurance company refuses to pay or does not cover the full amount.

Financial Issues

A pharmacy's business records are the key to good management practice. The pharmacy technician who can keep accurate financial records and who will conduct the nonclinical side of the practice in a business-like fashion is genuinely needed and appreciated. Financial records that are complete, correct, and current are essential for the following:

- Prompt billing and collection procedures
- Professional financial planning
- Accurate reporting of income to federal and state agencies

Purchasing

The complexity of the pharmacy department will dictate the level of involvement that a pharmacy has with the purchasing department. In pharmacies with intravenous infusion programs, central supply services, or other services, such as supplying orthopedic assistance, there will be continued involvement with purchasing in the buying of equipment and supplies. Pharmacies with limited services may have little involvement, particularly if purchasing medications is the pharmacy's responsibility. Regardless of the frequency of involvement, the purchasing department can provide valuable assistance to the pharmacy. The purchasing department in a hospital or retail pharmacy deals with sales representatives, negotiates contracts, purchases and stores supplies, and acts as a liaison between departments within the hospital or retail pharmacy and the manufacturers. The department provides expertise concerning quality of supplies. Although the selection of drugs must always remain with the pharmacist, the actual purchase orders may be prepared by the purchasing department.

Accounting

Accounting is a system of recording, classifying, and summarizing financial transactions for preparing a pharmacy budget. It is an important function that has to be carried out on an annual basis. Good accounting principles provide for an efficient department. The accounting department or section can be instrumental in supplying the pharmacy with data depicting expenses, revenues, dollar volume of inventory, cost per patient per day of pharmacy operations, and cost/revenue relationships to previous periods of operation. This will save the pharmacist a great deal of time when he or she is trying to justify new programs or when financial comparisons are needed.

Pricing

To understand the wide variations in prescription prices, it is important to understand various pricing mechanisms in the pharmacy setting. There are three basic pricing mechanisms:

- Percentage markup system
- Dispensing fee
- Markup fee system

Percentage Markup System

The oldest and probably least equitable pricing mechanism is the **percentage markup system.** In tying the price of the medication to the cost of the drug, one assumes that total operating expenses are directly related to the acquisition cost. This is not a valid assumption. Although the inventory cost of an expensive medication may be slightly greater than that of a less expensive drug, other operating expenses such as salaries, expendable supplies, and so forth, remain relatively stable. This system also relates the pharmacy charge directly to the product and does not consider the services involved. Another disadvantage of this system is that it does not separate different categories of operating expenses, such as dispensing cost, administrative cost, clinical cost, and others.

Dispensing Fee

The second, and probably the most commonly used pricing mechanism, is the **dispensing fee.** This fee is calculated by determining the operating expenses, including salaries, overhead, supplies, and equipment cost, which is **amortized** over a period of time. A desired profit margin is added to this figure. A unit charge is then calculated by adding the operating expenses and profit margin and dividing by the total work units, either unit doses or inpatient prescriptions. The end result is a dispensing fee that is added to the acquisition cost of the medication to determine the total price charged to the patient. The advantage of this system is its lack of a direct relationship between the price charged, the patient, and the acquisition cost of the medication. Thus, the system does not encourage the dispensing of a more expensive medication.

Markup Fee System

A third pricing mechanism that has been used to price medications in hospital pharmacies is a combination of the first two, namely, the **markup fee system.** In this system, the price charged to the patient is calculated by adding a percentage markup, in addition to a dispensing fee, to the acquisition cost of the drug. The sum of these costs yields the total charge to the patient for the medication. For example, if the acquisition cost of a medication is $1.00, the percentage markup is 20%, and the dispensing fee is $0.75, the total charge for the medication would be $1.95. As a result, this system may appear to provide the best of both worlds.

HEALTH INSURANCE

Health insurance is a contract between a policyholder and an insurance carrier or government program to reimburse the policyholder for all or a portion of the cost of medical care rendered by health care professionals. This care includes care that is medically necessary and preventative treatment. The purpose of health insurance is to help offset some of the high costs accrued from an injury or illness. Patients may receive coverage under different types of private, state, or federal programs. Each patient may have a different type of health insurance policy with various benefits. Therefore, the pharmacy technician should be familiar with different types of patient insurance coverage.

There are three ways in which a person can acquire health insurance:

1. Enrolling in a prepaid health plan
2. Obtaining insurance through a group plan
3. Paying the premium on an individual basis

Insurance Policy

An insurance policy is a legally enforceable agreement. It is also called an insurance contract, regardless of whether the contract is a group, individual, or prepaid contract. There is no standard health insurance contract; however, state laws regulate the way policies are written and minimum requirements of coverage.

Health Insurance Terminology

Pharmacy technicians should be familiar with the following terms that are commonly used in health insurance:

- **Assignment of benefits**: An authorization to an insurance company to make payment directly to the pharmacy or physician.
- **Co-payment**: Most policies have a coinsurance, or cost-sharing requirement, which is the responsibility of the insured.
- **Coordination of benefits**: This prevents duplicate payment for the same service. For example, if a child has coverage through both parents' insurance policies, a primary carrier is designated to pay benefits according to the terms of its policy, and the secondary plan may cover whatever charges are still left. If the primary carrier pays $145 of a $180 charge, the most the secondary carrier will pay is $35.
- **Deductible**: A specific amount of money must be paid each year before the policy benefits begin (e.g., $50, $100, $300, or $500). The higher the deductible is, the lower the cost of the policy, and the lower the deductible is, the higher the cost of the policy.
- **Dependents**: A policy might also include the spouse and children of the insured. These are called the dependents of the insured.
- **Eligibility**: This can be obtained by contacting the insurance company and verifying that the patient indeed has coverage. Contact may be done over the telephone, via a voice-automated system, by using computer software, over the Internet, or by checking an eligibility list for a managed care plan.
- **Overpayment**: Payment by the insurer or by the patient of more than the amount due.
- **Policy limitation**: There are some patients or individuals who have exclusion health insurance policies. Some exclusions are acquired immunodeficiency syndrome (AIDS), attempted suicide, cancer, losses due to injury on the job, and pregnancy.
- **Policy terms and financial obligations**: The policy becomes effective only after the company offers the policy and the person accepts it and pays the initial premium.
- **Preauthorization**: Many private insurance companies and prepaid health plans have certain requirements that must be met before they will approve diagnostic testing, hospital admissions, inpatient or outpatient surgical procedures, specific procedures, and specific treatment or medications.
- **Premium**: The premium is the cost of the coverage that the insurance policy contains and may vary greatly, depending on the age and health of the individual and the type of insurance protection.
- **Subscriber**: The individual or organization protected in case of loss under the terms of an insurance policy. The subscriber is known as an insured or a member, policyholder, or recipient.
- **Time limit**: The time limit is the amount of time from the date of service to the date (deadline) a claim can be filed with the insurance company. Each insurance program has specific time limits that must be adhered to, or the insured party will not be able to collect from the insurance company.
- **Waiting period**: A waiting period or elimination period is the period of time that an individual must wait to become eligible for insurance coverage (e.g., 30 days) before coverage commences or for a specific benefit (e.g., an employee must wait 9 months before seeking maternity benefits).

Types of Health Insurance

There are many forms of health insurance coverage in the United States. Health insurance may include private insurance, government plans, managed care contracts, and workers' compensation—all referred to as third-party payers. **Third-party payers** are groups or agencies that provide payment for services instead of the patient. There are three major third-party payers:

- Third-party full payment groups (private insurance companies)
- Third-party contractual payment groups (Blue Cross®, Medicare, and Medicaid)
- The cash payment group

Private Health Insurance

There are numerous private insurance companies across the United States that offer health insurance to individuals and groups. They offer a variety of managed care plans. Examples of private insurance include Blue Cross® Blue Shield®, Kaiser Foundation, various health maintenance organizations (HMOs), and workers' compensation.

The Blue Cross® Blue Shield® (BCBS) Association is a nationwide federation of local nonprofit service organizations that offer prepaid health care services to subscribers. Under a prepaid health coverage plan, the carrier will pay for specified medical expenses if premiums are paid in advance. The Blue Cross® of BCBS covers hospital services, outpatient and home care services, and other institutional care. Blue Shield® plans cover physician and dental services, vision, and other outpatient benefits. Now, however, both offer full health care coverage for their subscribers. In most states, they have become a single corporation, although in some they remain separate. A variety of plans are offered through Blue Cross® Blue Shield®, including individual and family, group, preventative care, and managed care plans. Some local BCBS organizations help the government administer Medicare, Medicaid, and TRICARE programs. There are 86 local BCBS plans in the United States, each with its own claim form. Plans make direct payments to member physicians, but payments may be made to the subscriber (patient) if the physician is a nonmember. Many small groups and individuals who may not be able to get coverage elsewhere can join a Blue Cross® Blue Shield® plan. Some plans offer coverage regardless of medical condition during special periods of time. Plans must get permission from the state to raise their rates.

Government Plans

Government plans sponsor insurance coverage for eligible individuals. The federal government provides coverage under Medicare, Medicaid, TRICARE or CHAMPUS, and CHAMPVA.

Medicare provides health insurance to citizens aged 65 and older and to younger patients who are blind or widowed or who have serious long-term disabilities such as kidney failure. There are two distinct parts (A and B) to the Medicare program. Medicare Part A covers hospital, nursing facility, home health, hospice, and inpatient care. Those who are eligible for Social Security benefits are automatically enrolled in Medicare Part A. Medicare Part B covers outpatient services, services by physicians, durable medical equipment, and other services and supplies. Medicare Part B coverage is optional and voluntary. Everyone eligible for Part A can choose to enroll in Part B by paying monthly premiums. Deductibles must be met in Parts A and B before payment benefits begin. Some federal employees and former federal employees who are not eligible for Social Security benefits and Part A may still enroll in Part B. Many Medicare enrollees also carry private supplemental insurance that pays the deductible and the 20% co-payment. If a patient has both Medicare and Medicaid, charges must be filed with Medicare first, and Medicaid is the secondary payer.

Medicaid is a health benefit program designed for low-income people (those receiving welfare payments or other forms of public assistance), the blind, the disabled, and members of families with dependent children deprived of the support of at least one parent and financially eligible on the basis of income and resources. Each state decides what services are covered and what the reimbursement will be for each service. Two types of co-payment requirements may apply to the Medicaid patient. Some states require a small fixed co-payment paid to the provider at the time of service (e.g., $1.00 or $2.00). This policy was instituted to help pay some of the administrative costs of physicians participating in the Medicaid program. There may be certain groups of patients that are exempt from this co-payment requirement (e.g., persons under 18 years of age or women receiving perinatal care).

The **TRICARE** program is a comprehensive health benefits program offering three (*tri*) types of plans for dependents of men and women in the uniformed services (military). Under the basic TRICARE program, individuals have the following three options:

- TRICARE standard: fee-for-service (cost-sharing plan)
- TRICARE extra: preferred provider organization plan
- TRICARE prime: health maintenance organization plan with a point-of-service option

TRICARE is a new program that replaced CHAMPUS. CHAMPUS stands for "Civilian Health and Medical Program of the Uniformed Services." CHAMPUS was a health care benefit for families of uniformed personnel and retirees from the uniformed services (the Army, Navy, Marines, Air Force, Coast Guard, Public Health Service, and the National Oceanic and Atmospheric Administration).

CHAMPVA stands for "Civilian Health and Medical Program of the Veterans Administration." It covers the expenses of the families of veterans with total, permanent, service-connected disabilities. It also covers the expenses of surviving spouses and dependent children of veterans who died in the line of duty. Eligibility is determined, and identification cards are issued by the nearest Veterans Affairs medical center. The insured persons are then free to choose their own private physicians. Benefits and cost-sharing features are the same as those for TRICARE beneficiaries who are military retirees or their dependents and dependents of deceased members of the military.

Workers' Compensation

All state legislatures have passed workers' compensation laws to protect wage earners against the loss of wages and the cost of medical care resulting from occupational accidents or disease. Compensation benefits include medical care benefits, weekly income replacement benefits for temporary disability, permanent disability settlements, and survivor benefits when applicable. The provider of service, such as doctors, hospitals, therapists, or pharmacies, accepts the workers' compensation payment as payment in full and does not bill the patient. Time limitations are set forth for the prompt reporting of workers' compensation cases. The employee is obligated to promptly notify the employer; the employer, in turn, must notify the insurance company and must refer the employee to a source of medical care. Individuals entitled to workers' compensation insurance coverage are private business employees, state employees, and federal employees such as postal workers, coal miners, and maritime workers. Workers' compensation insurance coverage provides benefits to employees and their dependents if employees suffer work-related injury, illness, or death.

Managed Care Programs

During the past 6 decades, there have been many reforms of the health care system. Medical practices have made transitions from rural to urban, from generalist to specialist, from solo to group practice, and from fee-for-service to capitated reimbursement. The expansion of health care plans to a number of different types of delivery systems that try to manage the cost of health care has resulted in managed care. Managed care organizations manage, negotiate, and contract for health care with the goal of keeping costs down. Managed care organizations sign up health care providers who agree to charge a fixed fee for services. These fixed fees are set by the managed care organization or by the government agency responsible for managed care.

Health maintenance organizations (HMOs) were the first type of managed care organizations developed to control the expenditure of health care dollars and manage patient care. The HMO contracts with employers to provide health service for their employees. The member of an HMO selects a primary care physician (PCP) from the medical group. The HMO is responsible for all but limited administrative needs of a PCP, including processing of capitation (a system of payment used by managed care plans in which physicians and hospitals are paid a fixed, per capita amount for each patient enrolled over a stated period of time, regardless of the type and number of services provided), and fee-for-service checks.

An **independent practice association (IPA)** is a closed-panel HMO. Instead of maintaining its own staff and clinic buildings, the IPA contracts with independently practicing physicians. The IPA may pay each doctor a set amount per patient in advance (capitation), or the fees charged for services to group members may be billed directly to the IPA rather than to the patient. Fees for services to nonmember patients are handled the same as any other fee for service. The physician may contract with several IPAs.

A **preferred provider organization (PPO)** is a type of managed care plan in which enrollees receive the highest level of benefits when they obtain services from a physician, hospital, or other health provider designated by their program as a preferred provider. Enrollees receive reduced benefits when they obtain care from a provider who is not designated as a preferred provider by their program. PPO patients may see specialists without prior authorization from their primary care physicians. HMOs offering point-of-service options are more like PPOs.

The Kaiser Foundation Health Plan is a type of prepaid group practice (HMO). The Kaiser Foundation was a pioneer of nonprofit prepaid group practice beginning in California in 1933. The plan owns the medical facilities and directly employs the physician and other providers.

Point of service is an option added to some HMO plans that allows patients to choose a physician outside the HMO network and to pay increased deductible and coinsurance fees.

WEB SITES OF INTEREST

Blue Cross® Blue Shield®: http://www.bcbs.com
Centers for Medicare & Medicaid Services: http://cms.hhs.gov
CHAMPVA: http://www.va.gov/hac/champva/champva.asp
Kaiser Insurance: http://www.kaiserinsurance.com
Medicare: http://www.medicare.gov
TRICARE: http://www.tricareonline.com

REVIEW QUESTIONS

1. If a person is covered under both Medicare and Medicaid, to which program should the claim be sent first?
A. Medicaid
B. Medicare
C. Both should get it at the same time
D. The Kaiser Foundation Health Plan

2. TRICARE is a health care benefit program for all of the following, except
A. the National Oceanic and Atmospheric Administration.
B. families of uniformed personnel.
C. families of veterans with service-related disabilities.
D. the Coast Guard.

3. An authorization to the insurance company to make payments directly to the physician is called
A. coordination of benefits.
B. service benefit plan.
C. tracker.
D. assignment of benefits.

4. Capitation is
A. fixed payment made for each enrolled patient rather than reimbursement based on the type and number of services provided.
B. payment at the time of service.
C. various payments for specific services.
D. fixed prospective payment for services provided.

5. Carol Smith goes to her participating HMO provider for a checkup and a flu shot. The allowed charge for a checkup is $65, and the physician's usual fee is $70. The allowed charge for the flu shot is $40, and the physician's usual fee is $25. Considering her co-pay is $25, and preventive care is a covered service under her plan, how much is Mrs. Smith charged for the visit?
A. $5
B. $10
C. $25
D. Nothing

Continues

6. Medicaid is
A. a governmental insurance plan with which all physicians must comply.
B. a secondary carrier when the patient has Medicare.
C. always the primary carrier.
D. a type of Medigap insurance policy.

7. Medicare Part B covers
A. nursing facility care.
B. hospice care.
C. hospital care.
D. outpatient services.

8. Which of the following is a federation of nonprofit organizations offering private insurance plans?
A. CHAMPVA
B. Medicare
C. Blue Cross and Blue Shield Association
D. TRICARE

9. TRICARE was formerly known as
A. CHAMPUS.
B. CHAMVA.
C. BCBS.
D. Medicaid.

10. The term *point of service* refers to
A. the preauthorization some HMOs require.
B. the geographic place where a medical service is performed.
C. an option added to some HMO plans that allows patients to choose physicians outside the HMO network.
D. a type of Medicare.

11. Which of the following pricing mechanisms appears to provide the best system?
A. Markup fee system
B. Percentage markup system
C. Dispensing fee system
D. None of the above

12. Financial records that are complete, correct, and current are essential for all of the following except
A. professional financial planning.
B. accurate reporting of income to federal agencies.
C. prompt finding of fraud and bankrupt.
D. prompt billing and collection procedures.

13. If a medical insurance policy has a deductible of $50
A. the patient may deduct this amount from the pharmacy's bill.
B. the patient does not have to pay the first $50 of service.
C. the pharmacist is reimbursed for $20 only.
D. the patient has to pay this amount.

14. The amount charged for a medical insurance policy is called a
A. claim.
B. premium.
C. beneficiary.
D. fee schedule.

15. Part B of Medicare is
A. voluntary.
B. compulsory.
C. free to the policy holder.
D. required for hospital benefits.

14 Safety in the Workplace

OUTLINE

Safety
- Occupational Safety and Health Administration Standards

Aseptic Technique
- Medical Asepsis
- Surgical Asepsis

Laminar Airflow Hoods

Employee Responsibilities

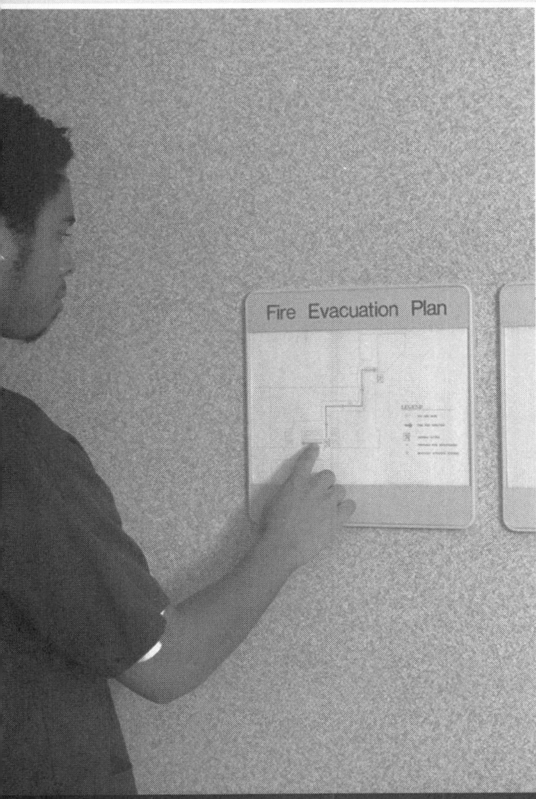

GLOSSARY

autoclave A sterilizing machine. An autoclave uses a combination of heat, steam, and pressure to sterilize equipment.

biohazard symbol An image or object that serves as an alert that there is a risk to organisms, such as ionizing radiation or harmful bacteria or viruses.

chemical sterilization A method of cleaning equipment used for instruments that cannot be exposed to the high temperatures of steam sterilization.

disinfection Destruction of pathogens by physical or chemical means.

dry heat sterilization A method of sterilization that uses heated dry air at a temperature of 320 to 356°F (160 to 180°C) for 90 minutes to 3 hours.

exposure control plan A written procedure for the treatment of persons exposed to biohazardous or similar chemically harmful materials.

fire safety plan A written procedure that includes fire extinguisher locations, fire alarm pull-box locations, sprinkler system location, exit signs, and clear directions to the quickest and safest way to exit a building during an emergency.

gas sterilization The use of a gas such as ethylene oxide to sterilize medical equipment.

hazard communication plan Use of warning labels for all hazardous chemicals.

laminar airflow hood A system of circulating filtered air in parallel-flowing planes in hospitals or other health care facilities. The system reduces the risk of airborne contamination and exposure to chemical pollutants in surgical theaters, food preparation areas, hospital pharmacies, and laboratories.

medical asepsis The destruction of organisms after they leave the body.

standard precautions A set of guidelines for infection control.

sterilization Complete destruction of all forms of microbial life.

surgical asepsis Complete destruction of organisms before they enter the body.

SAFETY

Safety issues are present in any place, and commonsense precautions need to be taken in the workplace, particularly in the pharmacy. The purpose of environmental protection measures is to minimize the risk of occupational injury by isolating or removing any physical or mechanical health hazards in any workplace. In 1970, the federal government passed the Occupational Safety and Health Act, the first national heath and safety law, with the goal of ensuring safe and healthful working conditions for all workers in the United States. The Act established the Occupational Safety and Health Administration (OSHA) in the Department of Labor. OSHA establishes safety regulations for employers and monitors compliance.

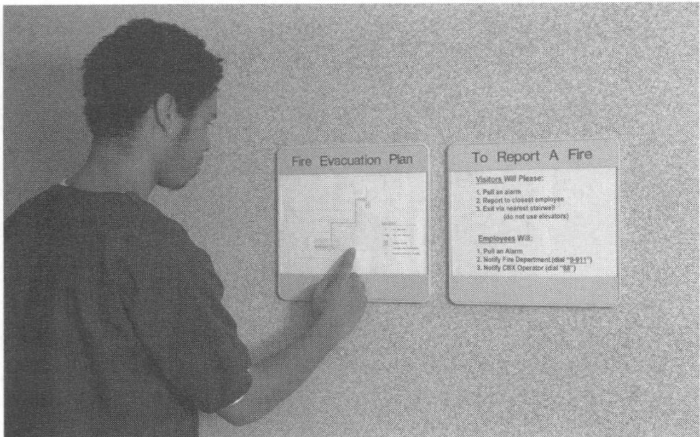

Figure 14-1. Emergency plans should include clearly posted and marked escape routes.

Occupational Safety and Health Administration Standards

OSHA establishes standards requiring employers to provide their workers with workplaces free from recognized hazards that could cause serious injury or death. In addition, employees must abide by all safety and health standards that apply to their jobs. OSHA regulates all workplace environments by enforcing protocols for the proper removal of hazards and fire safety and emergency plans. Two specific functions related to the pharmacy, specifically the hospital pharmacy, are protection of employees from exposure to disease and protections from exposure to chemicals. OSHA has the right to inspect private and public work sites to be sure all protocols and guidelines are being followed. The general health of the employee must be protected, and many standards require plans, training of employees, and monitoring of injuries with detailed records. In addition, the employer must provide general protective equipment (such as fire extinguishers and first-aid kits), as well as specialized protective equipment as needed. OSHA provides for research, information, education, and training in the field of occupational safety and health and authorized enforcement of OSHA standards.

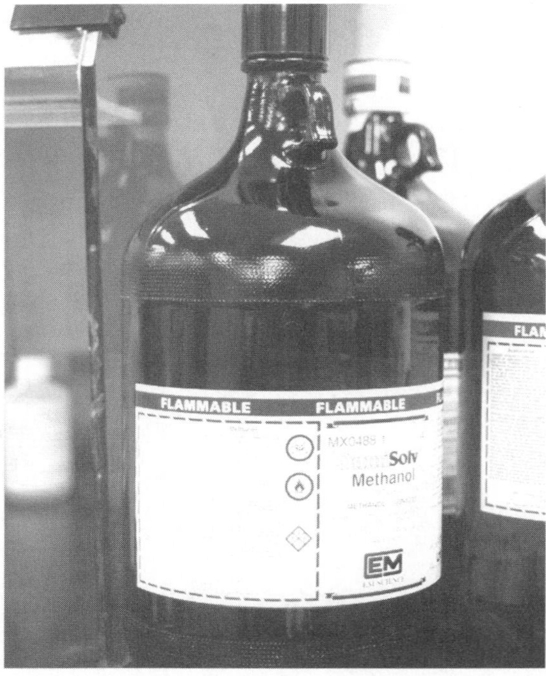

Figure 14-2. All hazardous chemicals found in a laboratory should be clearly marked with warning labels.

Fire Safety Plan

An OSHA-compliant **fire safety plan** must include written procedures. Exits must be marked and escape routes published (see Figure 14-1). Fire extinguishers and fire alarm pull boxes must be present, and the employer must provide fire prevention training, conduct fire drills, and test the fire alarm and sprinkler systems.

Hazard Communication Plan

A **hazard communication plan** protects the rights of employees to know what types of hazardous chemicals are present in the workplace and what health risks are associated with those chemicals. All hazardous chemicals must have warning labels, as shown in Figure 14-2.

Exposure Control Plan

The **exposure control plan** is designed to minimize risk of exposure to infectious material and bloodborne disease. The plan must be written and updated as necessary. OSHA also has regulations for or provides information about hazards associated with radioactive materials and use of lasers and latex allergies.

Standard Precautions

Standard precautions are a set of guidelines for infection control requiring the employer and employee to assume that all human blood and specified human body fluids are infectious for human immunodeficiency virus (HIV), hepatitis B virus, and other bloodborne pathogens (Table 14-1). Standard precautions should be used for blood, other body fluids containing visible blood, semen, vaginal secretions, cerebrospinal fluid, pleural fluid, synovial fluid, and any other body fluids. A health care worker should also use standard precautions for urine, feces, nasal secretions, sputum, breast milk, tears, saliva, and vomitus. In addition, a health care worker should use standard precautions when dealing with broken skin and the mucous membranes inside the mouth, nose, and body cavities. A health care worker must use appropriate personal protective equipment, such as gloves, gowns, masks, lab coats, and eyewear, to protect himself or herself from exposure to pathogens (disease-causing microorganisms). A health care worker must undertake proper disposal of hazardous waste containers, which are marked. OSHA regulations require that all health care workers be immunized against hepatitis B, because they are at risk for infection from bloodborne pathogens.

Disposal of Hazardous Waste

Any materials that have come into contact with blood or body fluids are treated as hazardous waste. Various containers are used to collect hazardous material. Waste containers are labeled with the **biohazard symbol** to ensure that all employees are aware of the contents (see Figure 14-3). Plastic bags are used for gloves, paper towels, dressings, and other soft material; rigid containers are used for sharps such as needles, glass slides, scalpel blades, or disposable syringes (see Figure 14-4).

TABLE 14-1. Standard Precautions for Infection Control

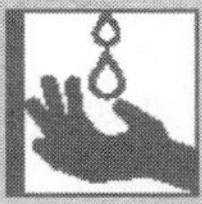

Wash Hands (Plain soap)
Wash after touching **blood**, **body fluids**, **secretions**, **excretions**, and **contaminated items**.
Wash immediately **after gloves are removed** and **between patient contacts**.
Avoid transfer of microorganisms to other patients or environments.

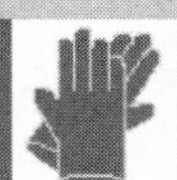

Wear Gloves
Wear when touching **blood**, **body fluids**, **secretions**, **excretions**, and **contaminated items**.
Put on **clean** gloves just **before touching mucous membranes** and **nonintact skin**.
Change gloves between tasks and procedures on the same patient after contact with material that may contain high concentrations of microorganisms. Remove gloves promptly after use, before touching noncontaminated items and environmental surfaces, and before going to another patient, and wash hands immediately to avoid transfer of microorganisms to other patients or environments.

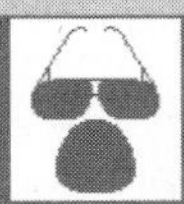

Wear Mask and Eye Protection or Face Shield
Protect mucous membranes of the eyes, nose, and mouth during procedures and patient-care activities that are likely to generate **splashes** or **sprays** of **blood**, **body fluids**, **secretions**, or **excretions**.

Wear Gown
Protect skin and prevent soiling of clothing during procedures that are likely to generate **splashes** or **sprays** of **blood**, **body fluids**, **secretions**, or **excretions**. Remove a soiled gown as promptly as possible and wash hands to avoid transfer of microorganisms to other patients or environments.

Patient-Care Equipment
Handle used patient-care equipment soiled with **blood**, **body fluids**, **secretions**, or **excretions** in a manner that prevents skin and mucous membrane exposures, contamination of clothing, and transfer of microorganisms to other patients or environments. Ensure that reusable equipment is not used for the care of another patient until it has been appropriately cleaned and reprocessed and single-use items are properly discarded.

Linen
Handle, transport, and process used linen soiled with **blood**, **body fluids**, **secretions**, or **excretions** in a manner that prevents exposures and contamination of clothing and avoids transfer of microorganisms to other patients or environments.

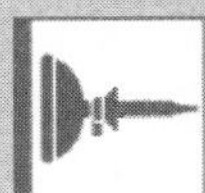

Use **resuscitation devices** as an alternative to mouth-to-mouth resuscitation.

(Courtesy of BREVIS Corporation.)

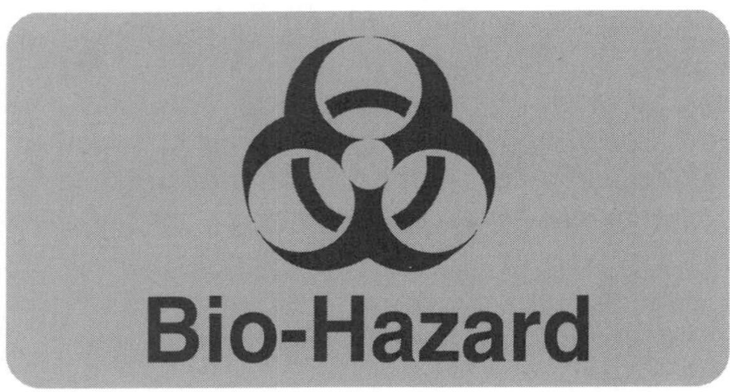

Figure 14-3. Biohazard symbols will appear on containers used to dispose of contaminated waste.

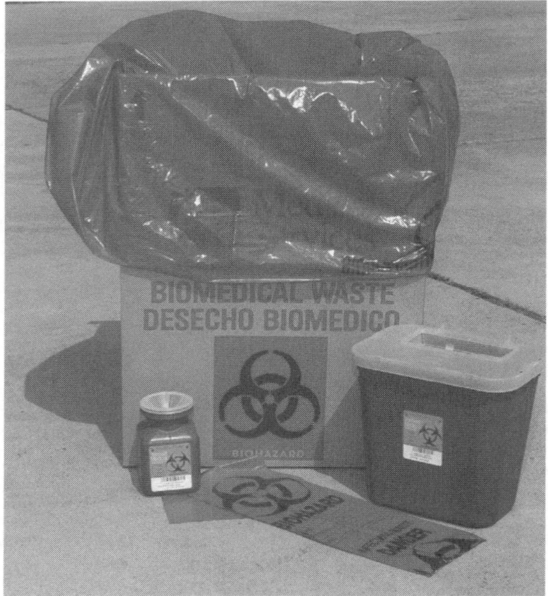

Figure 14-4. Red plastic biohazard bags are used to dispose of gloves, contaminated gowns, and bedding; hard plastic sharps containers are used to dispose of needles, glass slides, and scalpel blades.

Most facilities contract with a company that specializes in removal and disposal of hazardous waste. Cleaning staff should be instructed not to empty hazardous waste containers. When health care workers change hazardous waste bags, they must wear gloves, masks, and protective eyewear; close the bags securely; and put the bag inside a second hazardous waste bag (double bag) if there is any chance of leakage.

ASEPTIC TECHNIQUE

The most effective way to eliminate transmission of disease from one host to another is through asepsis, which means "sterile (free from microorganisms)." There are two types of asepsis: medical asepsis and surgical asepsis.

Medical Asepsis

Medical asepsis is the removal of pathogens to reduce transfer of microorganisms by cleaning any body part or surface that has been exposed to them. Medical asepsis benefits both the patient and the health care worker by preventing exposure to pathogens from other patients, from each other, or from other staff. Medical asepsis is also called *clean technique*.

Hand Hygiene

The single most important means of preventing the spread of infection is frequent and effective hand hygiene by all health care workers. Hands must be washed, using the correct technique. An extended scrub is not needed each time hands are washed, but the first scrub in the morning should be extensive, lasting 2 to 4 minutes, unless the hands are excessively contaminated. A good antimicrobial soap with chlorhexidine, such as Hibiclens®, which has antiseptic residual action that will last several hours, should be used. Even with this technique, the hands are still not sterile, because skin cannot be sterilized. Normal flora (nonpathogens) remain, but most pathogens have been removed. Proper handwashing depends on two factors: running water and friction. The water should be warm, because water that is too cold or too hot will cause the skin to become chapped. Friction involves the firm rubbing of all surfaces of the hands and wrists.

Cleaning and Sanitizing

Equipment and instruments need to be cleaned promptly after every use to remove visible residue. Microorganisms may hide under residue and survive the disinfection or sterilization process if residue is not removed. Items that cannot be cleaned at once are usually rinsed with cold water and placed in a soaking solution to prevent anyone from touching them and to prevent the residue from hardening.

Disinfection

Disinfection is the ability to kill microorganisms on the surface of various items. Disinfection can be accomplished by use of a chemical disinfectant or by boiling. Boiling is used for items that enter body cavities such as the mouth or anus, which are not sterile. Disinfection is also used for items that are sensitive to heat such as glass thermometers or rubber materials. Large equipment and counter surfaces that cannot fit into an autoclave for sterilization should be disinfected by use of chemical disinfectants. Boiling kills many microorganisms but does not kill bacterial spores. Directions for proper use are provided on labels of disinfectant solutions, including the proper length of time to soak items. Many pharmacies use commercial solutions or prepare solutions containing household bleach. A 1:10 solution of household bleach (1 part bleach to 10 parts water) provides disinfection. Small spills of blood or body fluids on counter surfaces can be cleaned with bleach solution and paper towels.

Surgical Asepsis

Surgical asepsis is the destruction of all microorganisms, pathogenic and nonpathogenic, on an object or instrument. The goal is to prevent any microorganisms from entering the patient's body through an open wound, especially during surgery. It is used when sterility of supplies and the immediate environment is required. Surgical asepsis requires sterile handwashing (surgical scrub), sterile gloves, special handling procedures, and sterilization of materials. Most dangerous microorganisms are destroyed at a temperature of 122 to 140°F (50 to 60°C).

Sterilization

Sterilization is the process of killing or destroying all microorganisms and their pathogenic products. Methods of sterilization include the application of steam under pressure, dry heat, gas, chemicals, and radiation. Sterilization can be achieved through the use of an **autoclave**, which generates steam under pressure (see Figure 14-5). When moist heat of 270°F (or 132°C) under pressure of 30 pounds is applied to instruments, all organisms will be killed in 20 minutes. Autoclaving is one of the most effective methods for destruction of all types of microorganisms. The autoclave must be cleaned after each load. **Dry heat sterilization** is another method of sterilization that uses heated dry air at a temperature of 160 to 180°C (320 to 356°F) for 90 minutes to 3 hours. The gas ethylene oxide is used for items that are sensitive to heat; this method of sterilization is called **gas sterilization**. It requires special equipment and aeration of materials after application of the gas. The gas is highly flammable and toxic. Gas sterilization is commonly used in hospitals that have room-sized gas sterilization chambers. Many prepackaged products for intravenous infusion and bandages are sterilized using this method. **Chemical sterilization** is used for instruments, and chemicals can be applied topically to the body for disinfection. Iodine, household bleach, Mercurochrome®, and alcohol are examples of disinfectants that can be used in this manner.

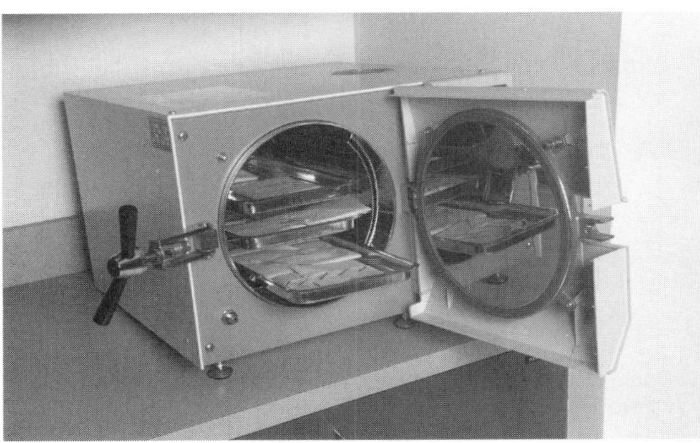

Figure 14-5. An autoclave is used to sterilize equipment.

LAMINAR AIRFLOW HOODS

A **laminar airflow hood** is a piece of equipment designed for the handling of materials whenever a sterile working environment is required (see Figure 14-6). This device uses a system of circulating filtered air in parallel flow planes. Because room air may be highly contaminated, the system reduces the risk of bacterial contamination or exposure to chemical pollutants in surgical theaters, hospital pharmacies, laboratories, and food preparation areas. Sneezing, for example, produces up to 200,000 aerosol droplets, which can attach to dust particles and stay in the air for weeks! Laminar airflow hoods are very effective for providing a clean area if they are operating properly.

There are two types of laminar airflow hoods: vertical and horizontal (see Figure 14-7). A horizontal airflow hood should be used for numerous types of parenteral medication preparations and sterile product mixtures. A vertical airflow hood is used for all chemotherapeutic agents, because of the

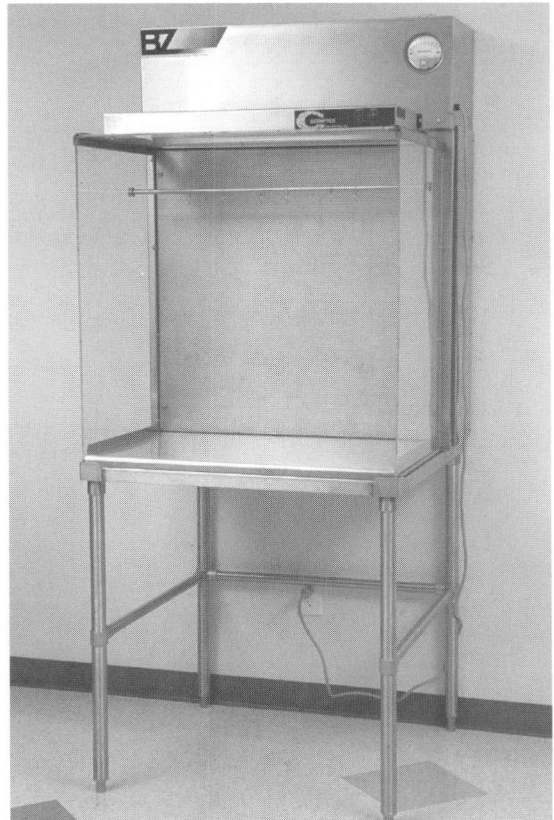

Figure 14-6. Laminar airflow hood.

direction of the airflow and the specifications of the hood. It can also be used to mix nonchemotherapeutic agents. However, chemotherapeutic agents should not be mixed in a horizontal airflow hood. The horizontal hoods used in hospital pharmacies must be inspected each year by an authorized inspector to ensure the effectiveness of the filtering system. Laminar airflow hoods basically have a box-like structure, with the top and sides made of Plexiglas, a transparent acrylic material. The work area is bathed by positive pressure (horizontal or vertical), flowing air called *laminar,* that has passed through a prefilter that removes lint and dust, and then through a high-efficiency particulate air (HEPA) filter. This filter, the most important part of the system, removes microorganisms and small particles of matter from room air, compressing and redistributing the now ultra clean air into air-flow streams that are parallel to each other. The air moves at a rate of 90 to 120 linear feet per minute, with very little turbulence, at a uniform velocity. This process removes nearly all of the bacteria from the air. The HEPA filter is located at the rear of the work area, with a removable, perforated metal diffuser further toward the front. HEPA filters cannot be cleaned or recycled and must be replaced every 3 to 5 years on average. The work area is illuminated by fluorescent lights.

The controlled area should be a limited-access area sufficiently separated from other pharmacy operations to minimize the potential for contamination that could result from the unnecessary flow of materials and personnel into and out of the area. The controlled air is a buffer from outside air that is needed because strong air currents from briefly opened doors, personnel walking past the laminar airflow workbench, or the air stream from the heating, ventilating, and air conditioning system can easily exceed the velocity of air from the laminar-airflow workbench.

Laminar airflow hoods should be left on 24 hours a day and require regular maintenance. If turned off for any reason, the unit should be turned on for at least 30 minutes and then thoroughly cleaned before reusing. Also, all items to be used in procedures under the hood should be cleaned thoroughly before work is begun, as should the operator's hands and arms. Excess dust must be avoided at all costs. The operator should remove any jewelry from the hands and wrists. Technicians should use gowns with knit cuffs and rubber gloves while doing work inside laminar airflow hoods. Masks are recommended because most personnel talk or may cough or sneeze. Personnel who have a sensitivity to latex should use powder-free, low-latex protein gloves or, if the allergy is severe, latex-free (synthetic) gloves are recommended. This

A
4.
Vertical hood
HEPA filter (exhaust)
HEPA filter (air supply)
2.
Glass shield
1.
Intake
Blower
3.

1. Room air enters the laminar airflow. This makes up about 30% of the air in the hood.
2. HEPA-filtered air enters and makes up 70% of the air in the hood.
3. Air from the work area is drawn down into the base and pulled back through the unit.
4. Air is exhausted after being filtered through carbon or HEPA filters.

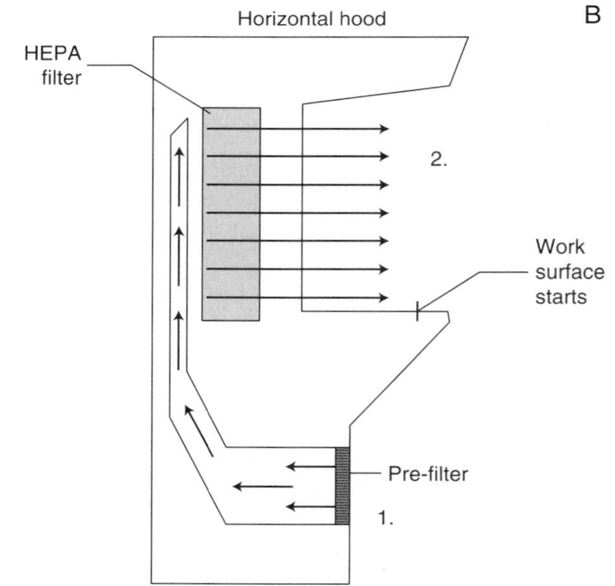

1. Room air enters, is filtered and drawn up to the top of the hood, where it is filtered through a HEPA filter.
2. Filtered air is directed out over the work surface.

Figure 14-7. (A) Direction of airflow in a vertical laminar airflow hood. (B) Direction of airflow in a horizontal laminar airflow hood.

minimizes the shedding of skin flora into the work area. Conventional lab coats are not sufficient, because their open cuffs allow entrapment of contaminated air between the technician's wrist and forearms and inside the sleeves. It is important for operators to keep their hands within the cleaned area of the hood as much as possible and not touch hair, face, or clothing. Only materials essential for preparing the sterile product should be placed in the laminar-airflow workbench or barrier isolator. The surface of ampules, vials, and container closures (e.g., vial stoppers) should be disinfected by swabbing or spraying with alcohol before placement in the workbench. All aseptic procedures should be performed at least 6 inches inside the front edge of the laminar-airflow workbench, in a clear path of unidirectional airflow between the HEPA filter and work materials (e.g., needles or closures). The operator should avoid spraying or squirting solutions onto the HEPA filter, always aiming away from the filter when opening ampules or adjusting syringes. In a horizontal hood, items should be placed away from the sides and HEPA filter, and nothing should touch the filter. Large objects should never be placed near the back of the hood, because they will contaminate everything downstream from them and disrupt the flow pattern of air. Work areas should be cleaned after each use. Before and after a series of IV admixtures are prepared (the preparation of sterile products) or any time something is spilled, the work surface of the laminar airflow hood should be thoroughly cleaned with alcohol. A long side-to-side motion should be used, starting at the back of the hood and then working forward. The acrylic plastic sides should also be cleaned periodically with solutions that can be used on them and following the directions closely. Disinfectants should be alternated periodically to prevent development of resistant microorganisms. The laminar airflow hood should be serviced and certified every 6 months. Active work surfaces in the controlled area (e.g., carts, compounding devices, and counter surfaces) should be disinfected. Refrigerators, freezers, shelves, and other areas where pharmacy-prepared sterile products are stored should be kept clean. The floors of the controlled area should be nonporous and washable to enable regular disinfection.

EMPLOYEE RESPONSIBILITIES

The U. S. Department of Labor web site states that "Although OSHA does not cite employees for violations of their responsibilities, each employee 'shall comply with all occupational safety and health standards and all rules, regulations, and orders issued under the Act' that are applicable. Employee responsibilities and rights in states with their own occupational safety and health programs are generally the same as those for workers in states covered by federal OSHA. An employee should do the following:

- Read the OSHA poster at the job site.
- Comply with all applicable OSHA standards.
- Follow all lawful employer safety and health rules and regulations, and wear or use prescribed protective equipment while working.
- Report hazardous conditions to the supervisor.
- Report any job-related injury or illness to the employer and seek treatment promptly.
- Exercise rights under the Act in a responsible manner."
- Cooperate with the OSHA compliance officer conducting an inspection if he or she inquires about safety and health conditions in the workplace.

WEB SITES OF INTEREST

Centers for Disease Control and Prevention: http://www.cdc.gov
Department of Labor: http://www.dol.gov
Occupational Safety and Health Administration: http://www.osha.gov

REVIEW QUESTIONS

1. If a needlestick injury occurs, you should take all of the following actions, except
   A. washing your hands.
   B. documenting and reporting the injury.
   C. sending the report to the local health department.
   D. notifying your supervisor.

2. A good, thorough handwashing time should be approximately
   A. 3 minutes.
   B. 5 minutes.
   C. 10 minutes.
   D. 15 minutes.

3. Destruction of all living microorganisms by specific means is called
   A. disinfection.
   B. sterilization.
   C. sanitization.
   D. ultrasonic cleaning.

4. Which of the following terms is used by OSHA to describe the use of physical or chemical means to remove, inactivate, or destroy bloodborne pathogens?
   A. *Decontamination*
   B. *Disinfection*
   C. *Distraction*
   D. *Sanitization*

Continues

5. Anytime that you are preparing a series of IV admixtures or anytime something is spilled, the work surface of the laminar airflow hood should be cleaned by
   A. cold water.
   B. hot water.
   C. alcohol.
   D. bleach.

6. Which of the following is used to destroy bloodborne pathogens in the hospital pharmacy?
   A. Phenol
   B. Alcohol
   C. Ammonium hydroxide
   D. Bleach

7. How often should an autoclave be cleaned?
   A. After each load
   B. Every day
   C. Every week
   D. Every 2 weeks

8. OSHA regulations require all health care workers who may be at risk to be vaccinated against which of the following diseases?
   A. Tuberculosis
   B. Acquired immunodeficiency syndrome (AIDS)
   C. Hepatitis B
   D. Hepatitis C

9. All of the following are examples of chemical sterilization, except
   A. household bleach.
   B. Mercurochrome®.
   C. mercury.
   D. iodine.

10. A horizontal airflow hood can be used for
    A. parenteral medication administration.
    B. parenteral medication preparation.
    C. mixing nonchemotherapeutic agents.
    D. both B and C.

11. Laminar airflow hoods must be replaced every
    A. 3 to 6 months.
    B. 1 to 3 years.
    C. 3 to 5 years.
    D. once in a while, but only after cleaning.

12. The most important part of a laminar airflow hood is
    A. the fluorescent light.
    B. a HEPA filter.
    C. spraying solutions onto the HEPA filter frequently.
    D. the acrylic plastic.

13. How far from the outside edge should work be performed in a laminar airflow hood?
    A. 2 inches
    B. 6 inches
    C. 12 inches
    D. 15 inches

14. Standard precautions are focused on
    A. avoiding contact with and touching patients with AIDS.
    B. avoiding contact with the body of a patient suspected of having hepatitis B.
    C. avoiding contact with terminally ill patients.
    D. avoiding contact with blood and body fluids.

15. To avoid contamination, when technicians work inside laminar airflow hoods, they must use all of the following, except
    A. conventional lab coat.
    B. rubber gloves.
    C. mask.
    D. gown with knit cuffs.

16. Many prepackaged products for intravenous infusion can be sterilized by
    A. dry heat sterilization.
    B. autoclaving.
    C. gas sterilization.
    D. all of the above.

17. After turning on a laminar airflow hood, it cannot be used until it has run for at least
    A. 5 minutes.
    B. 15 minutes.
    C. 30 minutes.
    D. 1 hour.

18. Laminar airflow hoods should be cleaned
    A. after each use.
    B. each shift.
    C. when spills occur.
    D. all of the above.

19. To allow for proper airflow in a horizontal flow hood, items are placed
    A. against the HEPA filter.
    B. against the sides of the hood.
    C. away from the sides and the HEPA filter.
    D. directly in front of each other.

20. All hazardous chemicals must
    A. be destroyed.
    B. have warning labels.
    C. have prescriptions.
    D. not be dispensed.

21. The laminar airflow hood should be serviced and certified
    A. every month.
    B. every 6 months.
    C. every year.
    D. none of the above.

Computer Applications in Drug-Use Control

15

OUTLINE

Computer Use in the Pharmacy
Computer Components
  Input and Output Devices
Computerized Systems in the Pharmacy Setting
  Benefits of Computer Use in the Pharmacy Setting
Confidentiality and Security

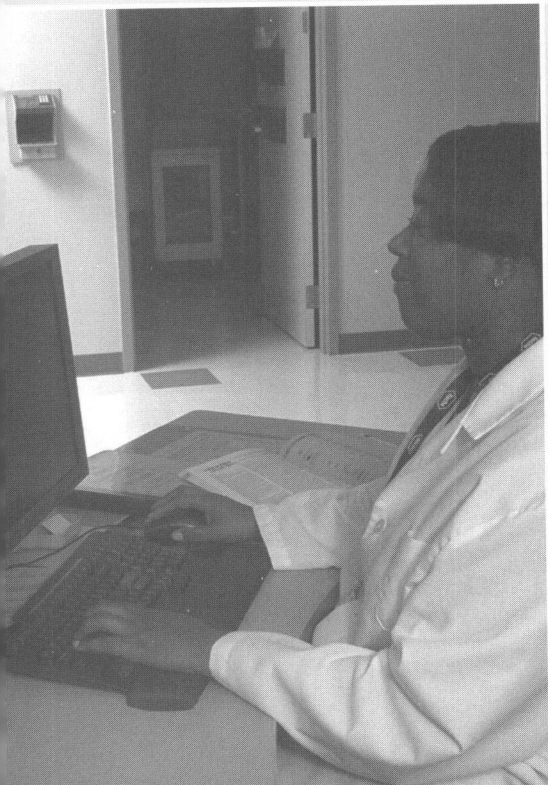

GLOSSARY

data The raw facts the computer can manipulate.
file A set of data or a program that has been given a name.
hardware The parts of the computer that you can touch.
modem A device used to transfer information from one computer to another.
programs A set of electronic instructions that tell the computer what to do.
software A set of electronic instructions that tell the computer what to do.

COMPUTER USE IN THE PHARMACY

Computers have revolutionized the world of pharmacy. Computer applications, which include programs for drug distribution, administration, clinical practice, and ambulatory care, have been developed in each retail pharmacy and for each segment of the hospital pharmacy. Development of programs related to administrative applications has been given the most attention because these programs have the most impact on the financial health of the pharmacy. Development of programs to improve drug distribution has also been a primary focus because this has been seen as the primary problem area in pharmacy practice. Computers now are a main component of pharmacy practice. If computers are used properly, they can significantly decrease the cost of any operation that involves the processing of information; therefore, it is essential for pharmacy technicians to be computer literate. In addition, the pharmacy technician must be aware of procedures to prevent compromising confidential pharmacy records.

COMPUTER COMPONENTS

A computer system consists of four parts: hardware, software, data, and users (people) (see Figure 15-1).

A pharmacy technician should be able to recognize the components and uses of a computer. The term **hardware** refers to the parts of the computer you can touch. It consists of interconnected electronic devices that control everything the computer does. When most people talk about a computer, they mean hardware. The hardware can be broken down into four types of physical components: processor (the central processing unit, or CPU), memory, storage, and input/output devices (see Figure 15-2).

The term **software** refers to sets of electronic instructions that tell the hardware what to do. These sets of instructions are also known as **programs,** and each of them has a specific purpose, such as entering, editing, and formatting data. Computer software can be classified into three groups: data, operating systems, and applications. All three are built from the same elements, with electronic instructions to the processor.

The term **data** refers to the raw facts the computer can manipulate. Data can consist of letters, numbers, sounds, or images. A computer **file** is simply a set of data or program instructions that has been given a name. A file containing data is often called a *document*, examples of which are addresses, medical records, insurance carriers, and transactions (received and outstanding payments, recorded in the form of charges, and adjustments). The last part of the computer system is the person who uses the computer. People are usually referred to as *users*.

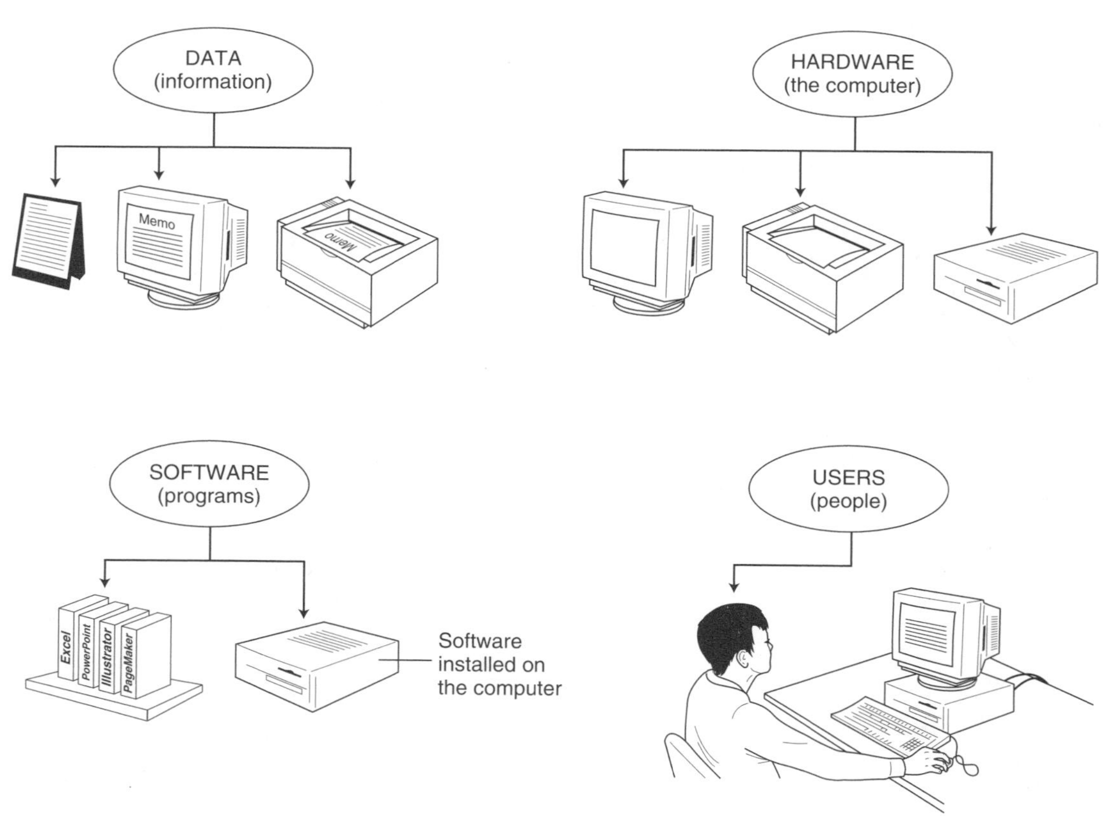

Figure 15-1. Components of a computer.

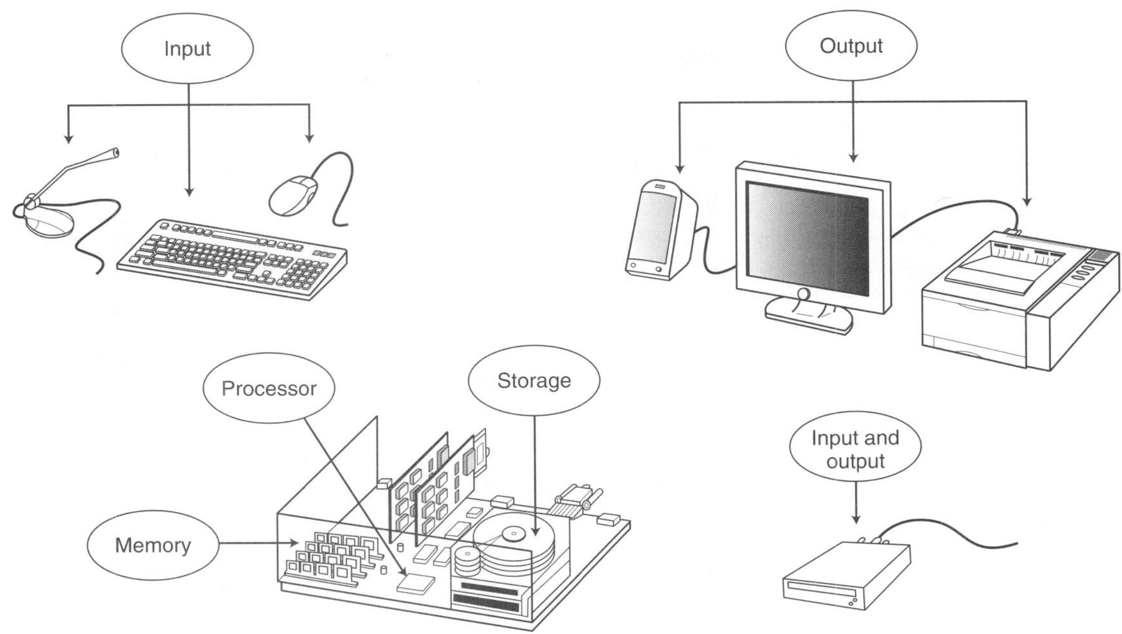

Figure 15-2. Hardware associated with a computer.

Input and Output Devices

Input and output devices consist of the keyboard, monitor, mouse, touch screen, scanner, modem, and printer. The keyboard is the most common device used to input information into the computer. It resembles a typewriter. The monitor is a device that resembles a television screen and is used by the computer to display information. The mouse is a device that enables the user to move a pointer around on the monitor to make selections or to place information. A monitor with a touch-sensitive surface, or a touch screen, enables the user to make a selection by simply touching the finger to the screen. A scanner is a device that can convert printed matter and images into information that can be interpreted by the computer. The **modem** is a device used to transfer information from one computer to another using telephone lines, cable lines, and servers. Modems allow access to the Internet and use of e-mail. A printer is a device used to produce a paper copy of information to be sent to pharmacies, vendors, insurance companies, and others.

COMPUTERIZED SYSTEMS IN THE PHARMACY SETTING

Today, almost all pharmacies (hospital or retail) in the United States are computerized. Computerization helps the pharmacist by providing a systematic method of order entry, development of patient profiles, label production, detection of patient's allergies and sensitivities, verification of dosage, and determination of interactions between drugs and food. The computer also offers the pharmacist or technician the ability to confirm the accuracy of drug use dosage, generic and trade names of drugs, contraindications, side effects, and other information that is essential to the well-being of the patient. Aside from the computer's clinical uses, it is also used to transfer charges to the patient's account, control inventory, and track unused drugs returned to the pharmacy.

The pharmacy technician is involved in all aspects of computerization of the pharmacy setting. The information in pharmacy systems is important to the management of the pharmacy. Hospitals and community pharmacies have been using information systems to improve productivity and the quality of pharmaceutical care for many years. Today, computerized systems create new opportunities for pharmacists and technicians in the health care delivery process. The network system in hospital pharmacy computers has created a need for pharmacy operations to link more closely with other departments within the hospital to communicate better and faster. In large retail pharmacies, networked computers have created much better communication and access to shared data or to the Internet. The processes of dispensing, record keeping, pricing, creating new prescriptions, and refilling prescriptions have become faster and easier. Computer applications are also helpful in drug use control. The processes of ordering, stocking, mixing medications, and preparing sterile intravenous medications all benefit from the use of computer applications.

Benefits of Computer Use in the Pharmacy Setting

Computer technology helps to make many aspects of work in the pharmacy—such as claims processing, billing for prescriptions, drug interactions, and cross referencing, among others—more efficient in many ways. In the future, computers may link the person preparing the prescription directly with the physician's office, increasing formulary compliance, simplifying pharmaceutical administration, and reducing dispensing or other errors related to illegible handwritten prescriptions. Use of computers will, most importantly, increase patient satisfaction. Also, the physician will be able to give and receive feedback about the patient's plan, the formulary used, prior authorization requirements, and treatment guidelines. By linking insurance companies with this system, the physician can also check on drugs preferred by the insurance company with just the click of a button. This new system would benefit doctors, pharmacists, and patients by reducing complications before the patient arrives, saving time from missed phone calls for prescription changes, and the like.

CONFIDENTIALITY AND SECURITY

Confidentiality and privacy are concepts associated with the rights of patients. Often there is a misconception about the meaning of these terms, and sometimes they are misused or interchanged. Privacy is usually understood to mean the right of individuals to limit access by others to some aspect of their personal information. For health data, the focus is on informational privacy. Confidentiality, on the other hand, is based upon special doctor-patient or pharmacist-patient relationships and refers to the expectation that the information collected will be used for the purpose for which it was gathered. With confidentiality, the patient has the expectation that information shared with a health care provider will be used for its intended purpose (diagnosis and treatment) and that this information will not be disclosed to others unless the patient is first made aware and consents to its disclosure. The pharmacy technician must understand the importance of the privacy and confidentiality of patients. The technician also must deal with the security of health information when working with computers. There are three principal goals for the security of patients' health information:

1. Protecting the informational privacy of patient-related data
2. Ensuring the integrity of information
3. Ensuring the availability of information to the appropriate individuals in a timely manner

Access to the computer system is limited by password or other security measures. Pharmacy technicians must follow security and confidentiality rules. Technicians are not allowed to provide information about treatment or patients to anyone unless specifically guided by the pharmacist in charge.

REVIEW QUESTIONS

1. A computer-related device that resembles a television is known as a
   A. mouse.
   B. scanner.
   C. monitor.
   D. modem.

2. Productivity and the quality of pharmaceutical care have been improved by which of the following elements?
   A. Computers
   B. Pharmacy technicians' experience
   C. Pagers
   D. Taking the National Certification Exam

3. Software refers to
   A. the part of the computer you can touch.
   B. the raw facts the computer can manipulate.
   C. people who are working with a computer.
   D. the set of electronic instructions that tell the hardware what to do.

4. Which device is used to transfer information from one computer to another using telephone lines and servers?
   A. Modem
   B. Mouse
   C. Monitor
   D. Scanner

5. All of the following are principal goals for security of patients' health information, except
   A. ensuring the availability of information to the appropriate individuals in a timely manner.
   B. ensuring the unavailability of information to the appropriate individuals.
   C. ensuring the integrity of information.
   D. protecting the informational privacy of patient-related data.

6. Access to the computer system is limited by which of the following?
   A. Modem
   B. Hardware
   C. Password
   D. Software

Continues

7. Which of the following parts of the computer is one that can be touched?
   A. Hardware
   B. Programs
   C. Software
   D. Modem

8. What is the most common device used to input information into the computer?
   A. Modem
   B. File
   C. Data
   D. Keyboard

9. Which of the following is a device that converts printed material and images into information that can be interpreted by the computer?
   A. Modem
   B. Monitor
   C. Scanner
   D. Printer

10. A computer file containing data is often called
    A. a document.
    B. a program.
    C. memory.
    D. storage.

Communications 16

OUTLINE

Communication
Methods of Communication
- Verbal Communication
- Written Communication
- Nonverbal Communication

The Communication Process
Technology and Communication
Barriers to Communication
- Environmental Factors
- Language Barriers
- Negative Communication
- Defense Mechanisms

Communicating with Staff Members
Communication in Special Situations
Professional Behavior
- Ethical Patient Care
- Autonomy
- Honesty
- Informed Consent
- Confidentiality
- Faithfulness

Sexual Harassment
Communication with Difficult People

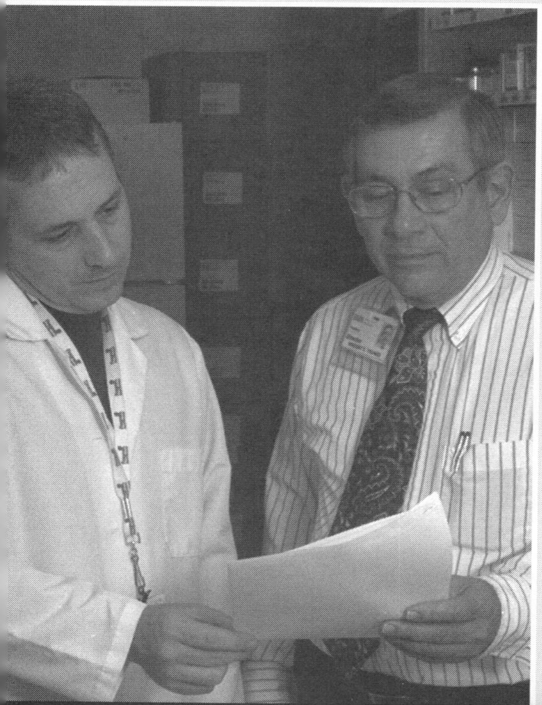

GLOSSARY

autonomy The right of an individual to make informed decisions for his or her own good.

body language The use of gestures, movements, and mannerisms to communicate something.

compensation An unconscious mechanism by which an individual tries to make up for fancied or real deficiencies.

displacement The transfer of impulses from one expression to another, such as from fighting to talking.

enunciation Clearly speaking and forming words.

informed consent A consent in which there is understanding of what treatment is to be undertaken and of the risks involved, why it should be done, and what alternative methods of treatment are available.

pitch The tone and level of one's voice.

projection A defense mechanism by which a repressed complex in the individual is denied and conceived as belonging to another person, such as when faults that the person tends to commit are perceived in or attributed to others.

rationalization A psychoanalytic defense mechanism through which irrational behavior, motives, or feelings are made to appear reasonable.

regression An unconscious defense mechanism involving a return to earlier patterns of adaptation.

repression A defense mechanism of removing from consciousness an unacceptable idea or impulse.

sublimation An unconscious defense mechanism in which unacceptable instinctual drives and wishes are modified into more personally and socially acceptable channels.

COMMUNICATION

Communication in the pharmacy setting is the foundation for all patient care and is of the utmost importance. Patients' satisfaction with their medical care is as much related to the effectiveness of the communication between themselves and their chosen health care provider as it is to the actual care itself. The business of pharmacy has become truly global and the electronic age has made immediate communication possible. The ability to keep up with changes and to understand them defines pharmacists' success as business professionals. However, communication is much more than just the spoken or written word. We use communication in every aspect of our lives: at work, with family and friends, and even with ourselves. Quality communication requires that we listen intensively to the needs and views of those we work with. Pharmacy technicians must listen to their customers, patients, co-workers, and supervisors.

METHODS OF COMMUNICATION

There are several ways that we can communicate with each other in our private, public, and professional lives. These various ways are verbal, written, and nonverbal or nonwritten (body language) forms of communication. Communicating in both verbal and nonverbal ways requires an exchange of information.

Verbal Communication

Communication is enhanced when it is coupled with an ability to know the impact of our actions and words. Verbal communication takes place when a message is spoken. Great communicators have an interactive style. True leadership is earned through personal and professional achievements and by the ability of the leader to motivate those around him or her. Verbal communication depends on words and sounds. Messages are conveyed by the use of language, which may be written or spoken. The **pitch** of the voice is a part of verbal communication. The tone of voice and choice of words also affect the message. The spoken word must be understood by all parties to the communication. For example, when two or more individuals are talking and a third person overhears their conversation, it is called verbal communication. **Enunciation** is the term that means to speak clearly and to articulate carefully. Pharmacy technicians must become aware of how they express themselves and how they affect the feelings of others.

Written Communication

Excellent written communication skills are also important in the pharmacy setting. The pharmacy technician should be concerned about his or her writing. Inaccurate or confusing writing in the pharmacy setting not only irritates others but also may lead to harmful patient care. The pharmacy technician will often be responsible for many kinds of writing, including memos, e-mail messages, ordering of supplies, and record keeping. These are some examples of written communication. Written communication can reinforce or back up oral instructions or explanations of possible side effects of medications and can clarify misunderstandings for others.

Nonverbal Communication

Nonverbal communication involves messages that are conveyed without the use of words. They are transmitted by body language, which is partly natural, partly trained, and partly imitative. Nonverbal communication, or **body language**, as it is sometimes called, involves training, dress, eye contact, facial expression, hand gestures, space, tone of voice, posture, the way one walks, ethnic customs, and much more. The face and eyes are probably the most noticed parts of the body, and their impact is powerful. For example, smiling cocktail waitresses earn larger tips than unsmiling ones. The influence of facial expressions and eye contact does not mean that nonverbal messages are always easy to read. Individuals are usually unaware of their own nonverbal signals and recognize only a small number of the signals in others. Appearance is a part of nonverbal communication. Posture can signal depression, excitement, anger, or even an appeal for help. It is important to remember the following points when communicating with others:

1. Anticipate different ideas in the communication process.
2. Try to be aware of unfair biases or prejudices about others, which may influence your perception of them, and be aware that others may have unfair biases or prejudices about you.
3. Ask for feedback from the receiver about your intended message.
4. Provide feedback to the sender to check your idea of the message and to make sure that you understood correctly.

THE COMMUNICATION PROCESS

Communication is the sharing of information, ideas, thoughts, and feelings. It involves not only the spoken word but also what is conveyed through inflection, vocal quality, facial expression, body posture, and other behavioral responses. As a first step toward communicating more effectively, pharmacy technicians must understand the communication process. The communication process consists of the communication cycle, which involves two or more individuals participating in an exchange of information. The cycle involves the sender, or source, communicating a message to the receiver through a chosen channel of

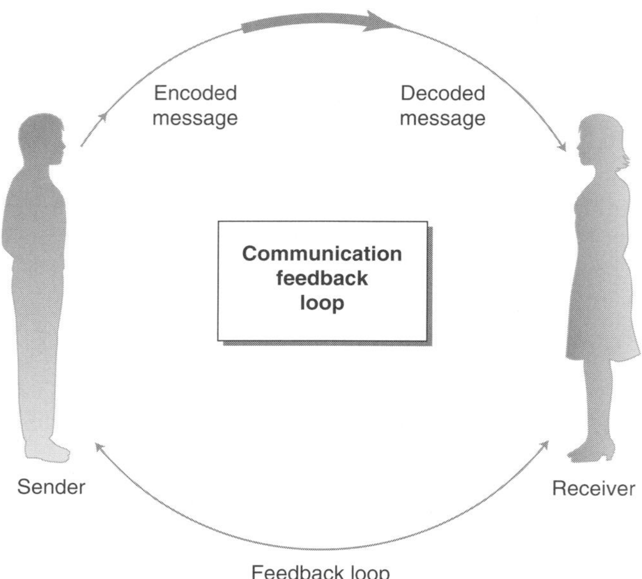

Figure 16-1. The communication process.

communication, to which the receiver responds with feedback (see Figure 16-1).

When a person wishes to share information with another, the sender must choose how to transmit that message. The medium of the message can be written, oral, nonverbal, or electronic. If the sender decides to transmit the message through words, the sender must encode the message by choosing words that best convey the intended meaning to the receiver.

After the information is encoded, the sender loses control of the message because its meaning comes from the receiver's decoding of it. If the receiver responds to the message, that response acts as feedback to the sender. This gives the sender an opportunity to clarify and correct any misunderstanding. This sequence of encoding, transmitting, and decoding messages continues as long as sender and receiver continue to communicate.

The communication cycle includes five basic elements:

- The sender or source
- The message
- The channel or mode of communication
- The receiver
- Feedback

The message must contain all necessary information (complete). The message must not contain any unnecessary information (concise). It must be free from obscurity and ambiguity (clear). The message must be organized and logical (cohesive). The message must be respectful and considerate of others (courteous). Strong communication skills can be built by using the techniques of active listening, questioning, positive feedback, timing, observation, and precise writing.

TECHNOLOGY AND COMMUNICATION

Face-to-face communication usually takes place through multiple nonverbal as well as verbal channels and is the mode of communication of choice in most workplaces. However, communication, in general, is accomplished through a broad spectrum of media. The use of technological devices is becoming more and more accepted as a means of communication. There are many methods of communication including, for example, mass media communication (TV and radio), small group communication (committee meetings and discussion groups), and large scale communication (lectures and speeches). Today new ways to communicate also exist. Technologies now used in the pharmacy in addition to telephones include fax machines, telecommunication conferences, e-mail, pagers, and laptop computers. These are all examples of ways in which communication is now faster. Computers are able to be linked together to form a network that communicates via satellites with offices in other parts of the community or even in other countries. If a pharmacy technician is expected to answer the phone, he or she should answer by the second or third ring.

BARRIERS TO COMMUNICATION

There are various factors that may obstruct the process of communication. These include environmental factors and language barriers. Removal of these barriers is a two-step process: recognizing that the barriers exist and taking appropriate action to overcome them. Nothing can be more disappointing than to realize that one is not communicating effectively with someone else.

Environmental Factors

Communication is obstructed by environmental barriers such as crowded, noisy prescription areas; the personal fears and anxieties of both pharmacy technicians and patients; administrative decisions; and lack of adequate time. The physical and psychological tension caused by certain events and situations can be a huge barrier to effective communication. Both positive and negative events can cause stress, and people react to stress in very different ways. In most daily situations, we learn to manage stress effectively. However, sometimes the amount of stress in our lives reaches a level at which we are unable to cope, and as a result, begins to affect our mental and physical health in negative ways.

The work of all health care workers, including pharmacy technicians, is often very stressful. They must use their physical, emotional, and mental abilities to the utmost each day to perform the job well.

Stress can negatively affect the ability to communicate with others. Tone of voice, words, and body language are all affected by stress level and emotional state. An angry tone of voice may confuse the receiver of the message, who may misunderstand the tone and think the pharmacy technician is upset about something the receiver has done.

Language Barriers

Pharmacy technicians may face a potential communication barrier with non–English-speaking patients. A major source of diversity among patients comes from their many cultural and language backgrounds. If a patient does not understand English, an interpreter should be present. However, if the patient has some understanding of English, certain strategies can be used to convey a message. Gestures and body language may help to convey a message. The technician should speak slowly and pronounce words distinctly, using formal English and avoiding slang. A demonstration of what the patient should do may help as well as the use of visual aids such as pictures, diagrams, and signs. Bias or unfair treatment of a person because of race, gender, religious affiliation, or handicap prevents effective communication. Written material may be used to reinforce oral information and to help answer questions and prevent misunderstandings.

Negative Communication

In some situations, communication practices may have a negative effect on others. Examples include the following:

- Mumbling
- Interrupting
- Showing boredom
- Bragging and confronting
- Forgetting common courtesies such as saying "please" and "thank you"
- Speaking too quickly or sharply
- Using negative body language such as frowning, slouching, and crossing one's arms
- Avoiding eye contact

Defense Mechanisms

Defense mechanisms may be used by certain individuals, causing an effect that can block the communication cycle. Pharmacy technicians should be aware of these mechanisms and avoid using them, because they do not lead to effective communication. Defense mechanisms may be used unconsciously by all individuals at one time or another. Some common defense mechanisms are the following:

- **Regression**: Moving back to a former stage (of development) to escape conflict or fear
- **Projection**: The act of placing one's own feelings upon another
- **Repression**: Pushing unpleasant thoughts or problems into the unconscious to avoid dealing with them
- **Rationalization**: Justifying problems or unacceptable behavior by giving acceptable reasons rather than real ones
- **Compensation**: The overemphasizing of characteristics to make up for a lacking quality or a handicap
- **Sublimation**: Redirecting a socially unacceptable impulse into one that is socially acceptable
- **Displacement**: Transferring negative feelings onto something or someone with no significance to the situation.

COMMUNICATING WITH STAFF MEMBERS

Cooperation is the ability to work with others effectively. It requires extending oneself to be helpful to others. It is important that the technician does not polarize an issue, seeing it only in black and white, but rather sees many possible alternatives and thinks outside the box. Many miscommunications arise not because people genuinely disagree, but because they use symbols to mean different things and make different assumptions. Behavior is influenced by the words and other symbols used to communicate with others. Working and writing in groups, as well as writing reports, are most useful for persuasion in difficult situations. As technicians write and speak, they need to get their meaning across to other people and staff members. Pharmacy technicians are expected to cooperate and communicate in many ways. Sharing ideas and listening when others are trying to help will facilitate communication as will working harmoniously with others to advance the interests of the pharmacy facility. Pharmacy technicians must communicate with other pharmacy personnel and technicians. They should be able to build strong communication with all internal and external customers. They must refer patients to the pharmacist for consultation. The pharmacy technician should communicate effectively with supervisors and the pharmacist.

COMMUNICATION IN SPECIAL SITUATIONS

Applying communication skills to pharmacy practice situations is not always easy. It can be somewhat difficult if patients have special communication needs. These situations or conditions require special sensitivities and unique strategies to ensure effective communication. The pharmacy technician needs special skills to deal with older adults, individuals with hearing and sight impairments, patients who are terminally ill, individuals with acquired immunodeficiency syndrome (AIDS), and patients with mental health problems.

PROFESSIONAL BEHAVIOR

The pharmacy technician needs to have the personal attributes of empathy, diplomacy, and courtesy, be well-organized, have a positive attitude, and show a professional appearance. These help contribute to the technician's commitment to excellence in caring for his or her patients and also help in communication with patients and other health care workers. Probably the most important character traits of a good pharmacy technician are honesty, reliability, and dependability. Technicians must always behave ethically and maintain confidentiality of patients and others. They need to be genuinely interested in helping people, warm and caring, and able to put the needs of others first. They must know how to perform necessary administrative activities effectively and efficiently. Sometimes they may face a special situation that requires them to stay calm and communicate with others effectively to solve the problem.

Ethical Patient Care

Pharmacists and pharmacy technicians, as health professionals, have obligations to patients and to society. They must understand general ethical principles and their applications in pharmaceutical care situations.

Autonomy

The principle of **autonomy** establishes a patient's right to self-determination. Autonomy is the ability to function in an independent fashion. The patient can choose what will be done to his or her body. This right is considered paramount even if a health professional may judge a patient's decision as being damaging to his or her health.

Honesty

The principle of honesty means that patients have the right to know the truth about their medical condition, the course of their disease, treatments recommended, and alternative treatments available.

Informed Consent

Both honesty and autonomy serve as foundations for the patient's right to give informed consent to treatment. The principle of **informed consent** ensures that patients have the right to full disclosure of all relevant aspects of care and that they must give explicit consent to treatment before it is initiated.

Confidentiality

Confidentiality assures patients that information about their medical conditions and treatment will not be given to third parties without their permission. Confidentiality is essential to preserving the patient's human dignity. Patients are expected to reveal the most personal details of their existence to virtual strangers. They must be able to trust that this information will not be shared with others who are not involved in their medical care.

Faithfulness

Faithfulness describes the right of patients to have health professionals provide services that promote the patient's interest rather than those that serve a competing or conflicting interest. A pharmacist or technician who encourages the use of vitamins the patient does not need may be promoting his or her financial well-being at the expense of the patient. Ethically, the responsibility of a health professional is, first and foremost, the welfare of the patient.

SEXUAL HARASSMENT

Sexual harassment is a form of sex discrimination that violates Title VII of the Civil Rights Act of 1964. Unwelcome sexual advances, requests for sexual favors, and other verbal or physical conduct of a sexual nature constitute sexual harassment. In particular, sexual harassment is present when submission to or rejection of this conduct explicitly or implicitly affects an individual's employment, unreasonably interferes with an individual's work performance, or creates an intimidating, hostile, or offensive work environment. Sexual harassment can occur in a variety of circumstances. The victim or the harasser may be a woman or a man. The victim does not have to be of the opposite sex.

The harasser can be the victim's supervisor, an agent of the employer, a supervisor in another area, a co-worker, or a nonemployee. The victim does not have to be the person harassed but could be anyone affected by the offensive conduct. Unlawful sexual harassment may occur without economic injury to or discharge of the victim. Instances of sexual harassment may be visual, verbal, or written communications, exchanges of employment benefits for sexual favors, or threats. Other types of harassment include verbal or physical abuse, interference with work or a hostile work environment, retaliation, and abuse via electronic media such as e-mail. The harasser's conduct must be unwelcome. It is helpful if the victim directly informs the harasser that the conduct is unwelcome and must stop. The victim should use any employer complaint mechanism or grievance system available. One of the best tools a company can have to help combat sexual harassment is a well-drafted, comprehensive sexual harassment policy. Appropriate use of a well-drafted policy can prevent sexual and other forms of harassment, increase awareness of activities that are considered harassment, and immediately improve the work environment. It should provide procedures for dealing with and reporting harassment, define disciplinary action in the event of harassment, and reduce the company's legal liability.

COMMUNICATION WITH DIFFICULT PEOPLE

Communication is not a skill that comes easily to everyone. Expressing feelings in an honest and open way is often difficult for individuals. When a crisis occurs, effective communication is much harder. A pharmacy technician must develop communication skills that can be used in times of trouble. There must be an understanding of why a patient, customer, or co-worker is unable to communicate.

Patience is important because people are not always at their best when they are concerned about their condition or that of a loved one. The technician should always remain calm when he or she deals with a person who is experiencing a traumatic event or has any depressive condition and remember that this individual may be reacting to emotions such as fear, anger, doubt, or inadequacy. The key is to listen to determine the best way to help the patient out of any immediate danger and help establish some type of support system.

REVIEW QUESTIONS

1. When greeting patients, a pharmacy technician should
A. tease them about the time they forgot to pick up their prescription.
B. ask personal questions.
C. make eye contact.
D. avoid using their names to preserve their privacy.

2. Instances of sexual harassment may be all of the following, except
A. ethical.
B. visual.
C. threats.
D. written.

3. Pharmacy technicians are expected to answer the phone
A. only if the answering service does not answer it first.
B. rarely, because it is not within their scope of training.
C. only if the call is personal.
D. by the second or third ring.

4. Speaking clearly and articulating carefully is known as
A. enunciation.
B. pronunciation.
C. intonation.
D. salutation.

5. When dealing with an angry patient or customer, you must learn how to
A. return to your work.
B. remain calm.
C. break off communication.
D. stop him or her from talking.

6. Steps toward having a positive attitude include all of the following, except
A. using positive statements.
B. saying something pleasant.
C. smiling.
D. accepting tips from patients.

7. The act of placing one's own feeling upon another is called
A. repression.
B. regression.
C. projection.
D. compensation.

8. A message from a sender to a receiver includes all of the following, except
A. writing.
B. feedback.
C. listening.
D. speaking.

9. Negative communication includes all of the following, except
A. eye contact.
B. crossing one's arms.
C. mumbling.
D. bragging.

10. The principle of autonomy establishes a patient's right to
A. be able to talk.
B. self-determination.
C. have the truth about their medical condition.
D. give informed consent to treatment.

11. The most important character traits of a good pharmacy technician include all of the following, except
A. honesty.
B. undependability.
C. organization.
D. reliability.

12. The ability to function in an independent fashion is called
A. faithfulness.
B. projection.
C. sublimation.
D. autonomy.

Continues

13. When individuals transfer their negative feelings onto something or someone with no significance to the situation, it is known as
A. sublimation.
B. projection.
C. displacement.
D. compensation.

14. Any person who makes intentional statements or actions that may cause another person to feel that his or her job is at risk is engaging in
A. regression.
B. repression.
C. sublimation.
D. sexual harassment.

15. Quality communication requires
A. intensive listening.
B. intensive writing.
C. intensive talking.
D. intensive smiling.

16. Ethically, the responsibility of a health professional is, first and foremost, to
A. reveal information to his or her family.
B. consider the welfare of the patient.
C. apply racial status to welfare patients.
D. A and C.

SECTION

IV

Drug Classifications

17 Biopharmaceutics

OUTLINE

Properties and Actions of Drugs
Pharmacokinetics
- Drug Absorption
- Drug Distribution
- Biotransformation (Metabolism) of Drugs
- Drug Excretion

Pharmacodynamics
- Drug Action
- Drug Bioavailability

Side Effects and Adverse Effects of Drugs
- Hypersensitivity or Allergy
- Anaphylactic Reaction

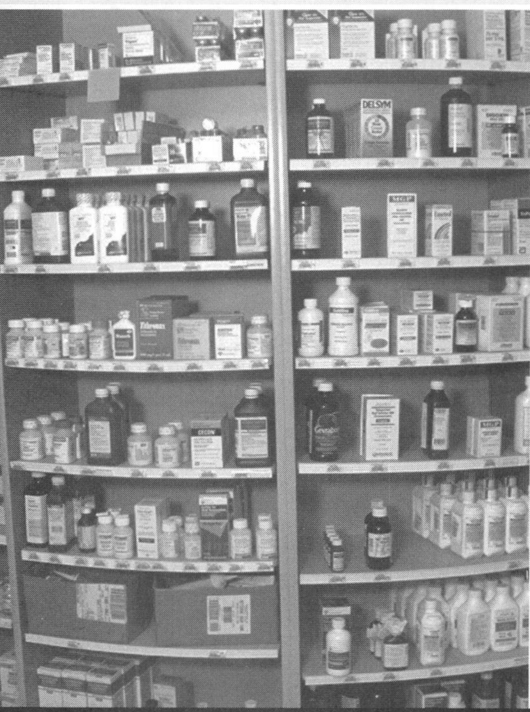

GLOSSARY

absorption The movement of a drug from its site of administration into the bloodstream.
agonist The drug that produces a functional change in a cell.
bioavailability Measurement of the rate of absorption and total amount of drug that reaches systemic circulation.
biotransformation The conversion of a drug within the body; also known as metabolism.
distribution The process by which blood leaves the bloodstream and enters the tissues of the body.
half-life The time it takes for the plasma concentration to be reduced by 50%.
hypersensitivity An unpredictable reaction to a drug due to the development of antibodies against it; also known as an allergy.
idiosyncratic reaction Experience of a unique, strange, or unpredicted reaction to a drug.
metabolism The conversion of a drug within the body; also known as biotransformation.
pharmacodynamics The study of the biochemical and physiological effects of drugs.
pharmacokinetics The study of the absorption, distribution, metabolism, and excretion of drugs.
placebo An inert substance given to a patient instead of an active medicine. Placebos are often given to people who participate in studies intended to evaluate the effectiveness of a medicine. Also called sugar pill.
receptor The cell to which a drug has an affinity.
specific affinity The attraction a drug has for particular cells.
tolerance Reduced responsiveness of a drug due to adaptation to it or when the body becomes increasingly resistant to a drug.

PROPERTIES AND ACTIONS OF DRUGS

The biochemical and physiological properties of drugs, as well as their mechanisms of action, differ widely. However, in clinical applications, drugs must penetrate, be absorbed by, and be distributed among the body tissues. The usual route of drug administration and mode of termination of their use should also be considered. There are certain general principles that help explain these differences. These principles have both pharmaceutic and therapeutic implications. For action, a drug must be absorbed, transported to the target tissue or organ, and then it must penetrate into the cell membranes and their organelles and alter the ongoing processes. The drug may be distributed to a number of tissues, bound or stored, and metabolized to inactive or active products. Then it must be excreted.

PHARMACOKINETICS

Pharmacokinetics is the study of the absorption, distribution, metabolism, and excretion of drugs.

Drug Absorption

The movement of a drug from its site of administration into the bloodstream is called **absorption**. In many cases, a drug must be transported across one or more biological membranes to reach the blood circulation. Drugs are transported across membranes by different processes. The most common and important mode of traversal of drugs through membranes is diffusion. This process depends upon the lipid solubility of the drug. Agents that are relatively lipid-soluble diffuse more rapidly than less lipid-soluble drugs. Generally, absorption takes place through the digestive system unless an agent is administered directly into the bloodstream by injection into the veins, arteries, muscles, and other sites of injectable administration. The digestive system is the most convenient, economical, and common route of administration and generally safe for most drugs. Lipid-soluble drugs and weak acids may be absorbed directly from the stomach. Weak bases are not normally absorbed from this site. The small intestine is the primary site of absorption because of the very large surface area across which drugs may diffuse. Acids are normally absorbed more extensively from the intestine than from the stomach, even though the intestine has a higher pH. The gastrointestinal tract absorption of drugs may be influenced by many factors. These factors include physical and chemical properties of the drugs, acidity of the stomach, presence of food, dosage of drugs, and the route of administration. Drugs can be administered under the tongue (sublingual), through the inner lining of the cheeks (buccal), or within the rectum (rectal). These routes are logical to protect the drugs from chemical decomposition, which might occur in the stomach or liver (the first-pass effect if the drug were given orally). The choice of the route of administration is crucial in determining the suitability of a drug for each patient. When the drug is injected directly into the bloodstream (vein or artery) and distributes throughout the body, it acts rapidly. The drug may be injected deeply into a skeletal muscle. The rate of absorption depends on the vascularity of the muscle site and the lipid solubility of the drug. If it is injected beneath the skin, drug absorption is less rapid, because the subcutaneous region is less vascular than the muscle tissues. Topical drugs may be absorbed through several layers of skin for local absorption. Drugs administered in high concentrations tend to be more rapidly absorbed than those administered in low concentrations. Sometimes, a drug may initially be administered in large doses that temporarily exceed the body's capacity to absorb them.

Drug Distribution

Distribution is the process by which a drug leaves the bloodstream and enters the tissues of the body. A drug diffuses across cellular membranes if its site of action is intracellular. Lipid solubility is important for effective distribution in this case. The initial rate of distribution of a drug is heavily dependent on the blood flow to various organs. Lipid-soluble drugs enter the central nervous system rapidly. Because of the nature of the blood-brain barrier, ionized drugs are distributed poorly to their desired site because they must pass through this barrier. The clinician must always consider the possibility that drugs administered to the mother may cross the placenta and reach the fetus. Drugs are often bound to plasma proteins, particularly albumin. Drugs that are bound to albumin are known as pharmacologically inactive drugs, whereas those that are unbound are called pharmacologically active drugs. If binding is extensive and firm, it will have a considerable impact upon the distribution and excretion of the drug in the body. A drug that is bound to a protein will not pass through the membrane in the bound form. Only the unbound form can pass among the various compartments of the body. Drug administration and its effect on drug action are shown in Figure 17-1.

Biotransformation (Metabolism) of Drugs

The overwhelming majority of drugs undergo **metabolism** after they enter the body. In most cases, biotransformation can terminate the pharmacological action of the drug and increase removal of the drug from the body. Most drugs are acted upon by enzymes in the body and are converted to metabolic derivatives during metabolism. The process of conversion is called **biotransformation**. The liver is the major site of biotransformation. Many biotransformations in the liver occur in the smooth endoplasmic reticulum of the hepatocytes. Numerous enzymes, which biotransform many drugs, are present in the endoplasmic reticulum. These

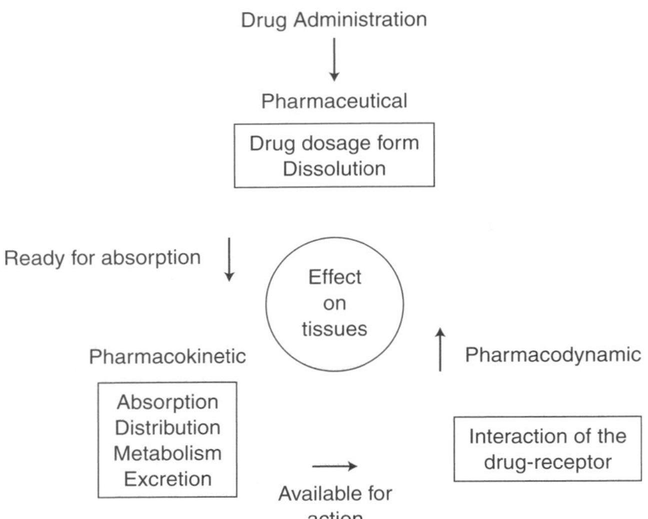

Figure 17-1. Drug administration and its effect on drug action.

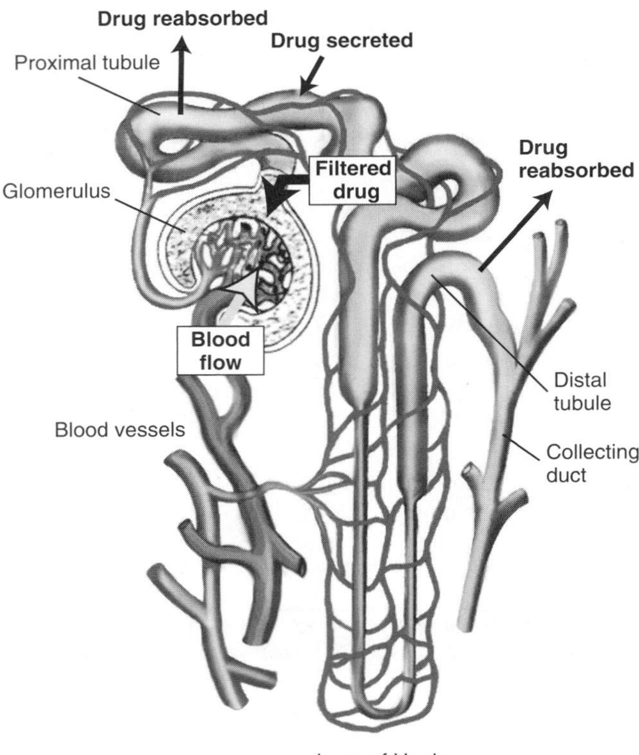

Figure 17-2. The excretion process of drugs.

drug-metabolizing enzymes are often called microsomal enzymes. One of these enzymes is cytochrome P-450, which has a very important role in drug metabolism. The reaction products that are produced by the action of these enzymes are known as metabolites. The majority of these metabolites are inactive and toxic. Biotransformations may be divided into four main categories: (1) oxidation, (2) reduction, (3) hydrolysis, and (4) conjugation. These occur primarily in the microsomal system of the liver.

Drug Excretion

Drugs may be excreted from the body by many routes, including urine, feces (unabsorbed drugs and those secreted in the bile), saliva, sweat, milk, lungs (alcohols and anesthetics), and tears. Any route may be important for a given drug, but the kidney is the major site of excretion for most drugs. Renal excretion of drugs and their metabolites may include three processes: (1) filtration, (2) secretion, and (3) reabsorption. The most common is the filtration of the agent through the glomerulus into the renal tubule (see Figure 17-2).

Approximately one fifth of the plasma reaching the kidney is filtered. The rate of filtration is referred to as the *glomerular filtration rate* and is normally 125 to 130 mL/min. Drugs bound to plasma proteins are not filtered. Secretion occurs primarily in the proximal convoluted tubule. This is an active process mediated by two carrier systems, one specific for organic acids and one specific for organic bases. Therefore, the pH of the urine may affect the rate of drug excretion by changing the chemical form of a drug to one that can be more readily excreted or to one that can be reabsorbed. Penicillins or barbiturates are weak acids and are available as sodium or potassium salts. These agents can be better excreted if the urine pH is less acidic. On the other hand, any drug that is available as a sulfate, hydrochloride, or nitrate salt, such as atropine or morphine, can be excreted better if the urine is more acidic. By altering the pH of urine, increased elimination of certain drugs can be facilitated, thus preventing prolonged action or overdosage of a toxic compound. Another technique to alter the rate of excretion of a drug is to produce a competitively blocking effect. For example, probenecid may be used to block the renal excretion of penicillin. This prolongs the effect of the antibiotic by maintenance of a higher therapeutic plasma level. Secretions of drugs are active transport systems. They require energy and may become saturated. Reabsorption may occur throughout the tubules of the nephrons. The mechanism is passive diffusion; therefore, only the un-ionized form of a drug is reabsorbed. Reabsorption depends upon its lipid solubility.

PHARMACODYNAMICS

The study of the biochemical and physiological effects of drugs is called **pharmacodynamics**. It is also defined as the study of the mechanisms of action of drugs. A basic understanding of the factors that control drug concentration at the site of action is important for the optimal use of drugs. This is the area of study referred to as pharmacokinetics, as discussed earlier. Blood represents the fluid most commonly sampled to characterize the pharmacokinetics of drugs. The drugs must dissolve before being absorbed. They must pass across many lipoid barriers and some metabolizing systems

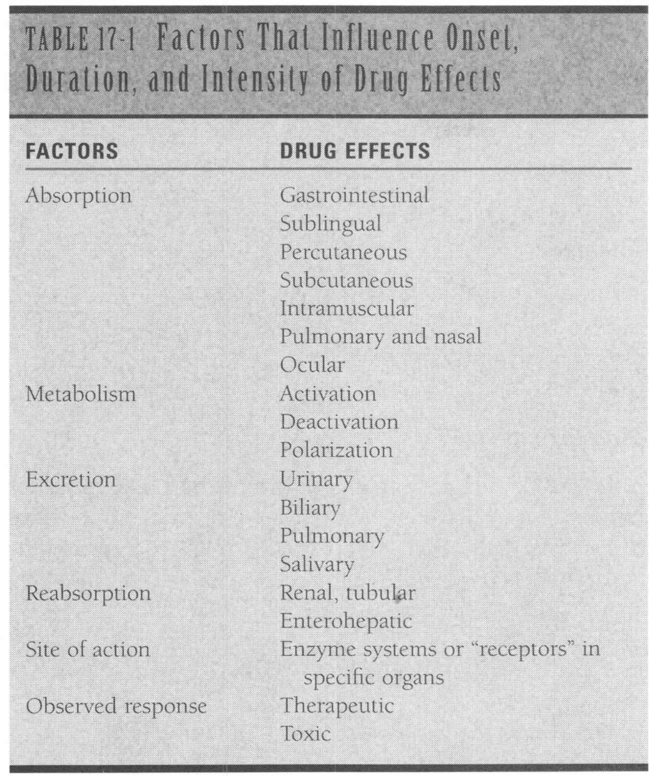

TABLE 17-1 Factors That Influence Onset, Duration, and Intensity of Drug Effects

FACTORS	DRUG EFFECTS
Absorption	Gastrointestinal Sublingual Percutaneous Subcutaneous Intramuscular Pulmonary and nasal Ocular
Metabolism	Activation Deactivation Polarization
Excretion	Urinary Biliary Pulmonary Salivary
Reabsorption	Renal, tubular Enterohepatic
Site of action	Enzyme systems or "receptors" in specific organs
Observed response	Therapeutic Toxic

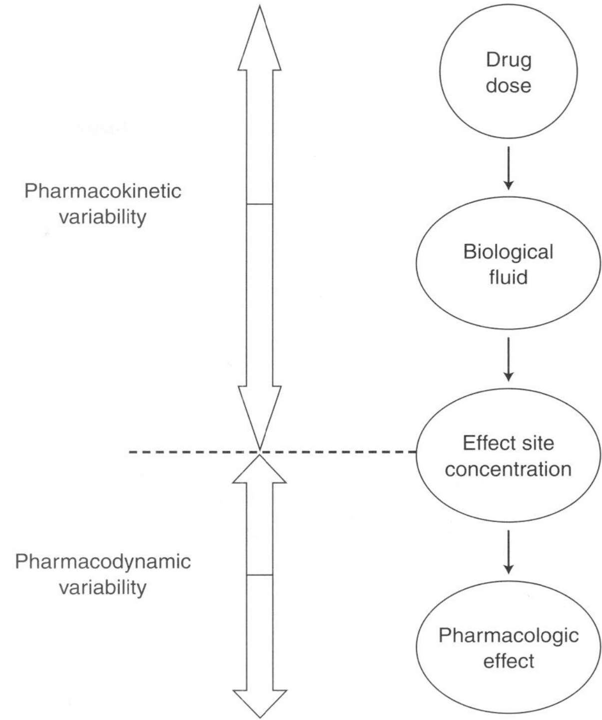

Figure 17-3. The dose-effect relationship.

before reaching the site of action. Table 17-1 shows the factors that may influence onset, duration, and intensity of drug effects.

Usually there are links between pharmacokinetics and pharmacodynamics that demonstrate the relationship between drug dose and blood or other biological fluid concentrations. The pharmacological response by itself does not provide information about some very important determinants of that response, for example, dose or drug concentration in plasma or at the site of action. Pharmacokinetics and pharmacodynamics can determine the dose-effect relationship (see Figure 17-3).

Drug Action

Drugs produce their effects by altering the normal function of the cells and tissues of the body. Correct cells are chosen because a particular drug has a **specific affinity** for a particular cell. The specific cell recipient is called a **receptor**, and the drug that has the affinity for it and produces a functional change in the cell is known as the **agonist**. Not all drugs that bind to specific cells cause a functional change in the cell. These drugs act as antagonists to the natural process and work by blocking a sequence of biochemical events. Some drugs may act by affecting the enzyme functions of the body. When drugs are metabolized in the liver, they produce antimetabolites.

Various factors are important in determining the correct drugs for a patient, such as the half-life of the drug; the age, sex, and body weight of the patient; the time of day of administration (diurnal); the presence of illnesses; psychological factors; tolerance; drug toxicity; idiosyncratic reactions; and interactions with other drugs.

Drug Half-Life

The **half-life** of a drug is the time it takes for the plasma concentration to be reduced by 50%. This is one of the most common methods used to explain drug actions. The half-life of each drug may be different; for example, a drug with a short half-life, such as 2 or 3 hours, will need to be administered more often than one with a long half-life, such as 8 hours. Another method of describing drug action is a graphic representation of the plasma concentration of the drug versus time (see Figure 17-4).

Age

Newborns and elderly individuals show the greatest effects of drugs. Because of their ages, they are more sensitive to medications that affect the central nervous system and are at risk for development of toxic drug levels. Drug dosages for these two groups must be carefully measured, and treatment usually starts with very small doses.

Sex

Men and women respond to drugs differently. Some medications pose a risk in pregnant women because of damage to the developing fetus. In addition, certain drugs may have

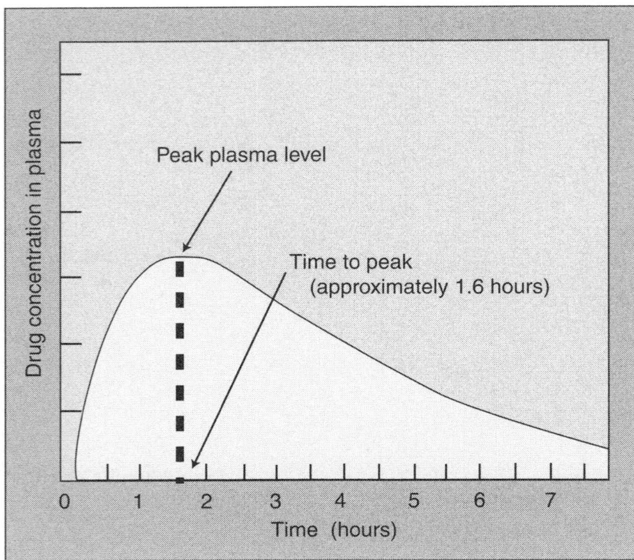

Figure 17-4. The half-life of a drug.

side effects that can stimulate uterine contractions, causing premature labor and delivery. Drugs administered intramuscularly are absorbed faster by men. They remain in women's tissues longer than in men's tissues because of higher body fat content.

Body Weight

Basically, the same dosage has less effect in a patient who weighs more and a greater effect in an individual who weighs less. Pediatric medications are designed for the body weight or body surface of children. If adult medications are used for children, the correct dosage must be calculated and adjusted for the child's body weight.

Time of Day

Diurnal (during the day) body rhythms play an important part in the effects of some drugs. For example, sedatives given in the morning will not be as effective as those administered before bedtime. On the other hand, the preferred time for corticosteroid administration is the morning, because this best mimics the body's natural pattern of corticosteroid production and elimination.

Presence of Illnesses

Patients with liver or kidney disease may respond to drugs differently, because the body is not able to detoxify and excrete chemicals properly.

Psychological Factors

Psychological factors involve how patients feel about the drug(s) prescribed for them and the different ways they respond to them. If an individual believes in the therapy, even a **placebo** (sugar pill or sterile water thought to be a drug) may help to bring relief. Some patients cooperate in following the directions for a specific drug, and a patient's mental attitude can reduce or increase an expected response to a drug.

Tolerance

Tolerance is the phenomenon of reduced responsiveness to a drug. The body becomes so adapted to the presence of the drug that it cannot function properly without it.

Drug Toxicity

Almost all drugs are capable of producing toxic effects. A range between the therapeutic dose of a drug and its toxic dose exists. This range is measurable by the therapeutic index, which is used to explain the safety of a drug. The therapeutic index is expressed in the form of a ratio:

$$\text{Therapeutic Index (TI)} = \frac{LD_{50}}{ED_{50}}$$

where LD_{50} is the lethal dose of a drug that will kill 50% of animals tested and ED_{50} is the effective dose that produces a specific therapeutic effect in 50% of animals tested.

The greater the therapeutic index, the safer a drug is likely to be. There are four general mechanisms by which drugs can change the physiology of the body's cells or tissues. They include the following:

1. Nonspecific chemical or physical interactions
2. Alterations in the level of the activity of enzymes
3. Action as antimetabolites
4. Interaction with receptors

The final effect of a drug may be removed from its site of action.

Idiosyncratic Reactions

An **idiosyncratic reaction** occurs when a patient has experienced a unique, strange, or unpredicted reaction to a drug. Idiosyncratic reactions may be caused by underlying enzyme deficiencies resulting from genetic or hormonal variation.

Drug Interactions

Plasma protein binding can be a source of drug interaction if several drugs compete for binding sites on protein molecules. Drug interactions may result in elevated concentrations of drugs by displacement of protein-bound drugs or by reduced rates of drug disposition that result in toxic drug concentrations (see Figure 17-5).

A drug interaction may also cause more rapid drug disappearance, with plasma concentrations decreasing to below minimum effective values. Drug interactions often take

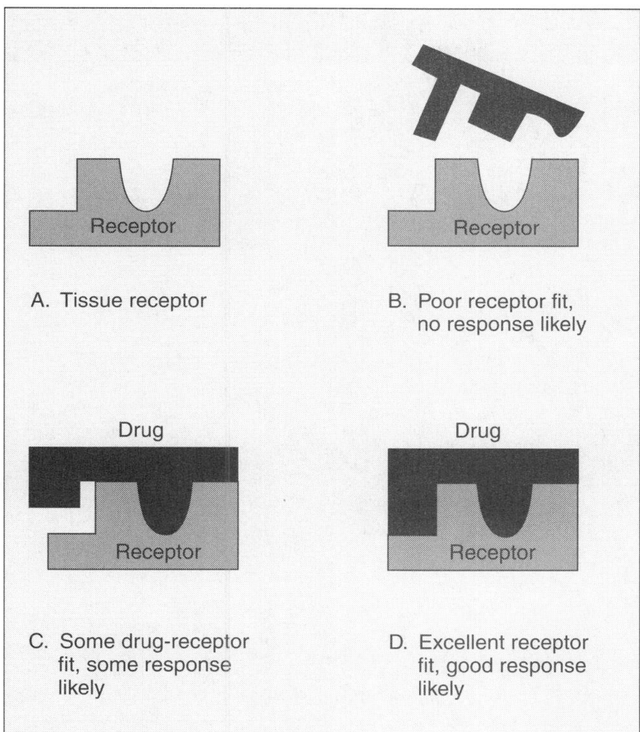

Figure 17-5. Drug interactions.

place during the process of metabolism in the liver and result from the cytochrome P-450 enzyme pathways each person inherits. Actions of many drugs may be altered by the cytochrome P-450 system when they are taken with other drugs. Examples include many antidepressants, cimetidine, ciprofloxacin, codeine, isoniazid, ketoconazole, morphine, phenobarbital, phenytoin, rifampin, tolbutamide, and warfarin. Some medications are given together because the drug interactions are helpful. For example, probenecid is given with penicillin to increase the absorption of penicillin. There are other drug interactions that may cause adverse effects. For example, some antibiotics make birth control pills less effective. Multiple-drug therapy should never be used without convincing evidence that each drug is beneficial beyond the possible detriments of combined administration or without proof that a therapeutically equivocal combination is definitely harmless.

Drug Bioavailability

Bioavailability is a term that indicates measurement of both the rate of drug absorption and total amount of drug that reaches the systemic blood circulation from an administered dosage form. The route of drug administration is essential for this measurement. If a drug is administered by intravenous injection, all of the dose enters the blood circulation. This is not true for drugs administered by other routes, especially for drugs given orally. Solid drugs such as tablets and capsules must dissolve. Thus, route of administration is a major source of difference in drug bioavailability. Poor solubility or incomplete absorption of a drug in the gastrointestinal tract and rapid metabolism of a drug during its first pass through the liver are other factors that influence bioavailability.

SIDE EFFECTS AND ADVERSE EFFECTS OF DRUGS

Side effects are mild, but annoying, responses to a medication. Adverse reactions or adverse effects usually are characterized as more severe symptoms or problems that develop because of a drug.

Adverse effects may require the patient to be hospitalized or may even pose a threat to the patient's life. Certain side effects such as nausea may disappear if the dosage of a drug is reduced. Some side effects such as drowsiness may go away after the patient takes the medication for a while. Occasionally, side effects are very problematic, and the dispensing of the drug to the patient is stopped or a different drug is used. Examples of problematic side effects are hyperactivity or inability to sleep, bleeding, nephrotoxicity, or hepatotoxicity.

Hypersensitivity or Allergy

Hypersensitivity is another unpredictable reaction caused in some patients by some drugs such as aspirin, penicillin, or sulfa products. Hypersensitivity reactions or allergies generally occur when a patient has received a drug that his or her body has developed antibodies against. After this process of antibody production, if the patient is re-exposed to the drug, the antigen-antibody reaction produces itching, hives, rash, or swelling of the skin. This is a common type of allergic reaction.

Anaphylactic Reaction

This response to a drug is a severe form of allergic reaction that is life threatening. The patient develops severe shortness of breath and may even have cardiac collapse. An anaphylactic reaction is a true medical emergency because the patient may suffer paralysis of the diaphragm, swelling of the oropharynx, and an inability to breathe.

REVIEW QUESTIONS

1. Which of the following statements correctly applies to the routes of administration?
   A. Sublingual: must take place in first-pass metabolism
   B. Intramuscular: generally offers poor absorption
   C. Rectal: poor compliance may limit
   D. Intravenous: complete (65%) bioavailability

2. Repeated administration of a drug may
   A. decrease its own metabolism.
   B. decrease the metabolism of other drugs.
   C. decrease the metabolism of endogenous compounds.
   D. induce the cytochrome P-450 enzyme system in the liver.

3. Decreasing the pH of the intestinal contents is more likely to increase the rate of absorption from the intestine of a drug that is a
   A. weak acid.
   B. weak base.
   C. neutral (not acidic or basic).
   D. strong acid.

4. The greater the therapeutic index, the more likely a drug will be
   A. more lethal.
   B. more safe.
   C. less safe.
   D. less expensive.

5. A term that indicates measurement of both the rate of drug absorption and the total amount of drug that reaches the bloodstream from an administered dosage form is called
   A. idiosyncratic reaction.
   B. drug toxicity.
   C. drug bioavailability.
   D. drug side effects.

6. Which of the following factors is the most important for effective distribution of a drug?
   A. Lipid solubility
   B. Water solubility
   C. Glomerular filtration rate
   D. Half-life of a drug

7. Renal excretion of drugs may involve all of the following processes, except
   A. secretion.
   B. absorption.
   C. filtration.
   D. reabsorption.

8. The most common and important mode of traversal of drugs through membranes is
   A. diffusion.
   B. filtration.
   C. pinocytosis.
   D. osmosis.

9. Which of the following is a sign of an anaphylactic reaction?
   A. Hypertension
   B. A fever
   C. Diarrhea
   D. Paralysis of the diaphragm

10. Probenecid is given with which of the following drugs to increase its absorption?
    A. Tetracycline
    B. Penicillin
    C. Aspirin
    D. Acetaminophen

Factors Affecting Drug Activity 18

OUTLINE

Factors Affecting Drug Activity
- Age
- Gender
- Weight
- Time and Route of Drug Administration
- Diet
- Pregnancy
- Psychological State
- Polypharmacy
- Diseases

Side Effects
- Hypersensitivity

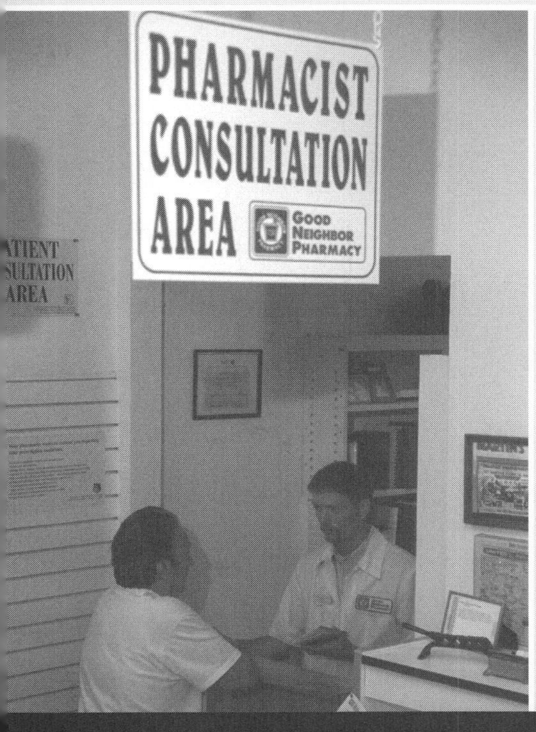

GLOSSARY

addition The combined effect of two agents, which is equal to the sum of the effects of each drug taken alone.

anaphylactic reaction A life-threatening allergic reaction that is characterized by a drop in blood pressure with difficulty breathing.

antagonism The combined effect of two drugs that is less than the effect of either drug taken alone.

Arthus reaction A severe local inflammatory reaction that occurs at the site of injection of an antigen in a previously sensitized individual.

cellular hypersensitivity reaction The result of the activity of many leukocyte actions. The T1 lymphocytes become sensitized by their first contact with a specific antigen. Subsequent exposure to an antigen stimulates multiple reactions aimed at destroying or inactivating the offending antigen.

cytotoxic reaction Severe damage to or destruction of cells by a substance.

dependence The total psychophysical state of one addicted to drugs or alcohol who must receive an increasing amount of the substance to prevent the onset of withdrawal symptoms.

first-pass metabolism The degree to which a drug is chemically altered as it circulates through the liver for the first time.

gray baby syndrome A disorder caused by administration of chloramphenicol to pregnant women or to neonates. The newborn baby exhibits an ashen-gray color within 24 hours after administration of the drug. The newborn may also have other signs and symptoms such as vomiting, irregular respiration, and cyanosis.

placebo An inert substance given to a patient instead of an active medicine. Placebos are often given to people who participate in studies intended to evaluate the effectiveness of a medicine.
placebo effect A decreased drug effect when the feeling of the patient toward the medication is negative.
potentiation An effect that occurs when a drug increases or prolongs the action of another drug, the total effect being greater than the sum of the effects of each used alone.
side effect An outcome other than that intended. Most commonly used in the context of drug therapy in which a side effect is an unwanted consequence of the drug in use.
synergism A combined action of two or more agents that produces an effect greater than would have been expected from the two agents acting separately.
tolerance Increasing resistance to the usual effects of an established dosage of a drug as a result of continued use.

FACTORS AFFECTING DRUG ACTIVITY

Certain factors may influence drug activity, such as age, gender, weight, time and route of drug administration (oral or parenteral routes), diet, pregnancy, psychological state, polypharmacy, and diseases. The prescribing physician must consider all of these factors when writing the prescription. The pharmacy technician must be familiar with these factors as well. The presence or absence of certain functional groups will determine the necessity, route, and extent of metabolism.

Age

The age of the patient may influence the effects of a drug. Infants and young children need to receive smaller doses of drugs than adults to avoid toxic side effects. Liver function is poorly developed in infants and young children. In older children, some drugs may be less active than in adults, particularly if the dosage is based on weight. This effect occurs because the liver develops faster than general body weight increases, and, thus, it represents a greater fraction of total body weight. In the elderly, the effectiveness of metabolizing enzyme systems declines. The lowered level of enzyme activity slows the rate of drug elimination, causing higher plasma drug levels per dose than in young adults.

Gender

Several hormones such as androgen, estrogen, and adrenocorticotropin might affect the activity of certain enzymes in men or women. Metabolism of prednisolone, acetaminophen, diazepam, and caffeine is slightly faster in women. Oxidative metabolism of lidocaine, propranolol, and some steroids is faster in men than in women. Men may require a larger dose of some drugs than women because many women are smaller than men.

Weight

In general, dosages are based on a weight of approximately 150 pounds, which is calculated to the "average" weight of men and women. A drug dose may sometimes be increased or decreased because the patient's weight is significantly higher or lower than this average. With narcotics, for example, higher or lower than average dosages, depending on the patient's weight may be necessary to produce relief of pain.

Time and Route of Drug Administration

During the night (nocturnal) plasma levels of drugs, such as theophylline and diazepam, are lower than plasma levels during the day (diurnal). The time of drug administration is an important factor that affects drug activity. Some drugs should be taken before or after meals. Some other medicines must be used in the early morning or before bedtime.

Oral Routes

Drugs administered orally are absorbed from the gastrointestinal tract and transported to the liver before they enter the systemic circulation. Thus, the drug is subject to hepatic metabolism before it reaches its site of action. This effect is known as **first-pass metabolism**, which is the degree to which a drug is chemically altered as it circulates through the liver for the first time. Most orally administered drugs are absorbed into the blood vessels within the intestinal tract. The blood in these vessels flows directly to the liver, the body's primary site for drug metabolism, before it goes anywhere else in the body. Some drugs are totally destroyed the first and only time they pass through, whereas other drugs are hardly affected at all. The oral route of administration is not suitable for most drugs for which a high degree of first-pass metabolism occurs because those drugs are quickly deactivated. Nitroglycerin tablets, for example, are dissolved under the tongue rather than being swallowed because nitroglycerin is completely inactivated during its first pass through the liver (see Table 18-1).

Parenteral Routes

Intravenous administration of drugs produces the most rapid drug action. Next in order of time of action is the intramuscular route, followed by the subcutaneous route.

TABLE 18-1. Examples of Drugs That Undergo First-Pass Metabolism

Acetaminophen	Nortriptyline
Alprenolol	Oxprenolol
Aspirin	Pentazocine
Cortisone	Progesterone
Cyclosporin	Propoxyphene
Estradiol	Propranolol
Imipramine	Salbutamol
Isoproterenol	Terbutaline
Lidocaine	Testosterone
Meperidine	Verapamil

With parenteral administration, drugs bypass the liver which causes a first-pass effect, because the drug is delivered directly to the bloodstream without being metabolized in the liver. The liver is also bypassed with sublingual and rectal administration.

Diet

Food can increase, decrease, or not affect the absorption of drugs. Diet can influence the bioavailability of a drug from a modified release dosage form. Absorption of the drug in the gastrointestinal tract with another food element is a common drug interaction that reduces the extent of drug absorption. For example, tetracycline complexes with calcium (found in milk products). Alcohol can increase or decrease the activity of hepatic drug-metabolizing enzymes. Chronic alcoholism can increase the rate of metabolism of tolbutamide, warfarin, and phenytoin. Acute alcohol intoxication can inhibit hepatic enzymes in individuals who are not addicted to alcohol.

Pregnancy

Drugs present in their active forms in the maternal circulation probably pass unchanged into the fetal circulation. In general, lipid-soluble drugs administered to pregnant women will usually pass through the placenta. The nicotine and carcinogenic substances in cigarettes will pass into the fetus through the bloodstream in pregnant women who smoke. Fetal metabolic activities vary and depend upon a number of factors including fetal age. A major deficiency in the fetus is lack of glucuronic acid-conjugating activity when a drug, which may have local or systemic effects, is applied to the surface of the body such as the skin. These drugs produce slow drug action both in the fetus and the neonate. The **gray baby syndrome** results from decreased chloramphenicol glucuronidation, and neonatal hyperbilirubinemia results from a decrease in bilirubin glucuronide formation. The gray baby syndrome includes symptoms such as vomiting, lack of sucking response, irregular and rapid respiration, abdominal distention, and cyanosis in newborn infants treated at birth with chloramphenicol or whose mothers were treated with chloramphenicol. An ashen-gray color is present for 24 hours.

Psychological State

The effect of drugs has been proven to depend on the positive or negative attitude of patients when they think about medications they have received. The more positive the patient feels about the drug he or she is taking, the more positive the physical response to the drug is. A decreased drug effect is possible when the feeling of the patient toward the medication is negative. This is called the **placebo effect**.

A **placebo** is an inactive substance, such as saline solution, distilled water, sugar, or a less than effective dose of a harmless substance, such as a water-soluble vitamin. Placebos are used in experimental drug studies to compare the effects of the inactive substance with those of the experimental drug. They are also prescribed for patients who cannot be given the medication they requested or who, in the judgment of the health care provider, do not need the medication. Health care professionals should realize that their attitudes and the impressions created at the time of drug discussion or administration may influence the therapeutic result.

Polypharmacy

The combined effect of drugs taken concurrently may result in antagonism or synergism and, consequently, may be lethal in some patients. It is important for health care professionals to be aware of the potential interactions of drugs that are prescribed as well as those that the patient may be self-administering. Many patients, especially elderly patients, may take several medicines each day. The chance for these individuals to develop an undesired drug interaction increases rapidly with the number of drugs used. It is estimated that if eight or more medications are being used, there is a 100% chance of interaction. One drug may interact with another to increase, decrease, or stop the effects of the other drug. The following terms are used to describe drug interactions:

- **Synergism**: A combined action of two or more agents that produces an effect greater than would have been expected from the two agents acting separately. For example, the combination of the antibacterial drugs trimethoprim and sulfamethoxazole is more effective for treating infections than either drug acting alone.
- **Antagonism**: The combined effect of two drugs that is less than the effect of either drug taken alone. For example, mutual opposition or contrary action may occur between muscles or medicines.
- **Potentiation**: An effect that occurs when a drug increases or prolongs the action of another drug with the total effect being greater than the sum of the effects of either drug used alone. For example, alcohol potentiates the sedating effects of the tranquilizer diazepam when the two drugs are ingested at the same time.

- **Addition**: The combined effect of two agents, which is equal to the sum of the effects of each drug taken alone. For example, psychological and physiological dependence on a chemical substance such as alcohol, heroin, or cocaine is additive.
- **Tolerance**: Increasing resistance to the usual effects of an established dosage of a drug as a result of continued use.
- **Dependence**: The total psychophysical state of one addicted to drugs or alcohol who must receive an increasing amount of the substance to prevent the onset of withdrawal symptoms.

Diseases

The presence of disease may influence the action of some drugs. Any disease or condition in the body and the severity of symptoms may affect the type and dose of drug administered. The presence of cardiovascular, hepatic (liver), or renal (kidney) dysfunctions will interfere with the normal processes of drug action. In liver disease, for example, the ability to metabolize or detoxify a specific type of drug may be impaired. If the average or normal dose of the drug is given, the liver may be unable to metabolize the drug at a normal rate. Therefore, the drug may be excreted from the body at a much slower rate than normal.

SIDE EFFECTS

A secondary response to a medication other than the primary therapeutic effect for which the drug was intended is called a **side effect**. Side effects can range from mild, which disappear when the drug is discontinued, to debilitating diseases that become chronic.

Hypersensitivity

A drug allergy is an altered state of reaction to a drug, resulting from previous sensitizing exposure and the development of an immunologic mechanism. Hypersensitivity reactions occur in nearly 10% of patients. All types of reactions from a simple rash to anaphylaxis can occur within 2 minutes or up to 3 days after administration. There are four different types of allergic drug reactions.

Type I—Anaphylactic

An **anaphylactic reaction** is an immediate reaction. An immediate reaction may be severe and may result in death if not treated quickly. Signs and symptoms of the most severe reactions include severe bronchospasm, vasospasm, hypotension, and rapid death. Drugs that may be associated with type I hypersensitivity include penicillins and cephalosporin.

Type II—Cytotoxic

A **cytotoxic reaction** is called an autoimmune response. It may cause hemolytic anemia (methyldopa- or penicillin-induced), thrombocytopenia (quinidine-induced) or systemic lupus erythematosus (procainamide-induced).

Type III—Arthus

An **Arthus reaction** (also known as serum sickness or Arthus phenomenon) is associated with an acute local inflammatory reaction, usually in the skin and marked by edema, hemorrhage, and necrosis, which occurs at the site of injection. Penicillins, sulfonamides, and phenytoin can cause this delayed reaction.

Type IV—Cellular Hypersensitivity

A cell-mediated or delayed hypersensitivity reaction is responsible for defense against certain bacterial, fungal, and viral pathogens or malignant cells. Allergic (contact) dermatitis is an example of a cell-mediated immune response. A type IV reaction is also called a **cellular hypersensitivity reaction**. Drugs produce their effects by altering the normal functions of the cells and tissues of the body via one of four general mechanisms:

1. Nonspecific chemical or physical interactions
2. Alteration in the level of enzyme activity
3. Action as antimetabolites
4. Interaction with receptors (neurotransmitters and hormones)

REVIEW QUESTIONS

1. The plasma level of diazepam or theophylline is lower in which of the following?
   A. Early morning
   B. At noon
   C. During the afternoon
   D. During the night
2. The first-pass effect means when the
   A. drug passes through the membrane wall of small intestine.
   B. drug enters the systemic circulation.
   C. drug is transported to the liver before entering the blood.
   D. drug plasma level disappears.

Continues

3. The gray baby syndrome is seen as a result of
A. decreased plasma protein.
B. decreased chloramphenicol glucuronidation.
C. increased chloramphenicol glucuronidation.
D. increased plasma protein.

4. The secondary response to a medication other than the primary therapeutic effect is called a
A. side effect.
B. drug interaction.
C. antagonism.
D. synergism.

5. Type III hypersensitivity is known as
A. cytotoxic reaction.
B. anaphylactic reaction.
C. serum sickness or Arthus reaction.
D. cellular hypersensitivity reaction.

6. An effect that occurs when a drug increases or prolongs the action of another drug is called
A. synergism.
B. tolerance.
C. dependence.
D. potentiation.

7. Which of the following hypersensitivities is called an autoimmune response?
A. Cellular hypersensitivity reaction
B. Cytotoxic reaction
C. Anaphylactic reaction
D. Arthus phenomenon

8. What is the reason that infants and young children need to receive smaller doses of drugs than adults?
A. Brain function is poorly developed.
B. Some drugs may be more active than in adults.
C. Liver function is not developed completely.
D. Metabolizing enzyme systems are increased compared with those of adults.

9. An inert substance given to a patient instead of an active medicine is called
A. complexation.
B. neutral substance.
C. plasma protein.
D. placebo.

10. Increasing resistance to the usual effects of an established dosage of a drug as a result of continued use is called
A. tolerance.
B. dependence.
C. placebo effect.
D. side effect.

11. Most elderly patients take several medicines each day. The term used for this action is
A. *polypodia.*
B. *polyploidy.*
C. *polypharmacy.*
D. none of the above.

12. Cellular hypersensitivities include which of the following types of allergic drug reactions?
A. Type I
B. Type II
C. Type III
D. Type IV

13. Allergic or contract dermatitis is an example of
A. a cell-mediated immune response.
B. the Arthus reaction.
C. an anaphylactic reaction.
D. a cytotoxic reaction.

14. Which of the following routes of drug administration usually has the first-pass metabolism?
A. Intramuscular
B. Sublingual
C. Rectal
D. Oral

15. In the elderly, the metabolizing enzyme system may
A. increase.
B. decrease.
C. sometimes decrease and at other times increase.
D. never change.

Antibiotics 19

OUTLINE

Antibiotics
Antibiotic Resistance
Bactericidal Agents
- Penicillins
- Cephalosporins
- Quinolones
- Aminoglycosides
- Vancomycin

Bacteriostatic Agents
- Sulfonamides
- Tetracyclines
- Macrolides

Miscellaneous Antibiotics
- Chloramphenicol
- Aztreonam
- Clindamycin
- Metronidazole

Antitubercular Drugs
- Isoniazid
- Ethambutol
- Rifampin
- Rifampin-isoniazid
- Pyrazinamide (PZA)
- Streptomycin

Antiparasitic Drugs
- Mebendazole
- Diethylcarbamazine
- Thiabendazole
- Niclosamide
- Piperazine
- Oxamniquine

Amebicides
- Iodoquinol
- Paromomycin
- Dehydroemetine
- Metronidazole
- Diloxanide

Antimalarial Agents
- Chloroquine
- Hydroxychloroquine
- Primaquine
- Quinine
- Mefloquine
- Pyrimethamine

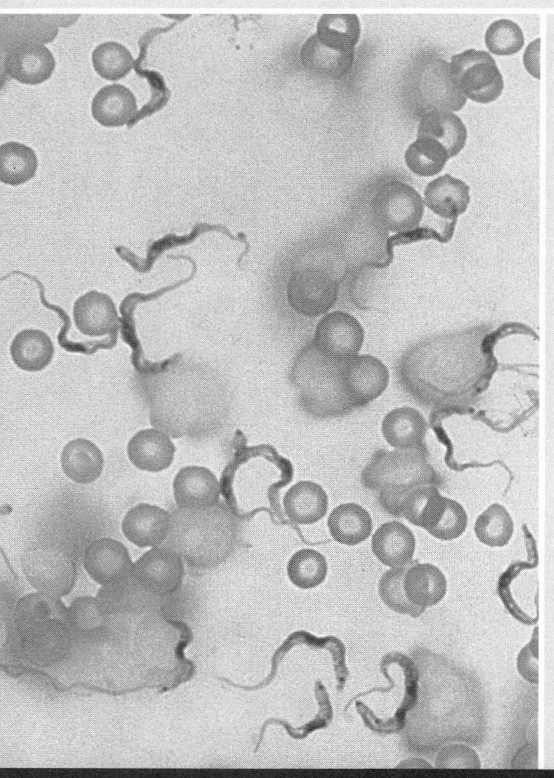

GLOSSARY

amebicides Drugs used to treat a protozoal infection.

aminoglycosides A group of potent bactericidal agents that are usually reserved for serious or life-threatening infections.

antibiotics Substances that have the ability to destroy or interfere with the development of a living organism.

antiparasitic Agents that are used to treat worms.

antitubercular Drugs that are used to treat tuberculosis.

bactericidal agents Antibiotic drugs that kill bacteria.

bacteriostatic agents Drugs that tend to restrain the development of the reproduction of bacteria.

broad-spectrum antibiotics A type of antibiotic that is used in the treatment of multiple organisms.

cephalosporins Semisynthetic antibiotics structurally and pharmacologically related to penicillins.

macrolides Broad-spectrum antimicrobials, which include erythromycins and erythromycin derivatives.

narrow-spectrum antibiotics A type of antibiotic that is effective against only a few organisms.

penicillins Natural or semisynthetic antibiotics produced by or derived from certain species of the fungus *Penicillium.*

quinolones Bactericidal agents that are effective against most gram-negative and many gram-positive bacteria.

sulfonamides Synthetic derivatives of sulfanilamide; these agents were the first drugs to prevent and cure human bacterial infections successfully.

tetracyclines Antibiotics and semisynthetic antibiotic derivatives obtained from cultures of *Streptomyces.*

ANTIBIOTICS

Antibiotics are substances that have the ability to destroy or interfere with the development of a living organism. They are natural substances derived from certain organisms (bacteria, fungus, and others) that are used against infections caused by other organisms. The body can overcome many simple infections, but more serious infections often require the assistance of antibiotics to kill pathogens.

Broad-spectrum antibiotics are used in the treatment of multiple organisms. This class of drugs is effective against both gram-negative and gram-positive bacteria. A broad-spectrum antibiotic usually is the most appropriate choice until the specific organism has been identified. In all patients, culture specimens must be obtained before therapy begins. **Narrow-spectrum antibiotics** are effective against only a few organisms.

The first major antimicrobial agents were the sulfonamides. The second group of antimicrobial agents (true antibiotics) were the penicillins.

ANTIBIOTIC RESISTANCE

By acquiring resistance to a specific antibiotic, a microorganism can survive in the drug's presence. Many gonococcal microorganisms, for instance, now are resistant to penicillin. Drug resistance is particularly common in geographic areas where a specific drug has been used excessively and perhaps improperly. Acquired resistance is a great concern because it can render currently effective antibiotics useless. This creates a continuous need for new antimicrobial agents. Several bacteria, such as *Staphylococcus aureus, Escherichia coli,* and *Mycobacterium tuberculosis,* now can cause serious clinical problems because of drug resistance. The frequent use of antibiotics promotes the emergence of drug-resistant microbes. The main reason for the development of drug-resistant microbes is the inappropriate use of antibiotics. The more an antibiotic is used, the faster drug-resistant microorganisms emerge. Inappropriate use and overuse of antibiotics increase the resistance of normal flora, turning them into possible pathogens. Patients contribute to this problem by failing to take the full ordered course of antibiotic treatment ordered by the physician. Every effort should be made to avoid the indiscriminate use of antibiotics in individuals and for viral infections.

BACTERICIDAL AGENTS

Bactericidal agents are antibiotic drugs that kill bacteria. Bactericidal agents include penicillins, cephalosporins, quinolones, aminoglycosides, and vancomycin. Bactericidal agents are generally used in the treatment of serious and life-threatening infections.

Penicillins

Penicillins are natural or semisynthetic antibiotics produced by or derived from certain species of the fungus *Penicillium.* Penicillins are the most widely used antimicrobial agents. However, cephalosporin usage has increased in the last decade.

The major cause of resistance to penicillin is production of β-lactamases (penicillinases). Common organisms that are capable of producing penicillinases include *S. aureus, E. coli, Pseudomonas aeruginosa,* and species of *Bacillus, Proteus,* and *Bacteroides.*

Penicillins are absorbed rapidly after parenteral administration and are distributed throughout body fluids. They penetrate cerebrospinal fluid (CSF) and ocular fluid to a significant extent only during inflammation. Most penicillins are excreted by the kidneys, predominantly via tubular secretion. Clearance can be slowed by administration of probenecid. (Probenecid is a uricosuric agent that inhibits the renal secretion of penicillins and cephalosporins. This effect is often taken advantage of in the treatment of infections because concomitant administration of probenecid will increase plasma levels of antibiotics.) The action of penicillins is usually bactericidal. Some must be administered parenterally (e.g., penicillin G, the drug of choice for many infections), because of instability in the presence of stomach acids. Others, such as ampicillin, are quite stable in gastric acid and may be administered orally. Parenteral administration of penicillin is more rapid and produces a higher concentration of penicillin in blood levels than when oral therapy is used. The most common types of penicillins are shown in Table 19-1.

Hypersensitivity occurs in nearly 10% of patients. Reactions from simple rash to anaphylaxis can be observed from within 2 minutes and up to 3 days after administration. Other adverse effects include direct irritation or pain at the injection site, gastrointestinal (GI) upset, and suprainfection (new infection that appears during the course of treatment for a primary infection). Penicillins are useful for the following microorganisms:

1. Gram-positive aerobes: pneumococcal, streptococcal (except *Streptococcus faecalis*), and non–penicillinase-producing staphylococcal infections
2. Gram-negative aerobes: gonococcal (non–penicillinase-producing) and meningococcal infections
3. *Treponema pallidum* (syphilis) and *Leptospira*

Penicillins are also used prophylactically for streptococcal infections and for bacterial endocarditis in patients with valvular heart disease who are undergoing dental or upper respiratory tract surgery. They are used to prevent recurrence of rheumatic fever.

TABLE 19-1. Common Penicillins

GENERIC NAME	TRADE NAME	ROUTE OF ADMINISTRATION
Narrow spectrum (first generation)		
penicillin G	Many trade names (Pentids®, Duracillin®, etc.)	IM, IV
penicillin V	Pen-VEE-K, V-cillin®K, Veetids®	Oral
Narrow spectrum antistaphylococcal		
methicillin	Staphcillin®	IM, IV
nafcillin	Nafcil®, Unipen®	Oral, IM, IV
oxacillin	Bactocill®, Prostaphlin®	Oral, IM, IV
cloxacillin	Cloxapen®	Oral, IM, IV
dicloxacillin	Dynapen®, Dycill®	Oral, IM, IV
Broad spectrum (second generation)		
ampicillin	Amcill®, Principen®, Omnipen®, Polycillin®	Oral
amoxicillin	Amoxil®, Trimox®, Polymox®	Oral
amoxicillin + clavulanate	Augmentin®	Oral
Extended spectrum (third generation)		
carbenicillin	Geocillin®, Geopen®	Oral, IM, IV
piperacillin	Pipracil®	IM, IV
Fourth generation		
mezlocillin	Mezlin®	IM, IV
azlocillin	Azlin®	IV

IM, intramuscular; IV, intravenous.

Penicillinase-Resistant Penicillins

Penicillinase-resistant penicillins are used predominantly for penicillinase-producing staphylococcal infections. Oxacillin, cloxacillin, dicloxacillin, and nafcillin sodium can be given orally. Methicillin is administered parenterally. Nafcillin is used parenterally for more serious infections.

Broad-Spectrum Penicillins

Broad-spectrum penicillins have greater activity than penicillin G against gram-negative bacteria. Ampicillin is useful for infections caused by *Haemophilus influenzae, Proteus mirabilis, E. coli,* and *Salmonella*. Although not absorbed well from the GI tract, they are usually administered orally. Ampicillin is most commonly used for otitis media. Amoxicillin is similar to ampicillin, with greater oral absorption. Carbenicillin is effective against *Pseudomonas, Enterobacter,* and certain *Proteus* species, which are often resistant to other penicillins.

TABLE 19-2. Classification of Cephalosporins

GENERIC NAME	BRAND NAME	ROUTE OF ADMINISTRATION
First generation		
cephradine	Velosef®	Oral, IM, IV
cephapirin	Cefadyl®	IM, IV
cephalexin	Keflex®	Oral
cefazolin	Ancef®, Kefzol®	Oral, IM, IV
cefadroxil	Duricef®	Oral
cephalothin	Ceporacin®	IM, IV
Second generation		
cefamandole	Mandol®	IM, IV
cefoxitin	Mefoxin®	IM, IV
cefaclor	Ceclor®	Oral
cefuroxime	Ceftin®, Zinacef®	Oral, IM, IV
cefotetan	Cefotan®	IM, IV
cefonicid	Monocid®	IM, IV
Third generation		
cefotaxime	Claforan®	IM, IV
moxalactam	Moxam®	IP
cefixime	Suprax®	Oral
ceftriaxone	Rocephin®	IM, IV
cefprozil	Cefzil®	Oral
cefdinir	Omnicef®	Oral
cefoperazone	Cefobid®	IM, IV
cefpodoxime	Proxetil®, Vantin®	Oral
ceftazidime	Fortaz®	IM, IV
ceftibuten	Cedax®	Oral
ceftizoxime	Cefizox®	IM, IV
Fourth generation		
cefepime	Maxipime®	IM, IV

IM, intramuscular; IV, intravenous; IP, intraperitoneal.

Cephalosporins

Cephalosporins are semisynthetic antibiotics that are structurally and pharmacologically related to penicillins. Cephalosporins are usually bactericidal in action, and they are resistant to β-lactamase. The antibacterial activity of the cephalosporins results from inhibition of mucopeptide synthesis in the bacterial cell wall. The cephalosporins are classified into four different "generations" and used as substitutes for penicillins in persons with drug-resistant bacteria or allergies and in the treatment of certain gram-negative bacterial infections (see Table 19-2).

Patients who are allergic to penicillin should be given cephalosporins with caution. Up to 25% of patients who are allergic to penicillin are also allergic to cephalosporins. Patients who have had anaphylactic reactions to penicillin should not receive cephalosporins.

Cephalosporins are the drugs of choice for the following conditions:

- Oral infections and dental work
- Neurosurgery

- Procedures and surgery of the female reproductive system
- Orthopedic surgery
- Upper respiratory system surgery
- Pneumonia
- Heart and pacemaker procedures

Side effects of cephalosporins are similar to those of penicillin.

First-Generation Cephalosporins

First-generation cephalosporins are similar to penicillinase-resistant penicillins with slightly greater coverage against gram-negative bacteria. They are effective against most gram-positive organisms and some gram-negative organisms. They are used mainly for *Klebsiella* and penicillin- and sulfonamide-resistant urinary tract infections.

Cephalothin, cephapirin, and cefazolin are used parenterally; others such as cephalexin and cefadroxil can be administered orally. Cephalosporins do not penetrate CSF.

Second-Generation Cephalosporins

Second-generation cephalosporins extend the spectrum of the first-generation cephalosporins to include *Haemophilus influenzae* and some *Proteus* infections. Second-generation cephalosporins are used primarily in the treatment of urinary tract, bone, and soft tissue infections (otitis media in children and respiratory tract infections) and prophylactically in various surgical procedures. All are administered parenterally except for cefaclor and cefuroxime, which may be given orally.

Third-Generation Cephalosporins

Third-generation cephalosporins have even broader activity against gram-negative bacteria and less activity against gram-positive bacteria than do second-generation agents. They are used for hospital-acquired infections. Because of their long half-life, these agents are also used in ambulatory patients, especially children. Third-generation cephalosporins include cefotaxime, moxalactam, which has a high potency against *H. influenzae, Neisseria gonorrhoeae,* and *Enterobacter.* The majority of third-generation cephalosporins are administered parenterally. Third-generation agents are used primarily for serious gram-negative bacterial infections, alone or in combination with an aminoglycoside.

Fourth-Generation Cephalosporins

Fourth-generation cephalosporins have the greatest action against gram-negative organisms among the four generations of cephalosporins and minimal action against gram-positive organisms. Fourth-generation cephalosporins are used for the treatment of urinary tract, respiratory tract, and integumentary (skin) infections. Cefepime is an example of this generation.

TABLE 19-3. Most Commonly Used Quinolones

GENERIC NAME	BRAND NAME	ROUTE OF ADMINISTRATION
nalidixic acid	NegGram®	Oral
cinoxacin	Cinobac®	Oral
ciprofloxacin	Cipro®, Ciloxan®	Oral, IM, IV
levofloxacin	Levaquin®	Oral, IV
sparfloxacin	Zagam®	Oral
trovafloxacin	Trovan®	Oral, IV
moxifloxacin	Avelox®	Oral
gatifloxacin	Tequin®	Oral, IM, IV
nitrofurantoin	Furadantin®	Oral
ofloxacin	Floxin®	Oral, IV
norfloxacin	Noroxin®	Oral, ophthalmic

IM, intramuscular; IV, intravenous.

Quinolones

Quinolones are bactericidal agents used in the treatment of infections caused by most gram-negative and many gram-positive bacteria. They cause DNA damage of the organisms and cell death. Quinolones are useful primarily as urinary tract antiseptics. Quinolones include nalidixic acid, cinoxacin, ciprofloxacin, nitrofurantoin, ofloxacin, and norfloxacin (see Table 19-3).

Quinolones are the drug of choice for urinary tract, upper respiratory tract, ophthalmic, and bone infections and some sexually transmitted diseases. Adverse effects include nausea, vomiting, dizziness, and an unpleasant taste. Quinolones should not be given with theophylline because of the increased risk of theophylline toxicity.

Quinolones may cause joint malformations. They should not be used in patients younger than 18 years of age nor in pregnant women.

Aminoglycosides

The **aminoglycosides** are a group of potent bactericidal agents that are usually reserved for serious or life-threatening infections. They inhibit bacterial protein synthesis (bactericidal). Generally, gram-negative bacilli are the main organisms sensitive to these drugs, but gram-positive microbes may also be affected. They are not absorbed orally and do not penetrate the CSF. Aminoglycosides are excreted by the kidneys. The most commonly used aminoglycosides are listed in Table 19-4.

A narrow therapeutic index may be necessary to monitor serum concentrations and individualize doses of aminoglycosides. Patients with impaired renal function, sepsis, burns, or fever, elderly or obese patients, and neonates are especially at risk. The major side effects of aminoglycosides are nephrotoxicity and ototoxicity. Toxic effects are seen more often in individuals with renal impairment. Damage related to toxicity may be permanent. Aminoglycosides should not be given with other ototoxic drugs such as ethacrynic acid or furosemide.

TABLE 19-4. Most Commonly Used Aminoglycosides

GENERIC NAME	BRAND NAME	ROUTE OF ADMINISTRATION
neomycin	Neobiotic®	Usually topical, oral
amikacin	Amikin®	IM, IV
gentamicin	Garamycin®	IM, IV, ophthalmic
streptomycin	Streptomycin®	Oral, IM
netilmicin	Netromycin®	Topical, oral
tobramycin	Nebcin®	IM, IV, ophthalmic
kanamycin	Kantrex®	Oral, IM, IV

IM, intramuscular; IV, intravenous.

Kanamycin is the most ototoxic of the aminoglycosides. Hypersensitivity reactions are rare. Neomycin, when applied topically, can cause contact dermatitis in as many as 8% of patients.

Streptomycin

Streptomycin is currently used only for plague, for severe cases of brucellosis, and as an adjunct treatment for recalcitrant mycobacterial infections. Streptomycin is often called by the trade name Trobicin®. Side effects are pain at the site of injection and hypersensitivity.

Gentamicin and Tobramycin

Gentamicin and tobramycin are active against *Enterobacter, Proteus, Pseudomonas, Klebsiella,* and other gram-negative organisms.

Amikacin

Amikacin is used in the treatment of severe gram-negative bacterial infections, especially those that are resistant to gentamicin or tobramycin.

Neomycin

Neomycin is too toxic for systemic use and is administered topically for minor soft tissue infections.

Netilmicin

Netilmicin is used for short-term treatment of serious infections caused by susceptible strains of *E. coli, Klebsiella pneumoniae,* and *Proteus mirabilis.*

Vancomycin

Vancomycin is usually the drug of last resort and should be reserved for severe infections caused by drug-resistant *Staphylococcus* and *Clostridium* infections. It inhibits bacteria by binding to a cell wall precursor and is bactericidal for many organisms. It can also inhibit RNA synthesis. Vancomycin is active against gram-positive organisms. It is administered parenterally, except in the treatment of enterocolitis. Vancomycin is eliminated unchanged by the kidneys. The most serious side effect is ototoxicity.

BACTERIOSTATIC AGENTS

Bacteriostatic agents are drugs that tend to restrain the reproduction of bacteria. Bacteriostatic agents include the sulfonamides, tetracyclines, macrolides (erythromycin), and lincomycin. For treatment of minor infections, there is little difference in the effectiveness of bactericidal or bacteriostatic antibiotics.

Lincomycin

Lincomycin is classified as lincosamide, an antibiotic that inhibits protein synthesis and causes cell death. It is used for the treatment of serious infections caused by staphylococcal, streptococcal, and Pneumococcal infections resistant to other antibiotics in penicillin-allergic patients, or when penicillin is inappropriate. It must be used cautiously in patients with hepatic or renal dysfunction. First, less toxic antibiotics, such as erythromycin or clindamycin, should be considered. It should be used in conjunction with other antibiotics.

Sulfonamides

Sulfonamides are synthetic derivatives of sulfanilamide, and these agents were the first drugs to be used successfully to prevent and cure human bacterial infections. Although their current use is limited because of the introduction of more effective antibiotics, sulfonamides remain the drugs of choice for certain infections. They are well absorbed from the GI tract. Sulfonamides readily penetrate the CSF. These agents are metabolized to various degrees in the liver and are eliminated by the kidneys. Sulfonamides most often are used to treat urinary tract infections caused by *E. coli,* including acute and chronic cystitis, and chronic upper respiratory tract infections. Sulfonamides may cause blood dyscrasias such as hemolytic anemia, aplastic anemia, and thrombocytopenia. Hypersensitivity reactions to sulfonamides probably result from sensitization and most commonly involve the skin and mucous membranes. Drug fever and serum sickness may also develop. Crystalluria and hematuria may occur, possibly leading to urinary tract obstruction. Sulfonamides should be used cautiously in patients with renal impairment. Sulfonamides are generally classified as short-acting, intermediate-acting, or long-acting. The classifications depend on the rate at which they are absorbed and eliminated (see Table 19-5).

TABLE 19-5. Classification of Sulfonamides

GENERIC NAME	TRADE NAME	ROUTE OF ADMINISTRATION
Short-acting sulfonamides		
sulfisoxazole	Gantrisin®	Oral
Intermediate-acting sulfonamides		
sulfamethoxazole	Gantanol®	Oral
sulfadiazine	Microsulfon®	Oral
Long-acting sulfonamides		
sulfasalazine	Azulfidine®	Oral
sulfadoxine	Fansidar®	Oral
Combination sulfonamides		
trisulfapyrimidines	Triple Sulfa®	Oral, vaginal
trimethoprim/ sulfamethoxazole	Bactrim®, Septra®, Cotrim®	Oral, IV

IV, intravenous.

Sulfisoxazole

Sulfisoxazole is a short-acting sulfonamide used to treat urinary tract infections, malaria, meningitis, and acute otitis media.

Sulfamethoxazole

Sulfamethoxazole is an intermediate-acting sulfonamide used for chronic and recurrent urinary tract infections, bacterial prostatitis, GI infections (particularly shigellosis), and traveler's diarrhea.

Sulfadiazine

Sulfadiazine is an intermediate-acting sulfonamide that is the best drug for the treatment of meningitis. Sulfadiazine should be used with care and with attention to adequate hydration.

Sulfasalazine

Sulfasalazine is a long-acting sulfonamide that is prescribed for the treatment of ulcerative colitis. Adverse effects include headache, insomnia, depression, orange-yellow discoloration of the skin, nausea, vomiting, and diarrhea. It can also cause orange-yellow urine, crystalluria, and hematuria.

Sulfadoxine

Sulfadoxine is a long-acting sulfonamide used in the treatment of chloroquine-resistant *Plasmodium falciparum* malaria.

Trisulfapyrimidines

Trisulfapyrimidines (triple sulfa) are sulfa drugs commonly used in combination to treat a variety of infections. At one time sulfonamides were widely used in the treatment and prevention of infection such as urinary tract infections, chlamydia, toxoplasmosis, and malaria. Triple sulfa is used in combination with pyrimethamine for the treatment of central nervous system toxoplasmosis in patients with acquired immunodeficiency syndrome (AIDS) and newborns with congenital infections. Adverse effects include hypersensitivity, rash, intense itching of the skin, photosensitivity, high fever, kidney damage, dizziness, mental depression, confusion, and insomnia.

Trimethoprim/Sulfamethoxazole

Trimethoprim/sulfamethoxazole is a combination of sulfonamides. It is used for the treatment of urinary tract infections caused by susceptible strains of bacteria and shigellosis enteritis. This agent is also used for the treatment of acute otitis media and acute or chronic bronchitis. Trimethoprim is commonly prescribed for treatment of traveler's diarrhea. Adverse effects are similar to those of other sulfonamide agents.

Tetracylines

Tetracyclines are antibiotics and semisynthetic antibiotic derivatives obtained from cultures of *Streptomyces*. They are bacteriostatic and are considered to be broad-spectrum agents. In general, tetracyclines are stable in acid solutions but are rapidly inactivated in neutral and alkaline solutions. Absorption of tetracycline is impaired by the stomach contents, especially milk and antacids, as a result of complex formation with ions, particularly magnesium, calcium, and aluminum. Tetracyclines are eliminated via renal and bilary routes; doxycycline is excreted almost entirely via feces, so it is the safest tetracycline to administer to individuals with impaired renal function.

Tetracyclines have a broad spectrum of activity and are effective against most *Rickettsia, Chlamydia, Mycoplasma, Spirochaeta,* and many gram-negative and gram-positive bacteria. The drugs are inactive against fungi and viruses.

Tetracyclines should not be used in children younger than 8 years of age unless other appropriate drugs are ineffective or are contraindicated. Use of the drugs in infants has resulted in retardation of bone growth. Because tetracyclines localize in the dentin and enamel of developing teeth, use of the drugs during tooth development may cause enamel hypoplasia and permanent yellow-gray to brown discoloration of the teeth.

Tetracyclines can cause fetal toxicity when administered to pregnant women (e.g., retardation of skeletal development). Liver toxicity has occurred after intravenous administration of tetracyclines to pregnant women. Oxytetracycline is the least hepatotoxic. Phototoxicity may occur in patients when they are exposed to strong sunlight (ultraviolet), especially with demeclocycline. Table 19-6 summarizes the types of tetracyclines.

TABLE 19-6. Classification of Tetracyclines

GENERIC NAME	TRADE NAME	ROUTE OF ADMINISTRATION
Short-acting		
tetracycline	Achromycin®, Sumycin®	Oral
chlortetracycline	Aureomycin®	Oral
oxytetracycline	Terramycin®	Oral, IM
Intermediate-acting		
demeclocycline	Declomycin®	Oral
Long-acting		
doxycycline	Vibramycin®	Oral
minocycline	Minocin®	Oral, IV

IM, intramuscular; IV, intravenous.

TABLE 19-7. Common Macrolides

GENERIC NAME	BRAND NAME	ROUTE OF ADMINISTRATION
erythromycin	Ilotycin®, Erythrocin®	Oral, IV
erythromycin estolate	Ilosone®	Oral
erythromycin succinate	E.E.S.®, EryPed®	Oral
erythromycin gluceptate	Ilotycin®	IV
azithromycin	Zithromax®	Oral
clarithromycin	Biaxin®	Oral
dirithromycin	Dynabac®	Oral
troleandomycin	Tao®	Oral, IM, IV

IV, intravenous; IM, intramuscular.

Macrolides

Macrolides are broad-spectrum antimicrobials, which include erythromycins and erythromycin derivatives (azithromycin, clarithromycin, dirithromycin, troleandomycin). Erythromycin is usually bacteriostatic, but it may be bactericidal in high concentrations or against highly susceptible organisms. The drug generally penetrates the cell wall of gram-positive bacteria more readily than that of gram-negative bacteria. The macrolides are used primarily for oral therapy of respiratory, urinary, skin, and soft tissue infections. These drugs are used particularly in patients who are allergic to penicillins, cephalosporins, or tetracyclines. They are the most effective drugs for Legionnaires' disease and *Mycoplasma* pneumonia.

Erythromycin is inactivated by stomach acid. Administered as enteric-coated tablets, erythromycins usually cause such severe GI distress that a "take with food" sticker is placed on the prescription bottle. Absorption is reduced by gastric contents. This medication penetrates all body fluids except CSF. Erythromycin is concentrated in the liver and is excreted predominantly via the bilary route. Hepatotoxicity is possible and requires cautious use of this medication in the presence of impaired hepatic function. Table 19-7 lists common macrolides.

Azithromycin

Azithromycin is in the class of macrolides antibiotics used in the treatment of lower respiratory tract infections, uncomplicated skin infections, otitis media, pharyngitis, and prevention and treatment of disseminated Mycobacterium avium complex in patients with advanced AIDS.

Clarithromycin

Clarithromycin is a macrolides antibiotic. Its indications include treatment of upper and lower respiratory infections. Treatment of active duodenal ulcer with H. pylori in combination with proton pump inhibitors, and treatment of disseminated mycobacterial infections due to M. avium. Clarithromycin should be used cautiously with colitis, hepatic or renal impairment, pregnancy, and lactation.

Dirithromycin

Dirithromycin is a macrolides antibiotic indicated for the treatment of acute bacterial exacerbations of chronic bronchitis, community-acquired pneumonia caused by Legionella pneumophila, Mycoplasma pneumoniae, and treatment of pharyngitis caused by Streptococcus pyogenes. It should be used cautiously with colitis, and hepatic or renal impairment.

Troleandomycin

Troleandomycin is a macrolides antibiotic used to treat many different types of bacterial infections, such as tonsillitis, bronchitis, sinusitis, and pneumonia. It is contraindicated in patients with liver disease, and it is not know if it is harmful to unborn babies.

MISCELLANEOUS ANTIBIOTICS

The following antibiotics are independent of other classes and each other due to structural differences.

Chloramphenicol

Chloramphenicol is a broad-spectrum antibacterial agent that inhibits protein synthesis in a bacterium. It is bacteriostatic to a wide variety of gram-positive and gram-negative organisms, although it may be bactericidal in large doses. Chloramphenicol is absorbed well from the GI tract and is metabolized in the liver. The unmetabolized drug is excreted by the kidneys. Chloramphenicol is the drug of choice for bacterial meningitis and *Salmonella* with septicemia. It can also be administered intravenously.

Adverse effects include bone marrow suppression, which may lead to irreversible aplastic anemia. This drug may cause gray baby syndrome, which occurs in neonates given large doses.

Aztreonam

Aztreonam is the first drug in the monobactam class of antibiotics. It is bactericidal, through its ability to bind to the bacterial cell wall. Aztreonam is used against gram-negative microorganisms, especially those involved in urinary tract infections, bronchitis, and gynecological infections. The adverse effects include nausea, vomiting, and diarrhea. Aztreonam should be avoided in patients with liver disease and impaired renal function.

Clindamycin

Clindamycin is prescribed for the treatment of certain serious infections and as a prophylactic agent preceding abdominal surgery. Clindamycin is a broad-spectrum antibiotic that inhibits protein synthesis. It has a special affinity for bone. It is extensively metabolized in the liver and is excreted in urine and bile. Clindamycin is a semisynthetic derivative of lincomycin and is used for bone and joint diseases, gynecological disease, skin and soft tissue infections, and septicemia. The adverse effects are mainly gastrointestinal disturbances and candidiasis.

Metronidazole

Metronidazole is a short-acting cytotoxic agent that is microbicidal. It is active against many anaerobic bacteria and protozoa. Also known by its brand name Flagyl®, it is well absorbed from the GI tract. High concentrations are achieved in the central nervous system. The drug is metabolized by the liver and eliminated via renal or hepatic routes. Metronidazole is prescribed primarily to treat intestinal amebiasis and amebic liver abscesses. It is also used to treat *Trichomonas* infections of the vagina and the male urethra. Metronidazole is active against *Giardia lamblia* infections of the intestine and is also the drug of choice for amebic dysentery and *Trichomonas* infections. Adverse effects include diarrhea, metallic taste, intolerance to alcohol, and rash. It may also discolor the urine. Alcohol and disulfiram should be avoided by patients taking metronidazole because it increases effectiveness of anticoagulants.

Table 19-8 shows miscellaneous antibiotics.

TABLE 19-8. Miscellaneous Antibiotics

GENERIC NAME	TRADE NAME	ROUTE OF ADMINISTRATION
chloramphenicol	Chloromycetin®	IV
aztreonam	Azactam®	IM, IV
vancomycin	Vancocin®	Oral
clindamycin	Cleocin®	Oral, IM, IV
metronidazole	Flagyl®	Oral, IV

IV, intravenous; IM, intramuscular.

ANTITUBERCULAR DRUGS

Antitubercular drugs are used to treat tuberculosis. They suppress or kill the slow-growing mycobacteria that cause this disease. Antitubercular agents fall into two main categories: primary and retreatment. Because the causative organisms tend to develop resistance to any single drug, combination drug therapy has become standard in the treatment of tuberculosis. Agents chosen for therapy must eradicate mycobacteria. Drugs available include ethambutol, isoniazid, streptomycin, rifampin, quinolones, pyrazinamide, and rifabutin. Agents showing the lowest incidence of resistance, such as isoniazid, rifampin, and streptomycin, are usually used in combination with ethambutol or pyrazinamide. The initial agents used in most patients are isoniazid, rifampin, and pyrazinamide. A fourth drug (ethambutol or streptomycin) is added if resistance is suspected.

Primary antitubercular drugs include isoniazid, ethambutol, rifampin, rifampin-isoniazid, pyrazinamide, and streptomycin. These drugs usually offer the greatest effectiveness with the least toxicity. In most patients, the combination of isoniazid, rifampin, and pyrazinamide is most effective.

Isoniazid

Isoniazid (INH) is the mainstay of antitubercular therapy. This drug should be included in all therapeutic regimens. It is bacteriostatic and bactericidal, yet its mechanism of action is unknown. Isoniazid is the most widely used antitubercular agent. Prophylactic isoniazid may be administered alone for up to 1 year in adults or children who have a positive tuberculin test result but lack active lesions. The most common adverse effects of isoniazid are skin rash, fever, jaundice, and peripheral neuritis.

Ethambutol

Ethambutol is a synthetic water-based compound. This agent is bacteriostatic. The mechanism of action is not known. Resistance to ethambutol may develop rapidly when it is used alone. Rarely, ethambutol causes optic neuritis, drug fever, abdominal pain, headache, dizziness, and confusion. Liver function, vision, and renal function should be periodically monitored.

Rifampin

Rifampin is a bactericidal drug. It should not be administered alone as an antitubercular agent because this can lead to drug-resistant organisms. Hepatotoxicity may result from rifampin therapy. Liver function tests should be routinely performed. Rifampin colors urine, sweat, tears, saliva, and feces orange-red.

Rifampin-isoniazid

Rifampin is an antibiotic that eliminates the bacteria that causes tuberculosis (TB). It is generally used in combination with other anti-tuberculosis agents, such as isoniazid, to prevent bacteria from becoming resistant to just one of the agents. Isoniazid may cause liver problems in patients over the age of 50. Severe side effects may occur in patients with seizures or epilepsy, history of gout, or severe kidney disease.

Pyrazinamide (PZA)

Pyrazinamide is an antituberculosis agent used along with other similar agents such as rifampin and isoniazid. It should not be used in patients with severe hepatic damage, acute or chronic gout, porphyria, diabetes, or renal failure. Risk to unborn babies cannot be ruled out, and it should be used in pregnant women only if the benefit outweighs the potential risk.

Streptomycin

Streptomycin is an antibiotic produced by a soil bacteria (*Streptomyces*) and is active against both gram-positive and gram-negative bacteria. It is commonly used in tuberculosis therapy, usually in combination with other anti-tuberculosis agents. Streptomycin acts by inhibiting protein synthesis and damaging cell membranes in susceptible microorganisms. Adverse effects include renal damage and nerve damage, which may result in dizziness or deafness.

Table 19-9 shows antituberculosis agents.

TABLE 19-9. Antituberculosis Agents

GENERIC NAME	BRAND NAME	ROUTE OF ADMINISTRATION
First-line agents		
isoniazid (INH)	Laniazid®	Oral
rifampin	Rimactane®, Rifadin®	Oral
rifampin-isoniazid	Rifamate®	Oral
pyrazinamide (PZA)		Oral
ethambutol	Myambutol®	Oral
streptomycin	(see Aminoglycosides)	IM
Second-line agents		
cycloserine	Seromycin®	Oral
capreomycin	Cepastat®	IM
p-aminosalicylic acid (PAS)		Oral

IM, intramuscular.

ANTIPARASITIC DRUGS

Antiparasitic drugs are used to treat infections with parasites. Parasites are unicellular or multicellular organisms that live on or within another organism and obtain nourishment from the host. They take only the nutrients they need and usually do not kill hosts. Examples of parasites that can produce an infection if they cause cellular damage to the host include helminths, such as pinworms and tapeworms. Helminths can infect the digestive system. The GI tract is a common site for the infections, with the lining, lymphatic system, and blood vessels also being involved. Early infestation may be asymptomatic, with severe problems appearing as the infection progresses. The most common types of parasitic worms are roundworms, tapeworms, and flukes. Roundworms include giant roundworms, pinworms, hookworms, whipworms, and threadworms. Tapeworms are found in beef, pork, and fish. Flukes are found in the blood, intestines, liver, and lungs. Antiparasitic drugs are dosed by weight.

Antiparasitic agents are used to rid the body of worms. Antihelmintic agents are among the most primitive types of chemotherapy. About one third of the world's population is infested with these parasites. The most common drugs used for the treatment of worms include mebendazole, diethylcarbamazine, thiabendazole, niclosamide, piperazine, and oxamniquine (see Table 19-10).

Mebendazole

Mebandazole is a vermicidal, inhibiting the formation of microtubules, and irreversibly blocking glucose uptake in the helminths, leading to death of the parasite. It is the drug of choice for intestinal roundworms, pinworms, hookworms, and great roundworms. Mebendazole is also used for treatment of trichuriasis (caused by pork roundworms). It is metabolized in the liver and excreted primarily in feces. This drug must be used with caution in patients with Crohn's disease and ulcerative colitis. The adverse effects are usually limited to diarrhea and abdominal cramping. With any treatment for pinworms, all household contacts of the patient should be treated at the same time.

TABLE 19-10. Antiparasitic Drugs

GENERIC NAME	TRADE NAME	ROUTE OF ADMINISTRATION
mebendazole	Vermox®	Oral
diethylcarbamazine	Hetrazan®	Oral
thiabendazole	Mintezol®	Oral
niclosamide	Niclocide®	Oral
piperazine	Entacyl®	Oral
oxamniquine	Vansil®	Oral

Diethylcarbamazine

Dietheylcarbamazine is a synthetic organic compound highly specific for several common parasites. This agent is active against *Filaria bancrofti, Ascaris, Loa loa,* and tropical eosinophilia.

Thiabendazole

The mechanism of action of thiabendazole is not known precisely. Thiabendazole inhibits the specific enzyme of helminths, fumarate reductase. It is vermicidal. This agent is used for the treatment of strongyloidiasis (threadworm), cutaneous larva migrans (creeping eruption), and trichinosis.

Niclosamide

Niclosamide inhibits the oxidative phosphorylation in the mitochondria of cestodes. It is used against *Taenia saginata* (beef tapeworm), *Diphyllobothrium latum* (fish tapeworm), and *Hymenolepis nana* (dwarf tapeworm). This agent may cause nausea, vomiting, dizziness, and drowsiness.

Piperazine

Piperazine causes paralysis of helminths by blocking the response of *Ascaris* muscle to acetylcholine. Piperazine is active against enterobiasis (caused by pinworms) and ascariasis (caused by roundworms). The most commonly reported reactions include GI tract and central nervous system effects. If these effects become significant, therapy should be discontinued. Piperazine should be taken on an empty stomach. Allergic or severe hypersensitivity reactions can occur.

Oxamniquine

Oxamniquine eradicates male and female schistosomes. This agent is active against *Schistosoma mansoni* infection, including acute and chronic phases, with hepatosplenic involvement. Convulsions may occur within a few hours of the first dose in patients with a previous history of seizures. This drug also may cause dizziness, drowsiness, nausea, and vomiting. It should be taken with food.

AMEBICIDES

Amebiasis is a protozoal infection of the large intestine. It is caused by *Entamoeba histolytica*. Transmission is usually via ingestion of cysts from contaminated water or food or from person-to-person contact.

Amebicides are crucial in the treatment of amebiasis, giardiasis, and trichomoniasis. These are the most common protozoal infections in the United States. The major amebicides include iodoquinol, paromomycin, dehydroemetine, metronidazole, and diloxanide (see Table 19-11).

TABLE 19-11. Antiprotozoal Agents

GENERIC NAME	TRADE NAME	ROUTE OF ADMINISTRATION
iodoquinol	Yodoxin®	Oral
paromomycin	Humatin®	Oral
dehydroemetine	Mebadin®	Oral
metronidazole	Flagyl®	Oral
diloxanide	Furamide®	Oral

Iodoquinol

Iodoquinol is effective against the *E. histolytica*. Its mechanism of action is not known. Poorly absorbed from the GI tract, it is excreted in urine and feces. It may produce optic atrophy and visual defects or peripheral neuropathy with high doses and prolonged use. Iodoquinol also can cause gastric distress, fever, headache, or hypersensitivity. It should not be prescribed for patients with liver or kidney disease.

Paromomycin

Paromomycin is an amebicide and also is effective against enteric bacteria such as *Salmonella* and *Shigella*. Paromomycin is not absorbed from the GI tract. This agent is indicated for acute and chronic intestinal amebiasis. It is not useful for extraintestinal amebiasis because it is not absorbed. Most of this drug is excreted in feces. Paromomycin may cause nausea, cramping, and diarrhea at high doses.

Dehydroemetine

Dehydroemetine is amebicidal and kills amoebae by inhibiting amebic protein synthesis. This drug is widely used to treat severe invasive intestinal amebiasis, amebic abscess, and amebic hepatitis. Dehydroemetine is usually administered in combination with another amebicidal agent.

Metronidazole

Metronidazole is useful in the treatment of anaerobic bacterial infections, amebiasis, giardia lamblia, trichomonas, and colitis. Metabolism of metronidazole may be increased and serum concentrations decreased by co-administration of phenobarbital or phenytoin. Adverse effects include nausea, vomiting, neutropenia, and rarely, seizures.

Diloxanide

Diloxanide is amebicidal; its mechanism of action is unknown. This agent is used to treat asymptomatic carriers of amebic and giardiac cysts. Diloxanide rarely causes serious adverse effects. Vomiting and flatulence have been reported.

ANTIMALARIAL AGENTS

Malaria is still a leading cause of illness and death in tropical and subtropical countries. Malaria results from infection by any of four species of the protozoal genus *Plasmodium*. Antimalaria drugs are selectively active during different phases of the protozoan life cycle. Major antimalarial drugs include chloroquine, hydroxychloroquine, primaquine, quinine, mefloquine, and pyrimethamine.

Chloroquine

The mechanism of action for chloroquine is unknown. This agent is used for the prevention and treatment of malaria for the four species of *Plasmodium*. Chloroquine is also prescribed to cure amebic liver abscesses. Because this drug concentrates in the liver, it should be used cautiously in patients with hepatic disease. Chloroquine may cause gastric distress, headaches, blurred vision, hair loss, and discoloration of skin, nails, or the inside of the mouth. It also may cause retinopathy, hypotension, cardiac dysrhythmia, and ototoxicity.

Hydroxychloroquine

The mechanism of action for hydroxychloroquine is inhibition of protozoal reproduction and protein synthesis. Hydroxychloroquine is used in the treatment of acute attacks of malaria caused by susceptible strains of plasmodia. It must be used cautiously with hepatic disease and alcoholism. Ototoxicity, emotional changes, nightmares, blood dyscrasias, nausea, vomiting, and diarrhea are the major adverse effects of hydroxychloroquine.

Primaquine

The mechanism of action for primaquine is unknown. It is active against liver forms of *Plasmodium vivax, Plasmodium ovale,* and the primary exoerythrocyte forms of *P. falciparum*. Primaquine is used for relapses in persons returning from regions where malaria is endemic. This agent is contraindicated in patients with rheumatoid arthritis and lupus erythematosus or those with bone marrow suppression. Primaquine may cause agranulocytosis, granulocytopenia, and mild anemia. Abdominal cramps, nausea, and vomiting may occur.

Quinine

In malaria, quinine has both suppressive and curative action against chloroquine-resistant strains of *Plasmodium*. Quinine is almost always given in combination with another antimalarial agent. Overdoses of or hypersensitivity reactions to chloroquine may be fatal. Manifestations of quinine poisoning include visual and hearing disturbances. It also may cause vomiting, fever, headache, and confusion.

Mefloquine

The exact mechanism of action of mefloquine is unknown. It is active against *P. falciparum* and *P. vivax*. It is indicated for the treatment of acute malaria, and the prevention of *P. falciparum* and *P. vivax* infections. Side effects include nausea, vomiting, diarrhea, headache, dizziness, insomnia, and visual disturbances.

Pyrimethamine

Pryimethamine is used for the treatment and prevention of malaria, as well as for AIDS-related diarrhea, and Toxoplasma gondii, a protozoal infection. It should be taken with food to reduce stomach irritation. Adverse effects include a painful, burning tongue, loss of taste, and anemia (in patients who have a folic acid deficiency). Other side effects can be skin rash, fever, nervousness, loss of appetite, nausea, vomiting, diarrhea, bone marrow depression, and jaundice.

REVIEW QUESTIONS

1. Clindamycin has a special affinity for which of the following organs?
   A. Brain
   B. Heart
   C. Bone
   D. Skin

2. Which of the following antibiotics should not be given if there is preexisting kidney damage?
   A. Streptomycin
   B. Erythromycin
   C. Kanamycin
   D. Nystatin

Continues

3. An antibiotic that should not be used in a patient known to be allergic to penicillin is
A. erythromycin.
B. cephalothin.
C. gentamicin.
D. tetracycline.

4. Which of the following include(s) penicillinase-resistant penicillins?
A. Methicillin
B. Tetracycline
C. Metronidazole
D. Nitrofurantoin

5. Second-generation cephalosporins include
A. ceftriaxone (Rocephin).
B. cefaclor (Ceclor).
C. Unipen.
D. azithromycin (Zithromax).

6. The macrolides are used particularly in patients who are allergic to
A. penicillins.
B. tetracyclines.
C. cephalosporins.
D. all of the above

7. Quinolones include which of the following agents?
A. Ciprofloxacin
B. Nitrofurantoin
C. Vancomycin
D. A and B

8. Which of the following antibiotics may lead to irreversible aplastic anemia?
A. Cephalosporins
B. Chloramphenicol
C. Penicillin
D. Erythromycin

9. Adverse effect(s) of metronidazole (Flagyl®) may include
A. discoloration of skin.
B. hypertension.
C. hepatitis.
D. metallic taste.

10. Which of the following antitubercular therapies may change the color of urine and tears to orange-red?
A. Isoniazid
B. Pyrazinamide
C. Rifampin
D. Ethambutol

11. The trade name of metronidazole is
A. Furamide®.
B. Flagyl®.
C. Mebadin®.
D. Humatin®.

12. Which of the following agents is carcinogenic and should not be used unnecessarily?
A. Metronidazole
B. Streptomycin
C. Penicillin
D. Rifampin

13. Manifestations of quinine poisoning include
A. dizziness.
B. visual and hearing disturbances.
C. aplastic anemia.
D. hypertension.

14. The generic name of Flagyl® is
A. clarithromycin.
B. azithromycin.
C. metronidazole.
D. nitrofurantoin.

15. The brand name of nalidixic acid is
A. Cinobac®.
B. Neg Gram®.
C. Furadantin®.
D. Floxin®.

16. Which of the following agents is currently used for giardiasis?
A. Isoniazid
B. Rifampin
C. Metronidazole
D. Gantrisin

17. First-generation cephalosporins include
A. Cephalexin.
B. Cefaclor.
C. Rifampin.
D. Metronidazole.

18. Which of the following antibiotics is contraindicated in children younger than 8 years of age?
A. Carbenicillin
B. Trimethoprim/sulfamethoxazole
C. Tetracycline
D. Penicillin V

19. The trade name of sulfisoxazole is
A. Gantrisin®.
B. Gantanol®.
C. Mebadin®.
D. Flagyl®.

20. The trade name of pyrazinamide is
A. Proxetil®.
B. Pipracil®.
C. Laniazid®.
D. Seromycin®.

Antivirals and Antifungals 20

OUTLINE

(Courtesy of Robert A. Silverman, M.D., Clinical Associate Professor, Department of Pediatrics, Georgetown University)

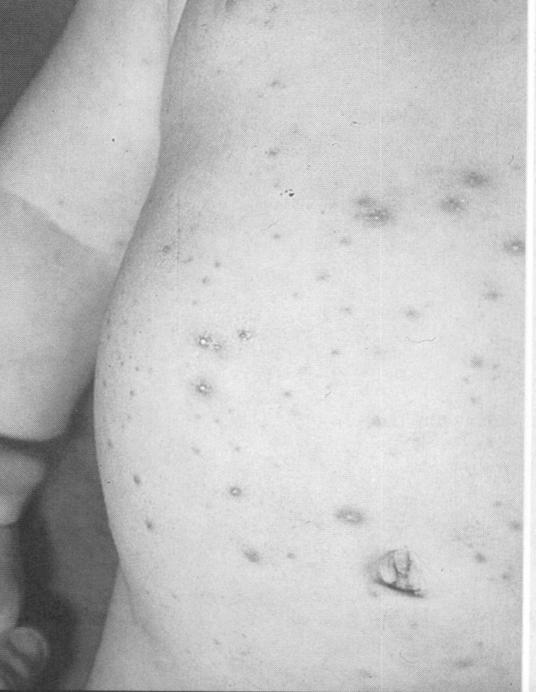

GLOSSARY

antiviral agents Substances used to treat viral infections by influencing viral replication.

black box warning A warning located in the *Physicians' Desk Reference* to alert physicians to high risks involved in administration of a particular drug.

highly active antiretroviral therapy (HAART) A substance that combines two reverse transcriptase inhibitors and one protease inhibitor in a cocktail that interrupts the human immunodeficiency virus in two different phases of its life cycle.

human immunodeficiency virus (HIV) The virus that causes acquired immunodeficiency syndrome.

lentiviruses A group of retroviruses that cause slow-developing diseases.

nucleoside reverse transcriptase inhibitors (NRTIs) Competitive inhibitors of the HIV enzyme that convert viral RNA into DNA and act as DNA chain terminators.

non-nucleoside reverse transcriptase inhibitors (NNRTIs) A substance that inhibits the action of the reverse transcriptase neuraminidase by preventing the formation of proviral DNA.

protease inhibitors A substance used to block the action of enzymes.

CHARACTERISTICS OF VIRUSES

Viruses are the smallest infectious agents. Because viruses lack independent metabolic activity and can replicate only within host cells, antiviral agents tend to injure host as well as viral cells. Unlike antibacterial agents, few antiviral drugs have been introduced over the years, and most are active against only one type of virus, either DNA or RNA viruses. A virus may infect the cells of animals, plants, or bacteria. Transmission of viruses can occur by direct contact, inhalation of airborne particles, or ingestion of contaminated food and water.

ANTIVIRAL AGENTS

Antiviral agents treat viral infections by influencing viral replication. Antiviral agents are the drug of choice for the following infections:

- Herpes simplex virus type 1 and 2
- Varicella-zoster virus
- Cytomegalovirus
- Influenza

The most commonly used agents against DNA viruses include acyclovir, amantadine, cidofovir, famciclovir, foscarnet, ganciclovir, oseltamivir, rimantadine, tenofovir, valacyclovir, valganciclovir, ribavirin, and zanamivir (see Table 20-1).

Acyclovir

Acyclovir is an antiviral agent that is used for initial and recurrent mucosal and cutaneous herpes simplex virus types 1 and 2 and herpes zoster infections in immunocompromised patients. Acyclovir is also used in herpes simplex encephalitis in patients older than 6 months of age and for acute herpes zoster (shingles) and chickenpox. It is contraindicated in patients allergic to this agent. Acyclovir should not be used in patients with seizures or renal disease or by women who are lactating. Adverse effects include headache, vertigo, depression, tremors, phlebitis at injection sites, and hair loss. Patients taking acyclovir may experience nausea, vomiting, diarrhea, or anorexia. Pharmacy technicians should have a basic understanding of herpes simplex and varicella-zoster infections.

TABLE 20-1. Most Commonly Used Antiviral Agents

GENERIC NAME	TRADE NAME
acyclovir	Zovirax®
amantadine	Symmetrel®
cidofovir	Vistide®
famciclovir	Famvir®
foscarnet	Foscavir®
ganciclovir	Cytovene®
oseltamivir	Tamiflu®
rimantadine	Flumadine®
tenofovir	Viread®
valacyclovir	Valtrex®
valganciclovir	Valcyte®
ribavirin	Virazole®
zanamivir	Relenza®

Amantadine

Amantadine is effective for influenza A viral infection. Influenza (also called the grippe or the flu), an acute, highly contagious infection of the respiratory tract, results from three different types of influenzae viruses. It occurs sporadically or in epidemics (usually during the colder months).

Although influenza affects all age groups, its incidence is highest in school children. However, its effects are most severe in very young patients, elderly patients, and those with chronic diseases. In these groups, influenza may even lead to death. Transmission of influenza occurs through inhalation of a respiratory droplet from an infected person or by indirect contact with a contaminated object, such as a drinking glass. Influenza viruses are classified into three groups: type A, type B, and type C.

Type A, the most prevalent, strikes every year, with new serotypes causing epidemics every 3 years. Type B and C are the genus of viruses of the family Orthomyxoviridae containing the agents of influenza B and C. Types A and B are responsible for epidemic disease, and among the influenza A viruses there are multiple subtypes (e.g., H1N1, H3N2). The occurrence of epidemic influenza type C virus is less common.

Amantadine inhibits replication of the influenza A virus by interfering with viral attachment and uncoating of the virus. This drug may also be used to treat some patients with parkinsonism. The most pronounced adverse effects of amantadine are nightmares, insomnia, ataxia, confusion, dizziness, headache, hypotension, dyspnea, urinary retention, edema, nausea, constipation, and dry mouth.

Cidofovir

Cidofovir suppresses cytomegalovirus (CMV) replication by selective inhibition of viral DNA synthesis. Use of this agent is limited to patients with acquired immunodeficiency syndrome (AIDS) and CMV retinitis. Cidofovir is contraindicated in patients with a history of severe hypersensitivity to probenecid or other sulfa-containing medications. It may cause nephrotoxicity and granulocytopenia. Cidofovir may also produce headache, palpitations, alopecia (loss of hair), nausea, vomiting, diarrhea, anorexia, dyspnea, chills, and fever. Probenecid must be administered with each cidofovir dose. The patient must be hydrated with 1 L of saline before infusion of cidofovir. Cidofovir is available only in intravenous form.

Famciclovir

Famciclovir is prescribed to treat acute herpes zoster (shingles), recurrent herpes simplex infection in immunocompromised patients, and genital herpes. Treatment is given for 5 to 7 days only. Common adverse effects include fatigue, nausea, diarrhea, vomiting, constipation, and anorexia. Other adverse effects may include nightmares, ataxia, coma, confusion, dizziness, headache, arrhythmia, hypertension or hypotension, rash, and alopecia.

Foscarnet

Foscarnet is a broad-spectrum antiviral agent and is the drug of choice for acyclovir- or ganciclovir-resistant infections. It is used to treat CMV infections in patients with human immunodeficiency virus (HIV) infection. Patients must be hydrated before foscarnet is infused. Intravenous foscarnet is highly nephrotoxic, causing acute tubular necrosis. It also may cause hypercalcemia, hypocalcemia, hypomagnesemia, and hyperphosphatemia. Other adverse effects include headache, seizures, tremor, ataxia, depression, confusion, insomnia, vision changes, taste abnormalities, nausea, vomiting, diarrhea, dry mouth, and melena (dark stool).

Ganciclovir

Ganciclovir is indicated for CMV infections, such as colitis, pneumonia, and retinitis. It is often prescribed for patients undergoing transplantation and for those with HIV infection. It is available in oral and intravenous formulations. The oral formulation is only approved for prevention and maintenance treatment of CMV infection. Ganciclovir has a **black box warning** concerning an increased potential for dose-limited neutropenia, anemia, and thrombocytopenia. (Black box warnings are prominently displayed in the *Physicians' Desk Reference* to alert practitioners to serious risks with certain drugs.) Solutions of ganciclovir are extremely alkaline. Direct contact with skin should be avoided.

Oseltamivir

Oseltamivir is an oral inhibitor of enzyme neuraminidase; it is indicated for the treatment of influenza A and B. It is not approved for use in children younger than 18 years of age or during pregnancy. The most common adverse effects are nausea and vomiting followed by vertigo and insomnia and also include nightmares, ataxia, coma, confusion, dizziness, and headache. Oseltamivir can also cause arrhythmia, hypertension, hypotension, nausea, vomiting, anorexia, diarrhea, and abdominal pain. Dosage adjustments are required for patients with impaired renal function.

Rimantadine

Rimantadine inhibits the early viral replication cycle, possibly inhibiting uncoating of the virus. Rimantadine is safe and effective in the prophylaxis against and treatment of infections caused by various strains of influenza A virus. The method of choice for prophylaxis against influenza is vaccination; however, in some patients use of the vaccine is contraindicated or it is not available. The most common adverse effects are nausea, vomiting, anorexia, insomnia, dizziness, and headache, which are less severe than those observed with amantadine. Dose reductions are recommended in patients with hepatic or renal dysfunction.

Tenofovir

Tenofovir is an antiviral agent that is used in the treatment of HIV-1 infection, in combination with other antiretroviral drugs. It is contraindicated in patients who are allergic to tenofovir, in those with renal insufficiency, and in women who are lactating. Tenofovir should be used cautiously in pregnant women and in patients with liver impairment. Adverse effects include headache, nausea, vomiting, diarrhea, anorexia, abdominal pain, and severe hepatomegaly.

Valacyclovir

Valacyclovir is active against herpes zoster in immunocompetent adults and is also used for genital herpes. An advantage of valacyclovir over acyclovir is that it can be given as an oral dose only once to three times daily. A disadvantage is that there is no intravenous form available. Valacyclovir is contraindicated in immunocompromised individuals such as those with advanced HIV infection or bone marrow transplant recipients. The most common adverse reactions are nausea, headache, anorexia, dizziness, and vomiting. Dosage adjustment is needed in patients with renal dysfunction.

Valganciclovir

Valganciclovir is an antiviral agent that may be used for the treatment of CMV retinitis in patients with AIDS. Valganciclovir is contraindicated in patients with hypersensitivity to this agent. It must be used cautiously in patients with impaired renal function, in pregnant women, and in elderly patients. Adverse effects include headache, insomnia, confusion, hallucinations, nausea, vomiting, diarrhea, fever, and anemia.

Ribavirin

Ribavirin is indicated for the treatment of respiratory syncytial virus. It is also used to relieve symptoms and speed recovery in young children with influenza A and B. It is absorbed systemically from the respiratory tract after nasal and oral inhalation. Ribavirin must be administered with a specific small-particle aerosol generator. Serious adverse effects include cardiac arrest, deterioration of pulmonary function, bacterial pneumonia, and apnea. It may also produce depression, suicidal behavior, nervousness, hypotension, rash, and anemia.

Zanamivir

Zanamivir is the first of a new class of antiviral agents called neuraminidase inhibitors. It is approved for the treatment of influenza A and B infections in patients who have been symptomatic for less than 48 hours. The drug is inhaled using a breath-activated plastic device called a Diskhaler. The recommended dosage is two inhalations daily, administered at 12-hour intervals for 5 days. It is not approved for use in children younger than 11 years of age or during pregnancy. The most common adverse effects are mild and include diarrhea, nausea, vomiting, headache, dizziness, anorexia, cough, rhinitis, bronchitis, and bronchospasm.

RNA VIRUSES

The most familiar of these viruses, called **lentiviruses,** is the **human immunodeficiency virus (HIV),** which causes AIDS. HIV infection is only one of a whole array of retroviruses associated with cancer and other diseases. With the sudden emergence of AIDS in the early 1980s, an enormous amount of public attention, research studies, and financial resources was focused on the HIV and the disease caused by it. The first patients with AIDS were seen by physicians in Los Angeles, San Francisco, and New York City. There are no conclusive answers to the question of where and how HIV originated. The first well-documented case of AIDS occurred in an African man in 1959. Today, AIDS has been reported in every country, and parts of Africa and Asia have been especially ravaged by it. Estimates of the number of individuals currently infected with HIV range from 35 to 40 million in the United States alone. Statistics show that AIDS in the United States is more common among males than females and that African Americans account for the most cases, followed by whites, Hispanics, and other groups. The average adult patient is about 35 years of age. AIDS is defined as a severe immunodeficiency disease arising from infection with HIV, accompanied by some of the following symptoms: life-threatening opportunistic infections, persistent fever, unusual cancers, chronically swollen lymph nodes, extensive weight loss, chronic diarrhea, and neurological disorders. So far, there is no cure for AIDS. None of the therapies do more than prolong life or diminish symptoms. Currently three classes of antiretroviral agents are approved for use in AIDS. These drugs are active against HIV and include the following:

- nucleoside reverse transcriptase inhibitors
- non-nucleoside reverse transcriptase inhibitors
- protease inhibitors

TABLE 20-2. Most Common Nucleoside Reverse Transcriptase Inhibitors

GENERIC NAME	TRADE NAME
abacavir	Ziagen®
zidovudine	Retrovir®
didanosine	Videx®
zalcitabine	Hivid®
stavudine	Zerit®
lamivudine	Epivir®, Epivir-HBV®

Nucleoside Reverse Transcriptase Inhibitors

The **nucleoside reverse transcriptase inhibitors (NRTIs)** include abacavir, zidovudine, didanosine, zalcitabine, stavudine, and lamivudine. The most commonly used NRTIs are shown in Table 20-2.

Abacavir

Abacavir is indicated for the treatment of HIV infection in both adult and pediatric patients. This agent is approved for use only in combination with other antiretroviral agents. Abacavir has good penetration into the CSF, unlike other agents in this class. The use of alcohol can increase the drug's toxicity, and patients must avoid alcohol entirely. Abacavir has a black box warning about a life-threatening hypersensitivity reaction that can lead to death. Adverse effects include headache, weakness, rash, diarrhea, anorexia, vomiting, dyspepsia, liver enlargement, dyspnea, pharyngitis, and severe hypersensitivity reactions.

Zidovudine

Zidovudine, formerly called azidothymidine (AZT), was the first available drug for the treatment of HIV infection in patients with AIDS and AIDS-related complex. Zidovudine is indicated for the prevention of maternal-fetal HIV transmission. It is used for the treatment of children older than 3 months of age and in combination with zalcitabine for the treatment of HIV infection. Zidovudine combined with lamivudine is prescribed for the prevention of HIV infection after a needlestick or sexual exposure. Zidovudine can cause severe bone marrow suppression. The most common adverse effects of this agent are headache, malaise, seizures, anxiety, fever, and rash.

Didanosine

Didanosine is approved for the treatment of patients with advanced HIV infection who cannot tolerate zidovudine or in whom zidovudine therapy has failed. Didanosine can cause reversible peripheral neuropathy and acute, lethal pancreatitis. Other adverse effects include headache, insomnia, hepatitis, and hyperuricemia. It must be taken on an empty stomach. Alcohol consumption will increase the risk of pancreatitis.

Zalcitabine

Zalcitabine is the least potent of the NRTIs and is not prescribed as often for HIV infections as the other NRTIs. The major clinical toxicity of zalcitabine is peripheral neuropathy. Pancreatitis may occur alone or in combination with zidovudine. Other adverse effects include esophageal ulcers, cardiomyopathy, anaphylactoid reactions, headache, insomnia, myalgia, dizziness, nausea, diarrhea, anorexia, vomiting, and oral ulcers.

Stavudine

Stavudine is indicated only for patients with advanced HIV infections who cannot tolerate other antiviral therapies. The major toxicity with stavudine is a dose-related peripheral neuropathy. Adverse effects may include headache, insomnia, myalgia, dizziness, peripheral neuropathy, nausea, diarrhea, anorexia, vomiting, dyspepsia, hepatomegaly, and pancreatitis. It may cause severe anemia, requiring transfusions.

Lamivudine

Lamivudine is indicated for use only in combination with zidovudine for the treatment of HIV infection with disease progression. It is also used for treatment of chronic hepatitis B. This agent must be taken exactly as prescribed. The adverse reactions are minor. Lamivudine has the fewest side effects of any of the NRTIs. The most common adverse reactions may include insomnia, headache, myalgia, dizziness, nausea, diarrhea, anorexia, vomiting, dyspepsia, pancreatitis, and hepatomegaly.

Non-Nucleoside Reverse Transcriptase Inhibitors

The **non-nucleoside reverse transcriptase inhibitors** (NNRTIs) include delavirdine, efavirenz, and nevirapine. They inhibit the action of the reverse transcriptase neuraminidase by preventing the formation of proviral DNA. These agents are indicated for use in adults and pediatric patients in combination with either NRTIs or protease inhibitors. Table 20-3 shows the most commonly used NNRTIs.

Delavirdine

Delavirdine is approved for use in the treatment of HIV infection in combination with other antiretroviral agents. It is a cytochrome P-450 inhibitor. It is important to review all medications before this agent is started because of its potential for numerous drug interactions. The most common adverse effects are minor and include headache, insomnia, malaise, dizziness, fatigue, nausea, diarrhea, vomiting, and dyspepsia. It also may cause anemia, arthralgia, and rash.

Efavirenz

Efavirenz is approved for use in combination with other antiretroviral agents for treatment of HIV infection in adults and pediatric patients older than 3 years of age. The most common adverse effects are insomnia, dizziness, drowsiness, nightmares, headache, depression, nausea, diarrhea, anorexia, vomiting, and liver impairment. It is only given once a day, preferably at bedtime. Individuals taking efavirenz should avoid high-fat meals.

Nevirapine

Nevirapine was the first NNRTI approved for use by the U.S. Food and Drug Administration (FDA) for the treatment of HIV infection. The most common adverse effects include rash, fever, nausea, vomiting, dry mouth, headache, and liver dysfunction. To decrease the occurrence of rash, nevirapine should be given at a low dose, which can then be increased to the appropriate therapeutic level.

Protease Inhibitors

Protease inhibitors include amprenavir, indinavir, nelfinavir, ritonavir, and saquinavir (see Table 20-4). These agents are either used together or in combination with other antiretroviral agents. Protease inhibitors are active against HIV protease. Saquinavir was the first protease inhibitor approved by the FDA. The most common adverse effects in

TABLE 20-3. Most Commonly Used Non-Nucleoside Reverse Transcriptase Inhibitors

GENERIC NAME	TRADE NAME
delavirdine	Rescriptor®
efavirenz	Sustiva®
nevirapine	Viramune®

TABLE 20-4. Most Commonly Used Protease Inhibitors

GENERIC NAME	TRADE NAME
amprenavir	Agenerase®
indinavir	Crixivan®
nelfinavir	Viracept®
ritonavir	Norvir®
saquinavir	Invirase®, Fortovase®

clinical trials were diarrhea, nausea, and abdominal discomfort. These agents can produce hyperglycemia.

Amprenavir

Amprenavir is a sulfonamide that has cross-sensitivity with other drugs in the sulfa class. Patients should not take supplemental vitamin E because there is a risk of vitamin E intoxication if taken with amprenavir.

Indinavir

Indinavir is an antiviral agent and is prescribed for the treatment of HIV infection when antiretroviral therapy is warranted. It may produce nausea, abdominal pain, headache, and diarrhea. It causes mild elevation of indirect bilirubin levels in patients, and kidney stones have been reported. Patients taking indinavir should drink at least 48 ounces of water daily to prevent nephrolithiasis.

Nelfinavir

Nelfinavir is used for the treatment of HIV infection when antiretroviral therapy is warranted. It has few adverse effects, with diarrhea being the major one.

Ritonavir

Ritonavir is used for treatment of HIV infection in combination with other antiretroviral agents. It can cause taste disturbance, anorexia, elevated triglyceride levels, peripheral paresthesias, headache, hypotension, syncope, tachycardia, and dry skin.

Saquinavir

Saquinavir should be administered with fatty foods to improve bioavailability. This agent is used for the treatment of HIV infection in combination with other antiretroviral agents. Side effects include headache, insomnia, myalgia, dizziness, fatigue, nausea, diarrhea, anorexia, vomiting, and dyspepsia.

Highly Active Antiretroviral Therapy

A regimen that has proved to be very effective in controlling AIDS and inevitable drug resistance is **highly active antiretroviral therapy (HAART)**. By combining two reverse transcriptase inhibitors and one protease inhibitor in a cocktail, the HIV is interrupted in two different phases of its life cycle. The therapy has been shown to successfully reduce viral loads to undetectable levels and to facilitate improvement of immune function. It has also reduced the rate of virus resistance to drugs and the incidence of deaths of patients with AIDS. Patients who are HIV-positive but asymptomatic can remain healthy with this therapy as well.

TABLE 20-5. The Combination Regimen Recommended for AIDS

COLUMN A	COLUMN B
Efavirenz (EFV)	Stavudine/Lamivudine (d4T/3TC)
Indinavir (IDV)	Zidovudine/Didanosine (AZT/ddI)
Nelfinavir (NFV)	Zidovudine/Lamivudine (AZT/3TC)
Ritonavir/Saquinavir (RTV/SQV)	Stavudine/Didanosine (d4T/ddI)

The primary drawbacks are high cost, toxic side effects, drug failure due to patient noncompliance, and the inability to completely eradicate the virus. Table 20-5 shows the initial regimen of combining two agents to control AIDS. In selection of the initial regimen, the recommendation is to include one agent from column A and one from column B.

AIDS Vaccine

From the very first years of the AIDS epidemic, the potential for a vaccine has been regarded warily, because the virus presents seemingly insurmountable problems for development of an effective vaccine. For example, it becomes latent in cells; its cell surface antigens mutate rapidly; and, although it does elicit immune responses, it is apparently not completely controlled by them. In view of the great need for a vaccine, none of those facts has stopped the medical community from moving ahead. Most of the 70 vaccines in various stages of development and testing are based on recombinant viruses and viral envelope or core antigens. The principal difficulties in human trials lie in determining the safety of the vaccine in volunteers and determining whether it stimulates effective cytotoxic T cells and neutralizing antibodies. One vaccine (AIDSVAX) that is currently being tested in Thailand is based on the surface antigen cloned in *Escherichia coli*.

CHARACTERISTICS OF FUNGI

Fungi are single-cell organisms similar to a human cell. There are three types of fungi: mushrooms, yeasts, and molds. Fungi lack chlorophyll. They produce spores. Human cell membranes contain cholesterol; fungi contain ergosterol. These organisms are able to cause systemic and local fungal (mycotic) infections.

Fungal Diseases

Some patients whose immune systems are weakened are susceptible to development of systemic fungal disease. The most common fungal agents and the diseases they cause are presented in Table 20-6.

TABLE 20-6. Most Common Fungi and Their Diseases

YEASTS	DISEASE
Candida	Thrush, vaginitis
Cryptococcus	Cryptococcosis (pneumonia, meningitis)
DIMORPHIC FUNGI	**DISEASE**
Histoplasma	Histoplasmosis
Blastomyces	Blastomycosis
Coccidioides	Coccidioidomycosis
MOLDS	**DISEASE**
Aspergillus	Aspergillosis (farmer's lung)
Mucor	Mucormycosis

TABLE 20-7. Most Commonly Used Antifungal Agents

GENERIC NAME	TRADE NAME	GENERIC NAME	TRADE NAME
amphotericin B	Fungizone®, Amphocin®	Amphotericin B	Amphotec®
flucytosin	Ancohon®	Butenafine	Mentax®
griseofulvin	Grisactin®, Fulvicin®	Ciclopirox	Loprox®
terbinafine	Lamisil®	Clotrimazole	Mycelex®, Lotrimin®
caspofungin	Cancidas®	Ketoconazole	Nizoral®
econazole	Spectazole®	Miconazole	Monistat®
fluconazole	Diflucan®	Nystatin	Nilstat®
itraconazole	Sporanox®	Terbinafine	Lamisil®
voriconazole	Vfend®		

Antifungal agents are classified in two groups: systemic agents and topical agents. The most common antifungal agents are listed in Table 20-7.

Systemic Antifungal Agents

Systemic fungal infections can occur throughout the body and usually have been growing for a period of time. There are two types of systemic infections: opportunistic infections of resident flora that cannot be fought by the body's immune system and occur in patients who are immunosuppressed, and nonopportunistic infections that can occur in any host.

Amphotericin B

Amphotericin B is a broad-spectrum antifungal agent. It is the most effective antifungal agent in the treatment of systemic fungal infections, especially in immunocompromised patients. It is the drug of choice for pulmonary *Aspergillus* infections; *Blastomyces* infections, which are life threatening in patients with AIDS; deep organ infections caused by *Candida;* and *Coccidioides* infections with severe pulmonary involvement. Amphotericin B is also effective against all *Cryptococcus* infections and disseminated *Histoplasma* infection. This agent may be used to treat coccidioidal arthritis. Topical preparations are given to eradicate cutaneous and mucocutaneous candidiasis. Amphotericin B can cause many serious adverse effects; it should be administered in a hospital setting, at least during the initial therapeutic stage. The drug must be infused slowly, not mixed with other drugs. Infusion reactions include fever, chills, hypotension, anorexia, nausea, vomiting, dyspnea, and tachypnea. Nephrotoxicity and electrolyte abnormalities occur often.

Caspofungin

Caspofungin is an anti-infective and antifungal agent used in the treatment of invasive aspergillosis in patients who cannot tolerate other antifungal therapies. It is contraindicated in patients with a known allergy to caspofungin and in pregnant and lactating women. Adverse reactions include phlebitis, thrombophlebitis, tachycardia, headache, insomnia, tremor, flushing, and rash. Patients who receive this agent may experience nausea, vomiting, abdominal pain, anorexia, and diarrhea. Other adverse reactions may include back pain, myalgia, fatigue, fever, and flu-like illness.

Econazole

Econazole is an antifungal agent used in the treatment of tinea pedis (athlete's foot), tinea corporis (ringworm), and cutaneous candidiasis. It is contraindicated in patients who have an allergy to this agent.

Fluconazole

Fluconazole is an antifungal agent that is used in the treatment of oropharyngeal, esophageal, and vaginal candidiasis. It is also prescribed for the treatment of cryptococcal meningitis. Therefore, fluconazole is indicated for local and systemic fungal infections. Prophylactic treatment is used to decrease the incidence of candidiasis in patients who have received bone marrow transplants. Fluconazole is contraindicated with in patients with hypersensitivity to this agent. It should be prescribed cautiously in patients with renal impairment. It is available as tablets, as a powder for oral suspension, and as an injection. Adverse effects include headache, nausea, vomiting, diarrhea, abdominal pain, and rash.

Flucytosine

Flucytosine is primarily active against *Cryptococcus* and *Candida.* It is most commonly used in conjunction with amphotericin B for severe systemic infections (for example, septicemia, endocarditis, pulmonary and urinary tract infections, and meningitis). Flucytosine should not be used alone. The most common side effects are rash and gastrointestinal upset.

Griseofulvin

Griseofulvin is effective for tinea infections of the skin, hair, and nails. This agent is given only for infections that do not respond to topical antifungal agents. It is available only in oral form. Griseofulvin can be used safely in children. The patient should avoid exposure to sunlight. The common side effects are headache, fatigue, dizziness, and drowsiness.

Itraconazole

Itraconazole is another systemic antifungal agent used in the treatment of blastomycosis and histoplasmosis in immunocompromised and nonimmunocompromised patients. It also is used in the treatment of aspergillosis in patients who cannot tolerate amphotericin B. Itraconazole is contraindicated in patients with hypersensitivity to this agent or in patients who have congestive heart failure. This agent must be used cautiously in patients with hepatic impairment. Adverse effects include headache, dizziness, nausea, vomiting, diarrhea, abdominal pain, anorexia, fever, and malaise.

Terbinafine

Terbinafine may be fungicidal or fungistatic depending on the drug concentration and species of fungus. Oral terbinafine is useful for infections of the toenail and fingernail. The topical form is used for treatment of athlete's foot and ringworm. It is applied to the affected area for at least 1 week. It should not be used vaginally. Adverse effects include headache, diarrhea, nausea, rash, dyspepsia, and taste disturbance.

Voriconazole

Voriconazole is an antifungal agent that may be prescribed for invasive aspergillosis or other serious fungal infections. Voriconazole is contraindicated in patients with hypersensitivity to the drug. It may cause severe hepatic dysfunction. Voriconazole also should not be used in patients taking the following drugs: ergot alkaloids, rifampin, carbamazepine, and long-acting barbiturates. It must be used cautiously in patients with known allergies to other azoles and in pregnant or lactating women. Adverse effects include headache, visual disturbance, hallucinations, dizziness, chest pain, and peripheral edema. Voriconazole may also cause nausea, vomiting, diarrhea, dry mouth, anemia, fever, and rash.

Topical Antifungal Agents

Topical fungal infections may be contracted from infected dust from soil, bird droppings, infected floors and showers, and the sharing of personal items such as hairbrushes and razors.

Amphotericin B

Amphotericin B is available as a 3% cream, lotion, or oral suspension. It is not absorbed through the gastrointestinal tract. It is used for oropharyngeal candidiasis, cutaneous and mucocutaneous candidal infections and in patients with progressive, potentially fatal infections such as cryptococcosis, blastomycosis, and histoplasmosis. It is contraindicated in patients with an allergy to this agent or those with renal dysfunction. Adverse effects include fever, headache, malaise, nausea, vomiting, dyspepsia, diarrhea, cramping, and weight loss. Amphotericin B may also cause hypokalemia, nephrocalcinosis (kidney stone), and anemia.

Butenafine

Butenafine is similar to terbinafine. The 1% cream is used in dermatophytoses. Butenafine should be applied to the affected area once a day for 4 weeks.

Ciclopirox

Ciclopirox is a synthetic antifungal agent that is chemically unrelated to any other antifungal agent. The drug is used either as a cream or as a "nail polish" to treat nail tissue infections. Local irritation is manifested by erythema, pruritus, burning, and blistering.

Clotrimazole

Clotrimazole is active against yeasts, dermatophytes, and some gram-positive bacteria. This agent is administered five times per day and is useful for treating oropharyngeal candidiasis. The cream, lotion, and solution are used to treat dermatophytosis, superficial mycoses, and cutaneous candidiasis. Intravaginal dosage forms are useful for treating vulvovaginal candidiasis. The troche is used for treatment of oropharyngeal candidiasis. It is contraindicated in patients who have an allergy to clotrimazole. Adverse effects include nausea, vomiting, and slight urinary frequency or irritation to the sexual partner.

Ketoconazole

Ketoconazole is an antifungal agent that is used for treatment of systemic fungal infections, such as candidiasis, chronic mucocutaneous candidiasis, oral thrush, blastomycosis, coccidioidomycosis, and histoplasmosis. It is also used for treatment of dermatophytosis. Ketoconazole is contraindicated in patients with an allergy to this agent and in women who are pregnant or breast feeding. The 2% topical cream or 2% shampoo may be used for treating fungal infection agents. The 2% shampoo is useful in reducing scaling due to dandruff. When combined with a steroid, ketoconazole is useful for treating atopic dermatitis, diaper rash, eczema, impetigo, and psoriasis. Adverse effects include abdominal pain, diarrhea, headache, dizziness, somnolence, fever, chills, and suicidal tendencies.

The topical cream may cause stinging, irritation, and pruritus. The shampoo may increase hair loss, irritation, and itching.

Miconazole

Miconazole is an antifungal agent used for local treatment of vulvovaginal candidiasis and for the treatment of tinea pedis and cutaneous candidiasis. The vaginal cream and vaginal suppositories are effective in treating vulvovaginal candidiasis. Topical creams may cause local irritation and burning, stinging, itching, pruritus, and pelvic cramps. It also produces headache and skin rash. The shampoo may increase hair loss, irritation, and itching. Miconazole nitrate is contraindicated in patients with an allergy to this agent. It should be used cautiously in women who are either pregnant or lactating. Adverse effects include abdominal pain, diarrhea, headache, dizziness, somnolence, fever, chills, and suicidal tendencies.

Nystatin

Nystatin is used primarily as a topical agent in vaginal and oral *Candida* infections. It is contraindicated in patients with an allergy to nystatin. It should be used cautiously in women who are pregnant or lactating. Adverse effects include nausea, vomiting, diarrhea, and vulvovaginal burning.

REVIEW QUESTIONS

1. For which of the following solution agents should direct contact with skin be avoided?
A. Oseltamivir
B. Ganciclovir
C. Amantadine
D. Acyclovir

2. Antiviral agents are the drug of choice for which of the following infections?
A. Cytomegalovirus
B. *Candida albicans*
C. Malaria
D. Aspergillosis

3. Which of the following fungi is classified as yeast?
A. *Histoplasma*
B. *Mucor*
C. *Aspergillus*
D. *Candida*

4. The trade name of amphotericin B is
A. Fungizone®.
B. Nilstat®.
C. Grisactin®.
D. Mentax®.

5. Which of the following antiviral agents was formerly called azidothymidine (AZT)?
A. Zalcitabine
B. Abacavir
C. Zidovudine
D. Lamivudine

6. Lamivudine is indicated in combination with zidovudine for the treatment of HIV infection and for which of the following diseases?
A. Chronic hepatitis B
B. Malaria
C. Chronic nephritis
D. Hepatitis A and C

7. The trade name of ketoconazole is
A. Nilstat®.
B. Lamisil®.
C. Loprox®.
D. Nizoral®.

8. Which of the following antifungal agents may be used for systemic and topical infections?
A. Butenafine
B. Ciclopirox
C. Amphotericin B
D. Ketoconazole

9. Which of the following antifungal agents may be useful as a shampoo in reducing scaling due to dandruff?
A. Nystatin
B. Ketoconazole
C. Terbinafine
D. Amphotericin B

10. Agents commonly used topically to treat topical fungal infections include
A. Flucytosine, ketoconazole, nystatin.
B. Nystatin, clotrimazole, butenafine.
C. Amphotericin B, clotrimazole, ketoconazole.
D. Moxalactam, mebendazole, miconazole.

Continues

11. Amantadine is effective against influenza A viral infection; it is also used to treat which of these diseases or conditions?
A. Parkinsonism
B. Insomnia
C. Anorexia
D. Hypotension

12. For which of the following antiviral agents must the patient be hydrated before infusion?
A. Zidovudine (AZT)
B. Amantadine
C. Nelfinavir
D. Foscarnet

13. *Candida* may cause
A. thrush.
B. Mucormycosis.
C. vaginitis.
D. A and C.

14. Which of the following is the trade of nystatin?
A. Monistat
B. Amphotec
C. Nilstat
D. Grisactin

Antineoplastic Drugs 21

OUTLINE

Neoplasms
Antineoplastic Agents
- Antimetabolites
- Hormonal Agents
- Antibiotics
- Alkylating Agents
- Mitotic Inhibitors (Plant Alkaloids)

Other Therapeutic Modalities
Toxicity
Specific Side Effects

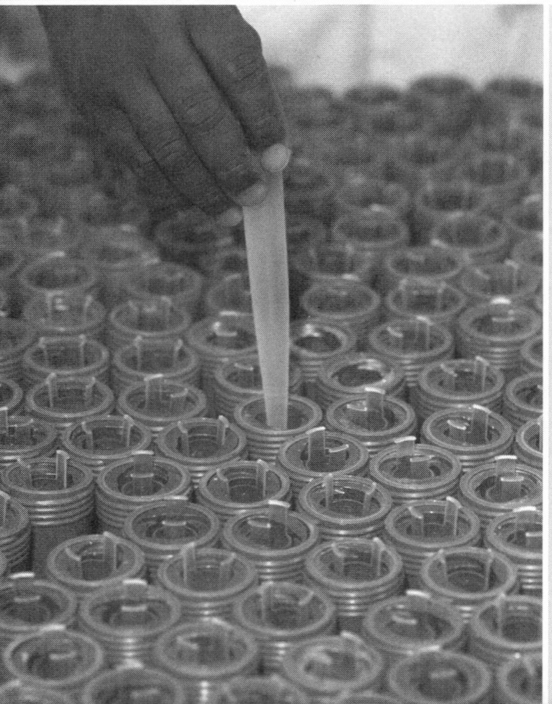

GLOSSARY

alkylating agents Antineoplastic drugs that affect cell growth.
antimetabolites Substances that prevent cancer growth by affecting DNA production.
antineoplastic agents Drugs used to treat cancers and malignant neoplasms.
benign Nonprogressive.
cardiac toxicity Adverse effects on the cardiovascular or hematopoietic systems that result from exposure to chemical substances.
extravasation Leakage of fluid from vessels into surrounding tissues.
hormonal agents Substances consisting of a heterogeneous compound that either blocks hormone production or blocks hormone action.
malignant Spreading.
metastasize Uncontrollable growth characteristic of cancer cells.
neoplasm A tumor.
nitrosoureas Newer forms of alkylating agents that are lipid soluble.
pulmonary toxicity Adverse effects on the functioning and structure of the pulmonary system that result from exposure to chemical toxins.

NEOPLASMS

A tumor, or **neoplasm**, arises from a single abnormal cell, which continues to divide indefinitely. The lack of growth controls, ability to invade local tissue, and ability to spread, or **metastasize,** are characteristics of cancer cells. These properties are not present in normal cells. Tumors are either **benign** (nonprogressive) or **malignant** (spreading). More than 100 different types of malignant neoplasms occur in humans. In treating cancers, multiple drug therapy is used to take advantage of drugs that have different mechanisms of action. To properly treat any type of cancer, the physician must think about two factors: the type of cancer and its stage. A biopsy or a blood specimen can determine the type of cancer. The extent of cancer progression is referred to as the stage.

ANTINEOPLASTIC AGENTS

Drugs used to treat cancers or malignant neoplasms are known as **antineoplastic agents**. There are many types of drug therapies for the treatment of cancer. The principal types of antineoplastic drugs are shown in Table 21-1.

Antineoplastic agents are also called chemotherapeutic agents. They interrupt the development, growth, or spread of cancer cells. Antineoplastic agents are used for malignant tumors. Treatment of cancer includes chemotherapy, surgery, and radiation therapy. Chemotherapy may reduce the size of malignant tumors and destroy the cancer cells. Antineoplastic agents do not kill tumor cells directly but interfere with cell replication. Each antineoplastic agent is effective at a specific stage of cell replication. It may inhibit DNA, RNA, and protein synthesis or cancer cells. Antineoplastic agents are most commonly given in combinations of two or more at a time. Many antineoplastic medications also have immunosuppressive properties that decrease the patient's ability to produce antibodies to attack infecting organisms. These medications are toxic to the body as a whole because they also destroy normal cells and decrease immunity.

Antimetabolites

Antimetabolites prevent cancer cell growth by affecting DNA production. They are only effective against cells that are actively participating in cell metabolism. The classes of antimetabolites include the following:

1. Folic acid antagonists: methotrexate
2. Purine antagonists: mercaptopurine
3. Pyrimidine antagonists: fluorouracil
4. Adenosine antagonists: fludarabine

Table 21-2 shows commonly used antimetabolites and routes of administration.

Methotrexate

Methotrexate (MTX) is one of the most versatile antineoplastic agents because it can be used for many malignancies. MTX is the only anticancer drug for which there is an antidote available to reduce toxicity. This antidote is leucovorin. Adverse effects include severe leukopenia, bone marrow aplasia, and thrombocytopenia.

Mercaptopurine

Mercaptopurine (6-MP) is an antimetabolite and antineoplastic agent that probably interferes with purine nucleotide synthesis to cause cell death. 6-MP is useful in maintenance

TABLE 21-2. Commonly Used Antimetabolites

GENERIC NAME	TRADE NAME	ROUTE OF ADMINISTRATION
methotrexate (MTX)	Rheumatrex®, Trexall®	Oral, IM, IV
mercaptopurine (6-MP)	Purinethol®	Oral
fluorouracil (5-FU)	Adrucil®, Efudex®, Fluoroplex®	IV, topical
fludarabine phosphate	Fludara®	IV

IM, intramuscular; IV, intravenous.

TABLE 21-1. Common Antineoplastic Agents

ANTIMETABOLITES	HORMONAL AGENTS	ANTIBIOTICS	ALKYLATING AGENTS	PLANT ALKALOIDS
Methotrexate	Corticosteroids	Doxorubicin	Nitrogen mustards	Vincristine
Mercaptopurine	Antiestrogens	Bleomycin	Nitrosoureas	Vinblastine
Fluorouracil	Antiandrogens	Dactinomycin	Busulfan	Vinorelbine
Fludarabine	Gonadotropin hormone	Mitomycin	Melphalan	Etoposide
		Plicamycin	Cyclophosphamide	
			Chlorambucil	

therapy of children with acute leukemia. It may cause anorexia, nausea, vomiting, hepatotoxicity, bone marrow depression, and hyperuricemia.

Fluorouracil

Fluorouracil (5-FU) is an antimetabolite and antineoplastic agent. It inhibits DNA synthesis and cell death. It penetrates cerebrospinal fluid well. 5-FU metabolizes in the liver to inactive compounds. It is therapeutically useful in certain types of carcinoma, such as carcinoma of the colon, rectum, breast, stomach, and pancreas. Topical application of 5-FU is useful for treatment of premalignant keratoses, superficial basal cell carcinomas, and severe psoriasis. 5-FU causes marked myelosuppression. It can also result in gastrointestinal tract disturbances, alopecia, dermatitis, and nail changes.

Fludarabine

Fludarabine is an antimetabolic and antineoplastic agent that inhibits DNA synthesis and prevents cell replication. It is used for chronic lymphocytic leukemia. Adverse effects include weakness, headache, hearing loss, sleep disorders, and depression. It may also cause bone marrow toxicity, pneumonia, dyspnea, nosebleed (epistaxis), and edema.

Hormonal Agents

Hormonal agents are a class of heterogeneous compounds that have varying effects on cells. These agents either block hormone production or block hormone action. Their action on malignant cells is highly selective. They are the least toxic of the anticancer medications. Hormones and their antagonists have various uses in the treatment of malignant diseases. Steroids are especially useful in treating acute lymphocytic leukemia. They are also used in conjunction with radiation therapy to reduce radiation edema. Sex hormones are used in carcinomas of the reproductive tract; for example, estrogen is given to a patient with testicular cancer or carcinoma of the prostate. Estrogen may also be administered to postmenopausal women with breast cancer. Androgens, male hormones, are prescribed for premenopausal women with breast cancer. Major side effects include masculization of the female and feminization of the male. Estrogen therapy may cause blood clots. Antiestrogens, such as tamoxifen, and antiandrogens are used to inhibit hormone production in advanced stages of cancer. Tamoxifen is prescribed for breast cancer and increases the risk of endometrial cancer; it must be used with caution. The most commonly used hormonal agents in cancer therapy are seen in Table 21-3.

TABLE 21-3. Most Commonly Used Hormones in Cancer

GENERIC NAME	TRADE NAME	ROUTE OF ADMINISTRATION
Androgens		
Fluoxymesterone	Halotestin®, Android-F®	Oral
Testolactone	Teslac®	Oral
Antiandrogens		
Flutamide	Eulexin®	Oral
Nilutamide	Nilandron®	Oral
Progestins		
Medroxyprogesterone acetate	Depo-Provera®	Oral, IM
Megestrol acetate	Megace®	Oral
Estrogens		
Diethylstilbestrol	Stilphostrol®	Oral, IV
Estramustine	Emcyt®	Oral
Polyestradiol	Estradurin®	IM
Antiestrogens		
Goserelin implant	Zoladex®	SC
Letrozole	Femara®	Oral
Tamoxifen	Nolvadex®	Oral
Toremifene	Fareston®	Oral
Gonadotropin-releasing hormone analog		
Leuprolide acetate	Lupron®	SC, IM
Corticosteroids		
Dexamethasone	Decadron®	Oral, IM, IV
Prednisone	Deltasone®, Orasone®	Oral

IM, intramuscular; IV, intravenous; SC, subcutaneous.

Antibiotics

Several antibiotics of microbial origin are very effective in the treatment of certain tumors. They are used only to treat cancer and are not used to treat infections. These antibiotics include bleomycin, doxorubicin, daunorubicin, mitomycin, and plicamycin. Their mechanism of action is to inhibit DNA and RNA synthesis. Table 21-4 shows generic names, brand names, and routes of administration of some antibiotics that affect cancer cells.

Bleomycin

Bleomycin is an antineoplastic and antibiotic agent. Bleomycin is among the commonly used anticancer drugs. It is a toxic drug with a low therapeutic index and is very cytotoxic. This antibiotic is widely used in combination with other chemotherapeutic drugs because it lacks significant myelosuppressive activity. Bleomycin is used in squamous cell carcinomas of the head, neck, penis, cervix, and vulva. It is also used for the treatment of lymphomas and testicular carcinoma. Adverse effects include ulcerations of the tongue and lips, nausea, vomiting, diarrhea, and weight loss. It may cause pneumonia and alopecia.

TABLE 21-4. Antibiotics That Affect Cancer Cells

GENERIC NAME	TRADE NAME	ROUTE OF ADMINISTRATION
bleomycin	Blenoxane®	SC, IM, IV
doxorubicin	Adriamycin®, Rubex®, Doxil®	IV
dactinomycin (actinomycin D)	Cosmegen®	IV
mitomycin	Mutamycin®	IV
plicamycin	Mithracin®, Mithramycin®	IV

IM, intramuscular; IV, intravenous; SC, subcutaneous.

TABLE 21-5. Alkylating and Alkylating-Like Drugs

GENERIC NAME	TRADE NAME	ROUTE OF ADMINISTRATION
nitrogen mustard (mechlorethamine)	Mustargen®	IV
cyclophosphamide	Cytoxan®, Neosar®	Oral, IV
chlorambucil	Leukeran®	Oral
busulfan	Myleran®	Oral
melphalan	Alkeran®	Oral

IV, intravenous.

Doxorubicin

Doxorubicin is the single most active agent against breast cancer. It is a cytotoxic antibiotic with a wide spectrum of antitumor activity and strong immunosuppressive properties. It is used in the treatment of acute lymphoblastic and myeloblastic leukemias, soft tissue and bone cancer, carcinomas of the breast and ovary, and lymphomas. It is generally used in combination with surgery, radiation, and immunotherapy. Doxorubicin may cause serious, irreversible myocardial toxicity, hypertension, and hypotension. It also produces nausea, vomiting, diarrhea, severe myelosuppression, and hypersensitivity or anaphylactoid reactions.

Dactinomycin

Dactinomycin is a potent cytotoxic antibiotic. It inhibits DNA, RNA, and protein synthesis. Dactinomycin is used as a single agent or in combination with other antineoplastic agents or radiation to treat carcinoma of the testes and uterus. Adverse effects include nausea, vomiting, abdominal pain, diarrhea, and ulceration of the tongue. Hepatitis and aplastic anemia may occur with use of dactinomycin.

Mitomycin

Mitomycin is a potent antibiotic, antineoplastic compound. It is effective in certain tumors that are nonresponsive to surgery, radiation, or other chemotherapeutic agents. Its mechanism of action is not known. Mitomycin is used in combination with other chemotherapeutic agents in palliative, adjunctive treatment of cancer of the breast, stomach, and pancreas. Adverse effects include nausea, vomiting, bone marrow toxicity, asthma, and pneumonia.

Plicamycin

Plicamycin is a cytotoxic, antibiotic, and antineoplastic agent. It appears to block the hypercalcemic action of vitamin D and may inhibit the effect of parathyroid hormone on bone cells (osteoclasts). Plicamycin may interfere with synthesis of various clotting factors. Its high toxicity and low therapeutic index limit its clinical use. Plicamycin is used to treat hypercalcemia or hypercalcinuria associated with advanced neoplasms and to treat testicular malignancy. Drowsiness, irritability, dizziness, headache, and mental depression are common side effects of plicamycin. It can also cause nausea, vomiting, diarrhea, and intestinal hemorrhage.

Alkylating Agents

Alkylating agents were the first group of antineoplastic agents. During World War I, chemical warfare using nitrogen mustard was introduced. After observation of the effects these gases had on cell growth, alkylating agents came to be used for cancer therapy. They are used to treat metastatic ovarian, testicular, and bladder cancers. They are also used for the palliative treatment of other cancers. The newer drugs in this category are **nitrosoureas,** lipid-soluble drugs used in treating brain tumors and testicular or ovarian cancers. The major side effects of the alkylating agents include nausea, vomiting, diarrhea, bone marrow suppression, hepatic and renal toxicity, and dermatitis. Subclassifications of alkylating agents are listed in Table 21-5.

Nitrogen Mustards

Nitrogen mustards are alkylating agents. The major cytotoxic and mustagenic effects of these agents may result from their interactions with DNA. Mechlorethamine is the most rapidly acting and must be freshly prepared and administered into a rapidly flowing intravenous line. If extravasated, it can cause severe local tissue damage. Its clinical use has been limited to the treatment of Hodgkin's disease. The dose-limiting toxicity of nitrogen mustards is bone marrow suppression. The major long-term toxicities of this drug, as with all akylating agents, are gonadal damage and an increased risk of secondary malignancies, in particular, acute leukemia.

Cyclophosphamide

Cyclophosphamide, unlike nitrogen mustard, has a wide spectrum of antitumor and immunosuppressive activity. It is used as part of combination therapy regimens to treat lymphoma, breast cancer, bladder cancer, and ovarian cancer. Long-term toxicity includes sterility and carcinogenesis.

Chlorambucil

Chlorambucil is a slow-acting nitrogen mustard. Chlorambucil is administered orally, and it is absorbed well. It is used primarily to treat chronic lymphocytic leukemia and low-grade lymphomas. Chlorambucil is well tolerated and usually does not cause nausea or vomiting.

Busulfan

The predominant effect of busulfan is bone marrow suppression, with little other pharmacological action. It is used exclusively to treat chronic myelocytic leukemia. This agent is well absorbed orally. Busulfan has some unusual side effects in addition to its bone marrow suppressive activity. It may cause generalized skin pigmentation, gynecomastia (enlargement of the male breasts), and pulmonary fibrosis.

Melphalan

Melphalan is well absorbed orally, and its major use has been for the treatment of multiple myeloma (a cancer of the white blood cells that causes abnormal plasma cells to develop), usually in combination with prednisone. It has also been used to treat breast cancer and melanoma. Nausea and vomiting are rare with this agent as is hair loss. The major toxicity is similar to that of other alkylating agents (i.e., bone marrow suppression).

Mitotic Inhibitors (Plant Alkaloids)

Mitotic inhibitors are derived from plants. The primary plant alkaloids are vincristine and vinblastine. Teniposide is an analog closely related to etoposide and is active against acute leukemias in children. Topotecan is a semisynthetic plant alkaloid, used for refractory ovarian cancer, and may have activity against small-cell lung cancer. Vinblastine is toxic to the bone marrow. Vincristine is toxic to the peripheral nerves. Most plant alkaloids may cause nausea and vomiting, particularly vinblastine. Examples of plant alkaloids are seen in Table 21-6.

Vinblastine

Vinblastine is a mitotic inhibitor and antineoplastic agent. It is used for the treatment of Hodgkin's disease, lymphoma, and advanced testicular carcinoma. Peripheral neuritis, mental depression, headache, seizures, and loss of hair are common adverse effects.

TABLE 21-6. Mitotic Inhibitors (Plant Alkaloids)

GENERIC NAME	BRAND NAME	ROUTE OF ADMINISTRATION
vinblastine	Velban®, Velsar®, Alkaban®	IV
vincristine	Oncovin®	IV
vinorelbine	Navelbine®	IV
etoposide	VePesid®	IV

IV, intravenous.

Vincristine

Vincristine is a mitotic inhibitor and antineoplastic agent. It is used for treatment of acute leukemia, Hodgkin's disease, and non-Hodgkin's lymphoma. Adverse effects include headache, convulsions, foot drop, optic atrophy, and photophobia. Vincristine can also cause constipation, oral ulcerations, vomiting, and diarrhea.

Vinorelbine

Vinorelbine is an antineoplastic and mitotic inhibitor agent. It is the first-line treatment for ambulatory patients with lung cancer. Adverse effects include numbness, headache, weakness, and dizziness. Nausea, vomiting, pharyngitis, diarrhea, constipation, and abdominal pain may also occur.

Etoposide

Etoposide is a mitotic inhibitor and antineoplastic agent. Etoposide is used for the treatment of refractory testicular tumors as part of combination therapy. Adverse effects include hypotension, fatigue, alopecia, nausea, vomiting, and liver toxicity.

OTHER THERAPEUTIC MODALITIES

For cancer treatment, other therapeutic modalities include surgery and radiation therapy.

The purpose of surgery may be diagnosis, such as a biopsy or exploratory laparotomy for a "second look," or therapy, such as tumor debulking or removal. Surgery is often combined with chemotherapy and/or radiation.

Radiation therapy involves application of high doses of ionizing radiation to the cancerous tissue. Radiation may be combined with surgery and/or chemotherapy, depending upon the area of the body being irradiated. Adverse reactions may include stomatitis (inflammation of the oral mucosa), nausea and vomiting, diarrhea, and bone marrow suppression.

TOXICITY

It is not possible to stop antineoplastic agents from attacking normal cells as well as tumor cells. The principles that apply to antitumor efficacy also apply to the toxicity of these agents. The bone marrow, lymphoblasts, mucous membranes, skin, and gonads are affected to a greater extent than other cells. Bone marrow depression is a major adverse effect of antineoplastic drugs. Skin toxicity includes alopecia (loss of hair), commonly seen in patients receiving chemotherapy. Local necrosis may result from **extravasation** of vesicant chemotherapy drugs during their administration. Cancer chemotherapy can also cause skin changes such as dryness and sensitivity to sunlight. Aspermia and amenorrhea (the absence of menstrual periods) are commonly caused by some antineoplastic agents. Immunosuppression makes the patient more vulnerable to infection. About 50% of patients with cancer die of intercurrent infections rather than from the terminal phases of the neoplastic disease. Certain antineoplastic drugs are mutagenic and carcinogenic, and the patient is subjected to the risk of future neoplasias. Hyperuricemia or renal damage may result from some antineoplastic agents. Massive destruction of certain leukemic cells may also cause an acute hypotensive crisis that is sometimes called anaphylaxis, even though it is not a true allergic response. Hypersensitivity reactions may occur with any chemotherapy agent. Life-threatening reactions, including anaphylaxis, appear to be more common with cisplatin, etoposide, paclitaxel, and teniposide. **Pulmonary toxicity** is generally irreversible and may be fatal. **Cardiac toxicity** includes irreversible congestive heart failure. Risk factors include chest irradiation and high cumulative doses of cardiotoxic chemotherapy agents.

TABLE 21-7. Specific Side Effects of Some Antineoplastic Drugs

ANTINEOPLASTIC DRUGS	SIDE EFFECTS
doxorubicin	Cardiotoxicity
bleomycin	Pneumonitis
cyclophosphamide	Hemorrhagic cystitis
vincristine	Peripheral neuropathy
cisplatin	Renal toxicity

SPECIFIC SIDE EFFECTS

Certain antineoplastic agents have specific effects on particular organs or systems in the body. Examples include doxorubicin (cardiotoxicity), bleomycin (pneumonitis), cyclophosphamide (hemorrhagic cystitis), vincristine (peripheral neuropathy), and cisplatin (renal toxicity) (see Table 21-7).

REVIEW QUESTIONS

1. The major side effect of bleomycin is
A. pneumonitis.
B. hemorrhagic cystitis.
C. renal toxicity.
D. peripheral neuropathy.

2. Drugs used to treat cancers are called
A. antipyretic agents.
B. antineoplastic agents.
C. anticoagulant agents.
D. antiemetic agents.

3. An example of a nitrogen mustard is
A. busulfan.
B. streptozocin.
C. carboplatin.
D. chlorambucil.

4. Mitotic inhibitors (plant alkaloids) include
A. mitomycin.
B. fluorouracil (5-FU).
C. bleomycin.
D. vincristine.

5. Which of the following is an example of an androgen?
A. Leuprolide
B. Prednisone
C. Testosterone
D. A and B

6. An adverse effect of methotrexate is
A. bone marrow aplasia.
B. alopecia.
C. hypertension.
D. hypothyroidism.

7. Busulfan has some unusual side effects in addition to its bone marrow suppressive activity. Which of the following side effects are caused by busulfan?
A. Skin pigmentation
B. Testicular cancer
C. Gynecomastia
D. A and C

Continues

8. The primary plant alkaloids include
A. topotecan.
B. vincristine.
C. paclitaxel.
D. etoposide.

9. The route of administration for methotrexate (MTX) is
A. oral.
B. intramuscular.
C. intravenous.
D. all of the above.

10. Most plant alkaloids may produce
A. nausea and vomiting.
B. internal bleeding.
C. hypertension.
D. gout.

11. Which of the following antimetabolites is useful in maintenance therapy for children with acute leukemia?
A. Fluorouracil (5-FU)
B. Methotrexate (MTX)
C. Mercaptopurine (6-MP)
D. Vincristine

12. A patient with testicular cancer may be given
A. testosterone.
B. estrogen.
C. progesterone.
D. estramustine.

Allergy and Respiratory Drugs 22

OUTLINE

Effects of Allergies on the Respiratory System
Allergic Rhinitis
Asthma
Histamine
Antihistamines
Antitussives
Anti-Inflammatory Agents
Bronchodilators
Asthmatic Prophylaxis
Leukotriene Antagonists
Xanthine Derivatives
β-Adrenergic Agents
Mucolytics and Expectorants
Decongestants
Intranasal Steroids
Drugs for Smoking Cessation

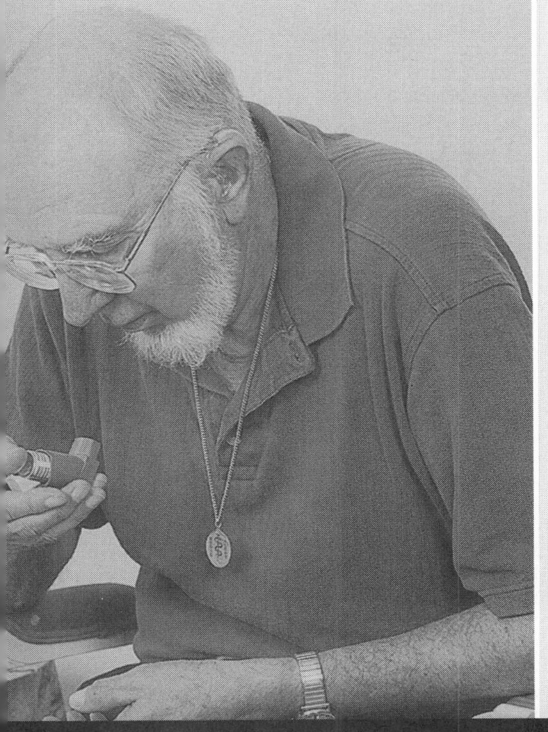

GLOSSARY

allergic rhinitis Inflammation of the nasal mucosa that is due to the sensitivity of the nasal tissue to an allergen.
allergy A state of hypersensitivity induced by exposure to a particular antigen.
antigen A substance that is introduced into the body and induces the formation of antibodies.
antihistamines Drugs that counteract the action of histamine.
antitussives Agents that relieve or prevent coughing.
asthma A chronic, reversible obstruction of the bronchial airways that is characterized by paroxysmal attacks of dyspnea or difficult respiration on expiration.
β-adrenergic agents A drug that works as both a cardiac and respiratory agonist.
bronchodilators Agents that relax the smooth muscle of the bronchial tubes.
corticosteroids The most potent and consistently effective anti-inflammatory agents that are currently available for relief in respiratory conditions.
decongestants Drugs that cause vasoconstriction of nasal mucosa and reduces congestion or swelling.
dry powder inhaler (DPI) A device used to deliver medication in the form of micronized powder into the lungs.
expectorants Agents that promote the removal of mucous secretions from the lung, bronchi, and trachea, usually by coughing.
histamine A chemical substance found in all the body tissues that protects the body from factors in the environment that produce allergic and inflammatory reactions.
leukotrienes Substances that contribute to the inflammation associated with asthma.

metered dose inhaler (MDI) A hand-held pressurized device used to deliver medications for inhalation.
mucolytic Destroying or dissolving the active agents that constitute mucus.
xanthine derivatives A substance that is effective for relief of bronchospasm in asthma, chronic bronchitis, and emphysema.

EFFECTS OF ALLERGIES ON THE RESPIRATORY SYSTEM

The most important function of the respiratory system is the inspiration of oxygen and the expiration of carbon dioxide. Therefore, the respiratory tract must exchange gases and supply oxygen to the body. The effectiveness of the respiratory system affects the body's ability to function correctly and be in homeostasis. Allergic reactions occur throughout the body, but they also commonly involve individuals who are suffering from respiratory tract disorders such as rhinorrhea and allergic bronchitis.

An **allergy** is a state of hypersensitivity induced by exposure to a particular **antigen** (a substance that is introduced into the body and induces the formation of antibodies), resulting in harmful immunologic reactions on subsequent exposure. The term is usually used to refer to hypersensitivity to an environmental antigen. There are varieties of allergic reactions such as allergic rhinitis, allergic conjunctivitis, allergic asthma, and allergic dermatitis. Because this chapter focuses on respiratory disorders and drug therapy, allergic rhinitis and allergic asthma will be discussed.

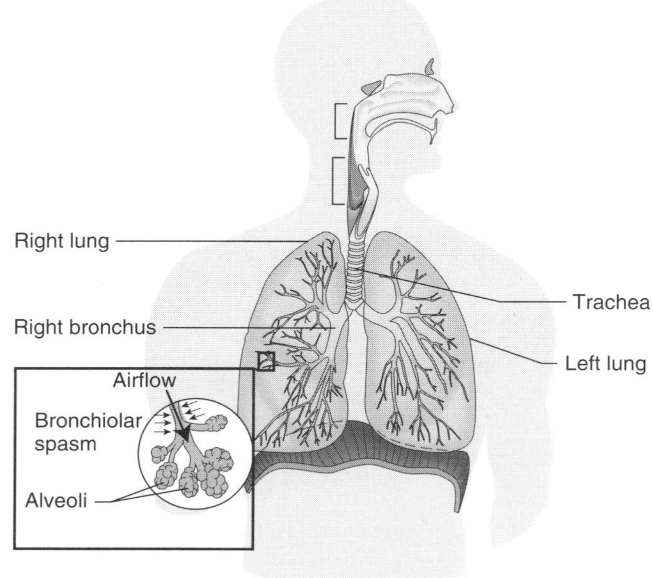

Figure 22-1. Asthma is a disease that involves bronchospasm and excessive airway secretions.

ALLERGIC RHINITIS

Allergic rhinitis is inflammation of the nasal mucosa that is due to the sensitivity of the nasal tissue to an allergen. It is usually associated with watery nasal discharge and itching of the nose and eyes, caused by a localized sensitivity reaction to house dust, animal dander, or an antigen, commonly pollen. The condition may be seasonal and is commonly known as "hay fever."

ASTHMA

Chronic obstructive pulmonary disease is a commonly used term for respiratory diseases such as asthma, emphysema, and chronic bronchitis. **Asthma** is a reversible lung disease characterized by obstruction or narrowing of the airways, which are typically inflamed and hyperresponsive to a variety of stimuli. It may resolve spontaneously or with treatment (see Figure 22-1).

Its symptoms range from mild wheezing and shortness of breath due to constriction of the bronchioles to life-threatening respiratory failure. Asthma is most commonly classified as allergic, exercise-induced, or caused by infections of the respiratory tract and salicylates. Symptoms include breathlessness, cough, wheezing, and chest tightness. The airway becomes inflamed with edema and mucous plugs, and hyperactivity of the bronchial tree adds to the symptoms. During asthma attacks, when bronchiole constriction and increased secretions are present, bronchodilators are used for relief. Anti-inflammatory drugs, such as corticosteroids and cromolyn, may be prescribed for relief of symptoms. The majority of medications for asthma are administered by inhalation. Antiasthma medications can be divided into two categories: long-term control and quick-relief medications.

HISTAMINE

Histamine is a chemical substance found in all the body tissues that protects the body from factors in the environment which produce allergic and inflammatory reactions. The greatest concentration of histamine is in the skin, lungs, and gastrointestinal tract. Histamine has several functions, including the following:

- Dilation of capillaries, which increases capillary permeability and results in hypotension
- Contraction of most smooth muscle of the bronchial tree and the gastrointestinal tract
- Induction of increased gastric secretion
- Acceleration of the heart rate

There are two types of histamines in our body, one that causes allergic reactions in the respiratory tract and another that works on the gastrointestinal tract (see Chapter 25). The free histamines play a role in the inflammatory process and defend exposed tissue from injury by damaging agents. Both H1 and H2 receptors mediate the contraction of vascular smooth muscle. Histamine has also been postulated to be a neurotransmitter in the central nervous system.

ANTIHISTAMINES

Drugs that counteract the action of histamine are called **antihistamines**. There are two types of antihistamines. The conventional ones, those used in allergies, block H_1 histamine receptors. The second type are block H_2 receptors, which are formed in the gastrointestinal tract. Antihistamines appear to compete with histamine for cell receptor sites on effector cells. Histamine-related allergic reactions and tissue injury are blocked or diminished in intensity. Antihistamines are used to relieve symptoms resulting from the release of histamine. Antihistamines are not effective against histamines that are already attached to the receptor sites, so the drug is most effective if taken before contact with the allergy-causing compounds. Therefore, these medications are more likely to be effective at the beginning of the allergy season. Allergic rhinitis is treated with antihistamines, decongestants, and nasal preparations. Antihistamines are also prescribed for relieving symptoms of allergies to insect bites and contact dermatitis. Some of these products are sedative agents, and one of the major side effects is drowsiness. Many over-the-counter (OTC) drugs contain antihistamines for sleeping aids (e.g., Nytol®). Other OTC antihistamines are used to relieve nausea, vomiting, and motion sickness. Antihistamines may cause drowsiness, dizziness, headaches, and photosensitivity. They may cause the respiratory tract to dry and mucus to thicken; therefore, the patient taking antihistamines should drink plenty of fluids to thin secretions and keep tissues moist. Table 22-1 shows classes of antihistamines.

TABLE 22-1. Classification of Antihistamines

GENERIC NAME	TRADE NAME	ROUTE OF ADMINISTRATION
First-generation Drugs		
azatadine*	Optimine®	Oral
brompheniramine†	Dimetane®	Oral
chlorpheniramine†	Chlor-Trimeton®	Oral
clemastine*,†	Tavist®	Oral
dexchlorpheniramine†	Polaramine®	Oral
dimenhydrinate*	Dramamine®	Oral
diphenhydramine*,†	Benadryl®	Oral
meclizine*,†	Antivert®, Bonine®	Oral
phenindamine†	Nolahist®	Oral
trimeprazine*	Temaril®	Oral
triprolidine/pseudoephedrine*	Actifed®	Oral
doxylamine*	Unisom®	Oral
Second-generation Drugs		
cetirizine*	Zyrtec®	Oral
fexofenadine*	Allegra®	Oral
loratadine†	Claritin®	Oral
Second-generation Drugs with Decongestant		
fexofenadine/pseudoephedrine	Allegra D®	Oral
loratadine/pseudoephedrine	Claritin D®	Oral

*Prescription drug.
†OTC drug.

ANTITUSSIVES

Agents that relieve or prevent coughing are called **antitussives**. The initial stimulus for cough probably arises in the bronchial mucosa, where irritation results in bronchoconstriction. Antitussives are classified into two major groups: opioid and nonopioid. The opioid cough suppressants decrease sensitivity of the central cough center to peripheral stimuli. They decrease mucosal secretions. An antitussive action occurs at doses that are lower than that required for analgesia. Examples of opiates are codeine, hydrocodone, and chlorpheniramine/hydrocodone. Side effects include constipation, nausea, and respiratory depression. Nonopioid cough suppressants do not have the gastrointestinal side effects of the codeine preparations and are nonaddicting. Examples of nonopioid cough suppressants are dextromethorphan, benzonatate, and diphenhydramine. Dextromethorphan is generally well absorbed and is the most effective of the nonopioid cough suppressants. This agent does not suppress respiration. Dextromethorphan causes less constipation than codeine. Benzonatate is chemically similar to procaine. It reduces the activity of peripheral cough receptors and also appears to increase the threshold of the central cough center. Diphenhydramine is sedating and has anticholinergic properties. The cough suppression comes with the sedation. Antitussives are also used to treat or prevent motion sickness, vertigo, and reactions to blood or plasma in susceptible patients. Cough suppression agents are classified in Table 22-2.

TABLE 22-2. Classification of Cough Suppressants

GENERIC NAME	TRADE NAME	ROUTE OF ADMINISTRATION
Opioids		
codeine*,†	Various with codeine	Oral
hydrocodone*	Hycodan®, Histussin®, Atuss HD®	Oral
chlorpheniramine hydrocodone	Tussionex®	Oral
Nonopioids		
dextromethorphan†	Sucrets Cough®, Benylin DM®, Robitussin DM®	Oral
diphenhydramine†	Benadryl®, Benylin®	Oral
benzonatate*	Tessalon®	Oral

*Prescription drug.
†OTC drug.

ANTI-INFLAMMATORY AGENTS

Corticosteroids are the most potent and consistently effective anti-inflammatory agents that are currently available for relief in respiratory conditions. These agents are administered by inhalation. There are three devices for inhalation administration: metered dose inhalers, dry powder inhalers, and nebulizers. Drug administration with a **metered dose inhaler (MDI)** is often accomplished with one or two puffs from a hand-held pressurized device (see Figure 22-2). **Dry powder inhalers (DPIs)** deliver medication in the form of micronized powder into the lungs. Medications such as cromolyn and albuterol are available for use this way. DPIs are breath-activated and are easier to use than MDIs. A nebulizer uses a small machine that converts a solution into a mist. The mist droplets are inhaled either through a face mask or through a mouthpiece (see Figure 22-3). Inhaled corticosteroids are preferred for the long-term control of asthma and are first-line agents for treatment of persistent asthma. Dosages for inhaled corticosteroids vary, depending on the specific agent and delivery device. Systemic corticosteroids are most effective for long-term asthma therapy. Long-term use of inhaled corticosteroids in children is not recommended because these agents may suppress growth and suppress production of hormones by the adrenal glands. Examples of inhaled corticosteroids are seen in Table 22-3.

Adverse reactions to corticosteroid inhalation include nasal irritation and dryness, headache, nausea, epistaxis, dizziness, hoarseness, and cough.

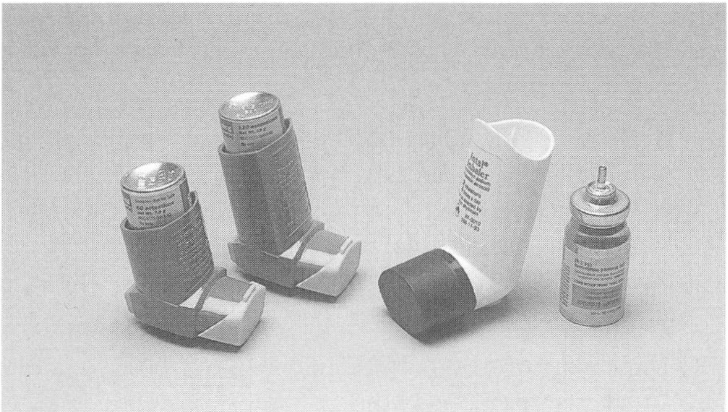

Figure 22-2. A metered dose inhaler allows aerosolization of a liquid for inhalation.

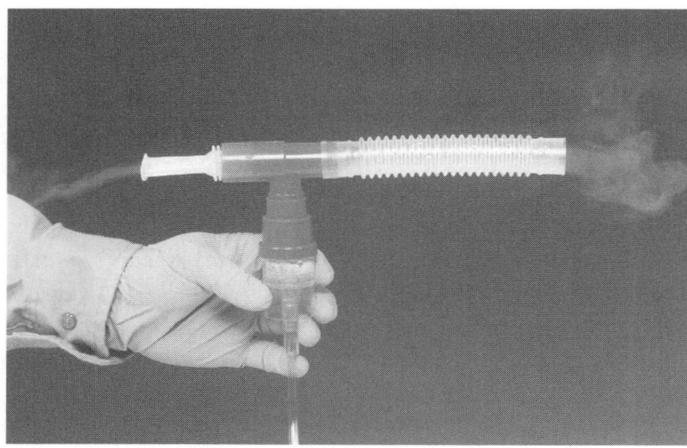

Figure 22-3. A nebulizer converts a solution into a mist for ease of inhalation.

TABLE 22-3. Corticosteroids for Treating Asthma

GENERIC NAME	TRADE NAME	ROUTE OF ADMINISTRATION
beclomethasone	Vanceril®, Beclovent®	MDI
dextromethasone	Decadron®	MDI, powdered inhaler
flunisolide	Nasalide®, Aerobid®	MDI
fluticasone	Flovent®	MDI
triamcinolone	Azmacort®	MDI
prednisone	Deltasone®	Oral
prednisolone	Prelone®	Oral

Note: All of the drugs listed above are prescription drugs.

BRONCHODILATORS

Bronchodilators relax smooth muscle of the bronchial tubes. They are the major drugs used to treat asthma (see Table 22-4).

TABLE 22-4. Classification of Bronchodilators

GENERIC NAME	TRADE NAME	ROUTE OF ADMINISTRATION
epinephrine*,†	Adrenalin®	Inhalation
	Bronkaid®, Medihaler®, Primatene®	Injection
ephedrine**	Vicks®, Vatronol®	Oral
isoproterenol*	Isuprel®	Oral, Sublingual
albuterol*	Proventil®	Oral, MDI
	Ventolin®	MDI, Nebulizer
bitolterol*	Tornalate®	MDI
isoetharine**	Bronkometer®	Nebulizer
terbutaline*	Brethaire®	MDI
	Brethine®	Oral
metaproterenol*	Alupent®	Inhalation
	Metaprel®	Oral
salmeterol*	Serevent®	MDI, DPI
Methylxanthines		
theophylline/ aminophylline*	Elixophyllin®, Slo-Phyllin®, Aminophyllin®	Oral
dyphylline*	Dilor®, Lufyllin®	Oral
Combination Bronchodilators		
ipratropium/ albuterol*	Combivent®	MDI
fluticasone*	Advair®	DPI

*Prescription drug.
†OTC drug.

ASTHMATIC PROPHYLAXIS

Cromolyn sodium and nedocromil are used to prevent asthma symptoms and improve airway function in patients with mild persistent asthma or exercise-induced asthma. Cromolyn suppresses inflammation but does not dilate the bronchial tree. It inhibits the release of histamines, so it acts as an antiallergenic. Cromolyn is the drug of choice as a prophylactic for moderate allergic asthma, especially in children, because of its safety and efficacy. It is also used to reduce the symptoms of seasonal allergic attacks. Adverse effects include coughing and wheezing on administration. Nedocromil is also anti-inflammatory and antiallergic. It has an unpleasant taste. Nedocromil may help reduce the dose requirements for inhaled corticosteroids. Table 22-5 shows the most common prophylactic drugs for asthma.

LEUKOTRIENE ANTAGONISTS

Leukotrienes contribute to the inflammation associated with asthma. Leukotriene antagonists block the bronchoconstriction, mucus production, and inflammation that occur with asthma. Zafirlukast was the first medication in this new class of anti-inflammatory agents. It is prescribed as maintenance therapy for patients with chronic asthma. Zafirlukast is a safe drug and has few side effects. A newer drug is zileuton. It is rapidly absorbed via oral administration. Zileuton is used in patients older than 12 years of age. Adverse effects include liver toxicity and dyspepsia. Montelukast is the latest addition to this class of drugs. Montelukast acts as a bronchodilator, respiratory stimulant, and leukotriene receptor antagonist. This medication should be given at night for maximum effectiveness. Montelukast is prescribed as a prophylactic drug for asthma attacks. It must not be used for acute asthma attacks. The main adverse effects are headaches and gastrointestinal symptoms.

TABLE 22-5. The Most Common Asthmatic Prophylactic Drugs

GENERIC NAME	TRADE NAME	ROUTE OF ADMINISTRATION
cromolyn	Aarane®, Intal®, Crolom®, Nasalcrom®	DPI, MDI, nebulizer, nasal spray
nedocromil	Tilade®	MDI
zafirlukast	Accolate®	Oral
zileuton	Zyflo®	Oral
montelukast	Singulair®	Oral

Note: All of the drugs listed above are prescription drugs.

XANTHINE DERIVATIVES

Xanthine derivatives (bronchodilators) are effective for relief of bronchospasm in asthma, chronic bronchitis, and emphysema. They relax the smooth muscles of the bronchial tree and stimulate cardiac muscle and the central nervous system. Methylxanthine is the base of xanthine derivatives, which must be converted to theophylline and aminophylline. These xanthine agents are used for the prevention and treatment of bronchial asthma and for the treatment of emphysema and bronchitis. Adverse effects include tachycardia, insomnia, nervousness, headache, and nausea. Patients with hypothyroidism, acute pulmonary edema, convulsive disorders, and heart disease cannot use xanthine derivatives. Aminophylline has a narrow therapeutic range and is not used as commonly today as theophylline. The β_2-adrenergic agonists (albuterol and terbutaline) are safer and more effective. Theophylline provides mild bronchodilation in asthmatic patients. This drug may also have important anti-inflammatory properties and enhance mucociliary clearance. Theophylline is the most widely-used oral xanthine derivative, and it is the preferred parenteral preparation. Adverse effects at therapeutic doses include insomnia, upset stomach, aggravation of dyspepsia, and difficulties with urination in elderly men with prostatism. Dose-related toxicities are common and include nausea, vomiting, tachyarrhythmias, headache, seizures, hyperglycemia, and hypokalemia.

β-ADRENERGIC AGENTS

β-adrenergic agents work as both cardiac and respiratory agonists. Their main action is on the smooth muscle of the bronchial tree and on the heart. A typical medication is isoproterenol, which may be taken orally or by injection. β_2-receptor agonists are the most effective medications for reducing acute bronchospasms and exercise-induced asthma. These agents provide bronchodilation by stimulating the β_2-receptors in the smooth muscle of the lung. The β_2 agonists relieve ongoing asthmatic attacks and may also be used prophylactically. Salmeterol is preferred for prophylaxis but is not effective for aborting an attack because of the slowness of its action. Salmeterol is the only agent of this class available in the United States and is indicated for long-term prevention of asthma symptoms and the prevention of exercise-induced bronchospasm. Salmeterol should not be used in place of anti-inflammatory therapy. Adverse effects include dizziness, headache, tremor, palpitations, and sinus tachycardia. Epinephrine and ephedrine are nonselective adrenergic agents. These agents are used to treat bronchial asthma and bronchitis and to prevent bronchospasm. Epinephrine and ephedrine have a rapid onset of action with a duration of 1 to 3 hours when used by inhalation or 1 to 4 hours when given parenterally. Common adverse effects include insomnia, tachycardia, nervousness, and anorexia. The cardiotoxic effects have led to the discovery and use of more specific respiratory agents that do not cause tachycardia or nervousness.

MUCOLYTICS AND EXPECTORANTS

Expectorants are agents that promote the removal of mucous secretions from the lung, bronchi, and trachea, usually by coughing. These medications are available OTC and by prescription. Expectorant drugs include acetylcysteine, guaifenesin, and dornase alfa. They are also **mucolytic** (destroying or dissolving the active agents that make up mucus). In many cases expectorants are added to other drugs, such as antitussives, decongestants, and antihistamines, to help remove mucus. Acetylcysteine is a mucolytic agent that decreases the viscosity of mucus. It is also an antidote for acetaminophen hepatotoxicity. Guaifenesin is safer and more effective. The contraindications for these expectorants are not significant. Dornase alfa is a specific expectorant for use in cystic fibrosis. It reduces the risk of respiratory infections. The drug works within 3 to 7 days of the start of treatment. It is available as a solution for inhalation by nebulizer (see Table 22-6).

TABLE 22-6. Mucolytics and Expectorants

GENERIC NAME	TRADE NAME	ROUTE OF ADMINISTRATION
acetylcysteine†	Mucomyst®	Inhalation
guaifenesin*,†	Hytuss®, Robitussin®, Dura-Tuss®	Oral
dornase alfa	Pulmozyme®	Inhalation

*Prescription drug.
†OTC drug.

DECONGESTANTS

Decongestants cause vasoconstriction of nasal mucosa and reduce congestion or swelling. These agents are available in both oral and nasal preparations. The majority of oral agents are adrenergic drugs that mimic the effects of the sympathetic nervous system. Decongestants should only be used by order of a physician for patients with glaucoma, prostate cancer, and heart disease. Decongestants may increase blood glucose levels in patients with diabetes mellitus. Warnings on the labels of OTC preparations include instructions for patients with hypertension, diabetes mellitus, ischemic heart disease, and hyperthyroidism. Decongestants may cause serious tachycardia, insomnia, nervousness, restlessness, blurred vision, and nausea or vomiting. Ephedrine is currently unavailable. Ephedrine is being reviewed and may be available as a controlled substance in the future. Table 22-7 shows decongestant agents.

INTRANASAL STEROIDS

Corticosteroids act by inhibiting the body's inflammatory response. They decrease vasodilation and edema of the mucous membranes and reduce inflammation. Corticosteroids have no antihistamine effect. They are administered intranasally to treat allergic and nonallergic rhinitis. The most commonly used intranasal steroids are listed in Table 22-8.

DRUGS FOR SMOKING CESSATION

Cigarette smoke contains chemical compounds that affect most organs of the human body. Cigarette smoking causes cancers of the mouth, pharynx, larynx, lungs, esophagus,

TABLE 22-7. Decongestant Agents

GENERIC NAME	TRADE NAME	ROUTE OF ADMINISTRATION
Nasal Decongestants		
ephedrine 0.5%	Vicks®, Vatronel®	Nasal drops
epinephrine 0.1%	Astham Haler Mist®, Primatene Mist®	Oral inhalation
naphazoline 0.05%	Allerest®	Nasal drops
phenylephrine 1%	Neo-Synephrine®, Sinex®	Nasal drops
tetrahydrozoline 0.1%	Tyzine®	Nasal drops
oxymetazoline 0.05%	Afrin®, Neo-Synephrine 12 hour®	Nasal drops and spray
Oral Decongestants		
pseudoephedrine	Sudafed®, Drixoral®	Oral
	Sudafed-SR®	Oral (sustained-release)
Combination Decongestants		
pseudoephedrine/chlorpheniramine	Aller-Chlor®, Chlor-Trimeton®, Chlo-Amine®, Chlor-Pro, Phenetron®, Sinutab Sinus Allergy®, Sudafed Plus®, Telachlor®, Teldrin®	Oral
pseudoephedrine	Afrin®, Allerest®, Cenafed®, Contac®, Decofed®, Dorcol®, Efidac/24®, PediaCare®, Sinutab®	Oral

Note: All of the drugs listed in this table are available OTC.

TABLE 22-8. Commonly Used Intranasal Steroids

GENERIC NAME	TRADE NAME	ROUTE OF ADMINISTRATION
beclomethasone	Beconase®, Vancenase®	Nasal spray
flunisolide	Nasalide®	Nasal spray
fluticasone	Flonase®	Nasal spray
mometasone	Nasonex®	Nasal spray
triamcinolone	Nasacort®, Tri-Nasal®	Inhaler, Nasal spray
budesonide	Rhinocort®	Nasal spray

Note: All of the drugs listed above are prescription drugs.

TABLE 22-9. Smoking Cessation Agents

GENERIC NAME	TRADE NAME	ROUTE OF ADMINISTRATION
bupropion*	Zyban®	Oral and patch
nicotine*,†	Nicorette®	Gum
	Nicoderm®	Patch
	Habitrol®	Patch
	Nicotrol® NS spray	Inhaler
	Prostep®	Patch

*Prescription drug.
†OTC drug.

TABLE 22-10. Adverse Effects of Nicotine

ADVERSE EFFECTS	SYSTEMS OF THE BODY
Headache, dizziness, light-headedness, insomnia, irritability, dependence on nicotine	Central nervous system
Arrhythmias, tachycardia, palpitations, hypertension	Cardiovascular system
Air swallowing, jaw ache, nausea, belching, salivation, anorexia, constipation, diarrhea, dyspepsia, vomiting, abdominal pain	Digestive system
Sore throat, cough, hiccups, hoarseness	Respiratory system
Erythema, pruritus, local edema, and rash	Skin

pancreas, kidney, bladder, and cervix. Cigarette smoking may also cause leukemia and may increase the risk of heart disease, lung disease, or stroke. Benefits of smoking cessation include better health and a longer life. The most commonly used drugs for smoking cessation are listed in Table 22-9.

Bupropion is an antidepressant; the dosage form for smoking cessation varies. For example, bupropion (Zyban®) is used as a tablet. Habitrol®, Nicoderm®, Nicotrol®, and Prostep® are available as transdermal patches. Nicorette® is used as a gum, and Nicotrol® NS must be used as a spray. Bupropion is the first non-nicotine drug for smoking cessation. It can be used alone or with the nicotine patch. Adverse effects of nicotine, nicotine polacrilex, and nicotine transdermal systems are summarized in Table 22-10.

REVIEW QUESTIONS

1. Histamine is found in all body tissue and particularly in which of the following blood cells?
   A. Erythrocytes
   B. Eosinophils
   C. Basophils
   D. Thrombocytes

2. Which of the following is an example of a nonopioid cough suppressant?
   A. Dextromethorphan
   B. Hydromorphone
   C. Codeine
   D. Budesonide

3. Which of the following is the drug of choice for asthma?
   A. Corticosteroids
   B. Cromolyn
   C. Theophylline
   D. Metaproterenol

4. A specific expectorant for cystic fibrosis is
   A. budesonide (Rhinocort Aqua).
   B. mometasone (Nasonex).
   C. diphenhydramine (Benadryl).
   D. dornase alfa (Pulmozyme).

5. Which of the following agents is the only one of value when taken prophylactically for asthma?
   A. Salmeterol
   B. Cromolyn
   C. Theophylline
   D. Antihistamine

6. Decongestants are contraindicated in patients with
   A. asthma.
   B. heart disease.
   C. pneumonia.
   D. encephalitis.

7. Allergic rhinitis is known as
   A. contact dermatitis.
   B. atopic allergy.
   C. allergen.
   D. hay fever.

8. The trade name of bupropion is
   A. Nicotrol®.
   B. Habitrol®.
   C. Zyban®.
   D. Nicoderm.®

9. A medication that is available in the form of a dry powder inhaler (DPI) is which of the following?
   A. Nicotrol®
   B. Salmeterol®
   C. Theophylline®
   D. Albuterol®

10. Xanthine derivatives are used for the prevention and treatment of
    A. nasal congestion.
    B. coughing.
    C. bronchial asthma.
    D. nausea.

11. Which of the following β-adrenergic agents has cardiotoxic effects?
    A. Ephedrine
    B. Estrogen
    C. ProStep®
    D. Diphenhydramine

12. Which of the following has no antihistamine effect?
    A. Nytol®
    B. Fexofenadine
    C. Guaifenesin
    D. Corticosteroids

13. Corticosteroids for treating asthma include
    A. prednisone.
    B. acetylcysteine.
    C. ephedrine.
    D. beclomethasone.

14. The generic name of Primatene®, a bronchodilator, is
    A. salmeterol.
    B. epinephrine.
    C. albuterol.
    D. prednisone.

15. Cromolyn, used as an asthmatic prophylactic, may be administered as a/an
    A. oral medication.
    B. suppository.
    C. injection.
    D. nasal spray.

16. The generic name for Robitussin® is
    A. acetylcysteine.
    B. guaifenesin.
    C. dornase alfa.
    D. ephedrine.

17. Oral decongestants include which of the following?
A. Primatene®
B. Sinex®
C. Sudafed®
D. Vicks®

18. Commonly-used intranasal steroids include
A. bupropion.
B. nicotine.
C. Flonase®.
D. Nicotrol®.

19. Adverse effects of nicotine include all of the following, except
A. headache.
B. arrhythmias.
C. nausea.
D. hair loss.

20. Antihistamines may cause the respiratory tract to become dry; therefore, one should
A. limit the intake of alcohol.
B. continue smoking in moderate amounts.
C. drink plenty of fluids.
D. use nasal sprays frequently.

23 Central Nervous System Drugs

OUTLINE

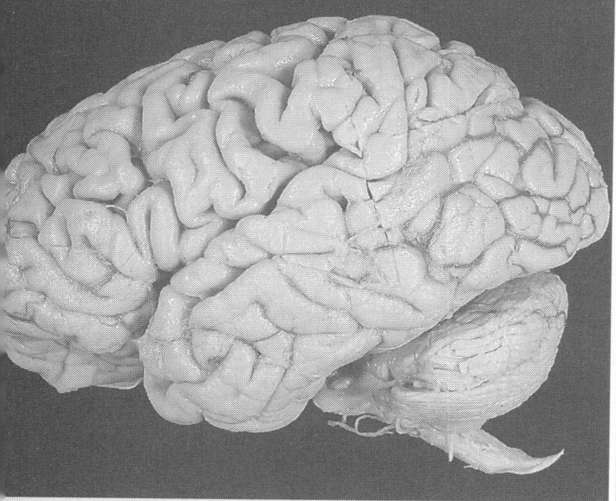

GLOSSARY

acetylcholine (ACh) A neurotransmitter that stimulates nerve endings of parasympathetic and sympathetic nervous systems.

Alzheimer's disease An illness characterized by progressive memory failure, impaired thinking, confusion, disorientation, personality changes, restlessness, speech disturbances, and inability to perform routine tasks.

anesthetics Agents that act on nervous tissue to produce a loss of sensation or unconsciousness.

barbiturates Chemical derivatives of barbituric acid that have a depressant effect on the central nervous system.

benzodiazepines Drugs used to treat anxiety that have a depressive action on the central nervous system.

convulsion Abnormal motor movements.

cross-dependence The ability of one drug to substitute for another drug in the same drug class to maintain a dependent state or prevent withdrawal.

cross-tolerance Tolerance to one drug conferring tolerance to other drugs in the same drug class.

dependence The total psychophysical state of one addicted to drugs or alcohol who must receive an increasing amount of the substance to prevent the onset of withdrawal symptoms.

drug abuse Nonmedical use of a drug that is deemed unacceptable by society.

endogenous depression Feelings of intense sadness, helplessness, and worthlessness that have no external cause and may be the result of genetic factors or biochemical changes in the brain.

epilepsy A group of disorders that are characterized by hyperexcitability within the central nervous system.
exogenous depression Feelings of intense sadness, helplessness, and worthlessness in response to a loss, disappointment, or illness.
hypnosis An increased tendency to sleep.
monoamine oxidase inhibitors (MAOIs) Drugs that reduce the activity of the enzyme monoamine oxidase and increase central nervous system activity.
neurohormones Neurotransmitters.
neuron The basic structure of a nerve consisting of dendrites, cell body, and axon.
nicotine A constituent of tobacco, along with various gases and particulate matter.
Parkinson's disease A disorder characterized by resting tremor, rigidity, or resistance to passive movement, akinesia, and loss of postural reflexes.
physical dependence The necessity to continue drug use to avoid a withdrawal syndrome.
psychological dependence The overwhelming need to take a drug to maintain a sense of well-being.
psychosis A mental illness accompanied by bizarre behavior and altered personality with failure to perceive reality.
sedation A state of consciousness characterized by decreased anxiety, motor activity, and mental acuity.
seizure An epileptic event.
selective serotonin reuptake inhibitor (SSRI) A type of antidepressant that blocks the reuptake and inactivation of serotonin in the brain.
tolerance A reduced drug effect with repeated use of a drug and a need for higher doses to produce the same effect.
tricyclic antidepressant (TCA) A drug that inhibits the uptake of norepinephrine and serotonin to result in stimulation of the central nervous system.

THE CENTRAL NERVOUS SYSTEM

The nervous system is composed of the brain, spinal cord, and nerves (see Figure 23-1). Neurons are the basic cells of the nervous system, carrying nerve impulses from one part of the body to another. The nervous system is divided into two sections: the central nervous system (CNS), consisting of the brain and spinal cord, and the peripheral nervous system (PNS), consisting of the nerves of the body. The PNS connects the CNS to various body structures (see Figure 23-2).

The **neuron** is the basic nerve cell of the nervous system and is able to conduct impulses. It consists of three parts: dendrites, cell body, and axons (see Figure 23-3). Dendrites are the receptors that carry information to the nerve cell body, and axons carry nerve information away from the nerve cell body. At the junction of neurons, the continuation of the messages is performed by neurotransmitters such as **acetylcholine (ACh)**, which stimulates the nerve endings, and cholinesterase, which inhibits ACh. There are some other neurotransmitters, or **neurohormones**, including the catecholamines (norepinephrine, epinephrine, and dopamine), serotonin, and endorphins. The nervous system is able to cope with different types of stressors at different times of life, which is part of normal living or mental health. Daily stressors may cause normal activities of the brain to become abnormal, resulting in a mental disorder.

DRUGS THAT ACT UPON THE NERVOUS SYSTEM

Many different medications are prescribed for a variety of conditions and disorders of the nervous system. These drugs are classified as sedatives and hypnotics, antipsychotic drugs (for bipolar disorder and schizophrenia), antianxiety drugs, and antidepressant drugs.

Sedative and Hypnotic Drugs

Sedatives and hypnotics are drugs that depress the CNS. Sedative medications are used to reduce the desire for physical activity and to produce a calming effect. **Sedation** is characterized by decreased anxiety, motor activity, and mental acuity. Sedation induces calmness or sleep. Hypnotic medication is used to induce or maintain sleep. Commonly prescribed sedative and hypnotic medications are listed in Table 23-1.

Barbiturates

Barbiturates are chemical derivatives of barbituric acid. All barbiturates exert a depressant effect on the CNS. The extent of their action ranges from mild sedation to deep anesthesia. Most patients using barbiturates may tolerate them quite well, but they may produce some adverse effects such as

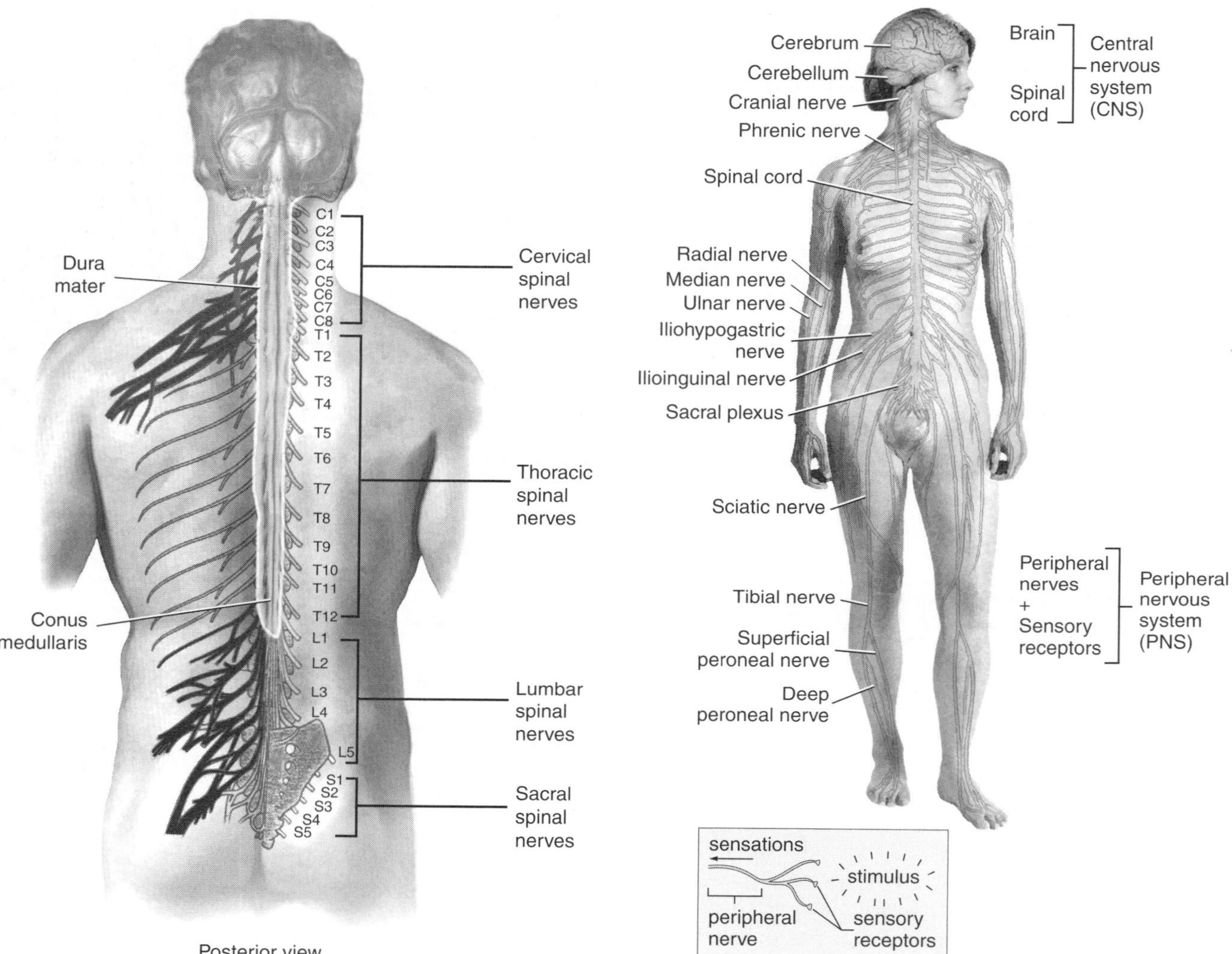

Figure 23-1. The central nervous system.

Figure 23-2. The peripheral nervous system.

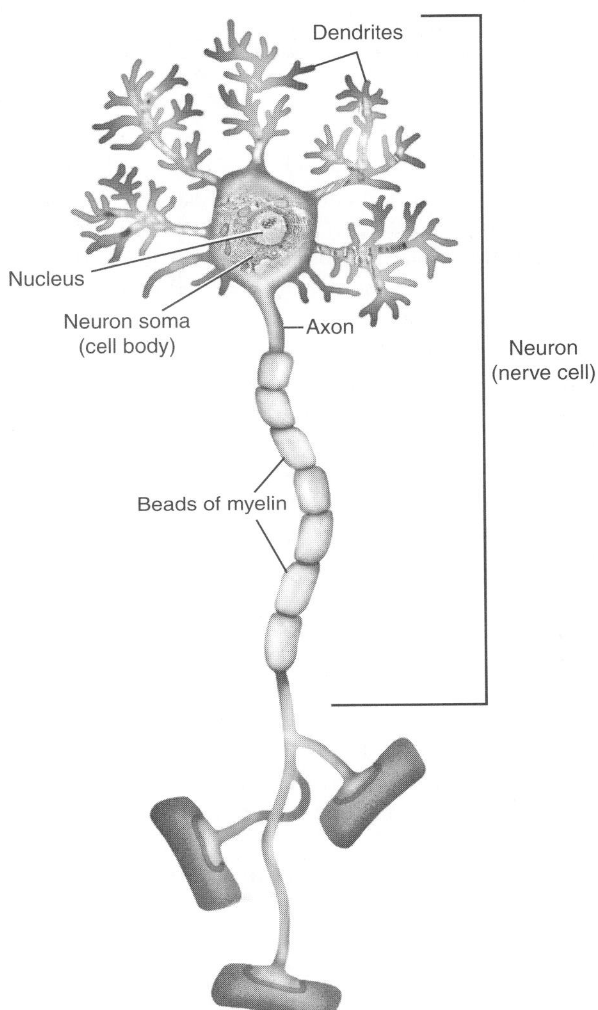

Figure 23-3. A neuron.

TABLE 23-1. Commonly Used Sedative and Hypnotic Drugs

GENERIC NAME	TRADE NAME	ROUTE OF ADMINISTRATION
Barbiturates		
amobarbital	Amytal®	Oral, IM
aprobarbital	Alurate®	Oral
butabarbital	Butisol®	Oral
mephobarbital	Mebaral®	Oral
pentobarbital	Nembutal®	Oral, IM, IV
phenobarbital	Luminal®	Oral, IM
secobarbital	Seconal®	Oral, IM, IV
Benzodiazepines: Short-acting		
alprazolam	Xanax®	Oral
lorazepam	Ativan®	Oral, IM, IV
quazepam	Doral®	Oral
temazepam	Restoril®	Oral
triazolam	Halcion®	Oral
Benzodiazepines: Long-acting		
chlordiazepoxide	Librium®	Oral
clonazepam	Klonopin®	Oral
chlorazepate	Tranxene®	Oral
prazepam	Centrax®	Oral
diazepam	Valium®	Oral, IM, IV
flurazepam	Dalmane®	Oral
Miscellaneous		
buspirone	BuSpar®	Oral
chloral hydrate	Noctec®	Oral
ethchlorvynol	Placidyl®	Oral
hydroxyzine	Atarax®, Vistaril®	Oral, IM
zolpidem	Ambien®	Oral

IM, intramuscular; IV, intravenous.

TABLE 23-2. Classification of Barbiturates

CLASSIFICATION	GENERIC NAME	TRADE NAME	ROUTE OF ADMINISTRATION
Ultra short-acting	thiopental	Pentothal®	IV
	methohexital	Brevital®	IV
	thiamylal	Surital®	IV
Short-acting	pentobarbital	Nembutal®	Oral, IM, IV
	secobarbital	Seconal®	Oral
Intermediate-acting (3-4 hours)	amobarbital	Amytal®	Oral
Long-acting (oral 10-16 hours)	phenobarbital	Bellatal®, Solfoton®	Oral, IM, SC, IV

excessive CNS depression, hypersensitivity reactions, and excitement. High doses of barbiturates tend to depress the respiratory and vasomotor centers of the medulla (in the brain), thereby causing respiratory depression and hypotension. In acute drug intoxication, death may result. Barbiturates also tend to exert a variety of effects on the liver. The barbiturates produce a dose-dependent continuum of CNS depression, leading ultimately to coma and death. Barbiturates are classified into four groups: ultra-short-acting, short-acting, intermediate-acting, and long-acting. Table 23-2 illustrates this classification of barbiturates.

Phenobarbital and mephobarbital are used for seizure disorders, congenital hyperbilirubinemia, and neonatal jaundice. Indications for intermediate-acting barbiturates are regional anesthesia, sedation, and **hypnosis**. Ultra-short-acting barbiturates are used for intravenous general anesthesia. Drowsiness, skin eruptions, and gastrointestinal disturbances are common adverse effects of barbiturates. Overdosage, such as that seen in suicide attempts, can cause tachycardia, respiratory depression, coma, cardiovascular collapse, and death.

Antipsychotic Drugs

Bipolar disorders are marked by severe pathological mood swings from hyperactivity and euphoria to sadness and depression. Bipolar disorders involve various symptom combinations. Type 1 bipolar disorder is characterized by alternating episodes of mania and depression, whereas type II is characterized by recurrent depressive episodes and occasional manic episodes. In some patients, bipolar disorder assumes a seasonal pattern, marked by a cyclic relationship between the onset of the mood episode and a particular 60-day period of the year. This disorder affects women and men equally, is more common in higher socioeconomic groups, and is associated with high levels of creativity. The cause of bipolar disorder is unclear, but hereditary, biological, and psychological factors may play a part.

Schizophrenia is characterized by disturbances (for at least 6 months) in thought content and form, perception, affect, sense of self, volition, interpersonal relationships, and psychomotor behavior. Schizophrenia may result from a combination of genetic, biological, cultural, and psychological factors. Severe mental illnesses, such as schizophrenia, psychotic depression, mania, or psychotic brain syndrome, are commonly treated with use of antipsychotic drugs.

Medications play an important role in modern psychotherapeutic care. These drugs are used to reduce or alleviate symptoms and allow the psychotic person an opportunity to participate in other psychotherapeutic treatment. Antipsychotic drugs do not cure mental disorders but are used to control the symptoms related to **psychosis**, a mental illness accompanied by bizarre behavior and altered personality with failure to perceive reality.

Antipsychotic drugs are also called *neuroleptics* (formerly called *major tranquilizers*). These agents may be used for acute and chronic psychosis. The most important classes of antipsychotic medications are the phenothiazines, butyrophenones, thioxanthenes, dibenzodiazepines, benzisoxazoles, and thienobenzodiazepines. They are used to decrease the symptoms of schizophrenia and other psychotic disorders. Their mechanism of action is unknown, but these agents are thought to act on dopamine and serotonin (neurotransmitters in the brain). The side effects of antipsychotic drugs include postural hypotension, tachycardia or bradycardia, and vertigo. Blurred vision, dry mouth, fever, constipation, and jaundice may also occur.

Phenothiazines

Chlorpromazine was the first antipsychotic agent and remains the typical phenothiazine. This agent possesses anticholinergic, antiemetic, antihistaminic, and α-adrenergic blocking effects, as well as antipsychotic actions. Adverse reactions to phenothiazines include orthostatic hypotension, tachycardia, confusion, drowsiness, insomnia, hyperglycemia, and gynecomastia. Overdosage of phenothiazines produce exaggerated CNS depression, coma, severe hypotension, seizures, and cardiac dysrhythmias.

Nonphenothiazines

Nonphenothiazines include butyrophenones, thioxanthenes, dibenzodiazepines, benzisoxazoles, and thienobenzodiazepines. The mechanism of action for these products is

TABLE 23-3. Selected Drugs Used to Treat Psychosis

GENERIC NAME	TRADE NAME	ROUTE OF ADMINISTRATION
Phenothiazines		
chlorpromazine	Thorazine®	Oral, rectal, IM
fluphenazine	Prolixin®	Oral, IM
mesoridazine	Serentil®	Oral, IM
perphenazine	Trilafon®	Oral, IM
prochlorperazine	Compazine®	Oral
promethazine	Phenergan®	Oral, rectal, IM
thioridazine	Mellaril®	Oral
trifluoperazine	Stelazine®	Oral, IM
Nonphenothiazines		
Butyrophenones		
haloperidol	Haldol®	Oral, IM
Thioxanthenes		
thiothixene	Navane®	Oral, IM
Dibenzodiazepines		
clozapine	Clozaril®	Oral
Benzisoxazoles		
risperidone	Risperdal®	Oral
Thienobenzodiazepines		
olanzapine	Zyprexa®	Oral

IM, intramuscular.

often not precisely understood. They are used mainly for schizophrenia. Table 23-3 shows selected drugs used to treat psychosis.

Lithium Therapy

Lithium is the primary drug used to treat patients in manic states. It is the drug of choice for the treatment of manic episodes such as those seen with bipolar disorder. Mania that is at some time severe enough to produce compromised functioning is necessary for diagnosis of bipolar disorder. This is a genetic disorder. The manic episode typically develops over days and may become uncontrolled and psychotic. The patient with bipolar disorder is depressed, with the depression usually being profound, but the disorder may present as a mild depressive syndrome. Attacks are usually separated by months or years, but they occasionally may cycle from one to the other over days or weeks. Bipolar disorder is a recurrent illness. A single attack is rare. The first manic episode often occurs before age 30, begins quickly, and resolves in 2 to 4 months if untreated. Suicide is the major risk during periods of depression. Drug therapy for bipolar disorder begins with lithium carbonate. The exact mechanism of action of lithium is unknown. Lithium is specifically used for patients with manic depressive psychosis who are in an acute manic phase. It can sometimes be useful for reducing excitement in patients suffering from schizophrenia. The therapeutic effect is seen in 2 to 3 weeks. Lithium normalizes mood in 80% of patients. It has no sedative, depressant, or euphoric actions, making it unique from all other psychiatric drugs. Adverse effects include diarrhea, tremor, anorexia, polydipsia, vomiting, polyuria, albuminuria, blurred vision, hyperglycemia, hypothyroidism, and weight gain. Overdosage may produce diarrhea, vomiting, muscle weakness, drowsiness, and ataxia.

Antianxiety Drugs

Agents used for the relief of anxiety may also be used as hypnotics and sedatives to promote sleep. The difference between using the agents as anxiolytics and hypnotics is based on dosage. Higher doses have hypnotic effects, and lower doses can relieve anxiety. Sometimes, a single medication may be prescribed for both uses (to lower anxiety and produce sleep). Antianxiety drugs may also be used as skeletal muscle relaxants for chronic muscle pain. Occasionally, minor tranquilizers are also used as antiseizure medications to reduce the number of convulsions and as adjunctive medications in alcohol withdrawal.

Benzodiazepines

The **benzodiazepines** are a chemical class of drugs widely used primarily for the treatment of anxiety. Their depressant action on the CNS appears to be closely related to their ability to potentiate γ-aminobutyric acid–mediated neural inhibition. For hypnosis and treatment of anxiety, the benzodiazepines are drugs of choice because of their great margin of safety. A new nonbenzodiazepine, buspirone, may specifically relieve anxiety without sedation, hypnosis, or general CNS depression. The classification of benzodiazepines is summarized in Table 23-4.

Indications for benzodiazepines include generalized anxiety disorders, panic disorders, agoraphobia (fear of open spaces), insomnia, seizures, and muscle relaxation. Adverse effects are drowsiness, ataxia, impaired judgment, rebound insomnia, and development of tolerance. Overdosage may result in CNS and respiratory depression as well as hypotension and coma. Gradual withdrawal of these drugs is recommended. Although the use of any of the benzodiazepines during pregnancy is likely to cause fetal abnormalities, flurazepam is entirely contraindicated during pregnancy.

Antidepressant Drugs

Depression is one of the most common psychiatric disorders. It is characterized by feelings of intense sadness, helplessness, and worthlessness and impaired functioning. There are two types of depression: endogenous and exogenous. **Endogenous depression**, or unipolar disorder, is characterized by depression that has no external cause and may be the result of genetic factors or biochemical changes

TABLE 23-4. Classification of Benzodiazepines

GENERIC NAME	TRADE NAME	ROUTE OF ADMINISTRATION
Short-acting		
alprazolam	Xanax®	Oral
lorazepam	Ativan®	Oral, IM, IV
quazepam	Doral®	Oral
temazepam	Restoril®	Oral
triazolam	Halcion®Oral	
Long-acting		
chlordiazepoxide	Librium®	Oral
clonazepam	Klonopin®	Oral
chlorazepate	Tranxene®	Oral
prazepam	Centrax®	Oral
diazepam	Valium®	Oral, IM, IV
flurazepam	Dalmane®	Oral
Miscellaneous Antianxiety Drugs		
buspirone	BuSpar®	Oral
hydroxyzine	Atarax®	Oral, IM

IM, intramuscular; IV, intravenous.

TABLE 23-5. Selected Drugs Used to Treat Depression

GENERIC NAME	TRADE NAME	ROUTE OF ADMINISTRATION
Tricyclic Antidepressants		
clomipramine	Anafranil®	Oral
desipramine	Norpramin®	Oral
nortriptyline	Aventyl®, Pamelor®	Oral
amitriptyline	Elavil®, Endep®	Oral
doxepin	Sinequan®, Adapin®	Oral
imipramine	Tofranil®	Oral
Second-generation Cyclic Antidepressants		
bupropion	Wellbutrin®, Zyban®	Oral
mirtazapine	Remeron®	Oral
nefazodone	Serzone®	Oral
trazodone	Desyrel®	Oral
Monoamine Oxidase Inhibitors		
phenelzine	Nardil®	Oral
Selective Serotonin Reuptake Inhibitors		
fluoxetine	Prozac®	Oral
citalopram	Celexa®	Oral
fluvoxamine	Luvox®	Oral
paroxetine	Paxil®	Oral
sertraline	Zoloft®	Oral
venlafaxine	Effexor®	Oral
Medications for Bipolar Disorder		
lithium carbonate	Eskalith®, Lithobid®	Oral
lithium citrate	Cibalith-S® (syrup)	Oral
carbamazepine	Tegretol®	Oral
valproic acid	Depakene®	Oral
valproate	Depakote®	Oral

in the brain. **Exogenous depression** is often a response to a loss or disappointment, such as the death of a loved one, loss of a job, or the presence of a debilitating illness. This type of depression is often called *the blues*. After a period of adjustment, the depression resolves, and life goes on. The main antidepressant drug classes are monoamine oxidase inhibitors, tricyclic antidepressants, and selective serotonin reuptake inhibitors. Drugs used to treat depression are shown in Table 23-5.

The therapeutic response rate for all antidepressants is similar. Selection of the proper agent depends on the side effects that the patient experiences from the drugs.

Monoamine Oxidase Inhibitors

Monoamine oxidase inhibitors (MAOIs) reduce the activity of the enzyme MAO. They increase CNS levels and activity of norepinephrine and serotonin. Their therapeutic effect is achieved in 3 to 5 weeks. MAOIs are rarely used for endogenous depression. They are generally used when tricyclic antidepressants are not effective. Another indication for MAOIs is narcolepsy. Adverse effects of MAOIs include orthostatic hypotension, drowsiness, inhibition of ejaculation, insomnia, headache, hallucinations, diarrhea, nausea, vomiting, fever, blurred vision, dry mouth, and incontinence. Overdosage produces restlessness, hypotension, tachycardia, mental confusion, seizures, respiratory depression, and shock. MAOIs may cause very serious reactions if taken with certain foods, such as those containing tyramine, or beverages. The patient must not eat foods such as chicken livers, cheese, yogurt, sour cream, bananas, raisins, and avocados. The patient must also avoid drinking wine.

Tricyclic Antidepressants

Tricyclic antidepressants (TCAs) inhibit the uptake of norepinephrine and serotonin in the CNS. TCAs are used primarily to relieve the symptoms of unipolar endogenous depression, resulting in elevation of mood, increased physical activity and mental alertness, increased appetite, increased sexual drive, and improved sleep patterns. They are effective in 70% of patients. They may also be used to treat mild exogenous depression, bipolar endogenous depression (with lithium), and nocturnal enuresis (only as a last resort and only for patients older than 6 years of age). Adverse effects of TCAs include delirium, confusion, manic reactions, sedation, weight gain, dry mouth, blurred vision, constipation, and difficulty in urination.

Selective Serotonin Reuptake Inhibitors

Selective serotonin reuptake inhibitors (SSRIs) are newer antidepressant drugs that block the reuptake and inactivation of serotonin in the brain. Unlike the TCAs, the SSRIs produce little blockage of cholinergic, adrenergic, or histamine receptors. Therefore, SSRIs produce fewer adverse effects, and they are now the most widely used antidepressant drugs. SSRIs should be administered in the morning because of the chance of nervousness and insomnia. They are used primarily to treat major depression. The adverse effects include sexual dysfunction, nausea, headaches, nervousness, insomnia, and anxiety. Examples of SSRIs are fluoxetine and citalopram hydrobromide. Fluoxetine was the first SSRI drug. This medication is the most widely prescribed antidepressant in the United States because it is as effective as TCAs, with fewer side effects, and is less dangerous when taken in overdosage. Citalopram hydrobromide is one of the newer SSRI-type medications. It does not produce a sympathomimetic response or anticholinergic activity. Its only use is for depression. This medication cannot be used with MAOIs and should not be given until 2 weeks after any MAOIs are stopped.

ALZHEIMER'S DISEASE

Alzheimer's disease is a devastating illness characterized by progressive memory failure, impaired thinking, confusion, disorientation, personality changes, restlessness, speech disturbances, and the inability to perform routine tasks. Unfortunately, the disease is incurable and newly affects about one quarter million individuals per year in the United States.

Treatment for Alzheimer's Disease

Alzheimer's disease is also called *primary degenerative dementia* and accounts for more than one half of all dementias. This disease is not found exclusively in the elderly population. Therapy consists of cerebral vasodilators, such as ergoloid mesylates, isoxsuprine, and cyclandelate, used to enhance the brain's circulation, and antidepressants if depression seems to exacerbate the patient's dementia. Tacrine, a centrally acting anticholinesterase agent, is given to treat memory deficits. The current pharmacotherapy is focused on improving cognitive functioning or limiting disease progression and symptom control. In Alzheimer's disease, the amount of ACh is decreased (this chemical substance is necessary for neurotransmission and for forming memories). There is no specific test for this disease; therefore, a definitive diagnosis is possible only upon autopsy. Tacrine (Cognex), rivastigmine tartrate (Exelon), and donepezil (Aricept) are the medications that have been approved by the U.S. Food and Drug Administration to improve memory deficits. There is significant risk of liver damage with use of tacrine, but the benefits are worth the risk because of the devastation caused by the disease. Adverse effects include nausea and vomiting, diarrhea, dyspepsia, myalgia, headache, and ataxia. The common adverse effects of donepezil are nausea and diarrhea. Unlike tacrine, donepezil does not damage the liver.

TABLE 23-6. Classification of Epileptic Events

I. FOCAL OR PARTIAL SEIZURES	II. GENERALIZED SEIZURES
A. Simple seizures	A. Nonconvulsive 1. Absence or petit mal seizures
B. Complex partial seizures	B. Convulsive 1. Tonic/clonic or grand mal seizures 2. Tonic/psychomotor seizures 3. Status epilepticus

EPILEPSY

Epilepsy is a group of disorders that are characterized by hyperexcitability within the CNS. The abnormal stimuli can produce many symptoms from short periods of unconsciousness to violent convulsions. Approximately 2.5 million Americans have epilepsy, and approximately one half are seizure-free with medication. **Seizure** is a term for all epileptic events, whereas **convulsion** relates to abnormal motor movements, such as the jerking movements of grand mal attacks. A classification of epileptic events is shown in Table 23-6.

Treatment for Epilepsy

Antiepileptic drugs prevent or stop a convulsive seizure. Seizures are characterized by an excessive discharge of cortical neuron activity, which can be measured by an electroencephalogram. Seizures are usually brief, with a beginning and an end. They may produce postseizure impairment. Seizures may result acutely from any of a number of neurological disorders, as well as from metabolic disturbances, trauma, and exposure to certain toxins. The most common diagnosis of chronic and recurring seizures is epilepsy, and its cause is often unknown. The terms *epilepsy*, *convulsions*, and *seizures* are commonly used

TABLE 23-7. Drug Treatment for Epileptic Events

GENERIC NAME	TRADE NAME	ROUTE OF ADMINISTRATION	INDICATIONS FOR USE
Barbiturates			Epilepsy—partial tonic/clonic seizures
phenobarbital			
mephobarbital			
Benzodiazepines			Myoclonic, absence, and status epilepticus
diazepam, clonazepam			
Hydantoins			
phenytoin	Dilantin®	Oral	Partial and tonic/clonic seizures when oral medications cannot be used
fosphenytoin	Cerebyx®	IM, IV	Partial, generalized tonic/clonic, absence seizures
lamotrigine	Lamictal®	Oral	Absence seizures
Oxazolidinediones			
paramethadione	Paradione®	Oral	
trimethadione	Tridione®	Oral	
Succinimides			Absence seizures
ethosuximide	Zarontin®	Oral	
phensuximide	Milontin®	Oral	
methsuximide	Celontin®	Oral	
Miscellaneous Antiseizure Agents			Partial and generalized
carbamazepine	Tegretol®	Oral	Tonic/clonic and mixed seizures
valproic acid	Depakene®	Oral	All generalized and partial seizures
valproate	Depakote®	Oral	As with valproic acid
primidone	Mysoline®	Oral	Psychomotor seizures
gabapentin	Neurontin®	Oral	Partial seizures
tiagabine	Gabitril Filmtabs®	Oral	Partial seizures
topiramate	Topamax®	Oral	Partial seizures

IM, intramuscular; IV, intravenous.

interchangeably, although each has a slightly different medical meaning.

Several major groups of medications are used to treat seizure disorders. The choice of medications varies according to individual patient conditions and physician preference. In treatment of epilepsy, it takes weeks to establish drug plasma levels and to determine the adequacy of therapeutic improvement. Monotherapy is usually the most effective with the least adverse effects. Drug treatment is not always necessary for the lifetime of the patient. Drugs used to treat epilepsy are listed in Table 23-7.

PARKINSON'S DISEASE

Parkinson's disease is characterized by resting tremor, rigidity or resistance to passive movement, akinesia, and loss of postural reflexes. Occasionally behavioral manifestations occur. It is caused by the progressive degeneration of dopamine neurons in the brain that leads to an imbalance in the activity of dopamine and ACh in the brain (basal ganglia). Parkinson's disease may also be drug induced. Because it is not possible to reverse the process of the disease, drugs are used to correct the imbalance of dopamine and ACh activity in the basal ganglia.

Treatment for Parkinson's Disease

There are several drugs that can be used for Parkinson's disease (see Table 23-8). In the following paragraphs, a few examples of antiparkinsonism drugs are discussed.

Levodopa

Levodopa is an antiparkinsonism and anticholinergic agent. It is a metabolic precursor of dopamine, a catecholamine neurotransmitter. Unlike dopamine, levodopa readily crosses the blood-brain barrier. The precise mechanism of action is unknown. Levodopa is prescribed for idiopathic Parkinson's disease and postencephalitic and arteriosclerotic parkinsonism. It is contraindicated in persons with a known

TABLE 23-8. Antiparkinsonism Drugs

GENERIC NAME	TRADE NAME	ROUTE OF ADMINISTRATION
levodopa	Dopar®, Larodopa®	Oral
carbidopa	Sinemet®	Oral
amantadine	Symmetrel®	Oral
bromocriptine	Parlodel®	Oral
benztropine	Apo-Benztropine®, Cogentin®	Oral, IV
trihexyphenidyl	Trihexy®	Oral
ropinirole	Requip®	Oral
pramipexole	Mirapex®	Oral
entacapone	Comtan®	Oral

IV, intravenous.

hypersensitivity to levodopa, in patients with narrow angle glaucoma, and in patients with acute psychoses and severe psychoneurosis. Adverse effects include increased hand tremor, grinding of teeth (bruxism), ataxia, numbness, fatigue, headache, and euphoria. Levodopa may also cause orthostatic hypotension, tachycardia, hypertension, nausea, vomiting, dry mouth, bitter taste, and hepatotoxicity.

Carbidopa

Carbidopa is an antiparkinsonism and anticholinergic agent. When levodopa is given alone, large doses must be administered. Carbidopa prevents peripheral metabolism (decarboxylation) of levodopa and thereby makes more levodopa available for transport to the brain. Carbidopa does not cross the blood-brain barrier and, therefore, does not affect metabolism of levodopa within the brain. It is effective in the management of symptoms of Parkinson's disease and parkinsonism of secondary origin and improves life expectancy. Contraindications and adverse effects of carbidopa are similar to those of levodopa.

Amantadine

Amantadine is an antiviral, anticholinergic, and antiparkinsonism agent. It reduces the rigidity associated with parkinsonian syndrome. Its mechanism of action in parkinsonism is not understood but may be related to the release of dopamine and other catecholamines from neuronal storage sites. Therapeutic effects, indications, and adverse effects are discussed in Chapter 20.

Bromocriptine

Bromocriptine is an autonomic nervous system and antiparkinsonism agent. It is a semisynthetic ergot alkaloid derivative. Bromocriptine activates the dopaminergic receptors of the CNS, which may explain its action in parkinsonism. It is used as an adjunctive to levodopa or levodopa/ carbidopa therapy to relieve symptoms of Parkinson's disease. Bromocriptine is contraindicated in patients who are hypersensitive to ergot alkaloids, in those with uncontrolled hypertension or pituitary tumor, and in lactating women. Adverse effects include headache, dizziness, vertigo, fainting, sedation, nightmares, and insomnia. It may also produce blurred vision, hypertension, palpitation, arrhythmias, nausea, vomiting, and diarrhea.

HEADACHES

Headaches, the most common complaint of patients seen by physicians, usually occur as a symptom of an underlying disorder. Of all headaches, 90% are vascular, muscular, or both, and 10% are due to underlying intracranial, systemic, or psychological disorders. Migraine headaches, probably the most intensively studied, are throbbing, vascular headaches that usually begin to appear in childhood or adolescence and recur throughout adulthood. Affecting up to 10% of Americans, they are more common in females and have a strong familial incidence.

Treatment for Headaches

Treatment depends on the type of headache. Analgesics used for headaches range from aspirin to codeine or meperidine and may provide symptomatic relief. Other measures include identification and elimination of causative factors and possibly psychotherapy for headaches caused by emotional stress. Chronic tension headaches may also require use of muscle relaxants.

For migraine headaches, ergotamine alone or with caffeine may be an effective treatment. However, these medications cannot be taken by pregnant women because they stimulate uterine contractions. These drugs and others, such as metoclopramide or naproxen, work best when taken early in the course of an attack. If nausea and vomiting make oral administration impossible, drugs may be given as rectal suppositories. Sumatriptan (Succinate) is considered to be the drug of choice for acute migraine attacks or cluster headaches. Other drugs that can help prevent migraine headaches include propranolol, atenolol, clonidine, and amitriptyline. Until 2000, the leading drug to combat migraine headaches was sumatriptan (Imitrex), but it has recently been superseded by almotriptan malate (Axert), which is as effective against migraines but with less side effects. Although both drugs relieve the devastating pain of a migraine, side effects may include nausea, dizziness, and sleepiness. A newer drug is frovatriptan succinate (Frova), which offers the additional benefit of helping to prevent migraines from coming back, at least in the short term. Most of these drugs activate serotonin receptors, narrowing the blood vessels of the brain and scalp.

INSOMNIA

Insomnia is a chronic inability to sleep. It is associated with and complicates a number of medical and psychiatric disorders. It may also be caused by stress, sleep schedule, medication and ingested substances, lifestyle, and primary sleep disorders.

Treatment for Insomnia

A number of classes of pharmacologic agents are used in the treatment of insomnia, including barbiturates, antipsychotic agents, antihistaminic compounds, and sedating antidepressants. However, many of these drugs have not been effective in the treatment of insomnia, are associated with unacceptable side effects, or both. Depression of the CNS reduces physical and mental activity; this is often related to the use of barbiturates, alcohol, and benzodiazepines. Zolpidem tartrate (Ambien) is the sleep aid prescribed most often in the United States. It is prescribed for people who have trouble falling asleep, who have trouble staying asleep, or who awake too early. This drug and the related drug zaleplon (Sonata) are in the class of drugs called sedative-hypnotic. Both of these substances are for short-term use only (less than 10 days). Longer-term use should only occur under close supervision of a physician.

NARCOTIC ANALGESICS

Opioid is the generic term for drugs with morphine-like activity that reduce pain and induce tolerance and physical dependence. They are also referred to as *narcotic analgesics*. *Opiate* is the generic term for drugs made from opium such as morphine and heroin, a powdered, dried exudate of the fruit capsule (poppy) of the plant *Papaver somniferum*. Opium alkaloids (e.g., thebaine) are used to make semisynthetic opioids.

Some opioids are prepared synthetically, such as meperidine and methadone. Narcotic analgesics are thought to change pain perception in the spinal cord, brain stem, thalamus, and limbic system. Opiate receptors in each of these areas interact with neurotransmitters of the autonomic nervous system, producing alterations in reaction to painful stimuli. The narcotic drugs relieve pain and produce sedation, euphoria, mental clouding, respiratory depression, meiosis, and constipation. They also cause depression of the cough reflex and orthostatic hypotension. Narcotic analgesics are used to treat moderate-to-severe acute pain. They are prescribed for acute coronary, pulmonary, hepatic, or renal vascular pain. Narcotic analgesics such as morphine are also used as preoperative medications and for severe diarrhea, persistent cough (codeine), pulmonary edema and its accompanying dyspnea, and post-surgical trauma. Adverse reactions to narcotic analgesics include hypotension, bradycardia, anorexia, constipation, dry mouth, euphoria, vomiting, itching, syncope, and shortness of breath. Overdosage may cause respiratory depression, deep sleep, coma, meiosis, cyanosis, hypotension, oliguria, and hypothermia. Table 23-9 shows the most common narcotic analgesics.

ANESTHESIA

Anesthesia, literally, is the unique condition of reversible unconsciousness or a loss of sensation. This condition is

TABLE 23-9. Narcotic Analgesics

GENERIC NAME	TRADE NAME	ROUTE OF ADMINISTRATION
fentanyl	Duragesic®	Transdermal patch
hydromorphone	Dilaudid®	Oral, SC, IM, IV
hydrocodone	Lortab®	Oral
meperidine	Demerol®	Oral, SC, IM
methadone	Dolophine®	Oral, SC, IM
morphine sulfate	Astramorph/PF®	Oral, SC, IM, IV
	Avinza®	
	Duramorph®	
	Infumorph 200®	
	Infumorph 500®	
	Kadian®	
	Morphine Sulfate®	
	MS Contin®	
	MS/L®	
	MS/L® concentrate	Oral
	Oramorph SR®	Oral, SC, IM, IV
	Roxanol®	Oral
	Roxanol SR®	Oral
	Morrhuate Sodium®	Oral
	Scleromate®	
	Statex®	
camphorated opium tincture	Paregoric	Oral
pentazocine	Talwin®, Talacen®	Oral, SC, IM
propoxyphene	Darvon®	Oral
codeine	Codeine®	Oral, SC, IM
oxycodone	OxyContin®	Oral

IM, intramuscular; IV, intravenous; SC, subcutaneous.

produced by certain chemical substances that have been called anesthetics. Anesthesia is characterized basically by four reversible actions: unconsciousness, analgesia, immobility, and amnesia. The critical factor is that no significant impairment of cardiovascular or respiratory functions, especially those supplying the brain and other vital organs with adequate blood, nutrients, and gases, should occur.

Anesthetics are agents that act generally on nervous tissue. General anesthetics produce a state affecting overall body function, but in anesthetic concentrations they do not produce detectable generalized effects on all nerves or all nerve cell membranes. Most of the major anesthetic agents in current use are listed in Table 23-10.

Stages and Planes of Anesthesia

The use of stages and planes helps to describe the levels and progression of anesthesia produced by anesthetics. There are four stages of anesthesia:

Stage I—Analgesia that begins when the agent is administered and lasts until loss of consciousness. Stage I is characterized by analgesia, euphoria, perceptual distortions, and amnesia.

Stage II—Delirium begins with loss of consciousness and extends to the beginning of surgical anesthesia. There may be excitement and involuntary muscular activity. The skeletal muscle tone increases and breathing is irregular. At this stage hypertension and tachycardia may occur.

Stage III—Surgical anesthesia lasts until spontaneous respiration ceases. It is further divided into four planes based on respiration, size of the pupils, reflex characteristics, and eyeball movements.

Stage IV—Medullary depression begins with cessation of respiration and ends with circulatory collapse. The pupils are fixed and dilated. There are no lid or corneal reflexes.

TABLE 23-10. General Anesthetics Currently in Use

ADMINISTERED BY INHALATION	ADMINISTERED INTRAVENOUSLY
Nitrous oxide	**Barbiturates**
halothane (Fluothane®)	thiopental (Pentothal®)
enflurane (Ethrane®)	methohexital (Brevital®)
isoflurane (Forane®)	**Benzodiazepines**
	diazepam (Valium)
	midazolam (Versed®)
	propofol (Diprivan®)
	ketamine (Ketalar®)

The most common route of administration for general anesthesia is inhalation, although some general anesthetics are given intravenously. The major intravenous drugs are used as an aid for induction of anesthesia or as preoperative medications.

Local Anesthetics

Local anesthetics are agents that act to produce a loss of sensation from a local area of the body. Local anesthetics act by depressing the excitability of excitable tissues. The objective of local anesthesia is to decrease pain. A primary site of action of local anesthetics is the nerve membrane. Local anesthetics can induce neuromuscular block and are either esters or amides. They produce a transient and reversible loss of sensation (analgesia) in a circumscribed region of the body without loss of consciousness. Local anesthetics may be administered topically, by infiltration into tissues, by injection directly around nerves, and by injection into epidural or subarachnoid spaces. At therapeutic doses all local anesthetics except cocaine are vasodilators. Examples of local anesthetics are shown in Table 23-11.

DRUGS OF ABUSE

Most drugs of abuse act on the CNS to modify the user's mental state. Chronic use leads to psychological or physical dependence or both. This may result in the development of tolerance. Complications related to drug administration by the parenteral route under unsterile conditions or to the coadministration of adulterants are extremely common. These complications include the transmission of viral hepatitis, acquired immunodeficiency syndrome (AIDS), and various bacteria and fungi, as well as the development of cellulites, thrombophlebitis, and local or systemic abscesses. The following terms are commonly used when one refers to drugs of abuse:

- **Drug abuse**: The use of a legal or an illegal drug that causes physical, mental, emotional, or social harm. These drugs may include narcotics, stimulants, depressants, antianxiety agents, and hallucinogens.

TABLE 23-11. Examples of Local Anesthetics

AMIDES	ESTERS
lidocaine (Xylocaine®)	procaine (Novocaine®)
mepivacaine (Carbocaine®)	chloroprocaine (Nesacaine®)
prilocaine (Citanest®)	cocaine
bupivacaine (Marcaine®)	tetracaine (Pontocaine®)
etidocaine (Duranest®)	dibucaine (Nupercaine®)
	benzocaine (Americaine®)

- **Tolerance**: A reduced drug effect with repeated use of a drug and a need for higher doses to produce the same effect.
- **Cross-tolerance**: Tolerance to one drug conferring tolerance to other drugs in the same drug class.
- **Dependence**: The psychological, physiological, or biochemical need to continue to take a drug.
- **Psychological dependence**: The overwhelming need to take a drug to maintain a sense of well-being.
- **Physical dependence**: The necessity to continue drug use to avoid a withdrawal syndrome.
- **Cross-dependence**: The ability of one drug to substitute for another drug in the same drug class to maintain a dependent state or prevent withdrawal.

Drugs of abuse may affect the CNS in several different ways such as depression, stimulation, and hallucination. Depressant drugs include benzodiazepines, barbiturates, marijuana, and ethanol. The benzodiazepines and barbiturates were discussed earlier in this chapter. Drugs that stimulate the CNS include amphetamines, cocaine, and nicotine. Drugs that cause hallucinations are called psychodysleptics (hallucinogens) and include lysergic acid diethylamide and phencyclidine.

Marijuana

Marijuana is classified as a CNS depressant, but can cause euphoria, sedation, and hallucinations. The resin from the female hemp plant *(Cannabis sativa)* is known as hashish, while the dried flower and leaves are called marijuana. Street names for marijuana include grass, weed, hemp, pot, and dope. Cigarettes made from marijuana are called joints, stogies, and reefers. Marijuana produces sedation, euphoria, and sometimes hallucinations. No other drug is able to produce all three of these responses. Marijuana increases heart rate, bronchodilatation, and cough. In males, sperm count and testosterone levels in the plasma are reduced. Females have a reduction in luteinizing hormone and prolactin, causing irregular menstrual cycles and sporadic ovulation. Estrogen levels are also reduced.

Ethanol (Ethyl Alcohol)

Alcohol is a CNS depressant. Its effects are dose dependent, with high doses causing depression of the medulla in the brain, and the basic functions of life. The most common concern is the nonmedical chronic use of alcohol by heavy drinkers, which causes atrophy of the cerebrum and a loss of intellectual functions. In extreme doses, alcohol may produce anesthesia that could be lethal.

The mechanism of action of ethanol is not known. It is used primarily as an antiseptic or as a solvent for other drugs. However, it is the most seriously abused drug. Ethanol depresses CNS activity (like other sedative-hypnotic drugs) and has antianxiety and sedative effects. It is rapidly absorbed from the stomach and small intestine and rapidly distributed in total body water. Absorption is delayed by food. The extreme dependence on excessive amounts of alcohol, associated with a cumulative pattern of deviant behaviors, is called *alcoholism*. Alcohol-related problems are common in males and peak in the 18- to 29-year-old age group, although they continue at a significant rate through middle age. Alcoholism is a maladaptive pattern of alcohol use, leading to a clinically significant impairment or distress, as manifested by three or more of the following occurring at any time in the same 12-month period:

1. Persistent desire for or one or more unsuccessful efforts to cut down or control drinking.
2. Characteristic withdrawal syndrome for alcohol.
3. Need for a markedly increased amount of alcohol to achieve intoxication.
4. Drinking in larger amounts.
5. Important social or occupational activities given up or reduced because of drinking.

For patients who drink more than the recommended amount, the medical history should be reviewed for evidence of alcohol-related problems, including hypertension, depression, and sleep disorders. Discontinuing alcohol consumption after chronic use results in a withdrawal syndrome, indicating the development of physical dependence. Symptoms occurring over 1 to 2 days include anxiety, hyperexcitability, weakness, intestinal cramps, confusion, visual hallucinations, delirium, and convulsions. The withdrawal syndrome can be life-threatening in debilitated individuals.

Amphetamines

Amphetamine and also methamphetamine, ephedrine, and mephentermine at low oral doses are able to increase wakefulness, alertness, self-confidence, and the ability to concentrate. They also decrease appetite. Intravenous administration results in intense euphoria and a feeling of mental alertness. Adverse effects, which usually occur after repeated intravenous administration or after overdosage, include anxiety, inability to sleep, hyperactivity, and sometimes dangerous behavior. Overdosage results in tachycardia, hypertension, hyperthermia, and tremor.

Cocaine

The use of cocaine is associated with atypical tolerance and withdrawal phenomena (like those for amphetamine). High-level use of this substance is characterized by episodes of repetitive self-administration that may last many hours or days, during which time the user remains continually awake and typically continues until supplies are exhausted. Use of cocaine as "crack" (more pure), by smoking, or by intravenous administration greatly increases the danger of overdosage and death. Cocaine (4% solution) is used therapeutically for local anesthetic and vasoconstrictor activity for surgery involving mucous membranes. Adverse effects are similar to those of amphetamine, but overdosage is more often fatal because of respiratory depression, seizures, and cardiac arrest. It also may cause cerebrovascular accidents, increased occurrence of spontaneous abortions, sexual dysfunction, and toxic psychosis.

Nicotine

Nicotine is a constituent of tobacco, along with various gases and particulate matter. It causes CNS stimulation and sedation. Nicotine may stimulate or inhibit heart rate and blood pressure. It is able to relax skeletal muscle and increase muscle tone. Nicotine increases secretion of the gastrointestinal tract. It is rapidly metabolized in the liver and is eliminated by the kidneys. It is also excreted into breast milk. Adverse effects include possible development of lung, oral cavity, bladder, and pancreatic cancer. Nicotine may cause obstructive lung disease, coronary artery disease, acceleration of arthrosclerosis, and abortion. Nicotine causes strong psychological dependence. A withdrawal-like syndrome occurs within 24 hours and persists for weeks or months. The symptoms include dizziness, tremor, hypertension, irritability, anxiety, restlessness, difficulty in concentration, drowsiness, headache, increased appetite, nausea, and vomiting.

Psychodysleptics or Hallucinogens

People who are hallucinating have a false sensory perception that occurs in the absence of a relevant sense of reality. People may be able to identify what is in fact not a real occurrence. The classic examples of true hallucinogens are lysergic acid diethylamide (LSD) and phencyclidine (PCP). LSD is an extremely potent synthetic drug that, taken orally, causes altered consciousness, euphoria, and increased sensory awareness ("mind expansion"). There is no physical dependence with use of LSD. Adverse effects include "flashback," panic reactions, misjudgment, suicide, and psychosis. PCP can be taken orally or intravenously. It also can be snorted or smoked. PCP produces euphoria, hallucinations, changed body image, and increased sense of isolation and loneliness. It impairs judgment and increases aggressiveness. Behavioral actions are thought to be related to increased activity of dopamine.

Marijuana

The active ingredient in marijuana, tetrahydrocannabinol, is now being made available as a Schedule II drug for use in lessening the nausea resulting from cancer chemotherapy. It may also be used therapeutically to decrease intraocular pressure for treatment of glaucoma or to stimulate appetite in patients with AIDS. Adverse effects with chronic use are similar to those of cigarette smoking. It impairs short-term memory and also disturbs the immune and reproductive systems.

REVIEW QUESTIONS

1. The rigidity of the parkinsonian syndrome may be reduced by
A. bromocriptine.
B. amantadine.
C. benztropine.
D. all of the above.

2. Morphine
A. relieves asthma attacks.
B. relieves dyspnea that accompanies pulmonary edema.
C. increases the sensitivity of the respiratory center to CO_2.
D. does all of the above.

3. Orthostatic hypotension is an occasional side-effect of
A. phenytoin.
B. trimethadione.
C. morphine.
D. lithium.

4. Which of the following is useful for treatment of tonic/clonic (grand mal) seizures?
A. Phenytoin
B. Lithium
C. Haloperidol
D. Morphine

5. Buspirone (BuSpar) is used for
A. general central nervous system depression.
B. sedation.
C. hypnosis.
D. anxiety.

6. The generic name of Librium® is
A. clorazepate.
B. chlordiazepoxide.
C. diazepam.
D. lorazepam.

Continues

7. All of the following are adverse effects of benzodiazepines, except
A. rebound insomnia.
B. development of tolerance.
C. vomiting.
D. drowsiness.

8. The primary drug used to treat patients in manic states is
A. valproic acid.
B. phenytoin.
C. prazepam.
D. lithium.

9. Which of the following is the trade name of promethazine?
A. Phenergan®
B. Compazine®
C. Valium®
D. Prolixin®

10. All of the following are amides except
A. Xylocaine®.
B. Duranest®.
C. Novocaine®.
D. Carbocaine®.

11. Which of the following is the stage of surgical anesthesia?
A. Stage I
B. Stage IV
C. Stage II
D. Stage III

12. Which of the following agents is administered by inhalation for general anesthesia?
A. Valium®
B. Fluothane®
C. Ketalar®
D. Pentothal®

13. Which of the following types of seizures is called *grand mal seizure*?
A. Tonic/clonic
B. Absence
C. Myoclonic
D. Atonic

14. All of the following drugs are central nervous system stimulants, except
A. nicotine.
B. cocaine.
C. ethyl alcohol.
D. amphetamine.

15. Which of the following drugs of abuse is now being made available as a Schedule III drug?
A. Cocaine
B. Marijuana
C. LSD
D. PCP

Cardiovascular and Renal Drugs

24

OUTLINE

- Heart Diseases
- Antianginal Drugs
  - Nitrates
  - β-Adrenergic Blockers
  - Calcium Channel Blockers
- Antidysrhythmic Agents
  - Class I—Drugs That Bind to Sodium Channels
  - Class II—β-Adrenergic Blockers Used for Arrhythmias
  - Class III—Antidysrhythmic Agents That Interfere with Potassium Outflow
  - Class IV—Calcium Channel Blockers for Dysrhythmias
- Myocardial Infarction
- Drug Effects on Congestive Heart Failure
  - Cardiac Glycosides
  - Diuretics
- Hypertension and Antihypertensive Drugs
  - Diuretics
  - Antiadrenergic Drugs
  - Calcium Channel Blockers
  - Vasodilators
- Antihyperlipidemic Drugs
  - Bile Acid Sequestrants
  - Statin Drugs
  - Miscellaneous Antihyperlipidemic Drugs

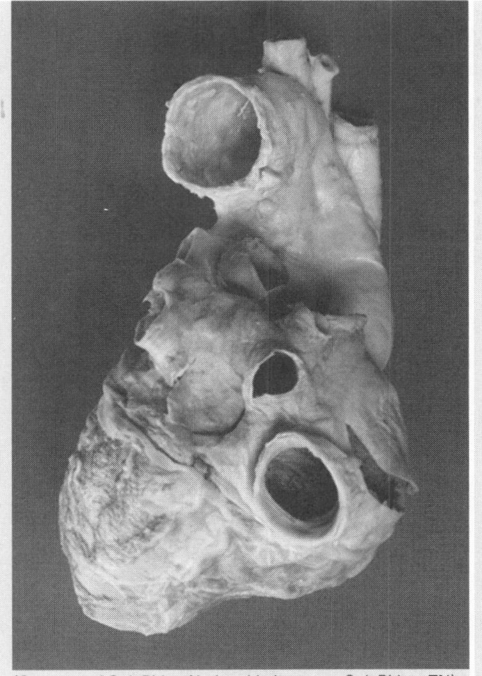

(Courtesy of Oak Ridge National Laboratory, Oak Ridge, TN)

GLOSSARY

angina pectoris An episodic, reversible insufficiency of oxygen to the heart muscle.

arrhythmia Loss of rhythm.

arteriosclerosis Hardening and narrowing of the arteries resulting from age.

atherosclerosis Narrowing of the arteries due to build up of plaque and fatty deposits on the walls of the arteries.

β-adrenergic blockers Drugs that reduce oxygen demand by decreasing heart rate and contraction of the myocardium while also decreasing arterial blood pressure.

bile acid sequestrants Drugs that are nonabsorbable and used for lowering cholesterol.

calcium channel blockers Drugs that prevent and reverse coronary spasm and decrease oxygen requirements, causing vasodilation.

cardiac glycosides Drugs derived from digitalis that increase cardiac output and renal blood flow.

congestive heart failure A condition in which the output of the heart is insufficient to supply adequate levels of oxygen for the body.

diuretics Drugs that reduce left ventricular pressure, decrease left ventricular volume, and lower oxygen demand.

essential (primary) hypertension A chronic cardiovascular disease with no known origins.

ischemic heart disease A condition in which there is insufficient blood supply to the myocardium.

myocardial infarction (MI) A condition in which a portion of the cardiac muscle suffers a severe and prolonged restriction of oxygenated coronary blood.

nitrates Antianginal drugs that relax vascular smooth muscles, dilating the vessels and lowering oxygen demand to decrease the work of the heart.
secondary hypertension A chronic cardiovascular disease related to an underlying abnormal condition.
statin drugs Drugs used to lower high blood cholesterol concentrations.
thrombolytic agents The agents that dissolve thrombi.

HEART DISEASES

Cardiovascular disease is the leading cause of death in the United States, with one of every five deaths being directly related to this disorder. Coronary artery disease occurs when insufficient blood flows through the coronary arteries. **Ischemic heart disease** is a condition in which there is an insufficient supply of oxygen to the myocardium (heart muscle tissue) so that oxygen demand exceeds oxygen supply. **Angina pectoris** is an episodic, reversible oxygen insufficiency. It is the most common form of ischemic heart disease. **Arteriosclerosis** is hardening and narrowing of the arteries, mainly due to aging. It causes decreased blood flow to the heart itself. Plaque from fatty deposits may develop in the arteries, called **atherosclerosis**. However, anemia, hyperthyroidism, hypotension, tachycardia, and arterial hypoxemia can all cause an oxygen imbalance. Angina pectoris involves spasms of the cardiac muscle as a result of insufficient blood flow to the myocardium (ischemia). The goal of therapy is to restore the balance between oxygen supply and demand in the ischemic region of the myocardium.

ANTIANGINAL DRUGS

Drugs to dilate blood vessels (vasodilators) are used for angina. There are three groups of medications that can be used for angina pectoris:

1. Nitrates
2. β-adrenergic blockers
3. Calcium channel blockers

Nitrates

The **nitrates** are the oldest and most commonly used antianginal drugs. The nitrates relax vascular smooth muscles. Dilation of all vessels occurs and, thus, lowers oxygen demand by decreasing the work of the heart. Nitrates are used during attacks of angina to relieve intense pain and are used prophylactically to prevent attacks (see Table 24-1). The most common route of administration is sublingual, with almost immediate onset of action (2 minutes) and a short duration of action (less than 30 minutes). Nitroglycerin is an example of this type of agent. It is the most widely used drug among the nitrates. The transdermal route is also available and is used to maintain blood levels. Nitroglycerin can be administered as a topical ointment, an aerosol, or an oral preparation. Adverse effects include vasodilation, resulting in orthostatic hypotension, tachycardia, and headache. Continuous exposure may lead to tolerance.

TABLE 24-1. Antianginal Agents

GENERIC NAME	TRADE NAME	ROUTE OF ADMINISTRATION
Nitrates		
nitroglycerin	Nitrostat®	Sublingual
	Nitrogard®	Transmucosal (tablets)
	Nitrong®	Oral
	Nitro-Bid®, nitroglycerin	Oral
	Transderm Nitro®, Nitro-Dur®, Nitro-Disc®	Transdermal patch
	Nitro-Bid®, Nitrol®	Transdermal ointment
isosorbide mononitrate	Monoket®, Imdur®	Oral
isosorbide dinitrate	Isordil®, Sorbitrate®	Sublingual
	Sorbitrate®	Oral chewable
	Dilatrate SR®	Oral
erythrityl tetranitrate	Cardilate®	Sublingual, oral
amyl nitrate		Inhalant
β-Adrenergic Blockers		
propranolol	Inderal®	Oral
Calcium Channel Blockers		
verapamil	Calan®, Isoptin®, Covera-HS®	Oral
nifedipine	Adalat®, Procardia®	Oral

β-Adrenergic Blockers

β-adrenergic blockers reduce oxygen demand, both at rest and during exertion, by decreasing the heart rate and contraction of the myocardium, which also decreases arterial blood pressure. β-blockers reduce the frequency and severity of exertional angina that is not controlled by nitrates. This prevents the development of myocardial ischemias and pain. Propranolol is often used for the treatment of angina (although other drugs may be used). β-blockers and their uses to treat other cardiac disorders will be discussed later in this chapter.

Calcium Channel Blockers

Calcium channel blockers are the newest group of drugs used to treat the pain of angina pectoris. These agents prevent and reverse coronary spasm and decrease oxygen requirements. The drugs cause coronary vasodilation. Calcium channel blockers are used for exertional angina that is not controlled by nitrates and β-blockers. Combination therapy may be the most effective. β-blockers are considered the drug of choice in treatment of angina at rest. Calcium channel blockers and their uses for treating other cardiac disorders are discussed later.

ANTIDYSRHYTHMIC AGENTS

The heart is a muscular pump divided into four chambers: two atria (located on the top of the heart) and two ventricles (located on the bottom). Each heartbeat in a normal person starts in the right atrium. Specialized groups of cells, called the sinus nodes (or natural pacemaker), send an electrical signal from the right atrium. This signal spreads throughout the atria to the atrioventricular (AV) node, located in an area between the two atria. The AV node connects to a group of pathways that conduct the signal to the ventricles. As the signal travels through the heart toward the ventricles, the heart contracts. These contractions occur as follows. First the atria contract, and blood is pumped into the ventricles. Just a fraction of a second later, the ventricles contract and send blood throughout the body. Figure 24-1 shows the conduction system of the heart. Usually, the entire heart contracts between 60 and 100 times per minute. Each contraction equals one heartbeat. An **arrhythmia** may occur for any of the following reasons:

- The heartbeat begins in another part of the heart rather than in the sinus node.
- The sinus node develops an abnormal rhythm or rate.
- A patient has a heart block.

An arrhythmia is a change in the regular heartbeat. The heart may seem to skip a beat, beat irregularly, beat very fast, or beat very slowly. Many arrhythmias occur in people who do not have underlying heart disease. Often there is no recognizable cause, although heart disease may cause arrhythmias. Other causes include stress, caffeine, tobacco, alcohol, diet pills, and cough and cold medicines. Arrhythmias do not cause harm in most people, and extensive examinations or special treatments are not needed. In those who do have heart disease, the heart disease itself and not the arrhythmia poses the greatest risk. In a very small number of people who have serious symptoms, the arrhythmias themselves may be dangerous and require medical treatment to keep the heartbeat regular. An example is a patient who has a very slow heartbeat (bradycardia), which causes lightheadedness or the feeling that he or she is about to faint. If arrhythmias are left untreated in this patient, the heart could stop beating and the patient could die.

Arrhythmias occur commonly in middle-aged adults. As patients age, they are more likely to experience arrhythmias. Types of arrhythmias that originate in the atria are as follows:

- Sinus arrhythmia
- Sinus tachycardia
- Premature supraventricular contractions
- Supraventricular tachycardia

Many different types of arrhythmias exist. They are identified by where they occur (the atria or the ventricles) and by what happens to the rhythm of the heart when they occur. Arrhythmias that arise in the atria are called atrial or supraventricular ("above the ventricles") arrhythmias. Those that begin in the ventricles are called ventricular arrhythmias. Ventricular arrhythmias caused by heart disease are generally the most serious. Many arrhythmias do not require treatment, although serious arrhythmias are treated using one or more of the following:

- Drugs
- Cardioversion (an electrical shock to the chest wall)
- Automatic implantable defibrillators
- Artificial pacemakers

Antidysrhythmic medications do not cure dysrhythmias, but they do attempt to restore normal cardiac function. These medications are found in four distinct classes, according to their effects.

Class I—Drugs That Bind to Sodium Channels

Class I drugs bind to the sodium channel and interfere with the sodium ion movement during heart excitation, which results in the heart being less excitable. Class I drugs include procainamide, disopyramide, lidocaine, and phenytoin (see Table 24-2).

Quinidine

Quinidine is used to treat abnormal heart rhythms. Do not confuse this medication with quinine, which, although related, has different uses. Quinidine is available only by prescription. It is used for atrial fibrillation, atrial flutter, and some ventricular dysrhythmias. Adverse effects include hypotension, severe headache, dizziness, blurred vision, nausea, vomiting, and diarrhea. Quinidine may also cause fatigue, weakness, and syncope.

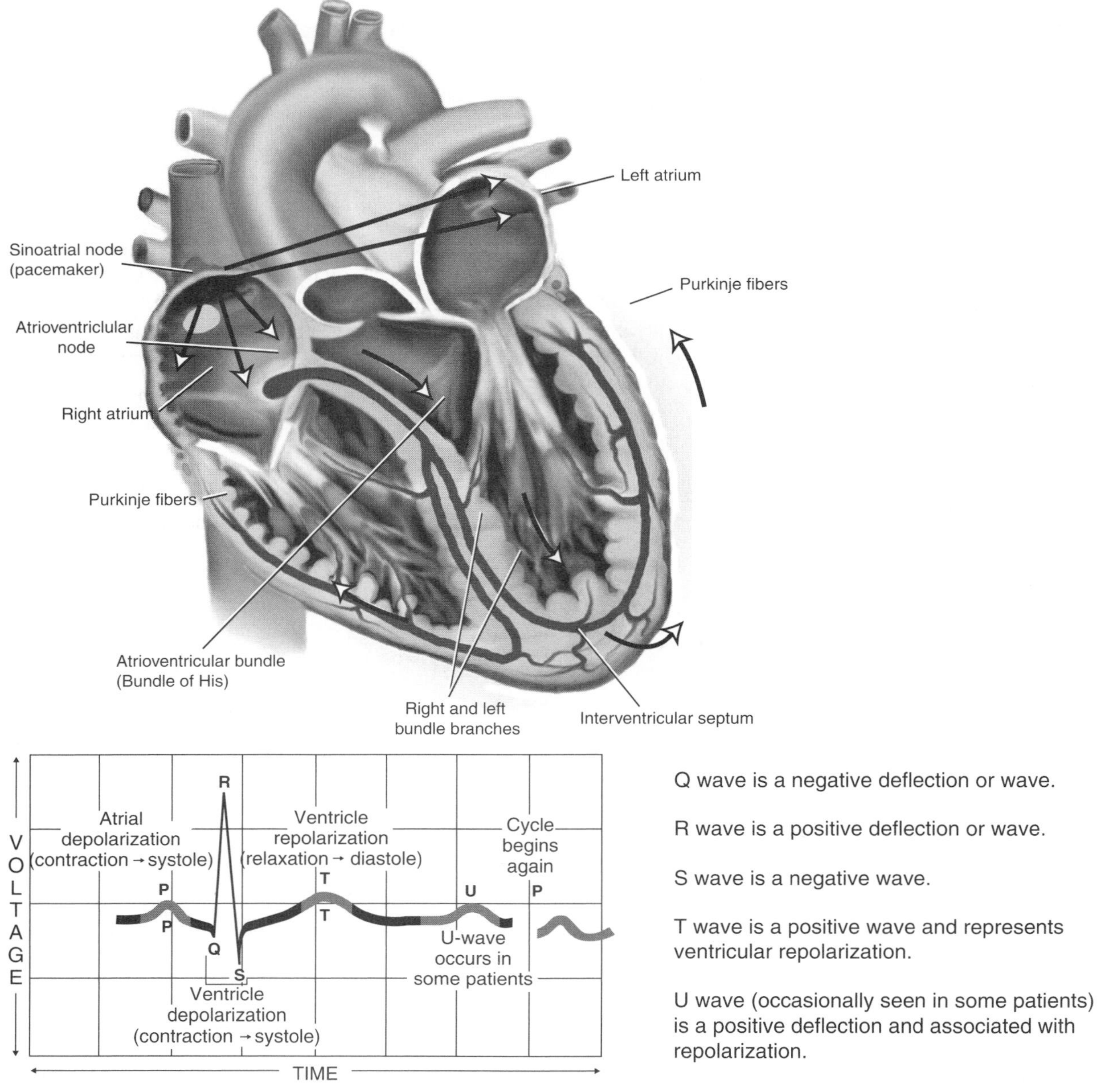

Figure 24-1. Cardiac conduction cycle.

Procainamide

Procainamide is related to procaine. It is used for treatment of ventricular arrhythmias that are life-threatening. Adverse effects of procainamide are the same as those of quinidine.

Disopyramide

Disopyramide is able to decrease cardiac excitability. Therefore, it is a cardiac depressant. Disopyramide is used for prevention of ventricular arrhythmias, which is considered to be life-threatening. Adverse effects include hypotension, edema, shortness of breath, syncope, and chest pain. Disopyramide may also cause dizziness, fatigue, headache, blurred vision, dry nose, dry eyes, and nausea.

Lidocaine

Lidocaine is an antidysrhythmic and a local anesthetic drug. It is used for ventricular arrhythmias and is given parenterally as a bolus (a dose of a medication preparation injected all at once, intravenously). Two agents that are chemically and therapeutically related to lidocaine have been modified for oral administration. These medications are mexiletine and tocainide. Adverse effects include hypotension, bradycardia, cardiovascular collapse, and cardiac arrest.

TABLE 24-2. Classification of Antidysrhythmics

GENERIC NAME	TRADE NAME	ROUTE OF ADMINISTRATION
Class I		
quinidine	Cardioquin®, Quinidex-SR®	Oral
procainamide	Pronestyl®, Pronestyl-SR®	Oral
disopyramide	Norpace®	Oral
lidocaine	Xylocaine®	IM, IV
mexiletine	Mexitil®	Oral
tocainide	Tonocard®	Oral
phenytoin	Dilantin®	Oral
Class II		
propranolol	Inderal®	Oral, IV
acebutolol	Sectral®	Oral
Class III		
amiodarone	Cordarone®	Oral, IV
sotalol	Betapace®	Oral
Class IV		
verapamil	Calan®	Oral
nicardipine	Cardene	
nifedipine	Pro-cardia	
diltiazem	Cardizem®, Tiazac®	Oral

IV, intravenous.

Phenytoin

Phenytoin is a medication for controlling grand mal epilepsy, which can alter nerve functions to act as an antidysrhythmic agent. Phenytoin is especially helpful in ventricular dysrhythmias induced by the use of digitalis. The adverse effects include hyperplasia of the gingiva (gums), mental confusion, insomnia, blurred vision, vertigo, and nystagmus.

Class II—β-Adrenergic Blockers Used for Arrhythmias

The β-adrenergic blockers reverse sympathetic activity that releases epinephrine and norepinephrine. The beta-blockers decrease the heart rate and the force of contraction, causing decreased oxygen use. This action prevents the development of myocardial ischemia and pain. Indications include restoration of blood pressure in certain acute hypertensive states and is used as an adjunct in treatment of cardiac arrest.

Propranolol

Propranolol is the most common β-blocker used as an antidysrhythmic agent. Adverse effects include hypotension, decreased heartbeat, mental confusion, and skin rashes.

Acebutolol

Acebutolol is a β-adrenergic blocker that primarily slows down the heart rate and decreases blood pressure. Acebutolol is used for management of hypertension and premature ventricular contractions. Adverse effects include hypotension, bradycardia, insomnia, fatigue, dizziness, and depression. Nausea, vomiting, diarrhea, dry mouth, impotence, and bronchospasm have also been reported.

Class III—Antidysrhythmic Agents That Interfere with Potassium Outflow

Class III medications are used in the treatment of dysrhythmias that interfere with potassium outflow during the resting phase of the heart (repolarization). This process results in decreasing the occurrence of heart failure.

Amiodarone

Amiodarone is an antidysrhythmic agent that prolongs action potential duration and the refractory period in myocardial cells. It may even block the exchange of sodium and potassium. Indications include treatment of life-threatening recurrent ventricular arrhythmias, for example, ventricular fibrillation and unstable ventricular tachycardia. This agent should only be used in patients with the indicated life-threatening arrhythmias because its use is accompanied by substantial toxicity. The adverse effects are dizziness, nausea, vomiting, anorexia, bitter taste, weight loss, numbness of the fingers and toes (paresthesias), and weakness.

Sotalol

Sotalol is an antidysrhythmic drug that is indicated for management or prevention of life-threatening ventricular arrhythmias. Adverse effects include sustained ventricular tachycardia or fibrillation. Depression, dizziness, lethargy, paresthesias, dry mouth, nausea, vomiting, and impotence are also seen.

Class IV—Calcium Channel Blockers for Dysrhythmias

Class IV agents are referred to as calcium channel blockers because they decrease the entry of calcium into the cells of the heart and blood vessels. The pacemaker cells—sinoatrial (SA) and AV nodes—require calcium for normal action. Calcium channel blockers reduce the amount of calcium on the SA node and the conduction velocity of the AV node. Therefore, these agents are effective in the treatment of supraventricular tachycardia. The calcium channel blockers also cause vasodilation by relaxing smooth muscle of the blood vessel walls. As a result of this effectiveness, these medications are used for angina treatment and hypertension.

Verapamil

Verapamil inhibits calcium ion influx through slow channels into cells of myocardial and arterial smooth muscle. Verapamil dilates coronary arteries and affects the SA node by decreasing its activity (decreasing the heart rate). It also decreases AV node conduction and is prescribed for AV node dysrhythmias. Verapamil is used for supraventricular tachyarrhythmias, angina, and essential hypertension. Adverse effects of verapamil include peripheral edema, hypotension, bradycardia, pulmonary edema, headaches, dizziness, nausea, and constipation.

Nicardipine

Nicardipine is a calcium entry blocker that inhibits the transmembrane influx of calcium ions into cardiac muscle and smooth muscle without changing calcium concentrations. Nicardipine may be used either alone or with β-blockers for chronic angina. It is also used either alone or with other antihypertensives for essential hypertension. Adverse effects are similar to those of other calcium channel blockers.

Nifedipine

Nifedipine is a calcium channel blocker that has a mechanism of action, indications, and adverse effects that are similar to those of nicardipine.

Diltiazem

Diltiazem is less potent than verapamil in decreasing the heart rate but is more potent as a vasodilator. Indications include treatment of angina pectoris caused by coronary artery spasm. It is essential for hypertension. Diltiazem is also useful for treatment of atrial fibrillation or flutter and supraventricular tachycardia.

MYOCARDIAL INFARCTION

In **myocardial infarction (MI)**, a portion of the cardiac muscle suffers a severe and prolonged restriction of oxygenated coronary blood. In the majority of patients, the cause of MI is an occlusive or near-occlusive thrombus or a ruptured atherosclerotic plaque. This results in cellular ischemia, tissue injury, and tissue necrosis (see Figure 24-2). Therapeutic agents include nitroglycerin, morphine, oxygen, and thrombolytic agents. Nitroglycerin helps to relieve chest pain. Controlling pain is crucial to relieving anxiety. Morphine is the drug of choice for MI pain and anxiety. Morphine can produce orthostatic hypotension, fainting, respiratory depression, bradyarrhythmias, nausea, vomiting, and severe constipation. Oxygen is required at 2 to 4 L/min via nasal cannula in any patient who has chest pain and who may have ischemia. **Thrombolytic agents** should be considered for all patients with an acute MI. Antithrombolytic agents include aspirin, heparin, warfarin, and antiplatelet agents.

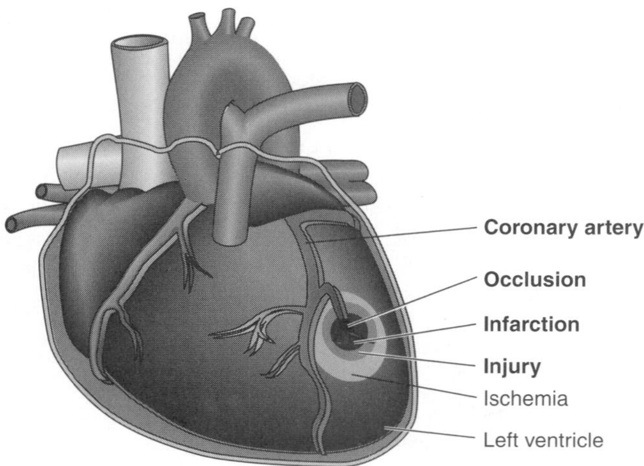

Figure 24-2. Myocardial infarction.

DRUG EFFECTS ON CONGESTIVE HEART FAILURE

Congestive heart failure (CHF) results when the output of the heart is insufficient to supply adequate levels of oxygen for the body. Impaired contractility and circulatory congestion are both components of failure. Therapy increases cardiac contractility and reduces left ventricular filling pressure and systemic vascular resistance. It also normalizes heart rate and rhythm. The principal drugs for heart failure change the force and the heart rate. Hypertension and coronary artery disease are risk factors for this disorder. The symptoms of CHF include tiredness, fatigue, shortness of breath, a rapid heart rate, and peripheral edema. Treatment for CHF includes bed rest, dietary controls, cardiac glycosides, diuretics, vasodilators, ACE inhibitors, β-adrenergic blocking agents, and calcium channel blockers.

Cardiac Glycosides

The oldest medications for CHF are the **cardiac glycosides**, digoxin and digitoxin, which are obtained from the plant leaves of digitalis. These glycosides provide benefits such as increased cardiac output and renal blood flow. They decrease cardiac filling pressure, venous and capillary pressure, heart size, fluid volume, and edema. After treatment with cardiac glycosides, the myocardium is able to increase the force of contractility, which improves blood circulation and reduces the congestion found with heart failure. The range between therapeutic and toxic doses is extremely narrow, and the patient must be watched closely. Dosing with digoxin is highly individualized, and each patient should be carefully evaluated until an effective dose has been established. A reduction in the dosage will usually relieve the symptoms of toxicity. Discontinuance of the glycoside may be necessary if the toxic symptoms continue. Adverse effects can be fatal. Digitalis induces virtually every type of arrhythmia. The major adverse effects are caused by overdose. The most common adverse effects of glycosides outside the heart occur in the gastrointestinal tract (anorexia, nausea, vomiting, and diarrhea). Disorientation, visual disturbances, headache, and slow pulse may also occur. All of the cardiac glycosides have similar properties; however, only digoxin has been deemed to be effective for the treatment of patients with chronic heart failure by the Food and Drug Administration (FDA) (see Table 24-3).

Diuretics

Diuretics reduce left ventricular filling pressure, decrease left ventricular volume, and lower oxygen demand. Diuretics are used in mild CHF and acute pulmonary edema. Body weight is an effective method of monitoring fluid losses and is best done on a daily basis by the patient. All diuretics increase urine volume and sodium excretion, but their pharmacologic properties differ. Diuretics used for the treatment of hypertension will be discussed later in this chapter.

HYPERTENSION AND ANTIHYPERTENSIVE DRUGS

In the past few decades, the definition of hypertension has changed drastically and seems to continue to change. It is presently recommended that antihypertensive therapy be started in patients who have "confirmed" hypertension, generally defined as a blood pressure exceeding 140/90 mm Hg. However, many more patients with blood pressure lower than 140/90 mm Hg have heart attacks, strokes, and other cardiovascular events than do patients with blood pressure greater than 140/99 mm Hg. Hypertension is a chronic cardiovascular disease affecting millions of Americans. It is known as a silent killer disease because 25% of the American population has hypertension. There are two types of hypertension, **essential (primary) hypertension** and **secondary hypertension**. Approximately 90% of cases of hypertension are essential, meaning that the causes are not known. Secondary hypertension is caused by another underlying abnormal condition, such as renal disease, complications of pregnancy, endocrine imbalances, obesity, arteriosclerosis, atherosclerosis, and brain injuries. The general principle of antihypertensive therapy is to reduce elevated blood pressure. Currently, there is no cure for primary hypertension. Antihypertensive therapy must begin with lifestyle modifications that are mostly nutritional and consist of weight loss for overweight patients, lowering of dietary sodium intake, modification of alcohol intake to at most two drinks per day, and maintenance of adequate dietary potassium, calcium, and magnesium intake. Regular physical activity for all hypertensive patients who have no conditions that would make exercise contraindicated are recommended. There is little doubt that many lifestyle factors, such as dietary salt intake, alcohol intake, exercise, and stress, can affect blood pressure and contribute to hypertension. Conversely, it has been well documented that blood pressure can be lowered by modifying lifestyle. For practicing physicians, these recommendations are often not very realistic. Once hypertension has been diagnosed, it should be treated with pharmacologic therapy. This statement does not mean that lifestyle modifications have no place in reducing hypertension because they can have profound effects. Drug therapy must start with β-adrenergic blockers and diuretics. If these drugs are not effective, treatment continues with antiadrenergic drugs other than β-blockers, calcium channel blockers, vasodilators, or a combination of drugs.

TABLE 24-3. Cardiac Glycosides

GENERIC NAME	TRADE NAME	ROUTE OF ADMINISTRATION
digoxin	Lanoxin®, Lanoxicaps®	Oral
digitoxin	Crystodigin®, Purodigin®	Oral

Diuretics

Diuretics increase sodium excretion by blocking the reabsorption of sodium and chloride. Because more fluid is retained in the kidney, excess water is excreted. The increase in urinary output is directly related to the degree to which reabsorption of sodium and chloride is blocked. Diuretics are the mainstays of hypertensive therapy and may be used alone or in combination with other antihypertensives. There are five major classes of diuretics: (1) thiazide diuretics, (2) loop diuretics, (3) potassium-sparing diuretics, (4) osmotic diuretics, and (5) thiazide-like diuretics (see Table 24-4).

Thiazide Diuretics

Thiazide diuretics are the most commonly used antihypertensive agents. These agents decrease blood volume and blood pressure. They increase the excretion of sodium, chloride, potassium, and water while increasing uric acid and glucose levels. Adverse effects are dehydration and loss of potassium. Hydrochlorothiazide is the most widely used of the thiazide diuretics.

Loop Diuretics

Loop diuretics are the most effective diuretics available, producing greater loss of fluids and electrolytes by acting on the loop of Henle (see Figure 24-3). Loop diuretics are not used routinely for hypertension but are used when diuresis is desired. Furosemide is the most commonly used loop diuretic. Its action is on reabsorption of sodium and chloride in the ascending loop of Henle. Adverse effects are loss of potassium, dehydration, increased uric acid and blood glucose levels, and hearing loss.

TABLE 24-4. Classification of Diuretics

GENERIC NAME	TRADE NAME	ROUTE OF ADMINISTRATION
Thiazide Diuretics		
chlorothiazide	Diuril®, Duragen®	Oral
hydrochlorothiazide	HydroDIURIL®, Esidrix®	Oral
cyclothiazide	Anhydron®	Oral
methyclothiazide	Enduron®	Oral
Thiazide-like Diuretics		
chlorthalidone	Hygroton®	Oral
metolazone	Zaroxolyn®	Oral
indapamide	Lozol®	Oral
quinethazone	Hydromox®	Oral
Loop Diuretics		
furosemide	Lasix®	Oral, IM, IV
torsemide	Demadex®	Oral, IV
ethacrynic acid	Edecrin®	Oral, IV
bumetanide	Bumex®	Oral, IV
Potassium-sparing Diuretics		
amiloride	Midamor®	Oral
spironolactone	Aldactone®	Oral
triamterene	Dyrenium®	Oral

IM, intramuscular; IV, intravenous.

Potassium-Sparing Diuretics

Potassium-sparing diuretics are able to produce diuresis while retaining potassium. They are used to avoid potassium depletion, especially when administered in the presence of cardiac glycosides. In hypertension, these agents are seldom used alone but are commonly used with primary drugs. Typical potassium-sparing diuretics are able to block aldosterone. Aldosterone is an agent that reabsorbs sodium in the distal part of nephrons.

Osmotic Diuretics

Osmotic diuretics contribute nonabsorbable osmolar particles to the tubule fluid and obligate water to remain with the extra solute. Mannitol is the most commonly used osmotic diuretic. Administration of mannitol results in increased total renal plasma flow. Urine flow increases as does excretion of sodium, potassium, chloride, bicarbonate, calcium, and magnesium. The major use of osmotic diuretics is related to increasing urine flow rate. They are used to prevent acute renal failure. The use of osmotic diuretics is contraindicated in a patient with congestive heart failure. Mannitol infusion should be terminated if a patient develops signs of progressive renal failure, heart failure, or pulmonary congestion. Otherwise, headache, nausea, and vomiting are relatively common complaints.

Thiazide-Like Diuretics

Thiazide-like diuretics are agents that inhibit reabsorption of sodium and chloride in the distal renal tubule, and increase excretion of sodium, chloride, potassium, and water by the kidney. Their indications for use are the same as thiazide diuretics. Adverse effects are dehydration, loss of potassium, orthostatic hypotension, cardiac dysrhythmias, headache, nausea, vomiting, hepatitis, and pancreatitis.

Antiadrenergic Drugs

Antiadrenergic drugs are the most effective of the antihypertensive medications. They are able to lower blood pressure by reducing peripheral resistance of blood vessels. Antiadrenergic drugs are also able to prevent serious cardiovascular complications. Antiadrenergic (sympatholytic) drugs include several different types, but all of these agents reduce blood pressure by inhibiting or blocking the sympathetic nervous system. They are classified by their site or mechanism of action and include the following:

- β-adrenergic blockers
- α/β-adrenergic blockers
- Peripherally acting adrenergic inhibitors
- Centrally acting adrenergic inhibitors
- Angiotensin-converting enzyme inhibitors
- Angiotensin II receptor antagonists

Table 24-5 shows classifications of antiadrenergic drugs.

β-Adrenergic Blockers

β-adrenergic blockers are especially useful in younger patients, in those with concurrent angina or vascular headaches, and in patients after myocardial infarction. The availability of a large number of different β-blockers with varying pharmacokinetic and pharmacodynamic variables can be confusing. However, the antihypertensive efficacy of all of them appears to be equal. Propranolol remains the gold standard because of the availability of inexpensive generic products. The longer-acting products (atenolol and nadolol) and those with relative β_1-receptor selectivity (atenolol and metoprolol) are widely used. The adverse effects include dizziness, vertigo, bradycardia, joint pain, bronchospasm, and sexual dysfunction. They are contraindicated in sinus bradycardia, asthma, and CHF.

α/β-Adrenergic Blockers

α/β-adrenergic blockers are similar to β-blockers and are prescribed for severe hypertension. The adverse effects are also similar to those of β-blockers, but postural hypotension, bronchospasm, dyspnea, and headache have also been reported. These agents cause vasodilation and decreased peripheral vascular resistance.

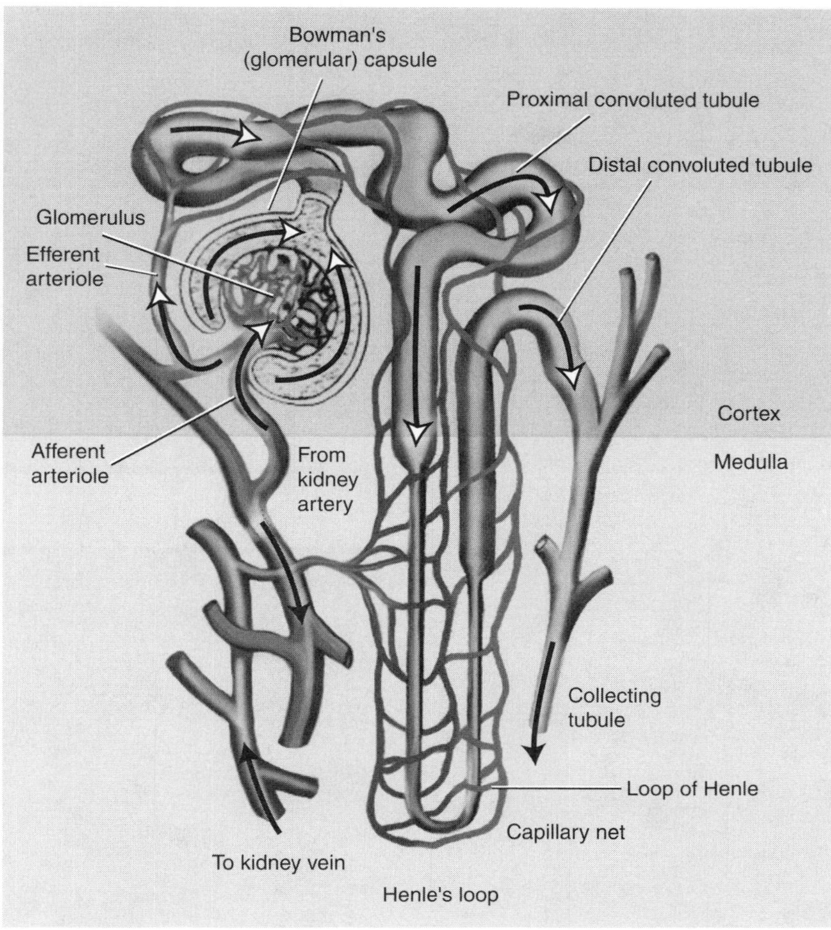

Figure 24-3. Structure of the nephron.

Peripherally Acting Adrenergic Inhibitors

Peripherally acting adrenergic inhibitors are potent antihypertensives. They interfere with the release of norepinephrine from nerve endings; therefore, these agents are able to decrease blood pressure by relaxing the smooth muscle of the vessels. The adverse effects include nausea, vomiting, dry mouth, depression, headache, and palpitations.

Centrally Acting Adrenergic Inhibitors

Centrally acting adrenergic inhibitors are effective antihypertensive agents, especially when used with a diuretic. Centrally acting adrenergic inhibitors reduce the hyperactivity in the medulla of the brain. Adverse effects include dizziness, dry mouth, anorexia, constipation, impotence, insomnia, nightmares, and CHF.

Angiotensin-Converting Enzyme Inhibitors

ACE inhibitors and calcium channel blockers are as effective as diuretics and β-blockers as first-line drugs. Their primary drawback is higher cost. These agents decrease the formation of angiotensin II, lower blood volume, and ultimately lower blood pressure. ACE inhibitors are used for the treatment of severe hypertension. ACE inhibitors are becoming the drug of choice in the first-line treatment of essential hypertension. Although these agents, as a group, are relatively free of side effects or toxicities in most patients, these do occur, and some can be life-threatening. The adverse effects include headaches, diarrhea, constipation, dry cough, dizziness, weakness, loss of taste, and joint pain. Table 24-6 shows ACE inhibitors used for hypertension.

Angiotensin II Receptor Inhibitors

The newest class of antihypertensive drugs is the angiotensin II receptor antagonists. This class of drugs has been approved for initial therapy for all grades of hypertension. One of the advantages of most angiotensin II receptor antagonists is that they can be given once a day and provide a smooth antihypertensive effect throughout a 24-hour period. Their efficacy is less pronounced in African Americans, in patients who are receiving volume expansion therapy, and in those taking nonsteroidal anti-inflammatory

TABLE 24-5. Classifications of Antiadrenergic Drugs

GENERIC NAME	TRADE NAME	ROUTE OF ADMINISTRATION
β-Adrenergic Blockers		
acebutolol	Sectral®	Oral
atenolol	Tenormin®	Oral
betaxolol	Kerlone®	Oral
bisoprolol	Zebeta®	Oral
carteolol	Cartrol®	Oral
metoprolol	Lopressor®	Oral
nadolol	Corgard®	Oral
pindolol	Visken®	Oral
propranolol	Inderal®	Oral
timolol	Blocadren®	Oral
α/β-Adrenergic Blockers		
labetalol	Normodyne®, Trandate®	Oral, IV
Peripherally Acting Adrenergic Inhibitors		
doxazosin	Cardura®	Oral
guanadrel	Hylorel®	Oral
guanethidine	Ismelin®	Oral
prazosin	Minipress®	Oral
reserpine	Serpalan®, Serpasil®	Oral
terazosin	Hytrin®	Oral
Centrally Acting Adrenergic Inhibitors		
clonidine	Catapres®	Oral, transdermal
guanabenz	Wytensin®	Oral
guanfacine	Tenex®	Oral
methyldopa	Aldomet®	Oral, IV
Angiotensin II Receptor Antagonists		
candesartan	Atacand®	Oral
irbesartan	Avapro®	Oral
losartan	Cozaar®	Oral
telmisartan	Micardis®	Oral
valsartan	Diovan®	Oral

drugs or cyclooxygenase-2 (COX-2) inhibitors. These drugs are the only antihypertensive drugs that have no specific adverse effects.

Calcium Channel Blockers

Calcium channel blockers are prescribed to treat angina, cardiac dysrhythmias, and hypertension. These medications decrease the influx of calcium in smooth muscles of the vascular walls, which results in relaxation of the muscles and lower blood pressure. The calcium channel blockers approved by the FDA for lowering blood pressure are shown in Table 24-7. The adverse effects include dry mouth, nausea, headache, dizziness, and tachycardia.

TABLE 24-6. Angiotensin-Converting Enzyme Inhibitors Used for Hypertension

GENERIC NAME	TRADE NAME	ROUTE OF ADMINISTRATION
benazepril	Lotensin®	Oral
captopril	Capoten®	Oral
enalapril	Vasotec®	Oral
fosinopril	Monopril®	Oral
lisinopril	Prinivil®, Zestril®	Oral
moexipril	Univasc®	Oral
perindopril	Aceon®	Oral
quinapril	Accupril®	Oral
ramipril	Altace®	Oral

TABLE 24-7. Most Commonly-Used Calcium Channel Blockers to Treat Hypertension

GENERIC NAME	TRADE NAME	ROUTE OF ADMINISTRATION
diltiazem	Cardizem®, Tiazac®	Oral
felodipine	Plendil®	Oral
mibefradil	Posicor®	Oral
nicardipine	Cardene®	Oral
nifedipine	Adalat®, Procardia®	Oral
nisoldipine	Sular®	Oral
verapamil	Calan®, Calan SR®, Isoptin®, Isoptin SR®	Oral

Vasodilators

Vasodilators relax the smooth muscle of the peripheral arterioles selectively and decrease their resistance. Vasodilator medications are used as second-line agents in patients with hypertension that is refractory to initial therapy with diuretics, β-blockers, or calcium channel blockers. The adverse effects are headache, dizziness, anorexia, hypotension, hyperglycemia, edema, and constipation. Table 24-8 lists the most commonly used vasodilators.

ANTIHYPERLIPIDEMIC DRUGS

Hyperlipidemia and atherosclerosis continue to be important medical concerns, especially with respect to their relevance as risk factors for coronary artery disease. Nicotinic acid and gemfibrozil are the current drugs of choice for the treatment of hypertriglyceridemia. Nicotinic acid or resin therapy reduces serum cholesterol and low-density lipoprotein

TABLE 24-8. Most Commonly Used Vasodilators

GENERIC NAME	TRADE NAME	ROUTE OF ADMINISTRATION
hydralazine	Apresoline®	Oral, IM, IV
minoxidil	Loniten®	Oral
nitroprusside	Nitropress®	IV
diazoxide	Hyperstat®	IV
tolazoline	Priscoline®	Oral

IM, intramuscular; IV, intravenous.

cholesterol (LDL-C) levels and has been shown to reduce the incidence of coronary events. Pravastatin and lovastatin are effective for reduction of serum cholesterol and LDL-C levels, but they have not been shown to decrease atherosclerotic events. Treatment of hyperlipidemia begins first with diet modification and exercise programs to reduce LDL-C to acceptable levels. Control of cholesterol levels can reduce the risk of atherosclerosis and subsequent cardiovascular disease. When medications are started, diet and physical activity must be continued. The antihyperlipidemic drugs are continued throughout the patient's lifetime because high levels of LDL-C will return if the medications are discontinued. Initial lowering of lipid concentrations should be accompanied by weight control, smoking cessation, moderate exercise, and blood pressure control. Because cholesterol concentrations become elevated in people as a result of diet, a basic recommendation for reducing the cholesterol concentration is to decrease caloric intake and lower the proportion of the diet composed of saturated fat. If diet alteration is attempted first and cholesterol levels are not lowered to acceptable concentrations, various pharmacological interventions are available. The argument for dietary change as the initial step is based on the following four considerations:

- It is the most physiological approach.
- The change should be lifelong.
- All drugs have known or potential adverse effects.
- Drug therapy is relatively expensive.

Antihyperlipidemic drugs are the group of medications used in adjuvant therapy to reduce elevated cholesterol and LDL levels in patients. There are two major classes of hypolipidemic drugs: bile acid sequestrants and statins (3-hydroxy-3-methylglutaryl-coenzyme A [HMG-CoA] reductase inhibitors). Other drugs that are also used for various effects on lipoproteins, but these two groups are the most specific. Classifications of antihyperlipidemic agents are listed in Table 24-9.

Bile Acid Sequestrants

Bile acid sequestrants are nonabsorbable drugs used for lowering cholesterol. Cholestyramine and colestipol are chloride salts of basic anion exchange resins. These resins are not

TABLE 24-9. Antihyperlipidemic Agents

GENERIC NAME	TRADE NAME	ROUTE OF ADMINISTRATION
Bile Acid–binding Resin		
cholestyramine	Questran®, Prevalite®	Oral
colestipol	Colestid®	Oral
Statins		
atorvastatin	Lipitor®	Oral
fluvastatin	Lescol®	Oral
lovastatin	Mevacor®	Oral
pravastatin	Pravachol®	Oral
simvastatin	Zocor®	Oral
Miscellaneous Antihyperlipidemics		
nicotinic acid (niacin)	Nicobid®, Niacor®	Oral
gemfibrozil	Lopid®	Oral
clofibrate	Atromid-S®	Oral
dextrothyroxine	Choloxin®	Oral

absorbed from the gastrointestinal tract. They bind bile acids by interrupting the enterohepatic circulation of bile acids. Therefore, the liver increases its utilization of cholesterol to bile acids, and the cholesterol level in the liver cells falls.

Cholestyramine

Cholestyramine is an antihyperlipidemic and a bile acid sequestrant agent. It binds bile acids in the intestine, allowing excretion in the feces. Cholestyramine is used as adjunctive therapy for reducing serum cholesterol levels in patients with primary hypercholesterolemia (elevated LDL levels). Adverse effects include headache, dizziness, fatigue, syncope, abdominal cramps, nausea, vomiting, and anorexia.

Colestipol

Colestipol is also an antihyperlipidemic and a bile acid sequestrant agent. Its mechanism of action, indications, and adverse effects are similar to those of cholestyramine.

Statin Drugs

Statin drugs are widely prescribed to lower high blood cholesterol concentrations and thus reduce the risk for heart disease. These drugs block cholesterol production in the body by inhibiting the enzyme HMG-CoA reductase in the early steps of its synthesis. One serious consequence of statin drugs is the inhibition of coenzyme Q10 synthesis. With long-term use, statin drugs can predispose patients to heart disease, the very condition these drugs are intended to prevent, by lowering the coenzyme Q10 levels.

Atorvastatin

Atorvastatin is an antihyperlipidemic agent and HMG-CoA reductase inhibitor. Therapeutic actions of atorvastatin include inhibition of HMG-CoA reductase. This enzyme is able to break down the first step of the cholesterol synthesis pathway, resulting in a decrease in serum cholesterol and serum LDL levels. HMG-CoA reductase inhibitors were introduced a little over a decade ago, and they have revolutionized the treatment of hyperlipidemia. For most hyperlipidemias, they are not only more effective than the older bile acid–binding resins, fibric acid derivatives, and niacin, but they are also more palatable and produce a much lower incidence of side effects and toxicities. Atorvastatin is used as an adjunct to diet for treatment of elevated total cholesterol, serum triglyceride, and LDL-C levels in patients with primary hypercholesterolemia. Adverse effects of atorvastatin are headache, abdominal pain, nausea, constipation, liver failure, and rhabdomyolysis (destruction of skeletal muscles), with acute renal failure and myalgia (muscle pain).

Fluvastatin

Fluvastatin is an antihyperlipidemic and statin agent that inhibits the enzyme HMG-CoA reductase, resulting in a decrease in serum cholesterol and serum LDL levels. Fluvastatin is prescribed an adjunct to diet in the treatment of elevated total cholesterol and LDL levels. The most common adverse effects include headache, blurred vision, insomnia, muscle cramps, and cataracts. Fluvastatin can also cause nausea, constipation, and abdominal pain.

Lovastatin

Lovastatin is an HMG-CoA reductase inhibitor that decreases serum cholesterol levels. It is used for the treatment of familial hypercholesterolemia and to slow the progression of atherosclerosis in patients with cardiovascular disease. Adverse effects are similar to those of fluvastatin.

Pravastatin

Pravastatin is another type of antihyperlipidemic agent and HMG-CoA reductase inhibitor. The action of this agent and its indications and adverse effects are similar to those of lovastatin.

Simvastatin

Simvastatin is one of the most commonly prescribed antihyperlipidemic agents and HMG-CoA reductase inhibitor. Therapeutic actions, indications, and adverse effects are similar to those of atorvastatin.

Miscellaneous Antihyperlipidemic Drugs

Some other agents are also used in the treatment of hyperlipidemia.

Nicotinic Acid

Nicotinic acid (niacin) is not only a vitamin but also is a therapeutic drug for hyperlipidemias. It may partially inhibit the release of free fatty acids from adipose tissue and increase lipoprotein activity. By this action, niacin could increase the rate of triglyceride removal from plasma, resulting in reduction of the total LDL and triglyceride levels. It is used as an adjunct to diet for the treatment of adults with very high serum triglyceride levels who present a risk of pancreatitis and who do not respond adequately to dietary control. Adverse effects include flushing and dry skin, which is common. Niacin may also cause headache, anxiety, arrhythmias, hypotension, peptic ulcer, abnormal liver function tests, hyperuricemia, and glucose intolerance.

Gemfibrozil

Gemfibrozil is an antihyperlipidemic drug that inhibits peripheral lipolysis and decreases the hepatic excretion of free fatty acids. This action reduces hepatic triglyceride production. Gemfibrozil is used for hypertriglyceridemia in adult patients with very high triglyceride levels, who are at risk of developing pancreatitis and whose hypertriglyceridemia is unresponsive to diet therapy. It is also used for reduction of the risk of coronary heart disease risk in patients whose condition has not responded to diet, exercise, and other agents. Adverse effects of gemfibrozil are similar to those of other antihyperlipidemics.

Clofibrate

Clofibrate is a drug for lowering cholesterol formation and LDL levels. It is prescribed in patients with very high serum triglyceride levels. Adverse effects include angina, dysrhythmias, phlebitis, thrombophlebitis, and pulmonary emboli. Clofibrate may also produce dry skin, alopecia, nausea, vomiting, diarrhea, gallstones (with long-term therapy), peptic ulcer, hepatic tumors, and impotence.

Dextrothyroxine

Dextrothyroxine is used to treat hypothyroidism in patients with heart disease. It increases the breakdown of LDLs. Common adverse effects include tremor, headache, irritability, and insomnia. It may also cause appetite changes, diarrhea, leg cramps, menstrual irregularities, fever, heat sensitivity, unusual sweating, and weight loss.

REVIEW QUESTIONS

1. Potassium-sparing diuretics are able to produce _______ while retaining potassium.
A. hypertension
B. diuresis
C. dysrhythmia
D. hyperkalemia

2. Which of the following is often used for the treatment of angina?
A. Potassium
B. Penicillin
C. Prednisone
D. Propranolol

3. Adverse effects of furosemide include
A. loss of potassium.
B. dehydration.
C. increased blood glucose levels.
D. all of the above.

4. Hydrochlorothiazide is the most widely-used of the
A. nonsteroidal anti-inflammatory drugs.
B. thiazide diuretics.
C. monoamine oxidase inhibitors.
D. diabetic medications.

5. The oldest agent used for congestive heart failure is
A. furosemide.
B. spironolactone.
C. diazepam.
D. digitalis.

6. The trade name of spironolactone is
A. Aldomet®.
B. Aldactone®.
C. Anhydron®.
D. Altace®.

7. The reason nitroglycerin is given sublingually is to
A. bypass the coronary circulation.
B. decrease renal excretion.
C. avoid hepatic first-pass metabolism.
D. decrease myocardial contractility.

8. The generic name of Lasix is
A. chlorothiazide.
B. atenolol.
C. furosemide.
D. ethacrynic acid.

9. Sotalol is a/an
A. diuretic.
B. antidysrhythmic.
C. antidiarrheal.
D. statin.

10. Digitalis toxicity is often associated with
A. nausea and slow pulse.
B. pleural effusions and pulmonary edema.
C. tinnitus and deafness.
D. hypertension and headache.

11. Which of the following is an adverse effect of clofibrate?
A. Dysrhythmias
B. Pulmonary emboli
C. Oily skin
D. Constipation

12. Hydralazine (Apresoline®) is a/an
A. vasodilator.
B. antihyperlipidemic agent.
C. diuretic.
D. calcium channel blocker.

13. The brand name of phenytoin is
A. Purinethol.
B. Dilantin®.
C. Tavist.
D. Atromid-S®.

14. β-adrenergic blockers are contraindicated in the presence of
A. congestive heart failure.
B. hypertension.
C. asthma.
D. A and C.

15. The symptoms of congestive heart failure (CHF) include
A. fatigue.
B. shortness of breath.
C. peripheral edema.
D. all of the above.

16. The most common route of administration for nitrates is
A. subcutaneous.
B. intradermal.
C. sublingual.
D. intramuscular.

17. Quinidine is used for
A. meningitis.
B. convulsion.
C. hemorrhage.
D. cardiac conditions.

18. Amiodarone is an antidysrhythmic agent in which of the following class?
A. I
B. II
C. III
D. IV

Continues

19. Which of the following is the drug of choice for myocardial infarction pain and anxiety?
    A. Nitroglycerin
    B. Thrombolytic agents
    C. Oxygen
    D. Morphine

20. The trade name of clonidine is
    A. Minipress®.
    B. Catapres®.
    C. Inderal®.
    D. Aldomet®.

Digestive System Drugs

25

OUTLINE

The Digestive System
Antacids
Histamine H_2 Receptor Antagonists
- Cimetidine
- Ranitidine
- Famotidine
- Nizatidine

Proton Pump Inhibitors
- Omeprazole
- Lansoprazole
- Rabeprazole
- Esomeprazole

Treatment for *Helicobacter pylori* with Ulcer
Antidiarrheal Agents
Laxatives and Cathartics
- Bulk-Forming Laxatives
- Fecal Softener Laxatives
- Hyperosmolar Laxatives
- Stimulant Laxatives
- Lubricant Laxatives

Antiemetics
Emetics

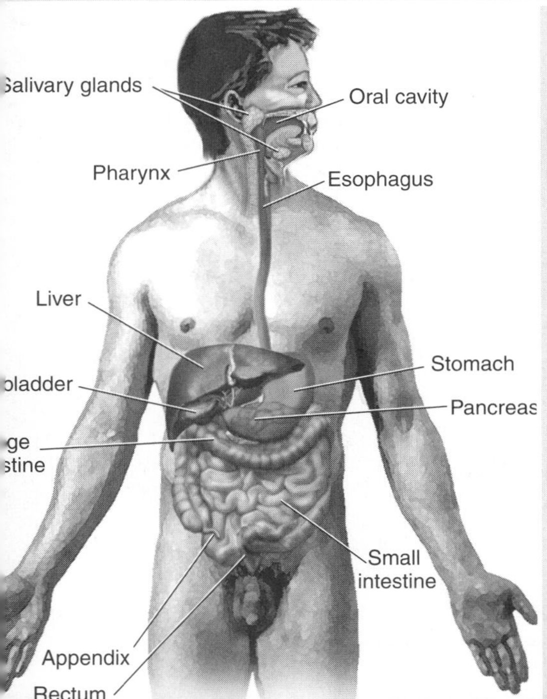

GLOSSARY

antacids Alkaline compounds used to neutralize hydrochloric acid in the stomach.

anticholinergics Medications that block acetylcholine.

antiemetics Drugs used to prevent or relieve nausea and vomiting that may be associated with many different disorders.

dopamine antagonists A major category of antiemetics.

emetics Agents used to promote vomiting.

histamine H_2 receptor antagonists Drugs that inhibit the interaction of histamine (H_2) at the H_2 receptors, which predominate in gastric parietal cells.

serotonin antagonists The most effective drugs for suppressing nausea and vomiting caused by antineoplastic drugs.

THE DIGESTIVE SYSTEM

The digestive system stores, digests, and absorbs nutrients and eliminates wastes. Regulation of the gastrointestinal (GI) organs is mediated by intrinsic nerves of the enteric nervous system, neural activity in the central nervous system, and an arrangement of GI hormones. Figure 25-1 is an illustration of the digestive system.

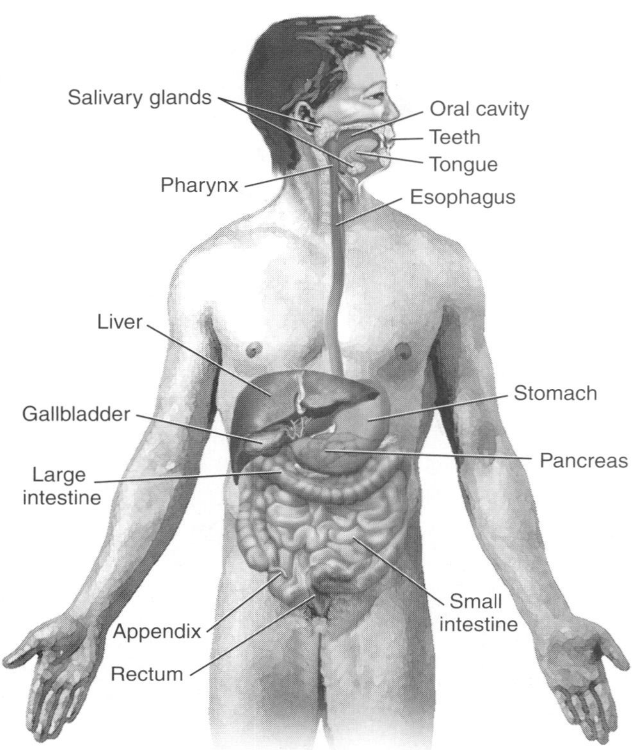

Figure 25-1. The digestive system.

The treatment of various conditions and disorders of the GI tract such as gastric peptic ulcer, delayed gastric emptying, constipation, diarrhea, vomiting, and infections must be carefully considered against potential adverse effects. Drugs for GI disorders work on muscular tissue and glandular tissue. They act either directly on these tissues or through the influence of the autonomic nervous system. These drugs may do any of the following:

1. Increase or decrease the function of the GI tract by changing muscle tone.
2. Change the rate of peristalsis (movement) of foods in the stomach and intestines.
3. Replace deficient enzymes.

ANTACIDS

Antacids are alkaline compounds used to neutralize hydrochloric acid in the stomach. The primary indication for antacids is peptic ulcer disease, but newer drugs are replacing these as the mainstays of ulcer therapy. Nonsystemic antacids containing aluminum and calcium cause constipation. Antacids containing magnesium have a laxative effect. Antacids are poorly absorbed with the exception of sodium bicarbonate (baking soda) and do not alter systemic pH when used as directed. Antacids are available as over-the-counter (OTC) drugs. They are classified by their formulation. The most common antacids are listed in Table 25-1.

TABLE 25-1. Common Antacids and Their Combinations

GENERIC NAME	TRADE NAME	ROUTE OF ADMINISTRATION
Selected Antacids		
aluminum compounds	Basaljel®	Oral
aluminum carbonate†	Alu-Cap®, Dialume®, Alu-Tab®	Oral
aluminum hydroxide†		Oral
magnesium compounds		
magnesium hydroxide†	Phillips'® milk of magnesia	Oral
magnesium oxide† and aluminum hydroxide†	Malox®, Mylanta®	Oral
calcium compounds		
calcium carbonate†	Tums®, Equilet®, Titralac®	Oral, IV
magaldrate†	Riopan®, Aludrox®, Gelusil®, Gaviscon®	Oral
sodium bicarbonate (baking soda)†	Alka Seltzer®	Oral
Other		
sucralfate*	Carafate®	Oral

*Prescription drug.
†OTC drug.

HISTAMINE H_2 RECEPTOR ANTAGONISTS

Histamine H_2 receptor antagonists inhibit the interaction of histamine (H_2) at the H_2 receptors, which predominate in the gastric parietal cells. Histamine H_2 antagonists are used to promote healing of gastric and duodenal ulcers and to treat hypersecretory conditions such as Zollinger-Ellison syndrome (a gastric acid-producing tumor that increases gastric and duodenal acid formation). These medications are not affected by food, so they may be taken with meals. Antacids and H_2 receptor antagonists should not be taken at the same time. Antacids should be taken 1 hour after cimetidine or ranitidine is taken. Histamine H_2 receptor antagonists are not recommended for use in nursing mothers or children younger than 16 years of age. Table 25-2 shows the classification of histamine H_2 receptor antagonists.

Cimetidine

Cimetidine is a histamine H_2 antagonist that is used to treat active duodenal ulcers, gastric ulcers, and pathological hypersecretory conditions (Zollinger-Ellison syndrome). Adverse effects include dizziness, sleepiness, confusion, diarrhea, impotence (reversible), gynecomastia (enlargement of breast in males with long-term treatment), and pain at the intramuscular injection site. Cimetidine can interact with warfarin and theophylline. It must be protected from moisture and strong light. It should not freeze.

Ranitidine

Ranitidine is a histamine H_2 antagonist that is 5 to 10 times more potent than cimetidine and requires less frequent dosing than cimetidine. Ranitidine also does not have antiandrogen activities and does not alter drug metabolism. This drug blocks daytime and nighttime basal gastric acid secretion, which is stimulated by histamine. Patients with hepatic and renal dysfunctions must be cautious when taking ranitidine. Side effects include a low incidence of headache and cutaneous rash.

TABLE 25-2. Histamine H_2 Receptor Antagonists

GENERIC NAME	TRADE NAME	ROUTE OF ADMINISTRATION
cimetidine	Tagamet®*, Tagamet-HB®†	Oral, IM, IV
ranitidine	Zantac®*,†	Oral, IM, IV
famotidine	Pepcid®*, Pepcid AC®†	Oral, IV
nizatidine	Axid®*,†	Oral

IM, intramuscular; IV, intravenous.
*Prescription drug.
†OTC drug.

Famotidine

Famotidine is a histamine H_2 antagonist. Indications for famotidine are similar to those for cimetidine and ranitidine. Adverse effects include headache, malaise, dizziness, insomnia, diarrhea, constipation, anorexia, and abdominal pain. Other side effects are muscle cramps, an increase in total bilirubin level, and sexual impotence.

Nizatidine

Nizatidine is also a histamine H_2 antagonist. Its indications and its adverse effects are similar to those of other histamine H_2 receptor antagonists.

PROTON PUMP INHIBITORS

Proton pump inhibitors suppress gastric acid secretion by inhibiting the H^+,K^+-adenosine triphosphatase enzyme system. In the parietal cells of the stomach, this enzyme acts as a pump to release acid onto the surface of GI mucosa. Proton pump inhibitors are widely used in the short-term therapy of duodenal and gastric ulcers. They are also used in gastroesophageal reflux disease as well as for long-term treatment of pathological hypersecretory conditions such as Zollinger-Ellison syndrome. Examples of proton pump inhibitors are shown in Table 25-3.

Proton pump inhibitors are a new class of drugs that work by inhibiting chemicals such as histamine, gastrin, and acetylcholine that are essential to the production of hydrochloric acid. These medications are for the short-term treatment of benign gastric ulcers. Proton pump inhibitors are effective when used in combination with antibiotics for *Helicobacter pylori* to promote ulcer healing and to prevent recurrence.

Omeprazole

Omeprazole is generally well tolerated. It is contraindicated for long-term use in patients with gastroesophageal reflux disease and duodenal ulcers and in lactating women. The most common adverse effects of omeprazole are headache, dizziness, fatigue, diarrhea, abdominal pain, nausea, hematuria,

TABLE 25-3. Proton Pump Inhibitors

GENERIC NAME	TRADE NAME	ROUTE OF ADMINISTRATION
omeprazole	Prilosec®	Oral
lansoprazole	Prevacid®	Oral
rabeprazole	AcepHex®	Oral
esomeprazole	Nexium®	Oral

and proteinuria. All proton-pump inhibitors should be used for only 4 to 8 weeks and then discontinued and should be prescribed only for confirmed active duodenal ulcers or erosive esophagitis.

Lansoprazole

Lansoprazole is one of the newest proton pump inhibitors used for gastric and duodenal ulcers. It is contraindicated in pregnant and lactating women and in patients who have severe hepatic impairment. Adverse effects are similar to those of omeprazole.

Rabeprazole

Rabeprazole is a proton pump inhibitor that suppresses gastric acid secretion. Indications for rabeprazole are similar to those for other proton pump inhibitors. Adverse effects are headache, dizziness, vertigo, insomnia, anxiety, dry skin, and alopecia. Rabeprazole may also cause diarrhea, abdominal pain, nausea, vomiting, constipation, dry mouth, and tongue atrophy.

Esomeprazole

Esomeprazole is a proton pump inhibitor that decreases gastric acid production in the stomach. Its indications and adverse effects are similar to those of the other proton pump inhibitors.

TREATMENT FOR *HELICOBACTER PYLORI* WITH ULCER

Peptic ulcer disease is believed to be caused by high gastric acid secretion. The bacterium *H. pylori* is found in 75% of duodenal ulcers. In chronic peptic ulcer, eradication of the bacterium has been found to prevent ulcer relapse in about 95% of patients. There is also a relationship between *Helicobacter* infection and adenocarcinoma of the stomach. Treatment for patients with peptic ulcers usually includes antacids, histamine H_2 receptor antagonists or proton pump inhibitors; other drugs are added as necessary. For eradication of *H. pylori* and healing of duodenal and gastric ulcers with drug therapy, special antibiotics must be added. The most common therapy for this condition includes the use of antibiotics (to reduce the risk of drug resistance) with bismuth salt (Pepto-Bismol®) to prevent the bacteria from attacking the stomach wall. The antibiotics of choice include amoxicillin (Amoxil®), clarithromycin (Biaxin®), tetracycline (Achromycin®), and metronidazole (Flagyl®). Bismuth products must also be added, such as bismuth subsalicylate (Pepto-Bismol®). Bismuth compounds are highly effective when combined with proton pump inhibitors and/or antibiotics. Eradication rates with these combinations are greater than 80%. Side effects with bismuth products include neurotoxicity, dark stools and tongue, headache, diarrhea, and abdominal pain. Treatment of *H. pylori* with ulcer antisecretory agents (proton pump inhibitors) should be included. Therefore, some medications for the treatment of *H. pylori* already exist as combinations. These combinations come in blister packs containing bismuth salicylate tablets, metronidazole tablets, and tetracycline, with a dose of one blister pack per day for 14 days, or ranitidine with bismuth citrate (Tritec®), omeprazole (Prilosec®), clarithromycin (Biaxin®) for short-term treatment. For long-term therapy for treatment of *H. pylori,* some combinations are listed below:

- Helidac® (bismuth, metronidazole, and tetracycline)
- Prevpac® (amoxicillin, clarithromycin, and lansoprazole)
- Tritec® (bismuth and ranitidine)

The goals of treatment of active *H. pylori*-associated ulcers are to relieve dyspeptic symptoms, to promote ulcer healing, and to eradicate *H. pylori* infection.

ANTIDIARRHEAL AGENTS

Antidiarrheal agents are used to treat diarrhea, which is a symptom of a disorder of the bowel associated with too rapid passage of intestinal content, gripping action, and frequent, watery stools. Diarrhea may be caused by certain medications, contaminated or spoiled food, maldigestion of food, intestinal infections, inflammatory bowel disorders such as Crohn's disease or ulcerative colitis, and chemicals such as lactate. Superinfections occurring during anti-infective

TABLE 25-4. Antidiarrheals

GENERIC NAME	TRADE NAME	ROUTE OF ADMINISTRATION
attapulgite†	Kaopectate®	Oral
bismuth subsalicylate†	Pepto-Bismol®	Oral
cholestyramine*	Questran®	Oral
activated charcoal†	CharcoCaps®	Oral
loperamide	Imodium®*,†	Oral
camphorated opium tincture (paregoric [Schedule III])*		Oral
difenoxin with atropine*	Motofen®	Oral
diphenoxylate with atropine*	Lomotil® (Schedule V)	Oral

*Prescription drug.
†OTC drug.

therapy are common causes of diarrhea. Diarrhea in children may become a medical emergency in as few as 24 hours because of the loss of electrolytes. The antidiarrheal agents are classified as absorbents and opioid or synthetic opioid medications. Selected agents used to treat diarrhea are shown in Table 25-4.

Opioid antidiarrheal agents are the most effective drugs for controlling diarrhea. Lomotil®, Motofen®, and Imodium® are commonly used antidiarrheal agents. Kaopectate® and Pepto-Bismol® also control diarrhea through absorbent action.

LAXATIVES AND CATHARTICS

Laxatives and cathartics are agents used to induce defecation (elimination of feces). Most of these medications are OTC preparations. These drugs are used for constipation, particularly in elderly patients. Constipation in elderly patients may lead to bowel obstruction or habituation to laxatives. Reasons that elderly patients have more constipation are polypharmacy and multiple chronic illnesses. Constipation is also common in children because of several factors such as emotions, dietary changes, fever, and new environments. Glycerin suppositories are the most appropriate treatment for constipation in children aged 10 years and younger. Laxatives produce the leisurely production of a soft-formed stool over a period of 1 to 2 days. Cathartics produce a fast, intense fluid evacuation from the bowel. The five major categories of laxatives are bulk-forming, fecal softener, hyperosmolar, stimulant and lubricant. They are often used in preparing patients for x-ray, obstetric, or surgical procedures. The rate of overuse of laxatives is high, and they destroy the body's natural emptying rhythm when used excessively. Bowel evacuations, or bowel cleaning solutions, are mixtures similar to body fluids so that water and electrolytes are neither absorbed nor secreted into the intestines. These agents can be used even in patients who are sensitive to electrolyte imbalance because water is not lost and electrolyte balance is maintained. Table 25-5 shows the most commonly used laxatives.

Bulk-Forming Laxatives

Bulk-forming laxatives increase peristalsis of the intestinal tract and are among the least harmful of the laxatives. These

TABLE 25-5. Laxatives and Cathartics

GENERIC NAME	TRADE NAME	ROUTE OF ADMINISTRATION
Bulk-forming Laxatives†		
methylcellulose	Citrucel®, Unifiber®	Oral
psyllium hydrophilic	Metamucil®, Perdiem®, Serutan®	Oral
polycarbophil	Mitrolan®, Fiber-Con®	Oral
Fecal Softener Laxatives†		
docusate sodium	Colace®	Oral
docusate potassium	Dialose®	Oral
docusate calcium	Surfak®	Oral
Hyperosmolar Laxatives†		
magnesium sulfate	Epsom salts	Oral
lactulose	Cephulac®	Oral
magnesium hydroxide	Phillips'® milk of magnesia, Phillips'® Chewable	Oral
sodium salts	Fleet® Enema®, Fleet® Phospho-Soda®	Rectal
Stimulant Laxatives†		
bisacodyl	Dulcolax®	Oral, rectal
senna	Purge®	Oral
cascara sagrada	Senokot®	Oral
Lubricant Laxatives†		
mineral oil	Kondremul®, Petrolagar®, Agoral®	Oral
glycerin	Sani-Supp®	Rectal
castor oil		Oral
Bowel Evacuants*		
electrolyte solution	Peg Lyte®	Oral
polyethylene glycol	Colyte®	Oral

*Prescription drug.
†OTC drug.

agents require large amounts of fluid to work properly. Laxation occurs after 2 to 4 days. The bulk-forming types are the laxatives of choice for pregnant patients. Their side effects are minimal.

Fecal Softener Laxatives

Fecal softener laxatives are drugs that lower the surface tension of the fecal mass, allowing intestinal fluids to penetrate and soften the stool. They are also called stool softeners.

Hyperosmolar Laxatives

Hyperosmolar laxatives directly stimulate the urge to defecate by their physical presence in the lower colon. These agents increase the amount of water in the colon and, thus, in the feces. Hyperosmolar laxatives can cause a substantial loss of fluids, and replacement is required. Because of the fluid retention, these laxatives should not be used in patients with edema, heart failure, and hypertension. Milk of magnesia is the mildest of the hyperosmolar laxatives.

Stimulant Laxatives

Stimulant laxatives are absorbed and, later, act directly on the intestinal mucosa to stimulate peristalsis. Examples are bisacodyl, senna, and castor oil. Cascara sagrada is the mildest of the laxatives in this group. If a patient uses senna, it may cause a yellow or yellow-green cast to feces, red-pink discoloration of alkaline urine, and a yellow-brown color in acid urine. The side effects are abdominal cramping, diarrhea, and flatulence.

Lubricant Laxatives

Lubricant laxatives coat fecal contents and thereby inhibit absorption of water. These laxatives do not increase bulk, but coat the surface of the stools and soften them to ease defecation. Mineral oil is used orally and is also given rectally as an enema for retention and softening. Side effects include decreased absorption of fat-soluble vitamins and lipoid pneumonia if aspirated.

ANTIEMETICS

Antiemetics are used to prevent or relieve nausea and vomiting that may be associated with many different disorders. The causes include infectious diseases that can directly irritate vomiting centers to inhibit impulses going to the stomach. Certain drugs, radiation, and chemotherapy may irritate the GI tract or stimulate the chemoreceptor trigger zone and vomiting center in the brain (medulla). After surgery, particularly abdominal surgery, nausea and vomiting are common. The main neurotransmitters that produce

TABLE 25-6. Common Antiemetic Agents

GENERIC NAME	TRADE NAME	ROUTE OF ADMINISTRATION
Serotonin Antagonists*		
ondansetron	Zofran®	Oral, IV
granisetron	Kytril®	Oral, IV
dolasetron	Anzemet®	Oral, IV
Dopamine Antagonists*		
promethazine	Phenergan®	Oral, IM, IV, rectal
perphenazine	Trilafon®	Oral, IM, IV
metoclopramide	Reglan®	Oral, IM, IV
Antihistamines and Anticholinergics*		
scopolamine	Transderm-Scop®, Transderm-V®	Transdermal patch
dimenhydrinate*,†	Dramamine®, Dramanate®	Oral, IM, IV
meclizine*,†	Antrizine®, Antivert®	Oral
cyclizine*,†	Marezine®	Oral
Corticosteroids*		
dexamethasone	Decadron®,* Deronil®	Oral
Benzodiazepines*		
lorazepam	Ativan	Oral
diazepam	Valium	Oral, IV

*Prescription drug.
†OTC drug.

nausea and vomiting include dopamine, serotonin, and acetylcholine. Vomiting may cause dehydration, imbalance of electrolytes, metabolic alkalosis, and arrhythmias. Antiemetics are divided into several classes, depending on how they work on the body. Examples of each class of the antiemetics are listed in Table 25-6.

Serotonin antagonists are the most effective drugs for suppressing nausea and vomiting caused by antineoplastic drugs. The adverse effects include diarrhea and headache. **Dopamine antagonists** are a major category of antiemetics. These medications suppress vomiting by blocking dopamine D_2 receptors. Adverse effects are headache, dizziness, dry mouth, and hypotension. **Anticholinergics** are medications that block acetylcholine. Antihistamines block acetylcholine and histamine and are used to treat motion sickness. Common adverse effects are sedation, dry mouth, urinary retention, and blurred vision. Corticosteroids are used to suppress nausea and vomiting from chemotherapy. Benzodiazepines are also used to suppress vomiting in patients receiving chemotherapy. Benzodiazepines are discussed in Chapter 23.

EMETICS

Emetics are agents used to promote vomiting. They usually are given for poisoning or drug overdose. The nearest poison control center should be called before using these medications. Ipecac is the OTC agent given to produce vomiting and should be in a home emergency kit. Ipecac stimulates the chemoreceptors of the vomiting center in the brain and irritates the stomach to induce vomiting. After taking ipecac, the person begins to vomit within 20 to 30 minutes. A full glass of water should be drunk after administration of ipecac to promote vomiting. If vomiting does not occur in 30 minutes, a second dose may be given. The effects of ipecac are stopped with activated charcoal.

REVIEW QUESTIONS

1. The trade name of nizatidine is
A. Zantac®.
B. Pepcid®.
C. Tagamet®.
D. Axid®.

2. Proton pump inhibitors are effective for *Helicobacter pylori* when used in combination with which of the following?
A. Histamines
B. Acetylcholine
C. Antibiotics
D. Antiemetics

3. Laxatives are used to induce
A. vomiting.
B. peristalsis.
C. defecation.
D. sleep.

4. An example of a bulk-forming laxative is
A. Polycarbophil.
B. Colace®.
C. Surfak®.
D. Purge®.

5. Which of the following drugs is a serotonin antagonist?
A. Promethazine
B. Metoclopramide
C. Scopolamine
D. Granisetron

6. Magaldrate (Riopan®) is a/an
A. proton pump inhibitor.
B. antacid.
C. antihistamine.
D. laxative.

7. Which of the following antiemetics are the most effective drugs for suppressing vomiting?
A. Dopamine antagonists
B. Anticholinergics
C. Antihistamines
D. Serotonin antagonists

8. Prevacid® is an example of a
A. laxative.
B. proton pump inhibitor.
C. histamine H_2 antagonist.
D. antidiarrheal agent.

9. The trade name of sodium bicarbonate is
A. Tums®.
B. Riopan®.
C. Alka Seltzer®.
D. Alu-Cap®.

10. Which of the following may be an adverse effect of cimetidine (Tagamet®)?
A. Constipation
B. Hypertension
C. Gynecomastia
D. Impairment of the kidneys

Continues

11. The trade name of rabeprazole is
    A. Nexium®.
    B. Prevacid®.
    C. AcepHex®.
    D. Prilosec®.

12. The route of administration for bisacodyl (Dulcolax®) is which of the following?
    A. Oral, intramuscular, intravenous, rectal
    B. Oral, intramuscular, rectal
    C. Oral, rectal
    D. Only oral

13. The most appropriate treatment for constipation in children younger than 10 years of age is
    A. glycerin.
    B. methylcellulose.
    C. bisacodyl.
    D. senna.

14. Ranitidine (Zantac®) may be administered by which of the following routes?
    A. Oral only
    B. Rectal only
    C. Oral, intravenous
    D. Oral, intramuscular, intravenous

15. Which of the following may produce a fast, intense fluid evacuation from the bowel?
    A. Laxatives
    B. Emetics
    C. Antidiarrheals
    D. Cathartics

Hormones of the Endocrine and Reproductive Systems

26

OUTLINE

- The Endocrine System
  - The Pituitary Gland
  - The Adrenal Glands
  - The Thyroid Gland
  - The Pancreas
- The Female Reproductive System
  - The Ovaries
  - Drugs Used During Labor and Delivery
- The Male Reproductive System
  - The Testes

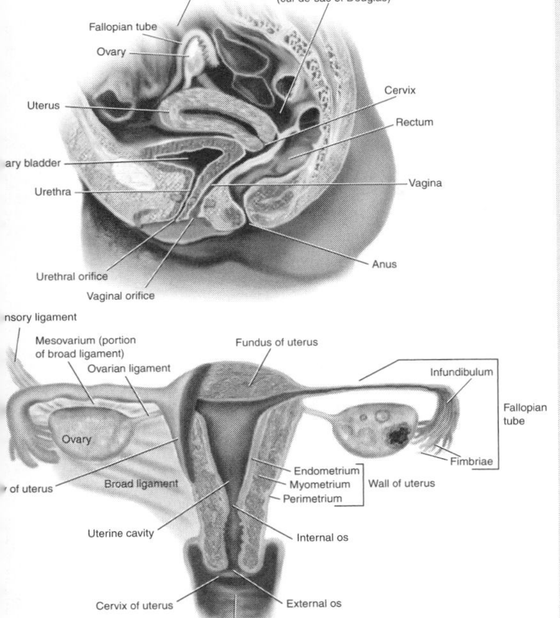

GLOSSARY

adrenal glands Glands that synthesize glucocorticoids, mineralocorticoids, and androgens.

anabolic steroids Synthetically produced androgens.

anabolism The metabolic process by which substances are converted into other chemical components of an organism's structure.

antithyroid agent A chemical agent that lowers the basal metabolic rate by interfering with the formation, release, or action of thyroid hormones.

diabetes mellitus A disorder of carbohydrate metabolism that involves either an insulin deficiency, insulin resistance, or both.

estradiol A chemical derivative of natural estrogen.

estrogen A female sex hormone produced by the ovaries and the placenta.

ethinyl A chemical derivative of natural estrogen.

glucocorticoids A hormone that increases the formation of glycogen from fatty acids and proteins rather than from carbohydrates, exerts an anti-inflammatory effect, and influences many body functions.

hormone A natural chemical secreted into the bloodstream from the endocrine glands to regulate and control the activity of an organ or tissues in another part of the body.

insulin A hormone synthesized and secreted by the pancreas.

medroxyprogesterone acetate A long-acting injectable drug that is a highly effective contraceptive.

mestranol A chemical derivative of natural estrogen.

mineralocorticoid A hormone that regulates sodium and potassium balance in the blood.
negative feedback A decrease in function in response to a stimulus.
pancreas An organ of digestion that lies behind the stomach and produces digestive juices, insulin, and glucagons.
pituitary gland A small gland situated at the base of the brain that secretes hormones that regulate other endocrine glands.
progesterone A hormone secreted by the corpus luteum at the time of ovulation.
tetraiodothyronine (T_4) A hormone produced by the thyroid that increases the rate of metabolism for most cells; also called thyroxine.
thyroxine A hormone produced by the thyroid that increases the rate of metabolism for most cells; also called tetraiodothyronine.
triiodothyronine (T_3) A hormone produced by the thyroid that increases the rate of metabolism for most cells.
uterine relaxants Drugs that inhibit the contractility of uterine smooth muscle and stop labor.

THE ENDOCRINE SYSTEM

The endocrine system is composed of endocrine glands, which are widely distributed throughout the body (see Figure 26-1). This system comprises glands that secrete chemical substances called hormones. A **hormone** is a natural chemical substance secreted into the bloodstream from the endocrine glands that regulates and controls the activity of an organ or tissues in another part of the body. A list of major hormones and endocrine glands is seen in Table 26-1. These hormones are important in maintaining homeostasis and vital functions in the body. The endocrine glands are referred to as the ductless glands because they secrete their hormones directly into the bloodstream, where they are carried to other organs or tissues in the body to affect, control, or regulate the activity of the organs or tissues.

Hormones from the various endocrine glands work together to regulate vital processes, such as the following:

1. Secretions of the digestive tract
2. Energy production
3. Composition and volume of extracellular fluid
4. Adaptation and immunity
5. Growth and development
6. Reproduction and lactation

Hormone secretion is controlled by a self-regulating series of events known as **negative feedback** (a decrease in function in response to a stimulus). Inactivation of hormones occurs enzymatically in the blood, liver, kidney, or target tissues. Hormones are secreted primarily via the urine and, to a lesser extent, the bile. In medicine, hormones generally are used in three ways: (1) for replacement therapy; (2) for pharmacological effects beyond replacement; and (3) for endocrine diagnostic testing.

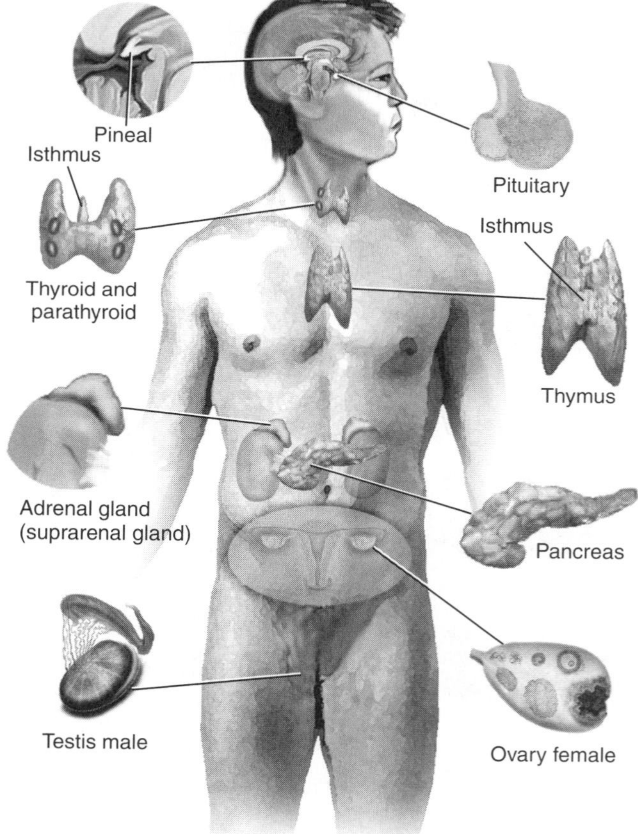

Figure 26-1. The endocrine system.

The Pituitary Gland

The **pituitary gland** (hypophysis) is a small gland situated at the base of the brain, which secretes hormones directly into the bloodstream to control and regulate the other

TABLE 26-1. Endocrine Glands and Their Hormones

GLAND	HORMONES
Hypothalamus	Releasing and inhibiting hormones such as GnRH, GHRH, TRH
Anterior pituitary	GH
	ACTH
	TSH
	LH
	Follicle-stimulating hormone (FSH)
	Prolactin
Posterior pituitary (hormone storage site)	Oxytocin
	Vasopressin (antidiuretic hormone)
Thyroid	Thyroid hormone (T_4 and T_3)
	Calcitonin
Thymus	Thymosin
Pancreas (islets of Langerhans)	Insulin
	Glucagon
Adrenal cortex	Cortisol (a glucocorticoid)
	Aldosterone (a mineralocorticoid)
	Androgens
Adrenal medulla	Epinephrine
	Norepinephrine
Testes	Testosterone
Ovaries	Estrogen
	Progesterone

ACTH, adrenocorticotropic hormone; FSH, follicle-stimulation hormone; GH growth hormone; GHRH, gonadotropin hormone-releasing hormone; GnRH, gonadotropin-releasing hormone; LH, luteinizing hormone; T_3, triiodothyronine; T_4, thyroxine; TRH, thyrotropin-releasing hormone; TSH, thyroid-stimulation hormone.

endocrine glands (see Figure 26-2). The pituitary gland is also called the *master gland.*

The pituitary gland consists of two lobes: anterior and posterior. The anterior lobe is particularly important in sustaining life. The anterior pituitary gland secretes at least six hormones. The major hormones secreted by the pituitary gland are growth hormone (GH), adrenocorticotrophic hormone (ACTH), thyroid-stimulating hormone (TSH), luteinizing hormone (LH), follicle-stimulating hormone (FSH), and prolactin (PRL). The anterior lobe is also called adenohypophysis because it is the glanular portion of the pituitary. Neurohypophysis is the posterior lobe of the pituitary gland. It consists largely of nerve fibers that originate in the hypothalamus. Specialized neurons in the hypothalamus produce the two hormones associated with the posterior pituitary—antidiuretic hormone (ADH) and oxytocin (OT). These hormones travel down from the hypothalamus and store them in the posterior lobe.

The Adrenal Glands

The **adrenal glands** consist of two parts: outer cortex and inner medulla. (see Figure 26-3). These two parts sit on top

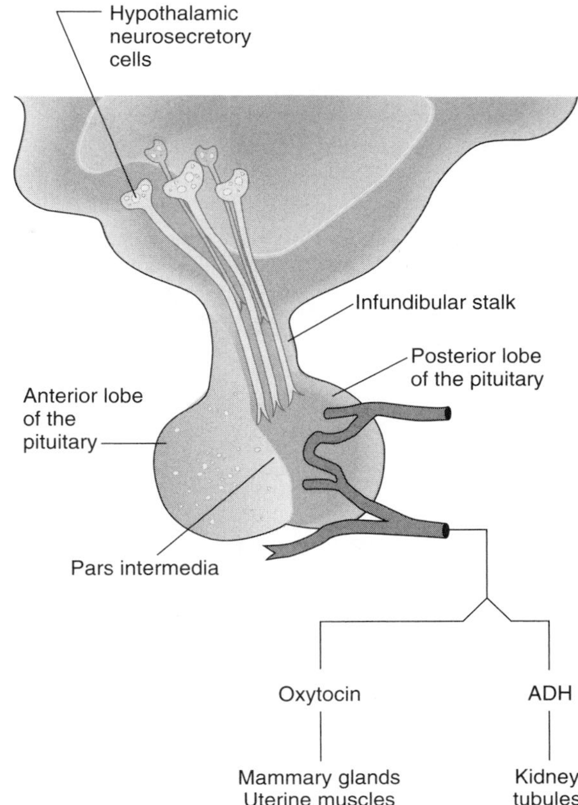

Figure 26-2. The pituitary gland.

of each kidney. The adrenal cortex synthesizes three important classes of hormones: glucocorticoids (cortisol), mineralocorticoids (primarily aldosterone), and certain sex hormones. These sex hormones are male types (adrenal androgens), but some are converted to female hormones (estrogen) in the skin, liver, and adipose tissue. Anabolic steroids are discussed later in this chapter.

Glucocorticoids

The **glucocorticoids** or adrenocortical steroid hormones increase formation of glycogen from fatty acids and proteins rather than from carbohydrates (gluconeogenesis), exert an anti-inflammatory effect, and influence many body functions. The glucocorticoids are under the control of ACTH from the pituitary gland. With stressful conditions such as trauma, major surgery, and infection, secretion of ACTH from the adrenal glands increases dramatically up to 300 mg daily (the basal production rate averages 30 mg every 24 hours). The glucocorticoids can be used to treat many different conditions or disorders, such as insect bites, exposure to poisonous plants, rheumatoid arthritis, asthma, life-threatening shock, and ulcerative colitis. They are also used with other antineoplastic drugs. Prolonged use of glucocorticoids may suppress the pituitary gland so that the body will not produce its own hormone. If these hormones are used for extended periods of time, they cannot be stopped abruptly.

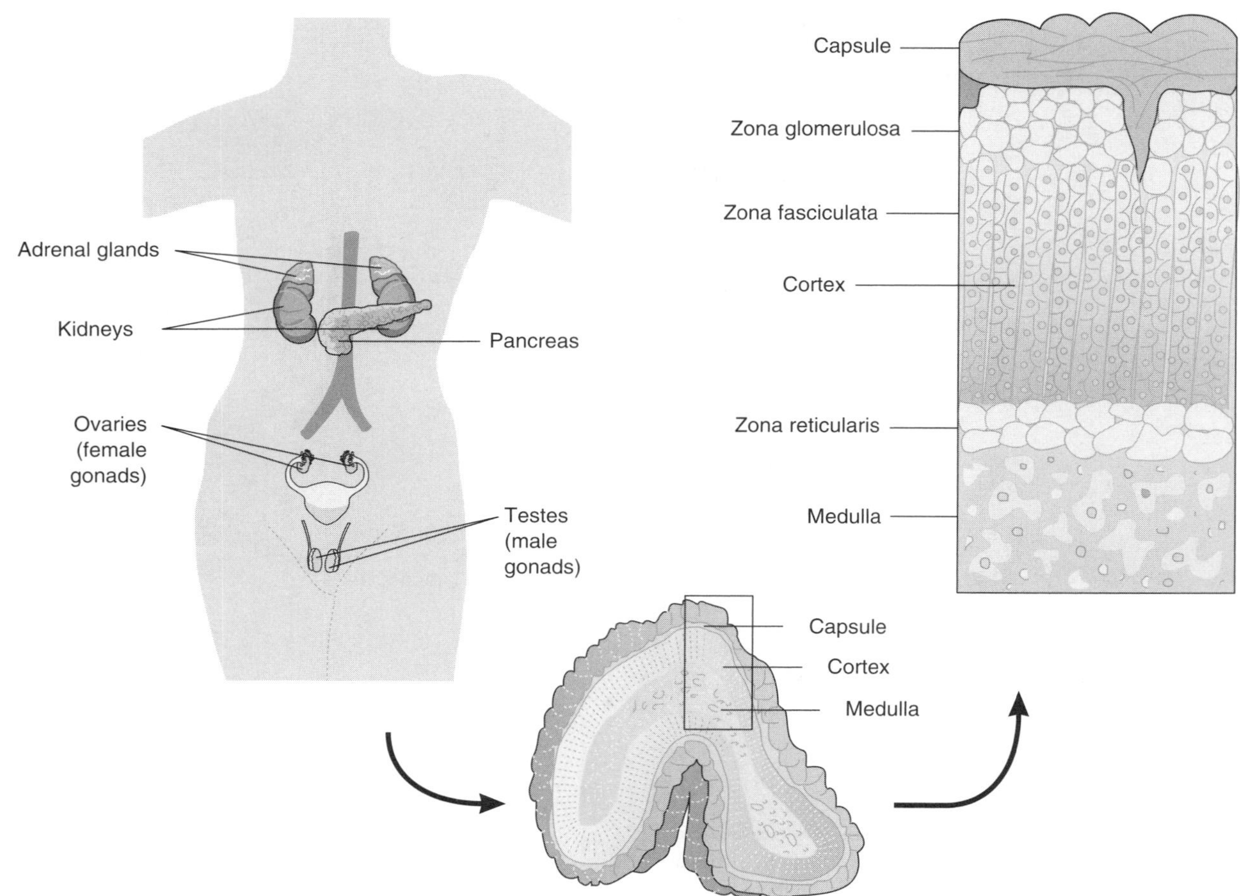

Figure 26-3. The adrenal glands.

A step-down dosage should be given to taper use of the hormone gradually. If corticosteroids are used for a prolonged period of time, they may cause the following side effects: atrophy of the adrenal cortex, delayed healing with infection, electrolyte imbalance, edema, hypertension, congestive heart failure, premature closure of bone plates in children (stunting growth), headache, insomnia, psychosis, and anxiety. Side effects of prolonged use of these hormones may be lack of menstruation in the female, hyperglycemia, and cushingoid state, and, in older women, osteoporosis and bone fractures. Table 26-2 shows some adrenal corticosteroids.

TABLE 26-2. Adrenal Corticosteroids

GENERIC NAME	TRADE NAME
cortisone	Cortone
dexamethasone	Decadron
fludrocortisone	Florinef
hydrocortisone	Cortef or Solu-Cortef
methylprednisolone	Medrol®, Solu-Medrol®
triamcinolone	Aristocort®, Kenalog®

Mineralocorticoids

Aldosterone is the primary **mineralocorticoid.** This hormone regulates sodium and potassium balance in the blood. It is secreted from the adrenocortical tissue. Aldosterone promotes sodium reabsorption in the kidneys to preserve extracellular fluid volume (blood). In the normal patient, aldosterone secretion is stimulated by a decrease in circulating volume such as loss of blood, excessive diuresis, low salt intake, and increased potassium levels. Aldosterone secretion is suppressed by an elevation of sodium levels in the blood (e.g., by excessive dietary salt intake). In adrenal insufficiency, an aldosterone deficit occurs, sodium reabsorption is inhibited, and potassium excretion decreases. Hyperkalemia and mild acidosis occur. The amount of aldosterone secreted by the adrenal cortex apparently is affected by the concentration of sodium in body fluids rather than by the stimulation of the adrenal cortex by ACTH.

Anabolic Steroids

Synthetically produced androgens are called **anabolic steroids**. **Anabolism** is the constructive metabolic process by which substances are converted into other chemical components of an organism's structure. In the human male, androgens as anabolic steroids function to build new body tissue and to increase muscle strength and endurance immeasurably. Androgens are given to men and women for various conditions for therapeutic purposes. In men, they are used to increase testosterone levels to correct hypogonadism (abnormally decreased gonadal function resulting in retarded sexual development) or cryptorchidism (undescended testes) and to increase sperm production in cases of infertility. In women, the main applications approved by the Food and Drug Administration are for the palliative treatment of metastatic breast cancer and as therapy for postpartum breast engorgement, endometriosis, and fibrocystic breast disease. Many athletes take anabolic (adrenergic) steroids to enhance athletic performance and increase the chance of winning in sports events. People also take these hormones to increase strength and body weight, and to "look good." There are many steroidal preparations available for oral or parenteral use, and these preparations have been prescribed, especially for underweight persons and for those wanting the athletic edge. The misuse of anabolic steroids is illegal and the Drug Enforcement Administration has withdrawn these agents from the noncontrolled market. Short-term effects of anabolic steroids may be an increase in aggressive behavior and some masculinization in females. Because of the misuses or abuses, steroids are Schedule III drugs in all states, with some states making these drugs Schedule II agents with a high potential for abuse or misuse. Anabolic steroids increase androgenic effects and cause increased amounts of body and facial hair and increased deepening of the voice. They also increase organ and muscle mass and protein synthesis. Adverse effects include hypercalcemia, edema of the feet or legs, liver impairment with jaundice, insomnia, nausea, vomiting, anorexia, and stomach pains. In the female, decreased breast size, ovulation, lactation, and menstruation are common. Unusual hair growth may be an irreversible effect. In the male, increased breast size with testicular atrophy, decreased sperm production, and impotence are seen.

The Thyroid Gland

The thyroid gland is composed of many secretory units called follicles. These follicular cells secrete two hormones, **triiodothyronine (T_3)** and **tetraiodothyronine (T_4 or thyroxine)**. Thyroid hormones regulate the metabolism of carbohydrates, proteins, and fats. In general, thyroid hormones increase the rate of metabolism of most cells. In addition to secreting T_3 and T_4, the thyroid gland also secretes a hormone called calcitonin that is secreted by the parafollicular cells found between the thyroid hormone. Calcitonin regulates plasma levels of calcium. The synthesis of T_3 and T_4 requires iodine. The iodine in the body comes from dietary sources. An iodine-deficient diet can result in low levels of T_3 and T_4 and can cause goiter formation and hypothyroidism. An iodine-deficient diet causes the thyroid gland to enlarge. Thyroid hormone deficiency (hypothyroidism) and excess (hyperthyroidism) are two conditions that are seen often. If an infant is born with no thyroid gland, a condition called cretinism develops. An infant with cretinism fails to develop both physically and mentally. Early diagnosis and prompt treatment with T_3, usually within 2 months after birth, can prevent further developmental delay. Hypothyroidism in an adult results in a condition called myxedema. Myxedema is a slowed-down metabolic state. An excess of thyroid hormone produces hyperthyroidism, a sped-up metabolic state. A common type of hyperthyroidism is Graves' disease. Hyperthyroidism is characterized by bulging eyes, a condition known as exophthalmia. Iodine is essential for thyroid hormone synthesis. About 1 mg of iodine is required per week, most of which is ingested in food, water, and iodized table salt. T_3 and T_4 are controlled by TSH from the anterior pituitary gland. Thyroid secretion is maintained by the TSH secretion. Decreased serum levels of T_3 and T_4 stimulate the release of thyrotropin-releasing hormone (TRH) from the hypothalamus, which stimulates the pituitary gland to secrete TSH. Then TSH stimulates the thyroid gland to release thyroxin and thyroglobulin. Calcitonin is a hormone that has a very important role in calcium metabolism. Normally calcitonin decreases the level of blood calcium; therefore, this hormone is used to treat hypercalcemia, osteoporosis, and Paget's disease.

Antithyroid Agents

An **antithyroid agent** is a chemical agent that lowers the basal metabolic rate by interfering with the formation, release, or action of thyroid hormones. A variety of compounds are known as antithyroid drugs. Iodine (iodide ions), radioactive iodine, and thioamide are the drugs of choice for antithyroid therapy. The side effects of these agents include nausea and vomiting, myalgia, fever, and rashes. These medications can cross the placenta and stop fetal thyroid development. They also pass through breast milk to affect the infant. Selected medications used as drugs for the thyroid gland are shown in Table 26-3.

The Pancreas

The primary hormones released by the **pancreas** are **insulin** and glucagon. When serum blood glucose levels decline, glucagon, which is synthesized in the α cells of the pancreatic islets, facilitates the breakdown of glycogen in the liver to glucose. The conversion of glycogen to glucose results in an increase in blood glucose levels. The release of glucagon stimulates insulin secretion, which then inhibits the release of glucagon. The most significant disease involving the endocrine pancreas is **diabetes mellitus**, a disorder of carbohydrate metabolism that is due to insulin deficiency, insulin resistance, or both. All causes of diabetes lead to hyperglycemia. The most common forms of diabetes are the following:

TABLE 26-3. Selected Medications Used as Drugs for the Thyroid Gland

GENERIC NAME	TRADE NAME	INDICATIONS FOR USE
Natural Thyroid Replacement		
desiccated thyroid (T_3 and T_4)	Armour Thyroid®	Hypothyroidism
Synthetic Thyroid Replacement		
thyroxine (T_4)	Levoxine®, Levoxyl®, Levothroid®, Synthroid®	Hypothyroidism
triiodothyronine (T_3)	Cytomel®	
Antithyroid Preparations		Hyperthyroidism
potassium iodide, iodine	Lugol's, SSKI Solution®	
thioamide derivatives		
propylthiouracil	Propyl-Thyracil®	
methimazole	Tapazole®	
Calcitonin		
calcitonin salmon	Miacalcin®	Paget's disease, hypercalcemia, osteoporosis, renal failure

1. Type 1 diabetes, previously called insulin-dependent diabetes mellitus (IDDM) because of complete or nearly complete insulin deficiency, which results from destruction of the pancreatic β cell mass on an immune or unknown basis.
2. Type 2 diabetes, previously called non–insulin-dependent diabetes mellitus (NIDDM), which results from insulin resistance and impairment of compensatory insulin secretion.
3. Secondary diabetes, which is caused by a variety of diseases and disorders of the exocrine pancreas such as cystic fibrosis, drugs, infections, and genetic syndromes.
4. Gestational diabetes, which is diabetes mellitus with onset or first recognition during pregnancy, usually during the second or third trimester. It often disappears after the end of the pregnancy, but many women with this condition develop permanent diabetes mellitus later in life. Although the disordered carbohydrate metabolism is usually mild, prompt detection and treatment are necessary to avoid fetal and neonatal morbidity and mortality.

Insulin Therapy

Insulin is normally synthesized and secreted by the β cells of the pancreas. Insulin is used for treatment of type 1 diabetes. Patients with type 1 diabetes do not produce enough insulin from the pancreas. Some patients with type 2 diabetes in whom sufficient concentrations of blood glucose are not maintained with dietary regulation and use of oral antidiabetic agents also need to receive insulin when they undergo surgery, have a fever, are under stress, have severe trauma, infection, serious renal or hepatic dysfunction, endocrine dysfunction, or gangrene, or are pregnant. Regular insulin must also be administered for emergency treatment of ketoacidosis or diabetic coma. Insulin must be given only by injection because it is destroyed by the digestive juices. The dosage of insulin is usually measured in units. Most of the insulin used today comes in unit sizes of 40, 80, and 100 U. Table 26-4 lists the new as well as the older agents currently available for clinical use and some of their properties. Table 26-5 shows dosages of regular insulin needed according to blood glucose levels.

Patients who will be using insulin need to be instructed on the rotation method of taking their medication. Insulin is absorbed more rapidly with administration in the arm or thigh, especially with exercise. The abdomen is used for more consistent absorption. Glucose levels should be checked per physician orders. All insulin must be checked for expiration date and clarity of the solution. Insulin should NOT be given if it appears cloudy. Vials should not be shaken but rotated in between the hands to mix contents. If regular insulin is to be mixed with NPH or lente insulin, the regular insulin should be drawn into the syringe first. Unopened vials should be stored in the refrigerator, and freezing should be avoided. The vial in use can be stored at room temperature. Vials should not be put in glove compartments, suitcases, or trunks. Humulin is a new type of insulin and is often the patient's preference because it can be taken orally. It is imperative that the physician be called if any adverse reactions to the medications are observed.

Oral Antidiabetic Agents

The goals of treatment for patients with type 2 diabetes are to restore metabolic abnormalities to values as near to normal as possible. In patients with type 2 diabetes, management of associated metabolic abnormalities is essential.

TABLE 26-4. Insulin Preparations

TYPE	PEAK (HR)	DURATION (HR)
Short-acting (regular)	2–4	4-6
Humulin R	2–4	4–6
Novolin R		
Rapidly Absorbed (lispro, aspart)	1–2	3–4
Humalog	1–2	3–4
Novolog		
Intermediate-acting (NPH, lente)	3–4	16–20
Humulin N	6–12	
Novolin N		
Long-acting (ultralente)	14–18	24
Humulin-U		
Daily (glargine)		
Lantus	None	24

TABLE 26-5. Dosages of Regular Insulin and Blood Glucose Levels

BLOOD GLUCOSE LEVEL (mmol/L)	DOSAGE OF REGULAR INSULIN (U)
>350	Call physician for dosage
301-350	12
251–300	8
200-250	5
<200	No insulin

Lipid and blood pressure control is even more important in patients with diabetes than in nondiabetic individuals. Thus, appropriate management of lipid and blood pressure abnormalities is essential in the treatment of type 2 diabetes. Patients with type 2 diabetes are treated with oral antidiabetic agents, diet, exercise, and when necessary, insulin. Today, three types of oral hypoglycemic agents are available: first- and second-generation sulfonylureas and a miscellaneous group, which contains agents that differ from insulin in mode of action. Table 26-6 shows some examples of hypoglycemic agents and their duration of action.

The advantages in using second-generation agents are that they have a long duration of action and cause fewer side effects. Of the first-generation agents, tolazamide also has advantages similar to those of the second-generation agents. Oral hypoglycemic agents are indicated for the treatment of uncomplicated type 2 diabetes in patients whose diabetes cannot be controlled by diet only. Side effects include nausea, vomiting, headache, blurred vision, sedation, confusion, anxiety, nightmares, and tachycardia. Oral hypoglycemic

TABLE 26-6. Hypoglycemic Agents

GENERIC NAME	TRADE NAME	DURATION OF ACTION (hr)
Sulfonylureas		
First-Generation		12–24
acetohexamide	Dymelor®	24–72
chlorpropamide	Diabinese®	12–24
tolazamide	Tolinase®	6–12
tolbutamide	Orinase®, Mobenol®	
Second-Generation		
glimepiride	Amaryl®	24
glipizide	Glucotrol®	12–24
glyburide nonmicronized	DiaBeta®, Micronase®	24
glyburide micronized	Glynase PresTab®	24
Miscellaneous		
acarbose	Precose®	NA
miglitol	Glyset®	NA
metformin	Glucophage®	6–12
repaglinide	Prandin®	NA
thiazolidinediones (glitazones)		
rosiglitazone	Avandia®	
pioglitazone	Actos®	

NA, not applicable.

agents are contraindicated in patients who are receiving sulfonamide- or thiazide-type diuretics, or who have a hypersensitivity to the medication, acidosis, severe burns, and severe diarrhea. These agents should not be used in patients with high fevers, severe infections, hyperthyroidism, or kidney function impairment.

THE FEMALE REPRODUCTIVE SYSTEM

The female reproductive system consists of two ovaries, two fallopian tubes, the uterus, and the vagina. Two hormones are responsible for the development of reproductive organs and secondary sex characteristics in the female: estrogen and progesterone.

The Ovaries

The ovaries are also called gonads. They produce ova and form endocrine secretions that initiate and maintain secondary sex characteristics in women. Gonadotropins from the pituitary gland are responsible for the development and maintenance of sexual gland functions. FSH stimulates the development of the ovarian follicles up to the point of ovulation. LH promotes the growth of the interstitial cells in the follicle and the formation of the corpus luteum.

Estrogen

Estrogen is a female sex hormone produced by the ovaries and placenta. Naturally occurring estrogens include estrone, estradiol, and estriol. These substances are synthesized by a variety of animals and plants and are found in the blood of both males and females. Most naturally occurring estrogens are not effective when administered orally, because they are rapidly inactivated by the liver. Chemical derivatives of the natural estrogens, such as **ethinyl estradiol** and **mestranol**, are only slowly inactivated by the liver and may be administered orally. Both natural estrogens and their derivatives may be administered by the intramuscular or subcutaneous route. Estrogen can be used for a variety of conditions such as for the treatment of amenorrhea and dysfunctional uterine bleeding. Replacement estrogen therapy is used in women who have had their ovaries removed during the reproductive years and in older women for the prevention and treatment of osteoporosis. Osteoporosis is a disorder characterized by abnormal loss of bone density. It occurs most often in postmenopausal women, immobilized individuals, and patients receiving long-term steroid therapy. In recent times, estrogen has been beneficial for maintaining healthy cardiac status in menopausal women. Estrogens are also used in primary ovarian failure, atrophic vaginitis, hypogonadism, and atrophic urethritis and as adjuvant therapy for prostate cancer. They *should not* be used in patients who have a sensitivity to any of the ingredients, are pregnant, or have breast cancer. They are also contraindicated in patients with undiagnosed abnormal uterine bleeding, thrombophlebitis, and thromboembolic disorders. The most common adverse effects are nausea, vomiting, breast swelling, fluid retention (weight gain), and thromboembolic disease. Table 26-7 shows selected estrogens and dosage forms.

Progesterone

Progesterone is secreted primarily by the corpus luteum at the time of ovulation during the female reproductive years. The corpus luteum secretes progesterone only during the last 2 weeks of the menstrual cycle. The greatest amount is secreted during the week after ovulation has taken place. Progesterone is responsible for changes in the uterine endometrium during the second half of the menstrual cycle, development of the maternal placenta after implantation, and development of the mammary glands.

It has become necessary to produce a synthetic form of progesterone by a chemical modification, because the natural type of the hormone is inactivated by the liver. The synthetic preparations are called progestins. Progesterone is used in the treatment of irregular uterine bleeding and is combined with estrogen for the treatment of amenorrhea. It is also used in cases of infertility and threatened or habitual abortion. The adverse effects of progestin include weight gain, stomach pain and cramping, swelling of the face and legs, headache, anxiety, weakness, rash, acne, and insomnia.

Progesterone is contraindicated in patients with a hypersensitivity to the medication or any of the ingredients, thrombophlebitis, liver disease, breast cancer, reproductive organ cancer, undiagnosed vaginal bleeding, and missed periods. Use during pregnancy and breast-feeding is not recommended. Table 26-8 shows the most commonly used progestins.

Oral Contraceptive Agents

Combinations of estrogens and progestins may be used as oral contraceptives in women. This method is nearly 100% effective when these drugs are used as directed to prevent pregnancy. Oral contraceptives contain various amounts of

TABLE 26-7. Selected Estrogens

GENERIC NAME	TRADE NAME	ROUTE OF ADMINISTRATION
estradiol (100)	Estrace®	Oral
	Estraderm®, Vivelle® (100)	Transdermal
	Climara®	Transdermal
	Estring® (100)	Vaginal ring
estradiol valerate	Delestrogen®	IM
estradiol, ethinyl	Gynogen LA®	IM
	Estinyl®	Oral
esterified estrogen (100)	Estratab, Menest®	Oral
esterified estrogen (100) with methyltestosterone	Estratest®	Oral
conjugated estrogens (100)	Premarin®	Oral, IM, IV, vaginal cream
esterified estrogen (100) with medroxyprogesterone	Prempro, Premphase (100)	Oral
estrone	Aquest®	IM
estropipate	Ogen®	Oral
chlorotrianisene	Tace®	Oral

IM, intramuscular; IV, intravenous.

estrogen and progestins. The estrogen inhibits ovulation by suppressing the normal secretion of FSH. The progestin inhibits pituitary secretion of LH, causes changes in the cervical mucus that make it an unfavorable for penetration by sperm, and alters the nature of the endometrium. The use of estrogen-progestin combinations in a cyclic fashion generally results in the inhibition of conception without prevention of menstruation. Most oral contraceptives are taken daily for 20 to 21 days, starting on the fifth day after menstrual bleeding begins. There are also 28-day pill cycles starting at the same time wherein a pill is taken every day of the cycle. Once started, the pill is not stopped. An inactive pill is taken during the week of menstruation, whereas with the 20- to 21-day pill there is a week without medication, and this is when menstruation takes place.

The use of oral contraceptives containing only a progestin has been advocated as a means of reducing some of the risk associated with the use of oral contraceptives. These products, which are sometimes referred to as "minipills," are generally taken continuously rather than cyclically. Because they contain no estrogen, they do not suppress ovulation. **Medroxyprogesterone acetate** is a long-acting injectable drug that is a highly effective and safe contraceptive with a failure rate of less than 1% per year. It provides birth control for 3 months when administered as a single injection of 150 mg. It has been proved to be safe and is relatively inexpensive. Many women find this method more convenient than taking oral contraceptives daily. Before a patient uses any hormonal type of contraception, a complete history should be obtained and a physical examination performed. The patient should be informed of the precautions, warnings, adverse effects, and possible side effects of the therapy. Patients should also be advised that smoking increases the risk of serious adverse effects on the heart and blood vessels from oral contraceptive use. The risk increases with age and with heavy smoking (15 or more cigarettes per day) and is quite marked in women older than 35 years of age. Women who use oral contraceptives should not smoke.

TABLE 26-8. Most Commonly-Used Progestins

GENERIC NAME	TRADE NAME	ROUTE OF ADMINISTRATION
medroxyprogesterone acetate (100)	Provera®, Amen®, Cycrin®	Oral
norethindrone (100)	Norlutin®, Micronor®	Oral
megestrol	Megace®	Oral
progesterone	Gesterol®, Crinone®	IM, vaginal gel
hydroxyprogesterone	Hylutin®	IM

IM, intramuscular.

Drugs Used During Labor and Delivery

Generally, two types of medications are used during labor and delivery: uterine stimulants and uterine relaxants. Uterine stimulants cause contractions of the myometrium during labor and delivery. Many agents are capable of stimulating the smooth muscle of the uterus, but only a few are selective and of use for the myometrium. These agents are known as oxytocic substances. Oxytocic agents are also used to control postpartum hemorrhage, to cause uterine contraction after cesarean section, or to induce therapeutic abortion after the first trimester. There are three types of oxytocic drugs: synthetic oxytocin, ergot derivatives, and prostaglandins.

Oxytocin (Pitocin®, Syntocinon®) is a hormone released from the posterior pituitary gland. Its primary effect is to stimulate the smooth muscle of the uterus and the mammary gland. When oxytocin is used to initiate or stimulate labor, it is generally administered by intravenous infusion. Ergot is a complex mixture of substances derived from fungus. Ergot alkaloids cause powerful contractions of the uterus. This action permits them to be used to control uterine bleeding. These agents are more suitable for use postpartum or after abortion to control bleeding and maintain uterine contraction. Their use is not advised for induction of labor, because ergot agents may damage the fetus. Prostaglandins are chemically related agents that exert wide-ranging effects in the human body. The effects of these agents are comparable to those of oxytocin when they are used as oxytocic agents. The prostaglandins currently approved as uterine stimulants are used for induction of second-trimester abortion.

Uterine Relaxants

Uterine relaxants inhibit contractility of uterine smooth muscle and stop labor. When labor begins before term, it may cause premature birth. The most common cause of neonatal deaths is premature birth. There are a variety of agents that have been used in the attempt to prevent premature labor, such as progesterone, ethanol, prostaglandin inhibitors, and β-adrenergic stimulants. Today, ritodrine and terbutaline sulfate are the drugs most commonly used for this purpose.

Ritodrine HCl Ritodrine (Yutopar®) is a uterine relaxant. It is used for management of preterm labor in suitable patients. Ritodrine is contraindicated before the 20th week of pregnancy, when continuation of pregnancy is hazardous to the mother or fetus, and in those with hypersensitivity to the drug or preexisting maternal conditions that would be seriously affected by the pharmacological properties of β-adrenergic stimulant agents. Adverse effects include chest pain, heart murmur, angina pectoris, myocardial ischemia, pulmonary edema, and drowsiness. Ritodrine may also cause tremor, headache, anxiety, or hyperventilation. Nausea, diarrhea, constipation, and vomiting are common side effects of this agent.

Terbutaline Sulfate Terbutaline sulfate (Brethine®) is also indicated for prevention of premature labor. This agent is also used for treatment of asthma to reverse bronchospasm and emphysema. Terbutaline sulfate is contraindicated in patients with cardiac arrhythmias associated with tachycardia. Adverse effects include palpitations, tachycardia, chest pain, arrhythmias, tremor, dizziness, headache, and weakness. It also can produce nausea, vomiting, sweating, and muscle cramps.

THE MALE REPRODUCTIVE SYSTEM

The male reproductive system consists of two testes, a system of ducts to carry sperm, accessory glands, and the penis. The male hormone responsible for development of the reproductive organs and secondary sex characteristics is testosterone.

The Testes

The FSH and LH or interstitial cell-stimulating hormone in males were listed in the section on pituitary gonadotropic hormones.They exert their actions on the gonads or reproductive organs. Gonads include the testes in the male and the ovaries in the female. Androgens are secreted mainly in the interstitial tissue of the testes in the male and secondarily in the adrenal glands of both sexes. Androgens include testosterone and androsterone. Inadequate production of androgens in the male may be due to pituitary malfunction. Testosterone stimulates the development of the male secondary sex characteristics, initiates the production of sperm, and enhances the functional capacity of the penis and the accessory sex organs. It is used for replacement therapy in androgen deficiency, for the treatment of hypogonadism and cryptorchidism, and for palliative treatment of certain metastatic breast carcinomas in women. Its use is contraindicated in patients with known hypersensitivity to any of its ingredients, in women during pregnancy and lactation, in men with cancer of the breast or suspected cancer of the prostate, in patients with pituitary insufficiency, a history of myocardial infarction, hypercalcemia, prostatic hyperplasia, hepatic dysfunction, and nephrosis, and in infants and young children. It should be used with caution in elderly patients, in diabetic patients, in those who have hypertension, coronary artery disease, renal disease, hypercholesterolemia, or gynecomastia, and in prepubertal males.

Adverse reactions in males include gynecomastia, excessive frequency and duration of penile erection, oligospermia, hirsutism, male pattern baldness, acne, increased or decreased libido, headache, anxiety, and depression. In females adverse reactions include amenorrhea, menstrual irregularities, inhibition of gonadotropin secretion, and virilization (deepening of the voice, clitoral enlargement, increased growth of facial and body hair, and male-type baldness).

REVIEW QUESTIONS

1. Which of the following is an example of a releasing hormone?
   A. TSH
   B. LH
   C. TRH
   D. FSH

2. Vasopressin is also known as
   A. prolactin.
   B. oxytocin.
   C. growth hormone.
   D. antidiuretic hormone.

3. The thymus gland secretes
   A. calcitonin.
   B. thymosin.
   C. prolactin.
   D. growth hormone.

4. An example of a mineralocorticoid hormone is
   A. testosterone.
   B. androgen.
   C. aldosterone.
   D. cortisol.

5. The pituitary gland is situated at the
   A. base of the brain.
   B. medulla.
   C. pons.
   D. frontal lobe of the brain.

6. The glucocorticoid hormones are under the control of
   A. LH.
   B. TSH.
   C. ACTH.
   D. FSH.

7. Which of the following is a side effect of corticosteroids?
   A. Delayed healing with infection
   B. Hypotension
   C. Weight loss
   D. Hypertrophy of the adrenal cortex

8. How many hormones are secreted by the thyroid gland?
   A. Only one
   B. Two
   C. Three
   D. Seven

Continues

9. Which of the following is the trade name of thyroxine (T_4)?
A. Synthroid®
B. Cytomel®
C. Armour Thyroid®
D. Proloid®

10. Which of the following endocrine glands secretes glucagons?
A. Liver
B. Pancreas
C. Ovaries
D. Thymus

11. Which of the following are necessary for menstruation?
A. Glucagons and metformin
B. Estrogen and progesterone
C. Oxytocin and ritodrine
D. All of the above

12. Synthetic preparations of progesterone are known as
A. fluoxetine
B. progestins.
C. primary.
D. follicles.

13. Progesterone is produced by __________ in the ovaries.
A. follicles
B. corpus luteum
C. ovulation
D. testes

14. Progesterone is responsible for changes in the uterus during the
A. second half of the cycle.
B. first half of the cycle.
C. time between the cycles.
D. none of the above.

15. Insulin is used mainly in which type of diabetes?
A. Type 1
B. NIDDM
C. IDDM
D. A and C

16. A new type of insulin, Humulin, is preferred because it is
A. cheaper.
B. taken orally.
C. similar to human insulin.
D. used topically.

17. FSH and LH are secreted from the
A. ovaries.
B. testes.
C. pituitary.
D. none of the above.

18. All of the following are side effects of oral hypoglycemic agents, except
A. confusion.
B. skin rashes.
C. nightmares.
D. tachycardia.

19. Which of the following is the trade name of chlorpropamide?
A. Diabinese®
B. Dymelor®
C. Tolinase®
D. Glucotrol®

20. Which of the following is the trade name of glipizide?
A. Tolinase®
B. Glucotrol®
C. Dymelor®
D. Glucophage®

Anticoagulants 27

OUTLINE

Blood Clotting
Anticoagulation
- Anticoagulant Agents
- Thrombolytic Agents
- Antiplatelet Agents

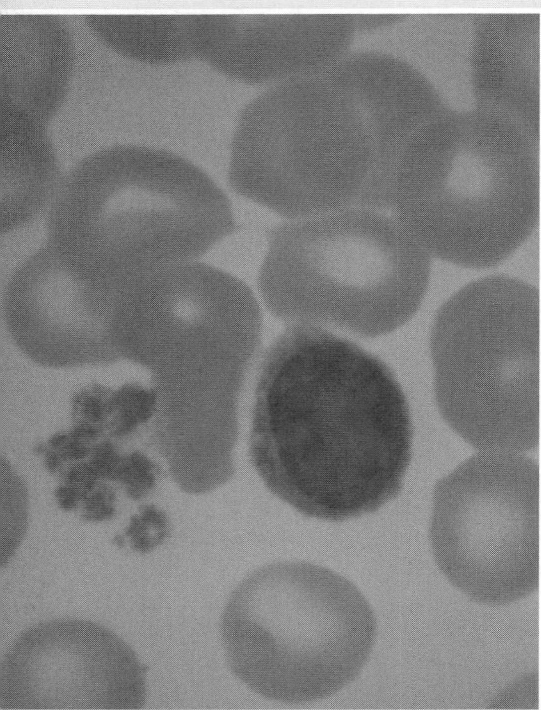

GLOSSARY

abciximab A platelet aggregation inhibitor.

anticoagulants Chemical substances that inhibit blood coagulation.

antiplatelet agent Any agent that destroys platelets or inhibits their function.

aspirin (acetylsalicylic acid) An analgesic, antipyretic, antirheumatic, and anti-inflammatory agent.

cilostazol A drug that inhibits platelet aggregation.

clopidogrel A drug that inhibits platelet aggregation.

coagulation The complex process that leads to the conversion of fibrinogen to fibrin to form a blood clot; also referred to as hemostasis.

coagulation factor One of 12 factors in the blood, the interactions of which are responsible for the process of blood clotting.

dicumarol A synthetic anticoagulant used for the prophylaxis and treatment of thrombosis and embolism.

dipyridamole A coronary vasodilator used for the long-term treatment of angina.

heparin sodium A mucopolysaccharide that enhances the effects of antithrombin III. It is used as an anticoagulant for laboratory testing and as a therapeutic agent.

protamine sulfate A heparin antagonist derived from fish sperm.

reteplase A human tissue enzyme produced by recombinant DNA techniques.

streptokinase A fibrinolytic activator that enhances the conversion of plasminogen to the fibrinolytic enzyme plasmin. It is produced by strains of streptococci and is used in the treatment of certain instances of pulmonary and coronary embolism.

thromboembolism A condition in which a blood vessel is blocked by an embolus carried in the bloodstream from the site of formation of the clot.

thrombolytic agents Agents that dissolve thrombi.

thrombus An aggregation of platelets, fibrin, clotting factors, and the cellular elements of the blood attached to the interior wall of a vein or artery, sometimes occluding the lumen of a vessel.

ticlopidine A platelet aggregation inhibitor used to reduce the risk of stroke. It works by preventing excessive blood clotting. Its trade name is Ticlid.

tissue plasminogen activator (TPA) A clot-dissolving substance produced naturally by cells in the walls of blood vessels. It is also manufactured synthetically by genetic engineering techniques. TPA activates plasminogen to dissolve clots and has been used therapeutically to dissolve blood clots blocking coronary arteries.

urokinase An enzyme produced in the kidney and found in urine that is a potent plasminogen activator of the fibrinolytic system.

warfarin An oral anticoagulant agent used for the prophylaxis and treatment of thrombosis and embolism.

BLOOD CLOTTING

Clot formation is essential for survival after injuries or surgery. Clots prevent further loss of blood from wounds. Stoppage of blood flow is necessary for homeostasis.

The process of transforming the blood into a solid clot, or **coagulation**, spontaneously stops bleeding from damaged blood vessels. Blood is normally fluid while circulating in the vessels, but with vessel injury, it rapidly clots at the site of injury. Each **coagulation factor** has been named and assigned a Roman numeral by an international committee. The numerical order does not, however, reflect the sequence of reactions. Roman numerals III, IV, and VI are not used. The interactions of these factors are responsible for the process of blood clotting. The coagulation factors are listed in Table 27-1.

TABLE 27-1. Standard Numeric Numbers of Coagulation Factors

DESIGNATION	NAME
I	Fibrinogen
II	Prothrombin
III	Tissue thromboplastin
IV	Calcium (Ca^{2+})
V	Labile factor
VII	Proconvertin
VIII	Antihemophilic factor
IX	Christmas factor
X	Stuart-Prower factor
XI	Plasma thromboplastin antecedent
XII	Hageman factor
XIII	Fibrin-stabilizing factor

ANTICOAGULATION

Occasionally, the body will form clots or thrombi that jam blood vessels, causing **thromboembolism**. A **thrombus** is a blood clot within a blood vessel, whereas an embolus is a mass of undissolved matter in the vessel. **Anticoagulants** are used to prevent venous clotting in patients with thrombohemolytic disorders. Antiplatelet drugs are used to keep platelets from clumping (aggregating) and are used on a regular basis in ambulatory care.

Anticoagulant Agents

Anticoagulant agents are used to prevent or delay abnormal blood clotting. The formation of a blood clot within blood vessels may result in a stroke, pulmonary embolism, or heart attack. These occurrences are serious and can be fatal. Anticoagulant drugs are prescribed to prevent blood clots (thrombi). These drugs are commonly known as "blood thinners." Blood clots may be caused from the following factors:

- Injury of blood vessel walls
- Stasis of blood flow
- Platelet adhesiveness
- Blood coagulation

Embolism is an abnormal circulatory condition in which a foreign body (such as fat, air, tumor tissue, or clot) travels through the bloodstream and becomes lodged in a blood vessel. The symptoms vary with the degree of occlusion that results, the character of the embolus, and the size, nature, and location of the occluded vessel. A thrombus usually arises from a peripheral vein (most commonly from the deep veins of the leg). Pulmonary embolism is difficult to distinguish from myocardial infarction and pneumonia. Pulmonary infarction often occurs within 6 to 24 hours after the formation of a pulmonary embolus. Two thirds of patients with a massive pulmonary embolus die within 2 hours. The formation of further emboli is prevented by the use of anticoagulants and sometimes streptokinase or urokinase.

Risk factors for deep-vein thrombosis include the following:

- Age older than 40 years
- Obesity
- Pregnancy
- Parturition
- Surgery
- Bed rest for longer than 4 days
- Estrogen therapy with cigarette smoking
- High-dose estrogen therapy
- Trauma and damage to wall of blood vessels

The two main groups of anticoagulant drugs are parenteral anticoagulant drugs and oral anticoagulant drugs. For effective anticoagulant therapy the manner of use for both groups is important.

Parenteral anticoagulants include heparin sodium, low-molecular-weight heparins, citrate dextrose solution, citrate phosphate dextrose (CPD) solution, and sodium citrate solution. Oral anticoagulants are agents that can be administered orally for use by ambulatory patients, have a longer duration of action, and are considerably less expensive. Oral anticoagulants include warfarin sodium and dicumarol.

Heparin Sodium

Heparin sodium is a naturally occurring mucopolysaccharide that acts in the body as an antithrombin factor to prevent intravascular clotting. Heparin is produced by basophils of the blood and mast cells of the lungs, liver, and intestinal mucosa. Its anticoagulant effect is monitored by clotting assays, such as activated partial thromboplastin time or prothrombin time or preferably with the international normalized ratio, to avoid thrombosis or hemorrhage due to under- or overcoagulation. Heparin is prescribed in the treatment and prophylaxis of a variety of thromboembolic disorders.

Heparin is preferred if rapid anticoagulation is necessary. It is also considered to be the drug of choice for sudden arterial occlusion because its action is immediate and can be readily reversed if surgery is necessary. Heparin does not cross the placental barrier and is not excreted in breast milk. Contraindications to heparin use are hypersensitivity to this drug. It is given only when frequent monitoring of the coagulation status of the patient's blood is possible. The most serious adverse reaction to heparin use is hemorrhage.

Heparin must be administered intravenously or subcutaneously. Distribution is limited to the vascular space. Anticoagulant therapy should be started with intravenous heparin, then overlapped a few days with warfarin, and then switched to warfarin only. Hypersensitivity and other adverse effects may occur. Manifestations include bronchospasms, rash, pruritus, chills, fever, and hair loss.

Low-Molecular-Weight Heparins

Several products consist of a mixture of low-molecular-weight fragments of heparin. Standard heparin forms a ternary complex with antithrombin III and thrombin, whereas the low-molecular-weight heparins form primarily binary complexes with antithrombin III. This results in enhanced inhibitor of factor X_a, with less inhibitory effect on thrombin. As with heparin, these agents also inhibit thrombin by binding to heparin cofactor II. Because small heparin molecules bound to antithrombin III react only slightly with platelets, deep vein thrombosis can be prevented or retarded without as much risk of hemorrhage as with standard heparin. Low-molecular-weight heparins include dalteparin, enoxaparin, and tinzaparin.

Dalteparin Dalteparin is indicated for the prophylaxis of deep-vein thrombosis in patients undergoing abdominal surgery who are at risk for thromboembolic complications. The major adverse event associated with its use is bleeding. In the event of serious bleeding, the drug should be discontinued, and a blood transfusion or other blood products may be administered. Because the agent includes sodium sulfite as a preservative, allergic-type reactions can occur with this drug.

Enoxaparin Enoxaparin is indicated for the prevention of deep-vein thrombosis in patients undergoing hip or knee replacement therapy as well as for patients undergoing abdominal surgery who are at risk for thromboembolic complications. This agent is administered by subcutaneous injection only. The incidence of hemorrhagic complications is lower than that with standard heparin; however, protamine sulfate is useful for treating patients who do experience hemorrhagic events.

Tinzaparin Tinzaparin inhibits thrombus and clot formation. It is used for treatment of deep-vein thrombosis with or without pulmonary emboli when given with warfarin sodium.

Anticoagulant Citrate Dextrose Solution

Anticoagulant citrate dextrose solution is a sterile solution of citric acid, sodium citrate, and dextrose in water for injection. The citrate chelates calcium ions and thus acts as an anticoagulant. The sterile solution is used mainly for the anticoagulation and preservation of whole blood for transfusion.

Anticoagulant Citrate Phosphate Dextrose Solution

Anticoagulant CPD solution is a sterile solution of citric acid, sodium citrate, sodium biphosphate, and dextrose in water for injection. CPD solution is the preferred anticoagulant for blood to be used for exchange transfusion.

Anticoagulant Sodium Citrate Solution

Anticoagulant sodium citrate solution is a sterile 4% solution of sodium citrate in water for injection. It prevents clotting of blood by forming an undissociated calcium citrate chelate. The sterile solution is used for preparation of blood for transfusion and for preparation of citrated human plasma.

Warfarin

Warfarin is an oral anticoagulant. Its effect on the liver prevents manufacturing of vitamin K–dependent clotting factors. Like heparin, it has no effect on existing clots, but it can prevent future clots. The onset of action is delayed (8 to 12 hours), because stores of the clotting factors must be depleted. The maximum anticoagulant effect of warfarin occurs after 1 week of administration. Because warfarin is effective when given orally, it is more useful than heparin for outpatients. The effects of the warfarin can be reversed with vitamin K. Foods with the highest amounts of vitamin K include green leafy vegetables, soybeans, beef liver, and green tea. Warfarin is the most widely used coumarin derivative. Warfarin should be taken without food. The patient must avoid foods high in vitamin K. The urine may turn red-orange. If the urine turns dark-brown or if red or tar-black stools occur, the patient must notify the physician. Table 27-2 lists the most commonly used anticoagulant drugs.

Warfarin is prescribed for the prophylaxis and treatment of thrombosis and embolism. Hemorrhage or known hypersensitivity to warfarin prohibits its use. The most serious adverse reaction with the use of warfarin is hemorrhage. Skin necrosis due to thrombosis of the microvasculature in skin can occur. Teratogenicity is possible, because warfarin readily crosses the placenta and affects the developing fetus. Many other drugs interact with this drug to increase or decrease its effects. Warfarin sodium and dicumarol have the most drug interactions of any commonly prescribed anticoagulant agent, as well as being affected by the nutritional and health status of the patient, all of which may lead to unpredictable results. Therefore, whenever a new drug regimen is introduced for a patient receiving this drug, an old drug may have to be withdrawn. An increased tendency for bleeding is seen with salicylates, chloral hydrate, phenylbutazone, clofibrate, disulfiram, chloramphenicol, metronidazole, cimetidine, ranitidine, cotrimoxazole, sulfinpyrazone, quinidine, quinine, oxyphenbutazone, thyroid drugs, glucagon, danazol, erythromycin, androgens, amiodarone, cefamandole, cefoperazone, cefotetan, moxalactam, cefazolin, cefoxitin, ceftriaxone, meclofenamate, mefenamic acid, famotidine, nizatidine, and nalidixic acid. Decreased anticoagulation effects may occur with barbiturates, griseofulvin, rifampin, phenytoin, glutethimide, carbamazepine, vitamin K, vitamin E, cholestyramine, aminoglutethimide, and ethchlorvynol. Altered effects occur with methimazole and propylthiouracil. Increased activity and toxicity of phenytoin occurs when it is taken with oral anticoagulants.

TABLE 27-2. Most Commonly-Used Anticoagulants

GENERIC NAME	TRADE NAME	ROUTES OF ADMINISTRATION
coumarin derivatives (Warfarin)	Coumadin®	Oral
dicumarol (bishydroxycoumarin)		Oral
heparin sodium	Hepalean®	IV, SC
dalteparin	Fragmin®	SC
enoxaparin	Lovenox®	SC
tinzaparin	Innohep®	SC

IV, intravenous; SC, subcutaneous.

Dicumarol

Dicumarol is a long-acting coumarin derivative. It interferes with blood clotting by depressing hepatic production of vitamin K–dependent coagulation factors II, VII, IX, and X. It has advantages over heparin for ambulatory and prolonged anticoagulant therapy because it is orally effective. It is unsuitable for short-term or emergency therapy because the maximal effect of a full initial dose does not occur for 48 to 96 hours after administration. During the period of onset of action, heparin may be given. Dicumarol is used for long-term therapy to a much greater extent than is heparin. This therapy must be monitored by frequent prothrombin tests, preferably with the international normalized ratio, to avoid thrombosis or hemorrhage due to under- or overcoagulation. Adverse effects include diarrhea, flatulence, nausea, vomiting, anorexia, hematuria, unusual hair loss, hypersensitivity, and fever. The precautions and drug interactions are the same as those for warfarin sodium.

Protamine Sulfate

Protamine sulfate is a heparin antagonist derived from fish sperm. It is an antidote for heparin; 1mg of protamine sulfate neutralizes 90 U of heparin activity derived from lung tissue or 115 U from intestinal mucosa. Protamine sulfate is prescribed to diminish or reverse the anticoagulant effect of heparin, particularly for a heparin overdose.

Pregnancy, allergy to fish, or known hypersensitivity to protamine sulfate prohibits its use. Among its more serious adverse reactions are hypotension, dyspnea, and bradycardia. Dosage greater than that needed to neutralize heparin causes the toxic and anticoagulant effects of protamine.

Thrombolytic Agents

Thrombolytic agents are used to dissolve thrombi. Thrombolytic drugs include tissue plasminogen activator, alteplase, urokinase, streptokinase, and reteplase. They are used to dissolve an arterial clot, such as a clot in a coronary artery in a patient with an acute myocardial infarction. Thrombolytic therapy is also used to dissolve clots (thrombus) in venous access devices. Thrombolytic drugs help the

TABLE 27-3. Most Commonly-Used Thrombolytic Agents

GENERIC NAME	TRADE NAME	ROUTES OF ADMINISTRATION
streptokinase	Streptase®	IV bolus, then IV infusion
urokinase	Abbokinase®	IV infusion
alteplase	Activase®	IV bolus, then IV infusion
anistreplase	Eminase®	IV injection
reteplase	Retavase®	IV bolus × 2 (30 min apart)

IV, intravenous.

TABLE 27-4. Antiplatelet Agents

GENERIC NAME	TRADE NAME
aspirin	Aspirin SR®, Ecotrin®, Ascriptin®, and many others
cilostazol	Pletal®
dipyridamole	Persantine®
reteplase	Retavase®
ticlopidine	Ticlid®
clopidogrel	Plavix®
abciximab	ReoPro®

conversion of plasminogen to plasmin, which dissolves the fibrin within a clot. The plasmin breaks down fibrin, thereby dissolving clots. The most common thrombolytic agents are shown in Table 27-3.

Thrombolytic agents are most commonly used to manage acute ischemic stroke in adults and also pulmonary embolism. Use of thrombolytic agents is prohibited in patients with active internal bleeding, a history of cerebrovascular accident (stroke), aneurysm, and severe uncontrolled hypertension. The window of opportunity for use of thrombolytic agents is a relatively short period of time. If given within the first 3 hours of a stroke, they may reduce permanent disability. If given within 12 hours of onset of a heart attack, the patient has a better chance of survival and recovery.

Hypersensitivity reactions, cerebral edema, bradycardia, cardiogenic shock, arrhythmias, pulmonary edema, heart failure, cardiac arrest, and pericarditis are contraindications for the use of thrombolytic agents.

Tissue Plasminogen Activator

Tissue plasminogen activator (TPA) is a clot-dissolving substance produced naturally by cells in the walls of blood vessels. It is also manufactured synthetically by genetic engineering techniques. TPA activates plasminogen to dissolve clots and has been used therapeutically to dissolve blood clots blocking coronary arteries. It is also used in the management of acute myocardial infarction, acute ischemic stroke, and pulmonary embolism.

Alteplase

Alteplase is an enzyme that has the property of fibrin-enhanced conversion of plasminogen to plasmin.

Urokinase

Urokinase is an enzyme produced in the kidney and found in urine that is a potent plasminogen activator of the fibrinolytic system. A pharmaceutic preparation of urokinase is administered intravenously for treatment of pulmonary embolism.

Streptokinase

Streptokinase is a fibrinolytic activator that enhances the conversion of plasminogen to the fibrinolytic enzyme plasmin. It is produced by strains of streptococci. It is used in the treatment of certain cases of pulmonary and coronary embolism.

Reteplase

Reteplase is a human tissue enzyme produced by recombinant DNA techniques. Reteplase converts plasminogen to the enzyme plasmin (fibrinolysin), which degrades fibrin clots. Therefore, it lyses thrombi and emboli. Reteplase is most active at the site of a clot and causes little systemic fibrinolysis. It is used for treatment of acute myocardial infarction to improve ventricular function.

Antiplatelet Agents

Any agent that destroys platelets or inhibits their function is called an **antiplatelet agent**. Venous thrombi consist mainly of fibrin and red blood cells. Arterial thrombi are composed mainly of platelet aggregates. Theoretically, anticoagulant drugs should be effective for reducing risks involved with venous thrombi formation and antiplatelet drugs should be more effective for reducing risks of arterial thrombi formation. The drugs most commonly used for their antiplatelet effects are seen in Table 27-4.

Aspirin

Aspirin (acetylsalicylic acid) is an analgesic, antipyretic, and antirheumatic agent. Aspirin inhibits cyclooxygenase, an enzyme that is essential for thromboxane A_2 synthesis. Thromboxane A_2 promotes platelet aggregation and vasoconstriction. Thus, aspirin can suppress the inhibition of cyclooxygenase.

Cilostazol

Cilostazol inhibits platelet aggregation induced by a variety of stimuli including thrombin, collagen, epinephrine, and arachidonic acid. Cilostazol produces vascular dilation in vascular beds with a specificity for the femoral vein. This agent reduces symptoms of a blood circulation problem in which too little blood flows into the leg muscles (intermittent claudication), allowing increased walking distance. Cilostazol is contraindicated in patients with an allergy to this drug and pregnant or lactating women.

Dipyridamole

Dipyridamole is a coronary vasodilator. It inhibits thromboxane A_2 formation and activates platelets and a platelet aggregation inhibitor. It is prescribed for long-term treatment of angina. The drug should be used with caution in patients with hypotension and in those receiving anticoagulant therapy.

Ticlopidine

Ticlopidine is a platelet aggregation inhibitor. Ticlopidine interferes with platelet membrane function by inhibiting adenosine diphosphate-induced platelet-fibrinogen binding. This drug decreases the risk of stroke related to a thrombosis. Ticlopidine can cause life-threatening hematological adverse reactions, including neutropenia and thrombotic thrombocytopenic purpura. It is contraindicated in persons with hemophilia and severe liver impairment.

Clopidogrel

Clopidogrel is chemically related to ticlopidine, which inhibits platelet aggregation. It is indicated for the reduction of atherosclerotic events including myocardial infarction, stroke, and vascular death in patients with documented atherosclerosis. The major adverse effects include chest pain, abdominal pain, joint pain, and purpura.

Abciximab

Abciximab is a platelet aggregation inhibitor that works by binding the glycoprotein receptor, which involves the pathway for platelet aggregation. It is prescribed as an adjunct to percutaneous transluminal coronary angioplasty or atherectomy. Abciximab should not be given to patients with active internal bleeding, recent gastrointestinal or urinary bleeding of significance, a history of stroke, thrombocytopenia, or recent major surgery. The side effects most often reported include bleeding, thrombocytopenia, pulmonary edema, and atrial fibrillation.

REVIEW QUESTIONS

1. Aspirin (ASA) is an example of an
A. anti-rheumatic.
B. analgesic.
C. antipyretic.
D. all of the above.

2. Which of the following may cause blood clots?
A. Hypertension
B. Hypotension
C. Platelet adhesiveness
D. Anemia

3. Which of the following agents can affect the liver by preventing the manufacture of vitamin K–dependent clotting factors?
A. Warfarin
B. Protamine sulfate
C. Urokinase
D. Aspirin

4. Prothrombin has a blood coagulation factor number of
A. I.
B. II.
C. VII.
D. X.

5. Which of the following is the antidote for heparin?
A. Vitamin K
B. Vitamin C
C. Protamine sulfate
D. Warfarin

6. Mary Smith is 38 years old and 5 months pregnant. While she was in the hospital, she developed a pulmonary embolism. The physician prescribed heparin sodium intravenously. Which of the following can be a major risk factor for her?
A. Hemorrhage
B. Hypertension
C. Hypotension
D. Myocardial infarction

7. Which of the following can cause embolism?
A. Clot
B. Air
C. Tumor tissue
D. All of the above

Continues

8. Heparin is produced by which of the following white blood cells?
   A. Neutrophils
   B. Eosinophils
   C. Lymphocytes
   D. Basophils

9. The most common indication for thrombolytic agents is
   A. pulmonary embolism.
   B. cerebral edema.
   C. aneurysm.
   D. severe uncontrolled hypertension.

10. Urokinase is an enzyme produced in which of the following organs?
    A. Liver
    B. Kidney
    C. Spleen
    D. Colon

11. All of the following are anti-platelet agents, except
    A. dipyridamole.
    B. ticlopidine.
    C. tissue plasminogen activator.
    D. abciximab.

12. An example of an oral anticoagulant is
    A. warfarin.
    B. ardeparin.
    C. heparin.
    D. enoxaparin.

13. Which of the following agents inhibits platelet aggregation?
    A. Dalteparin
    B. Tinzaparin
    C. Warfarin
    D. Clopidogrel

14. The brand name of warfarin is
    A. Refludan®.
    B. Heparin®.
    C. Coumadin®.
    D. Lovenox®.

15. The maximum anticoagulant effect of warfarin occurs after
    A. 1 hour.
    B. 1 day.
    C. 1 week.
    D. 2 weeks.

28 Skeletal Muscle Relaxants and Non-Narcotic Analgesics

OUTLINE

- The Musculoskeletal System
- Skeletal Muscle Relaxants
  - Centrally Acting Muscle Relaxants
  - Peripherally Acting Muscle Relaxants
- Anti-Inflammatory and Analgesic Drugs
  - Nonsteroidal Anti-inflammatory Drugs
  - Cyclooxygenase-2 Inhibitors
- Other Nonsteroidal and Nonsalicylate Anti-Inflammatory Drugs
  - Diclofenac
  - Misoprostol
  - Etodolac
  - Ibuprofen
  - Indomethacin
  - Naproxen
- Gouty Arthritis
  - Drugs for Gouty Arthritis
- Acetaminophen

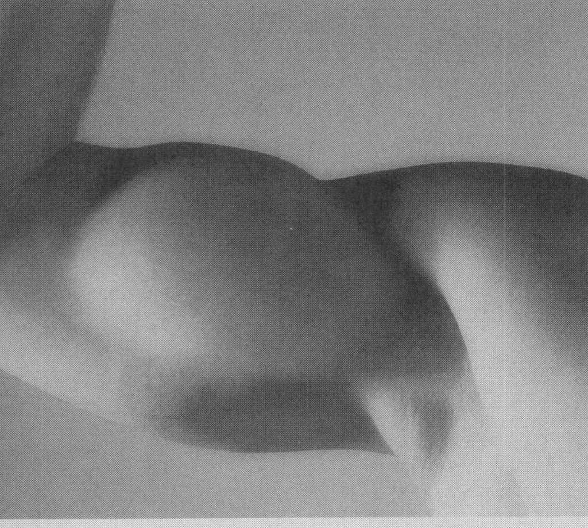

(Courtesy of PhotoDisc)

GLOSSARY

acetylcholine (ACh) A chemical substance released in the neuromuscular junction to help transmit nervous impulses.

analgesics Pain-relieving drugs.

antipyretics Fever-relieving drugs.

disease-modifying antirheumatic drugs (DMARDs) Immunosuppressive drugs useful in the treatment of lupus nephritis, seropositive progressive rheumatoid arthritis, and vasculitis syndromes.

motor nerve A nerve that originates in the spinal cord and stimulates several muscle fibers; also called somatic nerve.

neuromuscular junction The area where the motor nerve meets the muscle.

nonsteroidal anti-inflammatory drugs (NSAIDs) Drugs that inhibit the synthesis of the prostaglandin responsible for causing pain and inflammation.

salicylates Nonopioid analgesic and anti-inflammatory medications.

somatic nerve A nerve that originates in the spinal cord and stimulates several muscle fibers; also called motor nerve.

THE MUSCULOSKELETAL SYSTEM

Skeletal muscles cannot function unless they are stimulated by nerves (see Figure 28-1). They are generally attached to bone. Skeletal muscles can be controlled by choice. Therefore, they are called voluntary muscles. These muscles produce movement, maintain body posture, and stabilize joints (see Figure 28-2).

Skeletal muscle contraction can take place only if the muscle is first stimulated by a nerve. The type of nerve that supplies the skeletal muscle is a **motor nerve** or **somatic nerve**. A motor nerve comes from the spinal cord and supplies several muscle fibers with nerve stimulation. The area where the motor nerve meets the muscle is called the **neuromuscular junction**; at this site nerve endings release a chemical substance called **acetylcholine (ACh)**. Contraction of skeletal muscles requires ACh. Relaxation occurs when ACh is broken down by a special enzyme, called acetylcholinesterase.

SKELETAL MUSCLE RELAXANTS

Skeletal muscle injuries are usually self-limiting and are treated with rest, physical therapy, and possibly anti-inflammatory medications. Most injuries to muscles themselves are short-lived and respond to short-term muscle relaxant therapy in conjunction with rest and physical therapy. Centrally acting skeletal muscle relaxants are used for spasms that do not respond quickly to other therapy. These medications decrease local pain and tenderness, increase range of motion, and cause sedation. The choice of the skeletal muscle relaxant is usually determined by the preference of the physician and the response of the patient to the drugs. The most commonly used skeletal muscle relaxants are listed in Table 28-1.

Centrally Acting Muscle Relaxants

The exact mechanism of centrally acting muscle relaxants is unknown. They may act in the central nervous system (CNS) at various levels to depress polysynaptic reflexes, resulting in a sedative effect that may be responsible for relaxation of muscle spasms. The effectiveness of centrally acting muscle relaxants is erratic, owing to their limited selectivity. Orally, they are usually ineffective (the tolerated doses being much too low); intravenously, they have some established value in treating acute muscle spasms resulting from trauma or inflammation. They have little benefit for treating motor dysfunctions of the spinal cord or brain disorders.

Baclofen

Baclofen is a centrally acting skeletal muscle relaxant. It is prescribed for treatment of reversible spasticity or spinal cord injuries. The precise mechanism of its muscle relaxant

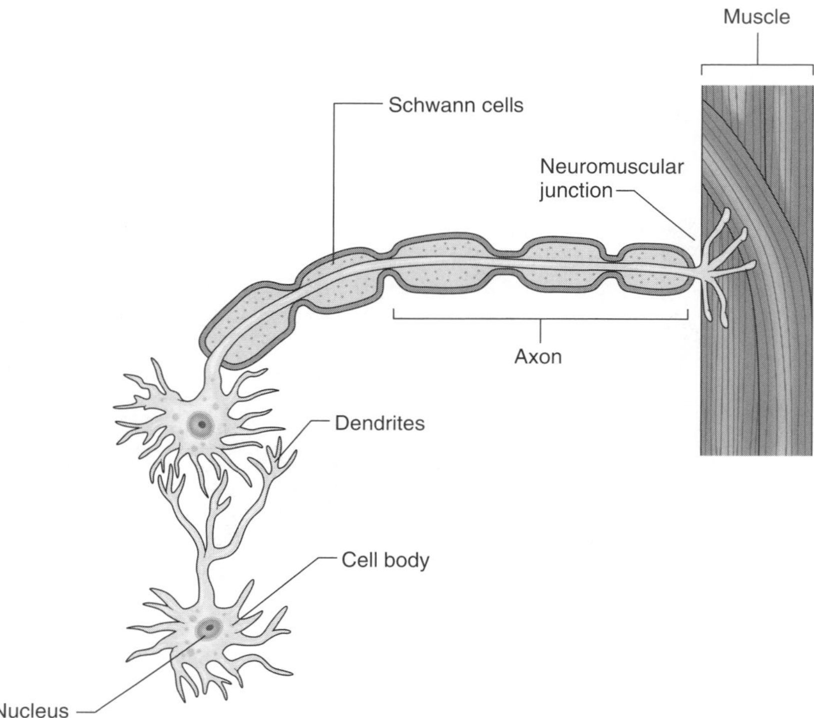

Figure 28-1. A neuron-stimulating muscle.

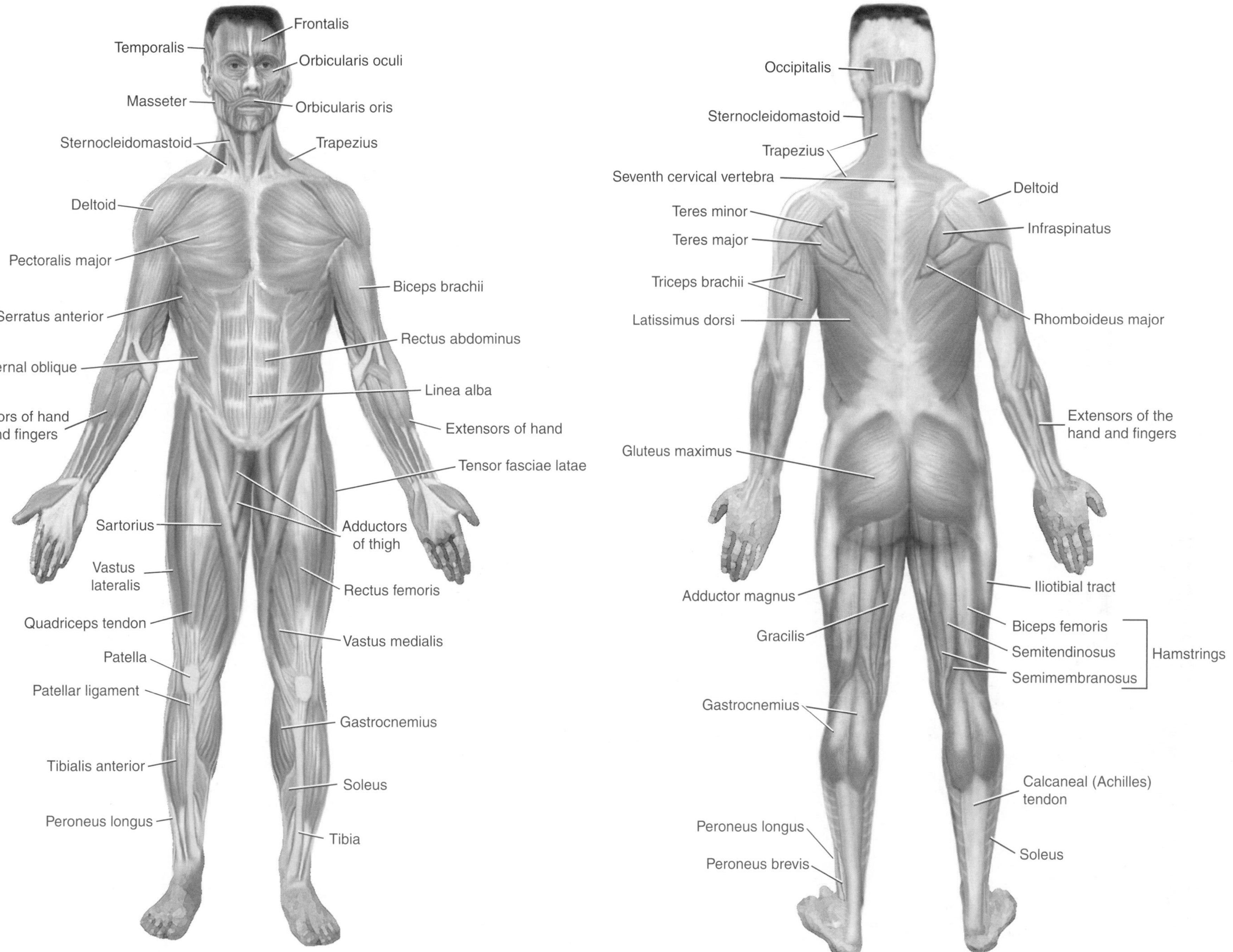

Figure 28-2. Principal skeletal muscles of the body.

TABLE 28-1. The Most Commonly-Used Skeletal Muscle Relaxants

GENERIC NAME	TRADE NAME	ROUTE OF ADMINISTRATION
Centrally Acting Muscle Relaxants		
baclofen	Lioresal®	Oral
carisoprodol	Soma®	Oral
chlorzoxazone	Parafon Forte®, Paraflex®	Oral
cyclobenzaprine	Flexeril®	Oral
diazepam	Valium®	Oral, IM, IV, rectal
methocarbamol	Robaxin®	Oral
orphenadrine	Anteflex®	Oral
	Norflex®	IM, IV
Peripherally Acting Muscle Relaxants		
dantrolene	Dantrium®	Oral, IV

IM, intramuscular; IV, intravenous.

properties is unknown. Its sedative and ataxic actions are consistent with such an action in the brain. It is also used for relief of painful spasticity in multiple sclerosis, for which it is more effective than diazepam. It is not indicated in musculoskeletal spastic disorders. Sedation is the most common adverse effect. It should not be used in combination with other CNS depressants. Consumption of alcohol (ethanol) should be avoided if possible. Other common side effects include dizziness, insomnia, pruritus, and rashes. Less common side effects include hypotension and mental confusion. Baclofen is contraindicated in pregnancy and if hypersensitivity to the drug exists. It is absorbed rapidly orally; absorption time is approximately 2 hours. More than 80% of the drug is excreted in the urine.

Carisoprodol

Carisoprodol is a sedative drug with muscle relaxant properties that result from CNS depression. It is used to treat muscle spasms of local origin, such as those resulting from strains, sprains, and lumbago. Part of its action may result from analgesia, sedation, and alleviation of anxiety. Adverse effects include sedation, weakness, ataxia, tachycardia, dizziness, confusion, depression, and syncope.

Chlorzoxazone

Chlorzoxazone is a muscle relaxant, and its effects may be due to sedation. It is used for treatment of acute, painful musculoskeletal conditions such as muscle spasms, sprains, and muscle strain. Chlorzoxazone should be used during pregnancy only if benefits clearly outweigh risks. It should be used with caution in patients with known allergies or a history of allergic reactions to drugs. Adverse effects include dizziness, drowsiness, and malaise. It may also produce allergic reactions (rare), discoloration of urine, and liver damage.

Cyclobenzaprine

Cyclobenzaprine is a skeletal muscle relaxant. It is related to the tricyclic antidepressants. This agent possesses both sedative and anticholinergic properties. Cyclobenzaprine is used as an adjunct to rest and physical therapy for relief of muscle spasms associated with acute and painful musculoskeletal conditions. It is not indicated for the treatment of spastic diseases or cerebral palsy. This drug should not be used during lactation or for children younger than age 15. Side effects include dry mouth, constipation, unpleasant taste, anorexia, and diarrhea. Cyclobenzaprine may also cause blurred vision, drowsiness, dizziness, and headache.

Diazepam

Diazepam is a centrally acting skeletal muscle relaxant. It acts on the spinal cord and the CNS. Diazepam is used as an adjunct for relief of reflex skeletal muscle spasm due to inflammation of muscles or joints, to trauma, or to spasticity caused by upper motor neuron disorders such as cerebral palsy and paraplegia. The common adverse effects are similar to those of other skeletal muscle relaxants, but, specifically, diazepam causes dependence with withdrawal syndrome when its use is discontinued.

Methocarbamol

Methocarbamol is classified as a centrally acting muscle relaxant. Its beneficial effects may be related to the sedative properties of the drug. Methocarbamol is prescribed as an adjunct for the relief of acute, painful sprains and strains of the muscles. It must be used with caution in patients with epilepsy and in women during lactation. Adverse effects include dizziness, drowsiness, vertigo, and headache. After intravenous use of methocarbamol, hypotension, bradycardia, and syncope have been reported.

Orphenadrine

Orphenadrine is a skeletal muscle relaxant. It is indicated for relief of pain in acute musculoskeletal conditions as an adjunct to rest and physical therapy. Adverse effects are headache, dizziness, confusion, hallucinations, memory loss, psychosis, and blurred vision. Orphenadrine also produces tachycardia, palpitation, and hypotension.

Peripherally Acting Muscle Relaxants

Peripherally acting muscle relaxants act directly on muscles to reduce skeletal muscle contractions. They are used to treat spasticity from stroke, spinal injury, cerebral palsy, and multiple sclerosis.

Dantrolene

Dantrolene is a skeletal muscle relaxant. It relaxes the spastic muscle directly but has no effect on smooth or cardiac muscles. The benefits of dantrolene may not be apparent for 1 week or more. It is also used to treat malignant hyperthermia. A major side effect of dantrolene is muscle weakness, which may limit therapy. Chronic use may result in hepatic toxicity, which may be fatal. Other side effects include drowsiness, dizziness, diarrhea, seizures, and pericarditis. It is contraindicated in patients with liver disease and respiratory muscle weakness.

ANTI-INFLAMMATORY AND ANALGESIC DRUGS

Anti-inflammatory drugs are used to treat inflammatory conditions of the musculoskeletal system. Joint diseases such as arthritis, bursitis, synovitis, spondylitis, gout, or muscle strains and sprains can cause inflammation (swelling, redness, heat, pain, and limited mobility.) Pain-relieving drugs are called **analgesics**. Many of the analgesics also reduce fever (**antipyretics**), and some of these drugs are anti-inflammatory agents. Analgesics may be classified as opioid (narcotics) or nonopioid medications. Narcotic drugs were discussed in Chapter 23. Nonopioid analgesics include **salicylates** and acetaminophen for relieving pain. Corticosteroids are used as anti-inflammatory agents for specific acute conditions, but they are not used for extended periods of time because of serious side effects. **Nonsteroidal anti-inflammatory drugs (NSAIDs)** including **salicylates** are commonly used medications for arthritic pain. Cyclooxygenase (COX) inhibitors are a newer class of antiarthritic drugs.

Nonsteroidal Anti-inflammatory Drugs

NSAIDs inhibit synthesis of prostaglandin, which is responsible for causing the inflammation and pain of rheumatic conditions, sprains, and menstrual cramps. There is no cure for rheumatic disorders, but NSAIDs are used to alleviate the pain and crippling effects. Antirheumatic drugs are classified into three categories: NSAIDs, **disease-modifying antirheumatic drugs (DMARDs)**, and glucocorticosteroids. NSAIDs are available over-the-counter (OTC) in lower doses and by prescription in higher doses; the difference between the OTC drugs and the prescribed drugs is the strength of the drug. DMARDs are more toxic and have a slower onset of action. These drugs require regular monitoring of the patient's condition, but they do delay progression of the disease. Glucocorticosteroids provide rapid relief of symptoms. They do not prevent the progression of the disease and are toxic with long-term use. Corticosteroids are used for severe and progressive rheumatoid arthritis, and they are usually recognized as agents of last resort. Corticosteroids occasionally may be used in elderly patients as alternatives that do not have the risks of second-line agents and in patients who cannot tolerate NSAIDs. Long-term administration may cause gastrointestinal (GI) bleeding, poor wound healing, myopathy, cataracts, hyperglycemia, hypertension, and osteoporosis.

TABLE 28-2. Salicylates (Nonsteroidal Anti-Inflammatory Drugs)

GENERIC NAME	TRADE NAME	ROUTE OF ADMINISTRATION
aspirin (acetylsalicylic acid)	(There are many examples: Bayer®, Bufferin®, Ecotrin®, etc.)	Oral
choline salicylate	Arthropan®	Oral
choline magnesium salicylate	Trilisate®	Oral
magnesium salicylate	Magan®, Mobidin®	Oral
salsalate	Disalcid®	Oral

Salicylates

Salicylates, such as aspirin, are the oldest of the nonopioid analgesics and NSAIDs. They are still often used as analgesics. Salicylates are effective and inexpensive drugs. Their actions are generally anti-inflammatory to give relief, but these agents also act as analgesics. Table 28-2 lists salicylates (NSAIDs).

Salicylates are prescribed for rheumatoid arthritis, osteoarthritis, and often for other inflammatory disorders. The top three NSAIDs prescribed are aspirin, ibuprofen, and naproxen. Aspirin is absorbed rapidly from the duodenum and stomach. Unmetabolized salicylates are excreted by the kidneys. The most common side effects of high doses of aspirin (70% of patients) include nausea, vomiting, diarrhea or constipation, dyspepsia, epigastric pain, bleeding, and ulceration in the stomach. Intolerance of aspirin is relatively common and symptoms include rash, bronchospasm, rhinitis, edema, or an anaphylactic reaction with shock that may be life-threatening. Use of aspirin and other salicylates to control fever during viral infections in children and adolescents (influenza and chickenpox) is associated with an increased incidence of Reye's syndrome (a combination of acute encephalopathy and fatty infiltration of the internal organs that may follow acute viral infections such as influenza B). This illness is characterized by vomiting, hepatic disturbances, and encephalopathy.

Cyclooxygenase-2 Inhibitors

NSAIDs inhibit both COX-1 and COX-2 in varying ratios. COX-2 is more specific for prostaglandin synthesis in response to an inflammatory event. COX-2 inhibitors are a new class of antiarthritic drugs used to suppress inflammation, while producing fewer side effects. Table 28-3 lists COX inhibitors.

Note: Prostaglandins are derived from prostanoic acid. In the body, prostaglandins are synthesized principally from

TABLE 28-3. Cyclooxygenase Inhibitors

GENERIC NAME	TRADE NAME	ROUTE OF ADMINISTRATION
celecoxib	Celebrex®	Oral
rofecoxib	Vioxx®	Oral

arachidonic acid (lipids), specifically by the enzyme COX. Its role appears to be the daily synthesis of prostaglandins that contribute to normal homeostasis.

Celecoxib

Celecoxib is an non-narcotic NSAID analgesic and specific COX-2 enzyme blocker. Celecoxib is an analgesic and anti-inflammatory agent. It is used for acute and long-term treatment of the signs and symptoms of rheumatoid arthritis and osteoarthritis. Adverse effects include headache, dizziness, somnolence, and insomnia. Celecoxib can also affect the GI tract and cause nausea, abdominal pain, and bleeding. Other side effects are peripheral edema and anaphylactic shock.

Rofecoxib

Rofecoxib is an NSAID analgesic and selective COX-2 enzyme blocker. Its analgesic and anti-inflammatory activities are related to the inhibition of COX-2 enzymes. It is used to relieve the signs and symptoms of osteoarthritis and rheumatoid arthritis. Adverse effects are similar to those of celecoxib.

Valdecoxib

Valdecoxib is another NSAID analgesic and anti-inflammatory drug that is a specific COX-2 enzyme blocker. Indications for valdecoxib and adverse effects are the same as those for the other COX inhibitors.

OTHER NONSTEROIDAL AND NONSALICYLATE ANTI-INFLAMMATORY DRUGS

Many patients tolerate effective doses of the NSAIDs better than high-dose aspirin therapy. However, the newer drugs are much more expensive. No clinical evidence has been found to prove that any one of these drugs is consistently more effective than another, but research shows that a condition that does not respond to one NSAID may respond to another. These drugs tend to cause less GI disturbance than aspirin. At present, many of these drugs are on the market.

TABLE 28-4. Other Nonsteroidal and Nonsalicylate Anti-inflammatory Drugs

GENERIC NAME	TRADE NAME	ROUTE OF ADMINISTRATION
diclofenac	Voltaren®	Oral
diclofenac with misoprostol	Arthrotec®	Oral
diflunisal	Dolobid®	Oral
etodolac	Lodine®	Oral
fenoprofen	Nalfon®	Oral
flurbiprofen	Ansaid®	Oral
ibuprofen	Motrin®, Advil®	Oral
indomethacin	Indocin®	Oral
meclofenamate	Meclomen®	Oral
naproxen	Naprosyn®	Oral
oxaprozin	Daypro®	Oral
piroxicam	Feldene®	Oral
sulindac	Clinoril®	Oral
tolmetin	Tolectin®	Oral
naproxen sodium	Anaprox®, Aleve®*	

OTC, over the counter.

They are used to treat not only arthritis but also other musculoskeletal disorders, such as tendonitis and bursitis. Table 28-4 lists other nonsteroidal and nonsalicylate anti-inflammatory drugs. In the following, some selected examples from Table 28-4 will be discussed.

Diclofenac

Diclofenac is an anti-inflammatory agent and NSAID. It inhibits prostaglandin synthetase to cause antipyretic and anti-inflammatory effects. Diclofenac is used for rheumatoid arthritis, osteoarthritis, and ankylosing spondylitis. Adverse effects include headache, dizziness, somnolence, insomnia, tiredness, renal impairment, and dysuria. Diclofenac may produce nausea, vomiting, diarrhea, constipation, and flatulence.

Misoprostol

Misoprostol is a synthetic prostaglandin used to treat gastrointestinal difficulties such as stomach ulcers. Misoprostol should not be used in pregnant women because it can induce labor, rupture the uterus, or cause an abortion of the fetus. This drug is used in combination with diclofenac as a NSAID.

Etodolac

Etodolac is an analgesic (non-narcotic), antipyretic, and NSAID. Its mechanism of action is similar to that of diclofenac. Etodolac is used for acute or long-term treatment of the signs and symptoms of osteoarthritis and rheumatoid arthritis. Adverse effects are the same as those for diclofenac.

Ibuprofen

Ibuprofen is an analgesic (non-narcotic) and NSAID. The mechanism of action, indications, and adverse effects are all similar to those of diclofenac and etodolac.

Indomethacin

Indomethacin is a NSAID. Its therapeutic actions are anti-inflammatory, analgesic, and antipyretic. It is used to relieve the signs and symptoms of moderate to severe rheumatoid arthritis and moderate to severe osteoarthritis. Indomethacin is also indicated for acute painful shoulder (bursitis or tendonitis) and acute gouty arthritis. It is not recommended as a simple analgesic or antipyretic because of the potential for severe adverse effects. The adverse effects are similar to those of other NSAIDs.

Naproxen

Naproxen is a NSAID and analgesic (non-narcotic) with antipyretic activities largely related to inhibition of prostaglandin; its exact mechanisms of action are not known. The indications for and adverse effects of naproxen are the same as those for other NSAIDs. It is contraindicated in patients with an allergy to naproxen and salicylates. It must be used cautiously in patients with asthma, chronic urticaria, hypertension, GI bleeding, and impaired hepatic or renal function.

GOUTY ARTHRITIS

Gouty arthritis, or gout, is a disease associated with an inborn error of uric acid metabolism that increases production of or interferes with the excretion of uric acid. Excess uric acid is converted to sodium urate crystals that precipitate from the blood and become deposited in the joints and other tissues. The great toe is a common site for the accumulation of urate crystals. The condition can cause exceedingly painful swelling of a joint and other signs of inflammation. The treatment goals are to end the attack as soon as possible, prevent recurrence of the acute condition, and decrease the possibility of complications from deposits of uric acid. The patient with gouty arthritis should avoid foods high in purines, such as red meat, tomatoes, oatmeal, cheese, fatty foods, shellfish, and alcohol.

Drugs for Gouty Arthritis

The drugs used to treat acute gout include colchicine, NSAIDs, and corticosteroids. Antigout drugs are listed in Table 28-5.

TABLE 28-5. Antigout Drugs

GENERIC NAME	TRADE NAME	ROUTE OF ADMINISTRATION
Acute Attacks		
colchicine	None	Oral, IV
Chronic Therapy		
allopurinol	Zyloprim®	Oral
probenecid	Benemid®	Oral
indomethacin	Indocin®	Oral
sulfinpyrazone	Anturane®	Oral

Colchicine

Colchicine is an anti-inflammatory agent and is the drug of choice for acute attacks of gout. It is used specifically for gout and is ineffective for any other disease. Colchicine interferes with white blood cells, reducing their mobility and joint phagocytosis, and also reduces uric acid production. This agent is not an analgesic; therefore, it does not relieve the symptoms of other conditions except gout. Adverse effects include nausea, vomiting, diarrhea, and abdominal pain. Colchicine should be prescribed with caution for elderly patients because of the dangers of GI, renal, hepatic, and cardiac diseases.

Allopurinol

Allopurinol is an antigout agent that inhibits the enzyme responsible for the conversion of purines to uric acid, thus reducing the production of uric acid with a decrease in serum and sometimes in urinary uric acid levels. Allopurinol relieves the signs and symptoms of gout. Adverse effects include headache, drowsiness, peripheral neuropathy, and neuritis. It may also cause nausea, vomiting, diarrhea, gastritis, hepatomegaly (enlargement of the liver), and jaundice.

Probenecid

Probenecid is an antigout and uricosuric agent. It inhibits the renal tubular reabsorption of urate and increases the urinary excretion of uric acid. Probenecid is used to treat hyperuricemia associated with gout and gouty arthritis. The adverse effects include headache, nausea, vomiting, urinary frequency, and exacerbation of gout and uric acid stones.

Sulfinpyrazone

Sulfinpyrazone is an antigout and uricosuric agent. It inhibits the renal tubular reabsorption of uric acid, decreasing serum uric acid levels and promoting the reabsorption of urate deposits. Sulfinpyrazone is used for chronic intermittent gouty arthritis. The adverse effects include upper GI disturbance, exacerbation of gout and uric acid stones, and renal failure.

ACETAMINOPHEN

Acetaminophen is another common nonopioid analgesic that is available as an OTC drug and is found in most households. Like aspirin, acetaminophen has analgesic and antipyretic actions. It can be used with relative safety in age groups from small children through older adults. Unlike aspirin, it does not have anti-inflammatory actions. The mechanism of action may be inhibition of prostaglandin in the peripheral nervous system, which makes the sensory neurons less likely to receive the pain signal. Acetaminophen is recommended as a substitute for treatment of fever of unknown etiology in children. Acetaminophen does not displace other drugs from plasma proteins. It causes minimal GI irritation. Acetaminophen has little effect on platelet adhesion and aggregation. It can be substituted for aspirin to treat mild to moderate pain or fever for selected patients who have the following:

- allergy to aspirin
- aspirin intolerance
- history of peptic ulcer or hemophilia
- anticoagulant use
- risk for complications (viral infection as a risk for Reye's syndrome)

Adverse effects include headache, chest pain, dyspnea, myocardial damage with high dosage, hepatic toxicity and liver failure, jaundice, acute kidney failure, and renal tubular necrosis.

REVIEW QUESTIONS

1. Long-term administration of corticosteroids may cause
   A. hypoglycemia.
   B. hypotension.
   C. gastrointestinal bleeding.
   D. asthma.

2. Which of the following is the drug of choice for acute gout attack?
   A. Probenecid
   B. Acetaminophen
   C. Acetylsalicylic acid (aspirin)
   D. Colchicine

3. The most common side effect of baclofen (Lioresal®) is
   A. sedation.
   B. seizures.
   C. osteoporosis.
   D. nosebleed.

4. The trade name of carisoprodol is
   A. Flexeril®.
   B. Valium®.
   C. Soma®.
   D. Lioresal®.

5. Which of the following agents is known as an anti-inflammatory, antipyretic, and analgesic?
   A. Prednisone
   B. Aspirin
   C. Acetaminophen
   D. Acetylsalicylic acid

6. Peripherally acting muscle relaxants include
   A. diazepam.
   B. dantrolene.
   C. baclofen.
   D. methocarbamol.

7. Which of the following is a major side effect of dantrolene that may limit therapy?
   A. Diarrhea
   B. Dizziness
   C. Drowsiness
   D. Muscle weakness

8. The adverse effects of acetaminophen include all of the following, except
   A. fever.
   B. chest pain.
   C. liver failure.
   D. renal tubular necrosis.

9. Disease-modifying antirheumatic drugs (DMARDS)
   A. are more toxic than NSAIDs.
   B. are more effective than NSAIDs.
   C. have a slower onset of action than NSAIDs.
   D. A and C.

10. By using aspirin to control fever during viral infections in children, the incidence of __________ may be increased.
    A. hepatitis
    B. renal failure
    C. Reye's syndrome
    D. heart failure

Continues

11. The trade name of rofecoxib is
A. Bextra®.
B. Vioxx®.
C. Benemid®.
D. Celebrex®.

12. Indomethacin is a/an
A. analgesic.
B. antipyretic.
C. anti-inflammatory.
D. all of the above.

13. The generic name of Advil® is
A. indomethacin.
B. ibuprofen.
C. naproxen.
D. aspirin.

14. Which of the following is a NSAID, non-narcotic drug, and *specific* COX-2 enzyme blocker?
A. Vioxx®
B. Ecotrin®
C. Tylenol®
D. Celebrex®

15. Probenecid is an antigout agent, and which of the following?
A. Narcotic
B. Uricosuric
C. Antipyretic
D. Antacid

Immunological Agents 29

OUTLINE

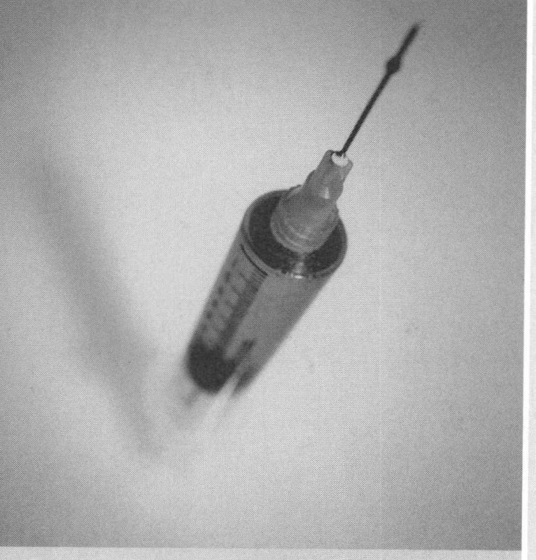

(Courtesy of PhotoDisc)

GLOSSARY

active immunity Immunity resulting from the development of antibodies within a person's body that renders the person immune; it may occur from exposure through a disease process or from immunizations.

anthrax A zoonotic disease caused by the anthrax bacillus that can infect humans in a number of ways and can be fatal.

antibody Protein that develops in response to the presence of an antigen in the body and reacts with the antigen on the next exposure. Antibodies may be formed from infections, immunization, transfer from mother to child, or unknown antigen stimulation.

Bacillus anthracis Bacteria causing anthrax with a cell shape that is cylindrical (longer than it is wide).

cell-mediated immunity The type of immune responses brought about by T cells (T lymphocytes).

contraindication A condition that increases the chance of a serious adverse reaction.

hepatitis Inflammation of the liver caused by microorganisms, especially viruses, or drugs such as alcohol and other poisons.

human rabies immune globulin A sterile solution of antirabies immune globulin for intramuscular administration. It is prepared from the plasma of human donors hyperimmunized with the rabies vaccine. It should be administered to patients as soon as possible after exposure to the disease.

humeral immunity Protective molecules (mostly B lymphocytes) carried in the fluids of the body.

hydrophobia A fear of water; a symptom caused by rabies as the disease progresses.

immunity An immunological reaction that destroys or resists antigens.

immunoglobulin A blood product that contains disease-specific antibodies for passive immunity.
inactivated vaccines Vaccines in which the infectious components have been destroyed by chemical or physical treatments.
live attenuated vaccines Vaccines containing living organisms or intact viruses that have undergone radiation or temperature conditioning to produce safe vaccinations which will help the patient become immune to a specific disease.
lymphocytes The second most common form of white blood cells.
Mantoux test An intradermal screening for tuberculin hypersensitivity. A red, firm patch of skin at the injection site greater than 10 mm in diameter, after 48 hours, is a positive result that indicates current or prior exposure to tubercle bacilli.
meningitis An inflammation of the meninges (membranes) that surround and protect the brain. It is often caused by bacteria.
meningococcal vaccine Vaccine aiding antibodies in the attacking of the gram-negative coccus bacteria that are responsible for meningitis.
passive immunity Immunity acquired from the injection or passage of antibodies from an immune person or animal to another for short-term immunity or immunity passed from mother to child.
precaution Specific warning to consider when medications are prescribed or administered.
rabies The only rhabdovirus that infects humans; it is a zoonotic disease characterized by fatal meningoencephalitis.
smallpox Acute viral disease that was essentially eradicated in 1979. It causes a disfiguring rash, headache, vomiting, and fever.
tine test In this test, the tuberculin antigen is injected just under the skin with a multipronged instrument. The antigen is located on the spikes (tines) that penetrate the skin. If positive, the skin around the injection site will be red and swollen like a mosquito bit, 48 to 72 hours after the injection. It is not as accurate as the Mantoux test.
tuberculin A glycerinated broth culture of *Mycobacterium tuberculosis* that is evaporated and filtered. Formerly used to treat tuberculosis, tuberculin is now used chiefly for diagnostic tests.
tuberculosis A chronic granulomatous infection caused by *Mycobacterium tuberculosis.* It is generally transmitted by the inhalation or ingestion of infected droplets and usually affects the lungs.
vaccination The process of immunization for prevention of diseases.

THE IMMUNE SYSTEM

The immune system protects the body against pathogenic organisms and other foreign bodies. The principal components of the immune system include the bone marrow, the thymus, the lymph nodes, the spleen, and the lymphatic vessels. The spleen is the largest organ in the system. The immune system protects the body initially by creating local barriers and inflammation. Local barriers provide chemical and mechanical defenses through the skin, the mucous membranes, and the conjunctiva. Inflammation draws leukocytes to the site of injury, where these phagocytes engulf the invading pathogens. If these first-line defenses fail or are inadequate to protect the body, the humeral immune response and the cell-mediated immune response are activated.

Immunity is an immunological reaction that destroys or resists foreign cells (antigens). An antigen is usually bacterial, viral, fungal, or rickettsial in the organs. There are two primary types of immunity: humeral and cell-mediated.

Humeral Immunity

Humeral immunity is a response to antigens, which is the result of the development and continuing presence of circulating antibodies carried in immunoglobulins (Igs) IgA, IgG, and IgM that are produced by the plasma cells (B cells).

Cell-Mediated Immunity

Cell-mediated immunity is the result of contact between T cells and antigens. Cellular immunity is involved in resistance to infectious diseases caused by viruses and some bacteria, delayed hypersensitivity reactions, some aspects of resistance to cancer, certain autoimmune diseases, graft rejection, and certain allergies. There are also two basic mechanisms for acquiring immunity: active and passive.

Active Immunity

Active immunity is protection that is produced by the person's own immune system. This type of immunity is usually permanent.

Passive Immunity

Passive immunity is protection by products produced by an animal or human and transferred to another human, usually by injection. Passive immunity often provides effective protection, but this protection disappears over time, usually in a few weeks or months.

LYMPHOCYTES

Lymphocytes play a major role in the maintenance of health and in the response to and recovery from disease. Lymphocytes are the primary cells of specific immune responses. There are two types: B and T lymphocytes. All B and T cells are antigen-specific because they have specific receptors as part of their plasma membranes. (The terms *B cell* and *T cell* are also used instead of *B lymphocyte* and *T lymphocyte*.)

Mononuclear T and B lymphocytes are able to mobilize and deploy antibodies and other responses to stimulation by an antigen. When they are activated by an antigen, they proliferate and produce a clone. Other leukocytes are also involved in the immune response. They are nonspecific cells that interact with lymphocytes to respond to the inflammatory process. B and T cells are able to recognize specific antigens and initiate the immune response. T lymphocytes from the bone marrow are transformed to maturity in the thymus gland and then migrate to lymphoid tissue. During contact with an antigen, T cells provide cellular immunity. B cells form antibodies that are able to identify and bind with specific antigens to provide humeral immunity.

ANTIBODIES AND IMMUNOGLOBULINS

The terms **antibody** and **immunoglobulin** are used interchangeably. Antibodies are produced by lymphocytes in response to bacteria, viruses, or other antigenic substances. An antibody is specific to an antigen. It is a type of protein called gamma globulin. Each class of antibody is named for its action. There are five classes of antibodies: IgG, IgA, IgM, IgD, and IgE.

Immunoglobulin G

The normal concentration of IgG in the blood is about 70% to 80% of the total antibodies. IgG is the only immunoglobulin that crosses the placenta and protects against red cell antigens and white cell antigens.

Immunoglobulin A

IgA is one of the most prevalent antibodies. It is found in all secretions of the body and is the major antibody in the mucous membrane in the intestines and in the bronchi, saliva, and tears. IgA combines with a protein in the mucosa and defends body surfaces against invading microorganisms.

Immunoglobulin M

IgM is the largest immunoglobulin in molecular structure. It is the first immunoglobulin the body produces when challenged by antigens and is found in circulating blood. IgM activates complement and can destroy antigens during the initial antigen exposure.

Immunoglobulin D

IgD is a specialized protein found in small amounts in serum. The precise function of IgD is not known, but its quantity increases during allergic reactions to milk, insulin, penicillin, and various toxins.

Immunoglobulin E

IgE is concentrated in the lungs, the skin, and the cells of mucous membranes. It provides the primary defense against environmental antigens and is believed to be responsive to IgA. IgE reacts with certain antigens to release certain chemical mediators (such as histamine) that cause type 1 hypersensitivity reactions characterized by wheal and flare. It can mediate the release of histamine in the immune response to parasites. Serum concentrations of IgE are low because the antibody is firmly fixed to the tissue surface.

VACCINATIONS

A **vaccination** is the act of giving an injection or other form of antibody to protect an individual from infectious disease. Vaccines are classified as live attenuated and inactivated. **Live attenuated vaccines** are produced from viruses or bacteria in a laboratory. Live attenuated vaccines available in the United States include live viruses and live bacteria. **Inactivated vaccines** can be composed of whole viruses, bacteria, or fractions of either. The more similar a vaccine is to the natural disease, the better the response is to the vaccine. Live attenuated vaccines are usually effective with one dose. They may cause severe reactions and may interfere with circulating antibodies. Table 29-1 shows some examples of live attenuated vaccines that are made from viruses or bacteria. Most vaccine preparations contain one of the following antigenic stimulants:

- Killed whole cells or inactivated viruses
- Live attenuated cells or viruses
- Antigenic components of cells or viruses
- Genetically engineered (recombinant) microbes or microbial antigens

TABLE 29-1. Examples of Live Attenuated Vaccines

VIRAL	BACTERIAL
MMR	BCG
Oral polio	Oral typhoid
Vaccinia	
Varicella	
Yellow fever	

Adverse Reactions after Vaccination

An adverse reaction is an untoward effect caused by a vaccine that is extraneous to the vaccine's primary purpose of production of immunity. Adverse reactions to vaccines fall into three general categories: local, systemic, and allergic. Local reactions are generally the least severe and most common. Allergic reactions are the most severe and least common.

Contraindication and Precautions

Generally, contraindications dictate circumstances in which vaccines will not be given. Most contraindications and precautions are temporary, and the vaccine can be given at a later time. A **contraindication** is a condition in a recipient that greatly increases the chance of a serious adverse reaction. A **precaution** is a condition in a recipient that may increase the chance of an adverse event. Permanent contraindications to vaccination include the following:

- Severe allergy to a prior dose of vaccine or to a vaccine component
- Encephalopathy after pertussis vaccine
- The recommended childhood immunization schedule is summarized in Figure 29-1. For a recommended schedule of vaccinations for adults, see Figure 29-2.

Table 29-2 lists currently licensed vaccines and toxoids available in the United States by type and recommended routes of administration.

HEPATITIS

Hepatitis is inflammation of the liver. Hepatitis may be caused by a drug or chemical toxin but more commonly is caused by a viral infection. Many forms of viral hepatitis are highly communicable and epidemics may be prevented by the use of vaccines.

Hepatitis A

Hepatitis A is caused by the hepatitis A virus. The virus may be spread through fecally contaminated food or water. Prophylaxis with immune globulin is effective for household and sexual contacts. A vaccine for immunization is available. Two inactivated whole virus vaccines for hepatitis A are available, both in pediatric and adult formulations. Neither vaccine is currently licensed for children younger than 2 years of age. More than 95% of adults will develop immunity. Both vaccines are highly effective for the prevention of clinical hepatitis A. Routine hepatitis A vaccination is recommended for children older than 2 years old. For children and adolescents, 0.5mL of vaccine should be administered intramuscularly into the deltoid muscle with a booster dose 6 to 12 months later. For adults, 1.0 mL of vaccine should be used.

Hepatitis B

Hepatitis B vaccines have been available in the United States since 1981. From 1981 until 1991, vaccination was targeted to people in groups at high risk of acquiring hepatitis B virus infection. However, the three major risk groups (heterosexuals with multiple partners in contact with infected persons, intravenous drug users, and male homosexuals) are not reached effectively by targeted programs. Recombinant hepatitis B vaccine was licensed in the United States in July 1986. Two manufacturers in the United States produce hepatitis B vaccine: Merck (Recombivax HB®) and SmithKline Beecham (Engerix-B®). Both vaccines are available in pediatric and adult formulations. Recommended dosage of the vaccine differs depending on the age of the recipient, certain exposure circumstances (e.g., perinatal), and the type of vaccine (see Table 29-3).

The schedule for hepatitis B vaccine is usually three doses at 0, 1, and 6 months. Infants whose mothers are hepatitis B surface antigen positive (carriers) should also receive hepatitis B immune globulin upon giving birth. Booster doses are *NOT* routinely recommended for any group. Indications for hepatitis B vaccine are as follows:

- Infants at birth to 2 months of age
- Adolescents 11 to 12 years of age
- Selected adults

The deltoid muscle is the recommended site for hepatitis B vaccination in adults and children, whereas the anterolateral thigh is the recommended site for infants and neonates.

Hepatitis C

Hepatitis C virus (HCV) accounts for a substantial proportion of cases previously designated as "non-A, non-B" hepatitis. HCV is transmitted primarily by the percutaneous route. Hepatitis C accounts for most cases of transfusion-associated hepatitis; however, only about 4% of all cases of hepatitis C are transfusion-associated. Up to 50% of cases of hepatitis C result from intravenous drug use, sometimes in the remote past. Sporadic cases of hepatitis C have also been described, although the exact route of transmission in these occurrences is unclear, because perinatal and sexual transmission of HCV is thought to be uncommon.

Acute hepatitis C is clinically silent in approximately 95% of individuals but is associated with a high rate of progression to chronic hepatitis. Patients with chronic HCV infection have a significant risk of developing cirrhosis, with an estimated incidence of more than 20% by 15 or 20 years, and such patients have an increased risk of developing liver carcinoma.

Currently there is little to offer an individual exposed to HCV that has been proven to reduce the risk of transmission.

Recommended Childhood and Adolescent Immunization Schedule — United States, 2003

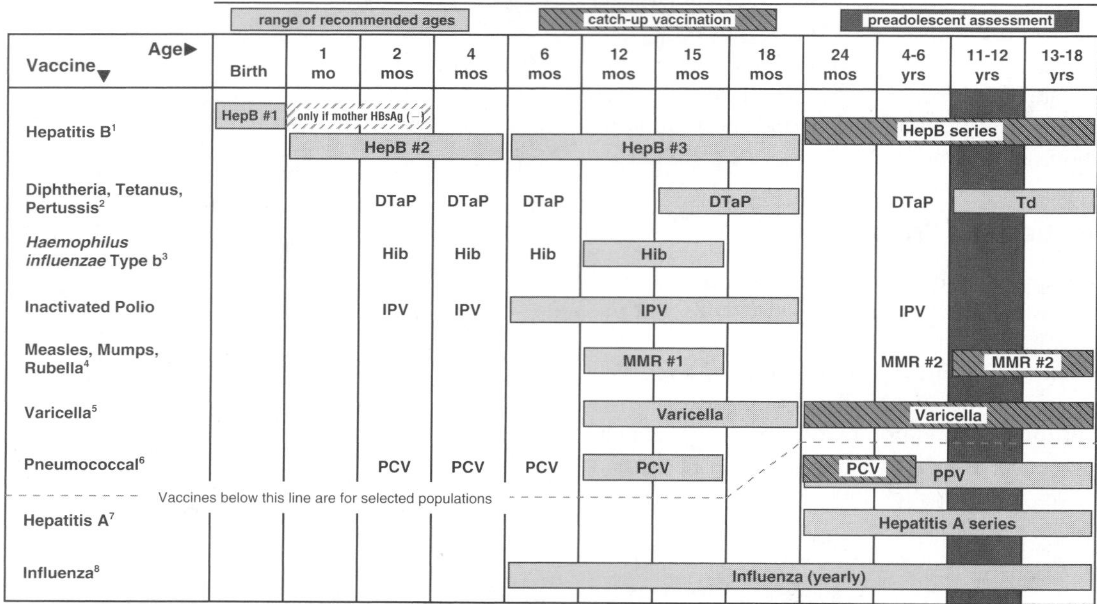

range of recommended ages | catch-up vaccination | preadolescent assessment

Vaccine ▼ / Age ▶	Birth	1 mo	2 mos	4 mos	6 mos	12 mos	15 mos	18 mos	24 mos	4-6 yrs	11-12 yrs	13-18 yrs
Hepatitis B[1]	HepB #1	only if mother HBsAg (−)							HepB series			
		HepB #2			HepB #3							
Diphtheria, Tetanus, Pertussis[2]			DTaP	DTaP	DTaP		DTaP			DTaP	Td	
Haemophilus influenzae Type b[3]			Hib	Hib	Hib	Hib						
Inactivated Polio			IPV	IPV	IPV					IPV		
Measles, Mumps, Rubella[4]						MMR #1				MMR #2	MMR #2	
Varicella[5]						Varicella			Varicella			
Pneumococcal[6]			PCV	PCV	PCV	PCV			PCV	PPV		
Vaccines below this line are for selected populations												
Hepatitis A[7]									Hepatitis A series			
Influenza[8]					Influenza (yearly)							

This schedule indicates the recommended ages for routine administration of currently licensed childhood vaccines, as of December 1, 2002, for children through age 18 years. Any dose not given at the recommended age should be given at any subsequent visit when indicated and feasible. ▨ Indicates age groups that warrant special effort to administer those vaccines not previously given. Additional vaccines may be licensed and recommended during the year. Licensed combination vaccines may be used whenever any components of the combination are indicated and the vaccine's other components are not contraindicated. Providers should consult the manufacturers' package inserts for detailed recommendations.

1. Hepatitis B vaccine (HepB). All infants should receive the first dose of hepatitis B vaccine soon after birth and before hospital discharge; the first dose may also be given by age 2 months if the infant's mother is HBsAg-negative. Only monovalent HepB can be used for the birth dose. Monovalent or combination vaccine containing HepB may be used to complete the series. Four doses of vaccine may be administered when a birth dose is given. The second dose should be given at least 4 weeks after the first dose, except for combination vaccines which cannot be administered before age 6 weeks. The third dose should be given at least 16 weeks after the first dose and at least 8 weeks after the second dose. The last dose in the vaccination series (third or fourth dose) should not be administered before age 6 months.

Infants born to HBsAg-positive mothers should receive HepB and 0.5 mL Hepatitis B Immune Globulin (HBIG) within 12 hours of birth at separate sites. The second dose is recommended at age 1-2 months. The last dose in the vaccination series should not be administered before age 6 months. These infants should be tested for HBsAg and anti-HBs at 9-15 months of age.

Infants born to mothers whose HBsAg status is unknown should receive the first dose of the HepB series within 12 hours of birth. Maternal blood should be drawn as soon as possible to determine the mother's HBsAg status; if the HBsAg test is positive, the infant should receive HBIG as soon as possible (no later than age 1 week). The second dose is recommended at age 1-2 months. The last dose in the vaccination series should not be administered before age 6 months.

2. Diphtheria and tetanus toxoids and acellular pertussis vaccine (DTaP). The fourth dose of DTaP may be administered as early as age 12 months, provided 6 months have elapsed since the third dose and the child is unlikely to return at age 15-18 months. **Tetanus and diphtheria toxoids (Td)** is recommended at age 11-12 years if at least 5 years have elapsed since the last dose of tetanus and diphtheria toxoid-containing vaccine. Subsequent routine Td boosters are recommended every 10 years.

3. *Haemophilus influenzae* type b (Hib) conjugate vaccine. Three Hib conjugate vaccines are licensed for infant use. If PRP-OMP (PedvaxHIB® or ComVax® [Merck]) is administered at ages 2 and 4 months, a dose at age 6 months is not required. DTaP/Hib combination products should not be used for primary immunization in infants at ages 2, 4 or 6 months, but can be used as boosters following any Hib vaccine.

4. Measles, mumps, and rubella vaccine (MMR). The second dose of MMR is recommended routinely at age 4-6 years but may be administered during any visit, provided at least 4 weeks have elapsed since the first dose and that both doses are administered beginning at or after age 12 months. Those who have not previously received the second dose should complete the schedule by the 11-12 year old visit.

5. Varicella vaccine. Varicella vaccine is recommended at any visit at or after age 12 months for susceptible children, i.e. those who lack a reliable history of chickenpox. Susceptible persons aged ≥13 years should receive two doses, given at least 4 weeks apart.

6. Pneumococcal vaccine. The heptavalent **pneumococcal conjugate vaccine (PCV)** is recommended for all children age 2-23 months. It is also recommended for certain children age 24-59 months. **Pneumococcal polysaccharide vaccine (PPV)** is recommended in addition to PCV for certain high-risk groups. See *MMWR* 2000;49(RR-9);1-38.

7. Hepatitis A vaccine. Hepatitis A vaccine is recommended for children and adolescents in selected states and regions, and for certain high-risk groups; consult your local public health authority. Children and adolescents in these states, regions, and high risk groups who have not been immunized against hepatitis A can begin the hepatitis A vaccination series during any visit. The two doses in the series should be administered at least 6 months apart. See *MMWR* 1999;48(RR-12);1-37.

8. Influenza vaccine. Influenza vaccine is recommended annually for children age 6 months with certain risk factors (including but not limited to asthma, cardiac disease, sickle cell disease, HIV, diabetes, and household members of persons in groups at high risk; see *MMWR* 2002;51(RR-3);1-31), and can be administered to all others wishing to obtain immunity. In addition, healthy children age 6-23 months are encouraged to receive influenza vaccine if feasible because children in this age group are at substantially increased risk for influenza-related hospitalizations. Children aged ≤12 years should receive vaccine in a dosage appropriate for their age (0.25 mL if age 6-35 months or 0.5 mL if aged 3 years). Children aged 8 years who are receiving influenza vaccine for the first time should receive two doses separated by at least 4 weeks.

For additional information about vaccines, including precautions and contraindications for immunization and vaccine shortages, please visit the National Immunization Program Website at www.cdc.gov/nip or call the National Immunization Information Hotline at 800-232-2522 (English) or 800-232-0233 (Spanish).

Approved by the Advisory Committee on Immunization Practices (www.cdc.gov/nip/acip), the American Academy of Pediatrics (www.aap.org), and the American Academy of Family Physicians (www.aafp.org).

Figure 29-1. Recommended childhood and adolescent immunization schedule—United States 2003. (Courtesy of the Centers for Disease Control and Prevention.)

Recommended Adult Immunization Schedule
United States, 2002-2003

Legend: For all persons in this group (solid) · Catch-up on childhood vaccinations (hatched) · For persons with medical/exposure indications (hatched)

Vaccine ▼ / Age Group ▶	19-49 Years	50-64 Years	65 Years and Older
Tetanus, Diphtheria (Td)*	1 dose booster every 10 years[1]		
Influenza	1 dose annually for persons with medical or occupational indications, or household contacts of persons with indications[2]	1 annual dose	
Pneumococcal (polysaccharide)	1 dose for persons with medical or other indications. (1 dose revaccination for immunosuppressive conditions)[3,4]		1 dose for unvaccinated persons[3] 1 dose for revaccination[4]
Hepatitis B*	3 doses (0, 1-2, 4-6 months) for persons with medical, behavioral, occupational, or other indications[5]		
Hepatitis A	2 doses (0, 6-12 months) for persons with medical, behavioral, occupational, or other indications[6]		
Measles, Mumps, Rubella (MMR)*	1 dose if measles, mumps, or rubella vaccination history is unreliable; 2 doses for persons with occupational or other indications[7]		
Varicella*	2 doses (0, 4-8 weeks) for persons who are susceptible[8]		
Meningococcal (polysaccharide)	1 dose for persons with medical or other indications[9]		

See Footnotes for Recommended Adult Immunization Schedule, United States, 2002-2003 on back cover.

*Covered by the Vaccine Injury Compensation Program. For information on how to file a claim call 800-338-2382. Please also visit www.hrsa.gov/osp/vicp To file a claim for vaccine injury write: U.S. Court of Federal Claims, 717 Madison Place, N.W., Washington D.C. 20005. 202 219-9657.

This schedule indicates the recommended age groups for routine administration of currently licensed vaccines for persons 19 years of age and older. Licensed combination vaccines may be used whenever any components of the combination are indicated and the vaccine's other components are not contraindicated. Providers should consult the manufacturers' package inserts for detailed recommendations.

Report all clinically significant post-vaccination reactions to the Vaccine Adverse Event Reporting System (VAERS). Reporting forms and instructions on filing a VAERS report are available by calling 800-822-7967 or from the VAERS wesite at www.vaers.org.

For additional information about the vaccines listed above and contraindications for immunization, visit the National Immunization Program Website at www.cdc.gov/nip/ or call the National Immunization Hotline at 800-232-2522 (English) or 800-232-0233 (Spanish).

Approved by the Advisory Committee on Immunization Practices (ACIP), and accepted by the American College of Obstetricians and Gynecologists (ACOG) and the American Academy of Family Physicians (AAFP)

Figure 29-2. Recommended adult immunization schedule—United States 2002 to 2003. (Courtesy of the Centers for Disease Control and Prevention.)

Continues

Recommended Immunizations for Adults with Medical Conditions, United States, 2002-2003

For all persons in this group | Catch-up on childhood vaccinations | For persons with medical/exposure indications | Contraindicated

Vaccine ► / Medical Conditions ▼	Tetanus-Diphtheria (Td)*	Influenza	Pneumococcal (polysaccharide)	Hepatitis B*	Hepatitis A	Measles, Mumps, Rubella (MMR)*	Varicella*
Pregnancy		A					
Diabetes, heart disease, chronic pulmonary disease, chronic liver disease, including chronic alcoholism		B	C		D		
Congenital immunodeficiency, leukemia, lymphoma, generalized malignancy, therapy with alkylating agents, antimetabolites, radiation or large amounts of corticosteroids			E				F
Renal failure/end stage renal disease, recipients of hemodialysis or clotting factor concentrates			E	G			
Asplenia including elective splenectomy and terminal complement component deficiencies			E, H, I				
HIV infection			E, J			K	

A. If pregnancy is at 2nd or 3rd trimester during influenza season.

B. Although chronic liver disease and alcoholism are not indicator conditions for influenza vaccination, give 1 dose annually if the patient is ≥50 years, has other indications for influenza vaccine, or if the patient requests vaccination.

C. Asthma is an indicator condition for influenza but not for pneumococcal vaccination.

D. For all persons with chronic liver disease.

E. Revaccinate once after 5 years or more have elapsed since initial vaccination.

F. Persons with impaired humoral but not cellular immunity may be vaccinated. *MMWR* 1999;48(RR-06):1-5.

G. Hemodialysis patients: Use special formulation of vaccine (40 μg/mL) or two 1.0 mL 20 μg doses given at one site. Vaccinate early in the course of renal disease. Assess antibody titers to hep B surface antigen (anti-HBs) levels annually. Administer additional doses if anti-HBs levels decline to <10 milliinternational units (mIU)/mL.

H. Also administer meningococcal vaccine.

I. Elective splenectomy: vaccinate at least 2 weeks before surgery.

J. Vaccinate as close to diagnosis as possible when CD4 cell counts are highest.

K. Withhold MMR or other measles containing vaccines from HIV-infected persons with evidence of severe immunosuppression. *MMWR* 1996;45:603-606, *MMWR* 1992;41(RR-17):1-19.

Figure 29-2, continued. Recommended adult immunization schedule—United States 2002 to 2003. (Courtesy of the Centers for Disease Control and Prevention.)

Footnotes for Recommended Adult Immunization Schedule, United States, 2002-2003

1. **Tetanus and diphtheria (Td)**—A primary series for adults is 3 doses: the first 2 doses given at least 4 weeks apart and the 3rd dose, 6-12 months after the second. Administer 1 dose if the person had received the primary series and the last vaccination was 10 years ago or longer. *MMWR* 1991; 40 (RR-10): 1-21. The ACP Task Force on Adult Immunization supports a second option: a single Td booster at age 50 years for persons who have completed the full pediatric series, including the teenage/young adult booster. *Guide for Adult Immunization*. 3rd ed. ACP 1994: 20.

2. **Influenza vaccination**—Medical indications: chronic disorders of the cardiovascular or pulmonary systems including asthma; chronic metabolic diseases including diabetes mellitus, renal dysfunction, hemoglobinopathies, immunosuppression (including immunosuppression caused by medications or by human immunodeficiency virus [HIV]), requiring regular medical follow-up or hospitalization during the preceding year; women who will be in the second or third trimester of pregnancy during the influenza season. Occupational indications: health-care workers. Other indications: residents of nursing homes and other long-term care facilities; persons likely to transmit influenza to persons at high-risk (in-home care givers to persons with medical indications, household contacts and out-of-home caregivers of children birth to 23 months of age, or children with asthma or other indicator conditions for influenza vaccination, household members and care givers of elderly and adults with high-risk conditions); and anyone who wishes to be vaccinated. *MMWR* 2002; 51 (RR-3): 1-31.

3. **Pneumococcal polysaccharide vaccination**—Medical indications: chronic disorders of the pulmonary system (excluding asthma), cardiovascular diseases, diabetes mellitus, chronic liver diseases including liver disease as a result of alcohol abuse (e.g., cirrhosis), chronic renal failure or nephrotic syndrome, functional or anatomic asplenia (e.g., sickle cell disease or splenectomy), immunosuppressive conditions (e.g., congenital immunodeficiency, HIV infection, leukemia, lymphoma, multiple myeloma, Hodgkins disease, generalized malignancy, organ or bone marrow transplantation), chemotherapy with alkylating agents, anti-metabolites, or long-term systemic corticosteroids. Geographic/other indications: Alaskan Natives and certain American Indian populations. Other indications: residents of nursing homes and other long-term care facilities. *MMWR* 1997; 47 (RR-8): 1-24.

4. **Revaccination with pneumococcal polysaccharide vaccine**—One time revaccination after 5 years for persons with chronic renal failure or nephrotic syndrome, functional or anatomic asplenia (e.g., sickle cell disease or splenectomy), immunosuppressive conditions (e.g., congenital immunodeficiency, HIV infection, leukemia, lymphoma, multiple myeloma, Hodgkins disease, generalized malignancy, organ or bone marrow transplantation), chemotherapy with alkylating agents, anti-metabolites, or long-term systemic corticosteroids. For persons 65 and older, one-time revaccination if they were vaccinated 5 or more years previously and were aged less than 65 years at the time of primary vaccination. *MMWR* 1997; 47 (RR-8): 1-24.

5. **Hepatitis B vaccination**—Medical indications: hemodialysis patients, patients who receive clotting-factor concentrates. Occupational indications: health-care workers and public-safety workers who have exposure to blood in the workplace, persons in training in schools of medicine, dentistry, nursing, laboratory technology, and other allied health professions. Behavioral indications: injecting drug users, persons with more than one sex partner in the previous 6 months, persons with a recently acquired sexually-transmitted disease (STD), all clients in STD clinics, men who have sex with men. Other indications: household contacts and sex partners of persons with chronic HBV infection, clients and staff of institutions for the developmentally disabled, international travelers who will be in countries with high or intermediate prevalence of chronic HBV infection for more than 6 months, inmates of correctional facilities. *MMWR* 1991; 40 (RR-13): 1-25. (www.cdc.gov/travel/diseases/hbv.htm)

6. **Hepatitis A vaccination**—For the combined HepA-HepB vaccine use 3 doses at 0, 1, 6 months). Medical indications: persons with clotting-factor disorders or chronic liver disease. Behavioral indications: men who have sex with men, users of injecting and noninjecting illegal drugs. Occupational indications: persons working with HAV-infected primates or with HAV in a research laboratory setting. Other indications: persons traveling to or working in countries that have high or intermediate endemicity of hepatitis A. *MMWR* 1999; 48 (RR-12): 1-37. (www.cdc.gov/travel/diseases/hav.htm)

7. **Measles, Mumps, Rubella vaccination (MMR)**—Measles component: Adults born before 1957 may be considered immune to measles. Adults born in or after 1957 should receive at least one dose of MMR unless they have a medical contraindication, documentation of at least one dose or other acceptable evidence of immunity. A second dose of MMR is recommended for adults who:
   - are recently exposed to measles or in an outbreak setting
   - were previously vaccinated with killed measles vaccine
   - were vaccinated with an unknown vaccine between 1963 and 1967
   - are students in post-secondary educational institutions
   - work in health care facilities
   - plan to travel internationally

   Mumps component: 1 dose of MMR should be adequate for protection. Rubella component: Give 1 dose of MMR to women whose rubella vaccination history is unreliable and counsel women to avoid becoming pregnant for 4 weeks after vaccination. For women of child-bearing age, regardless of birth year, routinely determine rubella immunity and counsel women regarding congenital rubella syndrome. Do not vaccinate pregnant women or those planning to become pregnant in the next 4 weeks. If pregnant and susceptible, vaccinate as early in postpartum period as possible. *MMWR* 1998; 47 (RR-8): 1-57.

8. **Varicella vaccination**—Recommended for all persons who do not have reliable clinical history of varicella infection, or serological evidence of varicella zoster virus (VZV) infection; health-care workers and family contacts of immunocompromised persons, those who live or work in environments where transmission is likely (e.g., teachers of young children, day care employees, and residents and staff members in institutional settings), persons who live or work in environments where VZV transmission can occur (e.g., college students, inmates and staff members of correctional institutions, and military personnel), adolescents and adults living in households with children, women who are not pregnant but who may become pregnant in the future, international travelers who are not immune to infection. Note: Greater than 90% of U.S. born adults are immune to VZV. Do not vaccinate pregnant women or those planning to become pregnant in the next 4 weeks. If pregnant and susceptible, vaccinate as early in postpartum period as possible. *MMWR* 1996; 45 (RR-11): 1-36, *MMWR* 1999; 48 (RR-6): 1-5.

9. **Meningococcal vaccine (quadrivalent polysaccharide for serogroups A, C, Y, and W-135)**—Consider vaccination for persons with medical indications: adults with terminal complement component deficiencies, with anatomic or functional asplenia. Other indications: travelers to countries in which disease is hyperendemic or epidemic ("meningitis belt" of sub-Saharan Africa, Mecca, Saudi Arabia for Hajj). Revaccination at 3-5 years may be indicated for persons at high risk for infection (e.g., persons residing in areas in which disease is epidemic). Counsel college freshmen, especially those who live in dormitories, regarding meningococcal disease and the vaccine so that they can make an educated decision about receiving the vaccination. *MMWR* 2000; 49 (RR-7): 1-20. Note: The AAFP recommends that colleges should take the lead on providing education on meningococcal infection and vaccination and offer it to those who are interested. Physicians need not initiate discussion of the meningococcal quadravalent polysaccharide vaccine as part of routine medical care.

Figure 29-2, continued. Recommended adult immunization schedule—United States 2002 to 2003. (Courtesy of the Centers for Disease Control and Prevention.)

TABLE 29-2. Licensed U.S. Vaccines and Toxoids with Recommended Routes of Administration

LICENSED U.S. VACCINES AND TOXOIDS	RECOMMENDED ROUTE OF ADMINISTRATION
Anthrax	Subcutaneous
Diphtheria-tetanus-pertussis (DtaP, DT, Td, TT)	Intramuscular
Haemophilus influenzae type b (Hib)	Intramuscular
Hepatitis A	Intramuscular
Hepatitis B	Intramuscular
Inactivated polio vaccine (IPV)	Either route
Influenza	Subcutaneous
Japanese encephalitis	Subcutaneous
Measles-mumps-rubella (MMR)	Subcutaneous
Meningococcal	Subcutaneous
Pneumococcal conjugate vaccine (PCV)	Intramuscular
Pneumococcal polysaccharide vaccine (PPV)	Either route
Rabies	Intramuscular
Typhoid	Intramuscular
Varicella	Subcutaneous
Yellow fever	Subcutaneous

Source: Centers for Disease Control and Prevention.

TABLE 29-3. Recommended Dose of Hepatitis B Vaccine

AGE GROUP	VACCINE	
	RECOMBIVAX HB® DOSE (mL)	ENGERIX-B® DOSE (mL)
Infants and children <11 years	0.5	0.5
Adolescents 11–19 years	0.5	0.5
Adults ≥20 years	1.0	1.0
Dialysis patients and other compromised persons	1.0	2.0

A 6-month course of interferon alfa-2b (Intron® A) for acute HCV infection leads to viral clearance and clinical recovery in a high proportion of patients. Clearly, development of an HCV vaccine would represent a major advance in eradication of the infection. Unfortunately, major obstacles have prevented the development of an effective vaccine against HCV.

PNEUMONIA

Pneumonia is an inflammation of the bronchioles and alveoli caused by infection by bacteria, virus, or other pathogens. The severity of pneumonia may range from mild to life-threatening. This disorder occurs more often in elderly, chronically ill, or immunosuppressed patients.

Pneumococcal Vaccines

The first polysaccharide pneumococcal vaccine was licensed in the United States in 1977. Two polysaccharide vaccines are available in the United States (Pneumovax® 23, manufactured by Merck, and Pnu-Immune® 23, manufactured by Lederle). Pneumococcal vaccine is given by injection and may be administered either intramuscularly or subcutaneously. Pneumococcal polysaccharide vaccine should be shipped in an insulated container with coolant packs, although it can be kept at room temperatures for a few days without deterioration. The vaccine should be stored at a refrigerated temperature of 2 to 8°C (35 to 46°F).

MENINGITIS

Meningitis is any infection or inflammation of the membranes covering the brain and spinal cord. The most common causes in adults are bacterial infection with *Streptococcus pneumoniae, Neisseria meningitidis,* or *Haemophilus influenzae.* Nonbacterial agents such as chemical irritants, neoplasms, or viruses may cause septic meningitis.

Meningococcal Vaccine

Meningococcal vaccine is not recommended for routine use because of its ineffectiveness in children younger than 2 years of age. Polysaccharide meningococcal vaccine is useful for controlling serogroup C meningococcal outbreaks. Two doses should be administered 3 months apart.

RABIES

Rabies is an acute, usually fatal, viral disease of the central nervous system of animals. It is transmitted from animals to people by infected blood, tissue, or, most commonly, saliva. In humans, it is also called **hydrophobia**. Local treatment of wounds infected by rabid animals may prevent the disease. The wound is cleansed with soap, water, and a disinfectant. A deep wound may be cauterized and rabies immune globulin injected directly into the base of the wound. For active immunization, a series of five intramuscular injections with a human diploid cell rabies vaccine are given. Studies conducted in the United States by the Centers for Disease Control and Prevention have shown that the regimen of one dose of **human rabies immune globulin** and five doses of vaccine over a 28-day period is effective. The recommended schedule of rabies vaccinations is as follows:

- first dose at 0 days
- second dose 3 days after the first
- third dose 7 days after the first
- fourth dose 14 days after the first
- fifth dose 28 days after the first

Rabies vaccine should be injected intramuscularly (deltoid muscle) after exposure. Subcutaneous injection should be used pre-exposure.

INDICATIONS FOR IMMUNE GLOBULINS AND ANTITOXINS

Immune globulin is administered for prophylaxis of many communicable infectious diseases. Antitoxins are used in some instances for treatment of specific conditions.

For more than two decades, intravenous administration of high doses of IgG pooled from the plasma of healthy donors (immune globulin therapy, also known as IVIg) has benefited patients with a variety of autoimmune disorders such as hepatitis B, tetanus, and rabies. Table 29-4 shows immune globulins and antitoxins that are available in the United States by the type of antibodies and their indications for use.

TABLE 29-4. Immune Globulins and Antitoxins

IMMUNIZING AGENT	TRADE NAME	ROUTE OF ADMINISTRATION
	SERUMS	
Tetanus immune human globulin	Tetanus Ig	IM
Pertussis immune human globulin	Pertussis Ig	IM
Mumps immune human globulin	Mumps Ig	IM
Hepatitis B immune globulin (HBIG)	H-BIG, Hep-B-Gammagee	IM
Rabies immune globulin	Imogam	IM
Respiratory syncytial immune globulin	RespiGam	IV
	ANTITOXINS	
Diphtheria antitoxin	Dip/Ser	IM, IV
Tetanus antitoxin	ActHIB	IM, SC, IV
Botulism antitoxin	Trivalent	See package insert

TUBERCULOSIS

Tuberculosis is a chronic granulomatous infection caused by *Mycobacterium tuberculosis*. It is generally transmitted by inhalation or ingestion of infected droplets and usually affects the lungs, although infection of multiple organ systems also occurs.

BCG Vaccine

The vaccine for tuberculosis, BCG vaccine, is an active immunizing agent prepared from bacilli Calmette-Guérin.

BCG vaccine is prescribed most commonly for immunization against tuberculosis. Vaccination should be considered for an infant or child who has negative tuberculin skin test results. BCG vaccination is not recommended for patients infected with human immunodeficiency virus or those who are using corticosteroids concomitantly. It is not given after vaccination for smallpox, nor is it given to patients with a positive tuberculin reaction or a burn.

Tuberculin Test

A tuberculin test can determine past or present *M. tuberculosis* based on a positive skin reaction, using one of several methods. A purified protein derivative of tubercle bacilli, called **tuberculin**, is introduced into the skin by scratch, puncture, or intradermal injection. If a raised, red, or hard zone forms surrounding the tuberculin test site, the person is said to be sensitive to tuberculin, and the test is read as positive. The most common tests are the **Mantoux test** and the **tine test**. The Mantoux test is performed by administration of 0.1mL of solution into the dermis using an intradermal needle and syringe. The test site must be examined within 48 to 78 hours. The tine test determines the presence of tubercle bacilli. It is performed by applying a device with multiple sharp prongs to the skin. The prongs penetrate the skin and inject tuberculin. A hardened raised area at the test site 48 to 72 hours later indicates the presence of the pathogens in the blood.

SMALLPOX

Smallpox is an acute infectious disease caused by the *Variola* virus. First described in the fourth century AD Chinese text, the vaccine was developed in the late eighteenth century. The last case of smallpox in the United States was reported in Texas in 1949. In June 1966, the World Health Organization initiated an intensified global smallpox eradication program. The last indigenous case of smallpox on earth occurred in Somalia in 1977. The World Health Assembly officially certified the global eradication of smallpox in May 1980.

Humans are the only natural host. There is no chronic carrier state, and no known animal reservoir. Most transmission results from face-to-face contact with infected persons. Transmission most often occurs during the first week of a rash.

Smallpox Vaccine

In 1796, Edward Jenner, a doctor in rural England, discovered that immunity to smallpox could be produced by inoculating a person with material from a cowpox lesion. Cowpox is a pox virus in the same family as *Variola.* Jenner called the material used for inoculation a vaccine. The smallpox vaccine is currently available in the United States as a live virus preparation of infectious vaccine virus. Approximately 15 million doses of the vaccine are available now in the United States. More than 200 million additional doses of vaccine are being produced to be available in case of an introduction of smallpox. The vaccine is administered by using a multiple-puncture technique with a special bifurcated needle, which first became available in 1965. In 1983, the smallpox vaccine was removed from the civilian market. The vaccine is currently available only from the Centers for Disease Control and Prevention under an investigational new drug protocol.

Neutralizing antibodies develop 10 days after primary vaccination and 7 days after revaccination. Antibody titers persist more than 10 years after the second dose is received and up to 30 years after three doses of vaccine are received. A high level of protection (nearly 100%) against smallpox persists for up to 5 years after the primary vaccination. Smallpox vaccine also provides protection if administered after an exposure to smallpox. The lowest disease rates are seen among persons vaccinated less than 7 days after exposure. The disease is generally less severe in persons receiving postexposure vaccinations.

Routine childhood smallpox vaccination was discontinued in the United States in 1971. Routine vaccination of health care workers was discontinued in 1976 and of military recruits in 1990. In 1980, smallpox vaccine was recommended for laboratory workers who had an occupational risk for exposure to the vaccine. The schedule for smallpox vaccine is one successful dose (i.e., a dose that results in a major reaction at the vaccination site). Under routine circumstances, the vaccine should not be administered to persons younger than 18 years of age. In an emergency (postrelease) situation, there would be no age limit for vaccination of persons exposed to a person with confirmed smallpox. Contraindications and precautions to smallpox vaccine in nonemergency situations and emergency (postrelease) situations are seen in Table 29-5.

TABLE 29-5. Contraindications and Precautions to Smallpox Vaccination

NONEMERGENCY SITUATIONS	EMERGENCY (POSTRELEASE) SITUATIONS
1. Severe allergic reaction to prior dose or vaccine component	1. Exposed persons—no contraindications
2. Immunosuppression or immunosuppressed household contact	2. Unexposed persons—same as nonemergency situations
3. Pregnancy	
4. Eczema, history of eczema, or household contact with eczema or history of eczema	
5. Other skin conditions	
6. Age younger than 18 years	

ANTHRAX

Anthrax is a zoonotic disease caused by the spore-forming bacteria ***Bacillus anthracis***. A live attenuated animal vaccine was developed and tested by Louis Pasteur in 1881. A human vaccine composed of cell-free culture filtrate was developed in 1954 and improved in 1970. Anthrax was first used effectively as a bioterrorist agent in 2001. *B. anthracis* is a gram-positive aerobic bacterium. Spores may remain viable in soil for years. Humans can become infected with *B. anthracis* by skin contact, ingestion, or inhalation of spores originating from animal products of infected animals or from the environment. Spores can be inactived by sufficient contact with paraformaldehyde vapor, 5% hypochlorite, or phenol solution or by autoclaving. The symptoms and incubation period of human anthrax are determined by the route of transmission of the organism. There are three clinical forms of anthrax: cutaneous (most common in natural exposure situations), gastrointestinal (rare), and inhalation. Anthrax bioterrorism attacks in the United States in 2001 totaled 22 (11 by inhalation and 11 cutaneously) in four states and Washington, DC. *B. anthracis* was sent through the U.S. mail. Most of the patients were exposed in mail-sorting facilities or had direct contact with a contaminated envelope.

Anthrax Vaccine

Louis Pasteur successfully attenuated *B. anthracis* and produced the first live attenuated bacterial vaccine for animals in 1881. An improved cell-free vaccine was licensed for use in the United States in 1970. The duration of immunity in humans after vaccination is unknown.

Primary vaccination consists of three subcutaneous injections at 0, 2, and 4 weeks, followed by doses at 6, 12, and 18 months. To maintain immunity, the manufacturer recommends an annual booster dose. The basis for the schedule of vaccinations at 0, 2, and 4 weeks and 6, 12, and 18 months, followed by the annual booster, is not well defined. Interruption of the vaccination schedule does not require restarting the entire series of anthrax vaccine injections or the addition of extra doses.

The most common adverse reactions are local reactions. No studies have documented occurrence of chronic diseases (e.g., cancer or infertility) after anthrax vaccination.

The vaccine is contraindicated in persons who had a severe allergic reaction after a previous dose or to a vaccine component. Anthrax vaccine is contraindicated in persons who have recovered from anthrax.

Moderate or severe acute illness is a precaution, and vaccination should be postponed until recovery. Pregnant women should be vaccinated against anthrax only if the potential benefits of vaccination outweigh the potential risks to the fetus. Vaccines and toxoids are licensed in the United States.

SEVERE ACUTE RESPIRATORY SYNDROME

Severe acute respiratory syndrome (SARS) is a viral respiratory illness that was first reported in Asia in February 2003. A global alert about the syndrome was quickly issued, but during the next few months it spread to more than 24 countries over most continents. Rather suddenly, in July 2003, new occurrences seemed to stop completely. According to the World Health Organization, approximately 8100 people became sick with SARS during the outbreak, and 774 of those died. SARS usually begins with a high fever, greater than 100.4°F. After 2 to 7 days, a dry, nonproductive cough develops, sometimes accompanied by hypoxia or leading to hypoxia, wherein the blood does not receive sufficient amounts of oxygen. Most patients develop pneumonia. SARS appears to spread by close person-to-person contact, and its virus is thought to be transmitted via respiratory droplets produced when someone who is infected coughs or sneezes. The incubation period is usually 2 to 7 days, although in some patients it has been as long as 10 days. No specific treatment is recommended at this time. Empiric therapy should include the types of therapy used for pneumonia, including agents that act against both typical and atypical respiratory pathogens. The severity of the illness should influence the type of treatment used. A consultation with an infectious disease specialist is suggested, and health care professionals evaluating patients suspected of having SARS should use standard precautions, which include proper handwashing and use of respirators, gowns, and gloves.

VACCINE HANDLING RULES AND STORAGE REQUIREMENTS

Vaccines should be refrigerated immediately after they are received. Some vaccines, such as oral polio and varicella, should be stored in a freezer. To avoid breakage, vaccine vials should not be put in the door of the refrigerator. The measles-mumps-rubella (MMR) vaccine should be protected from light at all times and kept cold. Vaccine stock should be rotated to avoid outdating. A safety lock-type plug should be used as a safeguard so that the refrigerator always stays plugged in. Proper temperatures of between 2 and 8°C (35 and 46°F) in the refrigerator and lower than −15°C (5°F) in the freezer should be maintained. The refrigerator and freezer should be checked twice a day, first thing in the morning and last thing at night, to verify correct temperatures. Kitchen-type thermometers can be kept in both the refrigerator and freezer to verify temperatures. The doors must shut tightly, and the plug must be firmly plugged into its outlet. Warning signs should be posted to instruct electricians and janitorial personnel about never unplugging the refrigerator/freezer or never turning off the electrical circuit that controls the unit.

ADMINISTRATION OF VACCINES AND TOXOIDS

Vaccines must be administered by the recommended route. Examples of subcutaneously administered vaccines or toxoids include anthrax, MMR, and varicella. Examples of intramuscularly administered vaccines or toxoids include diphtheria-tetanus-pertussis (DPT), hepatitis A, and influenza. For a more complete listing of vaccines and toxoids and their routes of administration, see Table 29-2.

Today, 31 states allow pharmacists to administer vaccinations in certain situations. The other 19 states require a nurse to administer vaccinations to pharmacy patients.

REVIEW QUESTIONS

1. Which active vaccine is recommended for health care workers, but is not routinely given to infants?
   A. MMR
   B. Influenza
   C. Diphtheria
   D. Pertussis

2. Which of the following diseases is also called hydrophobia?
   A. Smallpox
   B. Polio
   C. Anthrax
   D. Rabies

3. The first immunoglobulin produced by the body when challenged by antigens during the initial antigen exposure is
   A. IgG.
   B. IgA.
   C. IgM.
   D. IgE.

4. Which of the following is a live attenuated vaccine that is bacterial?
   A. Vaccinia
   B. Oral typhoid
   C. Oral polio
   D. Yellow fever

5. The vaccine that is allowed to be administered at birth is
   A. hepatitis B
   B. hepatitis C.
   C. rabies
   D. oral polio.

6. Which of the following antibodies is able to cross the placenta?
   A. IgA
   B. IgM
   C. IgG
   D. IgE

7. The total number of vaccines administered to an individual for anthrax is
   A. only one.
   B. three.
   C. five.
   D. six.

8. Under routine circumstances, which vaccine should not be administered to children younger than 18 years of age?
   A. Influenza
   B. Smallpox
   C. BCG
   D. MMR

9. The BCG vaccine against tuberculosis is not recommended for patients infected with
   A. human immunodeficiency virus.
   B. hepatitis B.
   C. syphilis.
   D. warts.

10. The last scheduled dose of rabies vaccines is given
    A. 1 week after the first.
    B. 2 weeks after the first.
    C. 4 weeks after the first.
    D. 6 months after the first.

11. In how many states are pharmacists currently allowed to administer vaccines to pharmacy patients?
    A. 19
    B. 31
    C. 42
    D. 50

12. Which of the following is the treatment choice for the hepatitis C infection?
    A. Hepatitis C vaccine
    B. A 6-month course of antibiotics
    C. A 6-month course of interferon
    D. Immune globulins and antitoxins

13. For which of the following vaccines is/are subcutaneous administration recommended?
    A. Hepatitis B
    B. Influenza
    C. Rabies
    D. MMR

14. The proper temperature for storing vaccines is which of the following?
    A. 10–15° F
    B. 5–15° F
    C. 15–25° F
    D. 35–46° F

15. Which of the following vaccines should be stored in a freezer?
    A. Varicella
    B. Rabies
    C. Hepatitis A
    D. Pneumonia

30 Poisons and Antidotes

OUTLINE

- Poisoning
  - Detection of Poisons
- Common Poisons
  - Acetaminophen
  - Acids
  - Alkalies
  - Antihistamines
  - Atropine
  - Benzene and Toluene
  - Bleaches
  - Carbon Monoxide (CO)
  - Cyanide
  - Detergents and Soaps
  - Ethylene Glycol
  - Fluorides
  - Formaldehyde
  - Iodine
  - Isopropyl Alcohol
  - Lead
  - Magnesium
  - Mercury
  - Methyl Alcohol
  - Opioids
  - Petroleum Distillates
  - Phenol
  - Phosphorus
  - Salicylates
- Antidotes
  - Cyanide Antidote Kit
- Poison Control Centers

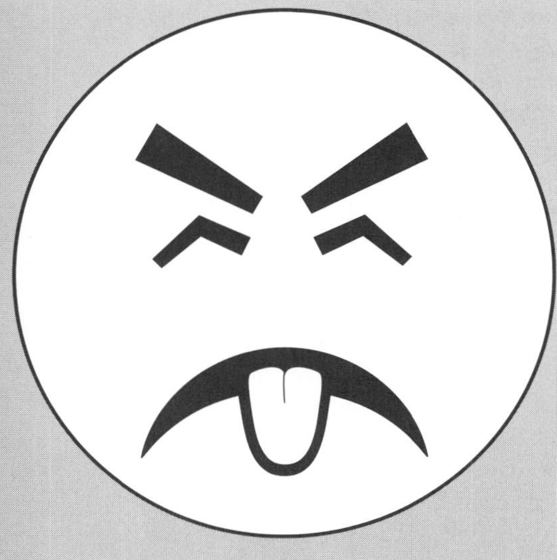

(Permission to reproduce Mr. Yuk has been granted by Children's Hospital of Pittsburgh.)

GLOSSARY

acetaminophen An analgesic and antipyretic commonly used instead of aspirin, particularly for patients who are allergic to aspirin, are taking anticoagulants, or have a peptic ulcer.

acid Any substance with a hydrogen ion that is released into a solution and reacts with metals to form salts; pH less than 7.

alkali Any of a class of compounds such as sodium hydroxide that form salts with acids and soaps with fats.

antihistamine A drug that counteracts the action of histamine.

atropine An anticholinergic alkaloid found in belladonna; it acts as a competitive antagonist of acetylcholine at muscarinic receptors.

benzene A liquid hydrocarbon obtained mainly as a by-product of the destructive distillation of coal. It is used as a solvent. Benzene is an irritant and is toxic and carcinogenic.

carbon monoxide (CO) A colorless, odorless, tasteless gas, formed by burning carbon or organic fuels with a scant supply of oxygen. It is the number one cause of unintentional poisoning around the world.

cyanide A binary compound that prevents tissue use of oxygen; most of its compounds are deadly poisons.

detergent An agent that purifies or cleanses.

ethylene glycol A chemical used in automobile antifreeze.

fluoride Any binary compound of fluorine.

formaldehyde A gaseous compound with strong disinfectant properties. It is used in a 37% solution (formol or formalin) as a disinfectant and as a preservative and fixative for pathological specimens. The gas is toxic and carcinogenic.

iodine A nonmetallic trace element that is an essential micronutrient of thyroid hormone.

isopropyl alcohol A transparent, volatile, colorless liquid used as a solvent and disinfectant and applied topically as an antiseptic. It is also called isopropanol.

lead A chemical element; excessive ingestion or absorption causes lead poisoning.

magnesium sulfate An anticonvulsant and electrolyte replenisher. It is also used as a laxative and local anti-inflammatory agent.

mercury A chemical element that can be absorbed by the skin and mucous membranes, causing chronic poisoning.

methyl alcohol A poisonous, colorless liquid used as a solvent and fuel; ingestion may cause blindness or death. It is also called methanol.

opioid Any synthetic narcotic that has opiate-like activities but is not derived from opium.

petroleum distillates Products made from the vaporization of natural oil.

phenol An extremely poisonous compound, used in dilute solution as an antimicrobial, anesthetic, and antipruritic agent.

phosphorus A nonmetallic chemical element occurring extensively in nature as a component of phosphate rock. Phosphorus is essential for the metabolism of protein, calcium, and glucose.

salicylism Toxic effects of overdosage with salicylic acid or salicylates, usually marked by tinnitus, nausea, and vomiting.

soap A kind of detergent used as a cleanser.

toluene An aromatic solvent similar to xylene. It is found in many paints and removers and is considered to be a neurotoxin.

POISONING

In the United States, accidental poisoning by chemical agents causes more than 5000 deaths each year, whereas suicides by chemical agents annually number more than 6000. In addition to the victims of fatal poisoning, a much greater number of persons are made seriously ill by chemical agents but recover after appropriate therapy. Unfortunately, some of these persons are left with permanent consequences of their intoxication. Accidental poisonings occur far more often in the home than through industrial exposure and the effects are usually acute; industrial intoxication is more often the result of chronic exposure. Accidental poisoning results most commonly from ingestion of toxic substances, and the majority of occurrences involve children. A poison is defined as any agent that in relatively small amounts can cause death or serious bodily harm. All drugs are potential poisons when used improperly or in excess dosage.

Detection of Poisons

Optimal management of the poisoned patient requires correct diagnosis. Although the toxic effects of some chemical substances are quite characteristic, most poisoning syndromes can simulate other diseases. Poisoning usually is included in the differential diagnosis of coma, convulsions, acute psychosis, acute hepatic or renal insufficiency, and bone marrow depression. Although it should be, poisoning may not be considered when the major manifestation is a mild psychiatric disturbance or neurologic disorder, abdominal pain, bleeding, fever, hypotension, pulmonary congestion, or skin eruption. Furthermore, patients may be unaware of their exposure to a poison, as with chronic insidious intoxications or after attempted suicide or abortion, or they may be unwilling to admit it. In every instance of poisoning, identification of the toxic agent should be attempted. Specific antidotal therapy is obviously impossible without such identification. Some poisons can produce clinical features characteristic enough to strongly suggest the diagnosis. Careful examination of the patient may reveal the unmistakable odor of cyanide, the cherry-colored flush of carboxyhemoglobin in skin and mucous membranes, or the pupillary constriction, salivation, and gastrointestinal hyperactivity produced by insecticides. Chemical analysis of body fluids provides the most definite identification of the intoxicating agent. Some common poisons, such as aspirin and barbiturates, can be identified and amounts even quantitated by relatively simple laboratory procedures. Others require more complex toxicological techniques. Chemical analyses of body fluids or tissues are of particular value in the diagnosis and evaluation of chronic intoxications.

COMMON POISONS

The most common poisons involving the general population are nonprescription drugs, household products, solvents, pesticides, and poisonous plants. The following discussions of specific poisons stress their action as well as the recognition or treatment of clinical poisoning.

Acetaminophen

Acetaminophen, a popular alternative to salicylates as an analgesic and antipyretic, is a common cause of poisoning. Although the toxic and lethal doses of acetaminophen may vary from patient to patient, hepatic damage may be expected if an adult has taken more than 8 g as a single dose. Clinical manifestations of acetaminophen poisoning are nonspecific. In the first few hours after ingestion, lethargy, nausea, vomiting, and diaphoresis may occur. Hepatic damage, the most important manifestation of acetaminophen toxicity, becomes evident 1 to 2 days after ingestion.

Treatment should begin with induction of emesis or gastric lavage followed by administration of activated charcoal. Treatment with acetylcysteine is most effective if started within 8 to 10 hours after ingestion.

Acids

Corrosive **acids** are used widely in industry and laboratories. Ingestion is almost always with suicidal intent. Toxic effects are due to their direct chemical action. Ingestion of acids may produce irritation, bleeding, severe pain, and severe burns in the mouth, esophagus, and stomach. Often, profound shock develops and may be fatal. Ingested acid should be diluted immediately with large amounts of water or milk. The danger of perforation contraindicates the use of emesis or gastric lavage. Diagnostic esophagoscopy, if performed, should be done in the first 24 hours after ingestion.

Alkalies

Strong **alkalies** such as ammonium hydroxide, potassium hydroxide (potash), potassium carbonate, sodium hydroxide (lye), and sodium carbonate (washing soda) are used widely in industry and in cleansers and drain cleaners. The toxic effects of alkalies are due to irritation and destruction of local tissues. Ingestion is followed by severe pain in the mouth, pharynx, chest, and abdomen. Vomiting of blood and diarrhea are common. Perforation of the esophagus or stomach may be immediate or delayed for several days. Treatment consists of immediate administration of large amounts of water or milk. Esophagoscopy should be done within the first 24 hours. Steroids usually are administered for about 3 weeks to decrease the incidence of stricture formation.

Antihistamines

There is a wide variation among patient tolerance to **antihistamines** and in the manifestations of poisoning. Manifestations of poisoning are central nervous system excitement or depression. In adults, drowsiness, stupor, and coma may occur. Treatment is supportive and is focused on removal of the unabsorbed drug and maintenance of vital functions. Convulsions may be controlled with phenobarbital or diazepam.

Atropine

Atropine is a widely prescribed drug. Young children are particularly susceptible to poisoning with this agent. Older persons appear to be more sensitive to the central nervous system effects of atropine. The most characteristic manifestations of atropine poisoning are dryness of mouth, thirst, dysphasia, hoarseness, dilated pupils, blurring of vision, flushing, tachycardia, hypertension, and urinary retention. Treatment includes emesis or gastric lavage followed by the administration of activated charcoal. If symptoms are severe, physostigmine salicylate should be given intravenously.

Benzene and Toluene

Benzene and **toluene** are solvents used in paint removers, dry-cleaning solutions, and rubber or plastic cements. Benzene is also present in most gasolines. Poisoning may result from ingestion or from the breathing of concentrated vapors. Toluene is an ingredient in some cements used by glue sniffers. Acute poisoning by these compounds causes central nervous system manifestations. Restlessness, excitement, euphoria, and dizziness, progressing to coma, convulsions, and respiratory failure, are common. Treatment of both acute and chronic poisoning is symptomatic.

Bleaches

Industrial strength bleaching solutions contain 10% or more sodium hypochlorite, whereas household products (e.g., Clorox®, Purex®, and Sanichlor®) contain 3% to 6%. The solution used for chlorinating swimming pools contains 20%. Their corrosive action in the mouth, pharynx, and esophagus is similar to that of sodium hydroxide. Treatment consists of dilution of the ingested bleach with water or milk.

Carbon Monoxide (CO)

Carbon monoxide (CO) is a colorless, odorless, tasteless, and nonirritating gas that is present in the exhaust of internal combustion engines in concentrations of 3% to 7%. CO is responsible for about 3500 accidental deaths and suicides in the United States annually. The toxic effects of CO are the result of tissue hypoxia. The most characteristic sign of severe CO poisoning is the cherry color of the skin and mucous membranes. Treatment of CO poisoning requires effective ventilation in the presence of high oxygen (O_2) tensions and in the absence of CO. If necessary, ventilation should be supported artificially. Pure O_2 should be administered. Cerebral edema should be treated with diuretics and steroids.

Cyanide

The **cyanide** ion is an exceedingly potent and rapid-acting poison, but one for which specific and effective antidotal therapy is available. Cyanide poisoning may result from the inhalation of hydrocyanic acid or from the ingestion of soluble inorganic cyanide salts. Parts of many plants also contain substances such as amygdaline, which release cyanide upon digestion. Cyanide poisoning is a true medical emergency. However, treatment is highly effective if given rapidly. The chemical antidotes should be immediately available wherever emergency medical care is dispensed. The diagnosis may be made by the characteristic "bitter almond" odor on the breath of the victim. The objective of treatment is the production of methemoglobin by the administration of nitrite. Supportive measures, especially artificial respiration with 100% oxygen, should be instituted as soon as possible.

Detergents and Soaps

These substances fall into three groups: anionic, nonionic, and cationic. The first group contains common **soaps** and household **detergents**. They may cause vomiting and diarrhea but have no serious effects, and no treatment is required. However, some laundry compounds contain phosphate water softeners whose ingestion may cause hypocalcemia. The ingestion of nonionic detergents also requires no treatment. Cationic detergents are commonly used for bactericidal purposes in hospitals and homes. These compounds are well absorbed from the gastrointestinal tract and interfere with cellular functions. The fatal oral dose is approximately 3 g. Ingestion produces nausea, vomiting, shock, coma, and convulsions and may cause death within a few hours. Treatment after ingestion of diluted preparations consists of minimizing gastrointestinal absorption by emesis and gastric lavage with ordinary soap solution, which rapidly inactivates cationic detergents. Activated charcoal should be administered.

Ethylene Glycol

Ethylene glycol and diethylene glycol are chemicals used in automobile antifreeze preparations. Symptoms in mild intoxication may resemble those of alcohol intoxication but without the breath odor produced by alcoholic beverages. Vomiting, carpopedal spasm, lumbar pain, renal failure, respiratory distress, convulsions, and coma may also occur. Treatment may include emesis, gastric lavage, establishment of electrolyte balance, and hemodialysis. In some cases, ethanol may be given because it impedes the metabolism of ethylene glycol.

Fluorides

Fluorides are used in insecticides. The gas fluorine is used in industry. Fluorine and fluorides are cellular poisons. Fluorides also form an insoluble precipitate with calcium and cause hypocalcemia. Ingestion of 1 to 2 g of sodium fluoride may be fatal. Inhalation of fluorine or hydrogen fluoride produces coughing and choking. After 1 or 2 days, fever, cough, cyanosis, and pulmonary edema may develop. Ingestion of fluoride salts is followed by nausea, vomiting, diarrhea, and abdominal pain. The Federal safe standard for ingestion of fluoride is 4 ppm (per day); however, most toothpaste contains 500 to 1500 ppm (per each pea-sized "dose"). Toothpaste should never be swallowed for this reason. The fluoride content of fluoridated water is lower, usually only 0.1 ppm (per serving). With a fluoride overdose, death results from respiratory paralysis or circulatory collapse. Treatment of acute fluoride poisoning consists of immediate administration of milk, limewater, or calcium lactate solution to precipitate calcium fluoride. Gastric lavage or emesis can be used, and charcoal can be given.

Formaldehyde

Formaldehyde is a gas available as a 40% solution (formalin), which is used as a disinfectant, fumigant, or deodorant. Poisoning by formalin may be diagnosed by the characteristic odor of formaldehyde. This agent reacts chemically with cellular components and depresses cellular functions. The fatal dose of formalin is about 60 mL. Ingestion of formalin immediately causes severe abdominal pain, nausea, vomiting, and diarrhea. This may be followed by collapse, coma, severe metabolic acidosis, and anuria. Death is usually the result of circulatory failure. Because any organic material can inactivate formaldehyde, milk, bread, and soup should be administered immediately unless activated charcoal is available.

Iodine

The traditional antiseptic **iodine** tincture is an alcoholic solution of 2% iodine and 2% sodium iodide. Strong iodine solution (Lugol's solution) is an aqueous solution of 5% iodine and 10% potassium iodide. The fatal dose of tincture of iodine is approximately 2 g. Iodides are less toxic, and no fatalities have been reported. The diagnosis of iodine poisoning is suggested by brown staining of the oral mucous membranes. The effects largely result from the corrosive effects of the compound on the gastrointestinal tract. Burning abdominal pain, nausea, vomiting, and bloody diarrhea may occur soon after ingestion. Fever, delirium, stupor, and anuria also have been observed. Treatment consists of the immediate administration of milk, starch, bread, or activated charcoal.

Isopropyl Alcohol

Isopropyl alcohol is used as a sterilizing agent or as rubbing alcohol. Ingestion produces gastric irritation and raises the danger of vomiting with aspiration. The systemic effects of isopropyl alcohol are similar to those of ethyl alcohol, but it is twice as potent as the latter. Emesis should be induced, or gastric lavage should be performed.

Lead

Lead poisoning can occur where there are old buildings or old paint or lead pipes. Even vegetable gardens can be a source of lead. Lead poisoning in adults is rare, but unfortunately it is one of the most common and preventable childhood health problems today. It can be a problem for those who lick or eat flakes of old paint containing lead. Lead can also contaminate water flowing through old lead pipes, slowly poisoning those who drink it. Lead poisoning causes severe damage to the brain, nerves, red blood cells, and digestive system. Symptoms of acute poisoning include a metallic taste in the mouth, abdominal pain, vomiting, diarrhea, collapse, and coma. Large amounts directly affect the nervous system and cause headache, convulsions, coma, and death. Treatment usually includes the administration of medicines (called chelating agents) to help the body rid itself of lead. For mild poisoning, the chelating agent penicillamine may be used alone; for chronic poisoning, it may be used in combination with edetate calcium disodium and dimercaprol. For acute poisoning, gastric lavage is performed.

Magnesium

Magnesium sulfate is used intravenously as a hypotensive agent and orally as a cathartic. The magnesium ion is a profound depressant of the central nervous system. Poisoning after oral or rectal administration is unlikely in the presence of normal renal function. In the presence of impaired renal function, an oral dose of 30 g may be fatal. Oral ingestion of this solution may cause gastrointestinal irritation. Systemic poisoning can cause paralysis, hypotension, hypothermia, coma, and respiratory failure. Treatment of magnesium poisoning therefore includes the intravenous administration of 10 mL of a 10% solution of calcium gluconate.

Mercury

Acute **mercury** poisoning usually occurs by ingestion of inorganic mercuric salts or inhalation of metallic mercury vapor. Ingestion of mercuric salts causes a metallic taste, salivation, thirst, a burning sensation in the throat, discoloration and edema of oral mucous membranes, abdominal pain, vomiting, bloody diarrhea, and shock. Direct nephrotoxicity causes acute renal failure. Inhalation of high concentrations of metallic mercury vapor may cause acute chemical pneumonia. There is no effective specific treatment for mercury vapor pneumonitis. Ingested mercuric salts can be removed by lavage, and activated charcoal should be administered. For acute ingestion of mercuric salts, dimercaprol can be given, unless the patient has severe gastroenteritis. In treating chronic poisoning, the person must be removed from exposure. Neurological toxicity is not considered to be reversible with chelation. With the advent of many alternate types of thermometers made for home use, the use of mercury thermometers should become a thing of the past. Mercury in all its forms is toxic and can result in permanent brain and kidney damage. A broken thermometer easily releases the toxic substance. It takes only 1 g of mercury to contaminate all the fish in a 20-acre lake. There are approximately 0.7 g of mercury in the average home thermometer, an amount that is surely toxic to an individual exposed to it. Many major retailers have already stopped selling mercury thermometers as a result. The medical instrument industry advises that digital thermometers should be purchased, and old mercury thermometers should be disposed of by contacting the local environmental health or public works department. (Disposal sites for household hazardous wastes are often listed in the city or county government section of the white pages of a local telephone directory.)

Methyl Alcohol

Methyl alcohol, also called wood alcohol or methanol, is the simplest of alcohols and is used as a solvent and in antifreeze and paint remover. Methyl alcohol poisoning results almost entirely from its ingestion as a substitute for ethanol or from the drinking of denatured ethyl alcohol. The toxic dose is quite variable: death has occurred after a dose of 20 mL, but 250 mL has been ingested with survival. Ingestion of as little as 15 mL of methanol has caused permanent blindness. Symptoms of methanol poisoning usually do not appear until 12 to 24 hours after ingestion, when sufficient toxic metabolites have accumulated. Manifestations include headache, dizziness, nausea, vomiting, central nervous system depression, and respiratory failure. In the treatment of methyl alcohol intoxication, emesis and gastric lavage are of use only within the first 2 hours after ingestion. Intravenous administration of large amounts of sodium bicarbonate combats acidosis. Intravenous ethanol therapy should be used.

Opioids

Opioids include morphine, heroin, and codeine. These drugs have widely varying potencies and durations of action. All of these agents decrease central nervous system and sympathetic nervous activity. Mild intoxication is characterized by euphoria, drowsiness, and constricted pupils. More severe intoxication may cause hypotension, bradycardia, hypothermia, coma, and respiratory arrest. Death is usually due to apnea or pulmonary aspiration of gastric contents. If the patient arrives for medical care shortly after ingestion, the stomach should be emptied by emesis or gastric lavage and activated charcoal should be administered. Naloxone is a specific opioid antagonist that can rapidly reverse signs of narcotic intoxication.

Petroleum Distillates

Diesel oil, gasoline, kerosene, and paint thinner are all liquid **petroleum distillates**. Kerosene is used widely as a fuel and as a vehicle for cleaning agents, furniture polishes, insecticides, and paint thinners. Petroleum distillates are central nervous system depressants; they damage cells by dissolving cellular lipids. Pulmonary damage manifested by pulmonary edema or pneumonitis is a common and serious complication. Inhalation of gasoline or kerosene vapors induces a state resembling alcoholic intoxication. Headache, nausea, and a burning sensation in the chest may be present. The oral ingestion of petroleum distillates causes irritation of the mucous membranes of the upper part of the intestinal tract. In the treatment of poisoning by petroleum distillates, extreme care must be used to prevent aspiration. When large amounts have been ingested, gastric emptying is indicated. In the alert patient, emesis may be induced. Oxygen therapy should also be given.

Phenol

Phenol and related compounds (creosote, cresols, hexachlorophene, Lysol®, and tannic acid) are used as antiseptics, caustics, and preservatives. The approximate fatal oral dose ranges from 2 mL for phenol and cresols to 20 mL for tannic acid. Ingestion of these agents produces erosion of mucosa from mouth to stomach. Vomiting of blood and bloody diarrhea may occur. Hyperpnea, pulmonary edema, stupor, coma, convulsions, and shock are seen. Emesis and lavage are indicated for treatment in the absence of significant corrosive injury to the esophagus. Activated charcoal should be administered.

Phosphorus

Phosphorus occurs in two forms: a red, nonpoisonous form, and a yellow, fat-soluble, highly toxic form. The yellow form of phosphorus is used in rodent and insect poisons and in fireworks. Yellow phosphorus causes fatty degeneration and necrosis of tissues, particularly of the liver. The lethal ingested dose of yellow phosphorus is approximately 50 mg. Ingestion of yellow phosphorus may cause pain in the upper part of the gastrointestinal tract, vomiting, diarrhea, and a garlic odor to the breath. Patients may also develop hepatomegaly, jaundice, hypocalcemia, hypotension, and oliguria. Treatment includes emesis or gastric lavage and administration of activated charcoal and an osmotic cathartic.

Salicylates

Each year, 30 million pounds of aspirin are consumed in the United States, and salicylates can probably be found in most American households. Aspirin is found in many compound analgesic tablets. The ingestion of 10 to 30 g of aspirin or sodium salicylates may be fatal to adults, but survival has been reported after an oral dose of 130 g of aspirin. Salicylate intoxication may result from the cumulative effect of therapeutic administration of high doses. Toxic symptoms may begin at dosages of 3 g/day or may not appear when 10 g/day is given. Therapeutic salicylate intoxication is usually mild and is called **salicylism**. The earliest symptoms are vertigo and impairment of hearing. Further overdosage causes nausea, vomiting, sweating, diarrhea, fever, drowsiness, and headache. The central nervous system effects may progress to hallucinations, convulsions, coma, cardiovascular collapse, pulmonary edema, hyperthermia, and death. Treatment of salicylate poisoning consists initially of inducing emesis or of gastric lavage, after which activated charcoal and then an osmotic cathartic are administered. Respiratory depression may require artificial ventilation with oxygen. Convulsions may be treated with diazepam or phenobarbital. Peritoneal dialysis and hemodialysis are also highly effective in removing salicylates from seriously poisoned patients.

ANTIDOTES

Specific antidotal therapy is available for only a few poisons. Some systemic antidotes are chemical and exert their therapeutic effect by reducing the concentration of the toxic substance. They may do this by combining with the poison or by increasing its rate of excretion.

TABLE 30-1. Poisons and Antidotes

POISON	ANTIDOTES
Acetaminophen	N-Acetylcysteine
Benzodiazepines	Flumazenil
Carbon monoxide	Oxygen
Cyanide	Amyl nitrate
Iron	Deferoxamine
Methanol	Ethanol
Opiates	Naloxone
Organophosphates	Atropine or pralidoxime

Other systemic antidotes compete with the poison for its receptor site. Specific antidotes are listed in Table 30-1.

Cyanide Antidote Kit

Most cyanide antidote kits consist of the following:

- 2 ampoules of sodium nitrate injection (USP 300 mg in 10 mL of sterile water)
- 1 vial of sodium thiosulfate injection (intraperitoneal, 25 g in 50 mL of sterile water)
- 12 Durules of amyl nitrate inhalant (0.3 mL)
- 1 sterile 10-mL plastic disposable syringe with 22-gauge needle
- 1 sterile 50-mL plastic disposable syringe with 22-gauge needle
- 1 stomach tube
- 1 nonsterile 50-mL syringe
- 1 set of instructions for the treatment of cyanide poisoning

Sodium nitrite reacts with hemoglobin to form methemoglobin. The latter removes cyanide ions from various tissues and couples with them to become cyanmethemoglobin, which has a relatively low toxicity. Sodium thiosulfate converts cyanide to thiocyanate via an enzyme known as rhodanase. The combination of sodium nitrite and sodium thiosulfate is the best therapy against cyanide and hydrocyanic acid poisoning. The two substances injected intravenously, one after the other (the nitrite followed by the thiosulfate), are capable of detoxifying approximately 20 lethal doses of sodium cyanide as tested in dogs and are effective even after respiration has stopped. As long as the heart is still beating, the chances of recovery with use of this method are very good.

POISON CONTROL CENTERS

A network consisting of more than 600 poison control centers exists in the United States. Through this network, poison treatment information is available free of charge, 24 hours a day. The first poison control center was established in Chicago under the leadership of the Illinois chapter of the American Academy of Pediatrics. A few months later, the Duke University Poison Control Center was begun in North Carolina. With the appearance of these two centers, the idea of poison control centers spread across the country. In 1957, the Food and Drug Administration established the National Clearinghouse for Poison Control Centers to coordinate activities at poison control centers across the United States. The Clearinghouse collected and standardized product toxicology data, reproduced this information on large file cards, and distributed them nationwide to poison control centers.

REVIEW QUESTIONS

1. Which of the following is the most important in every case of poisoning?
A. Looking for the cherry-colored flush in the skin
B. Evaluation of chronic intoxication
C. Recognition of the antidote for intoxication
D. Identification of the toxic agent

2. Which of the following is contraindicated in persons who have ingested acid?
A. Dilution with large amounts of water
B. Gastric lavage
C. Oxygen therapy
D. Dilution with large amounts of milk

3. The most characteristic manifestations of atropine poisoning include all of the following, except
A. dysphagia.
B. hypotension.
C. dryness of mouth.
D. blurring of vision.

4. Household bleach products such as Clorox® contain __________ sodium hypochlorite.
A. 6%
B. 10%
C. 20%
D. 45%

5. Which of the following types of poisoning is a true medical emergency?
A. Detergent or soap
B. Lead
C. Phenol
D. Cyanide

6. The chelating agents that may be used for lead poisoning include
A. penicillamine.
B. promethazine.
C. penicillin.
D. phenol.

Continues

7. A garlic odor to the breath is a result of ingesting
   A. salicylate.
   B. mercury.
   C. yellow phosphorus.
   D. magnesium.

8. Treatment for magnesium poisoning is
   A. formalin.
   B. calcium gluconate.
   C. active charcoal.
   D. atropine.

9. The toxic effects of carbon monoxide (CO) are the result of
   A. hypotension.
   B. anemia.
   C. hypoglycemia.
   D. tissue hypoxia.

10. The specific antidote for methanol posioning is
   A. naloxone.
   B. ethanol.
   C. atropine.
   D. pralidoxime.

11. Accidental poisonings occur more commonly in the
   A. laboratory.
   B. pharmacy.
   C. home.
   D. workplace.

12. The differential diagnosis of poisoning usually includes all of the following, except
   A. convulsions.
   B. coma.
   C. acute myocardial infarction.
   D. acute psychosis.

13. Hepatic damage may be expected if an adult has taken acetaminophen in a single dose of more than
   A. 2 g.
   B. 4 g.
   C. 8 g.
   D. 25 g.

14. Manifestations of antihistamine poisoning involve which of the following human body systems?
   A. Gastrointestinal
   B. Respiratory
   C. Urinary
   D. Central nervous

15. A fatal dose of formalin is about
   A. 25 mL.
   B. 45 mL.
   C. 60 mL.
   D. 75 mL.

Nutrition 31

OUTLINE

- Nutrition
  - Protein
  - Carbohydrates
  - Lipids (Fats)
- Vitamins
  - Fat-Soluble Vitamins
  - Water-Soluble Vitamins
- Minerals and Electrolytes
  - Calcium
  - Phosphorus
  - Chloride
  - Sodium
  - Potassium
  - Magnesium
  - Iron
  - Iodine
  - Zinc
  - Fluoride
  - Copper
  - Mineral Deficiencies
- Hyperalimentation or Total Parenteral Nutrition
- Malnutrition
  - Marasmus
  - Kwashiorkor
  - Obesity

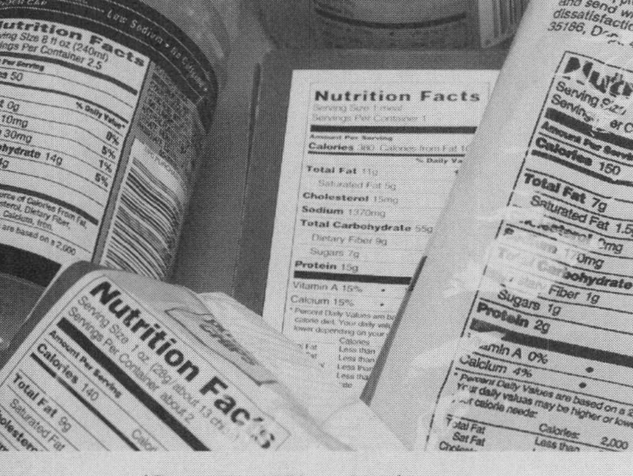

(Courtesy of PhotoDisc)

GLOSSARY

beriberi A disease of the peripheral nerves caused by a deficiency of or an inability to assimilate thiamine.

calcium An alkaline earth metal element. The body requires calcium ions for the transmission of nerve impulses, muscle contraction, blood coagulation, cardiac functions, and other processes.

carbohydrate The major source of energy for all body functions.

chloride An anion of chlorine. The most common form is sodium chloride (table salt).

cholesterol A waxy lipid found only in animal tissues. A member of a group of lipids called sterols, it is widely distributed in the body.

copper A metallic element that is a component of several important enzymes in the body and is essential to good health.

electrolyte A compound that dissociates into ions when dissolved in water.

fat A substance composed of lipids or fatty acids and occurring in various forms.

fatty acid Any of several organic acids produced by the hydrolysis of neutral fats.

fluoride Any binary compound of fluorine.

hypervitaminosis An abnormal condition resulting from excessive intake of toxic amounts of one or more vitamins, especially over a long period.

iodine A nonmetallic trace element that is an essential micronutrient of thyroid hormone.

iron A common metallic element essential for the synthesis of hemoglobin.

kwashiorkor An acute process associated with protein deficiency and impaired immune function.

magnesium A silver-white mineral element. It is the second most abundant cation of the intracellular fluids in the body and is essential for many enzyme activities.
malnutrition A disease resulting from unbalanced, insufficient, or excessive diet.
marasmus A chronic disease that develops as a result of a deficiency in caloric intake.
menadione A water-soluble injectable form of the product of vitamin K_3.
mineral An inorganic substance occurring naturally in the earth's crust, having a characteristic chemical composition.
neutral fat Consists of about 95% triglycerides or triacylglycerols.
nutrition The sum of the processes involved in the taking in of nutrients and their assimilation and use for proper body functioning and maintenance of health.
obesity A condition of excessive fatness.
pantothenic acid A member of the vitamin B complex. It is widely distributed in plant and animal tissues and may be an important element in human nutrition.
phospholipid A phosphorus-containing lipid.
phosphorus A nonmetallic chemical element occurring extensively in nature as a component of phosphate rock. Phosphorus is essential for the metabolism of protein, calcium, and glucose.
potassium An alkali metal element. Potassium salts are necessary to the life of all plants and animals. Potassium in the body helps to regulate neuromuscular excitability and muscle contraction.
protein A complex organic nitrogenous compound composed of large combinations of amino acids.
sodium One of the most important elements in the body. Sodium ions are involved in acid-base balance, water balance, transmission of nerve impulses, and contraction of muscles.
triglycerides A simple fat compound consisting of three molecules of fatty acid and glycerol. Triglycerides make up most animal and vegetable fats and are the principal lipids in the blood, where they circulate within lipoproteins.
vitamin An organic compound essential in small quantities for normal body functioning.
vitamin A A fat-soluble vitamin essential for skeletal growth, maintenance of normal mucosal epithelium, reproduction, and visual acuity; also known as retinol.
vitamin B complex A group of water-soluble compound vitamins.
vitamin B_1 A water-soluble, crystalline compound of the B complex; also known as thiamin. It is essential for normal metabolism and health of the cardiovascular and nervous systems
vitamin B_2 One of the heat-stable components of the B complex; also known as riboflavin. It is involved as a coenzyme in the oxidative processes of carbohydrates, fats, and proteins.
vitamin B_3 A compound made up of two enzymes that regulate energy metabolism; also known as niacin.
vitamin B_6 A water-soluble vitamin that is part of the B complex; also known as pyridoxine. It acts as a coenzyme that is essential for the synthesis and breakdown of amino acids.
vitamin B_7 A water-soluble B complex vitamin that acts as a coenzyme in fatty acid production and in the oxidation of fatty acids and carbohydrates; also known as biotin.
vitamin B_9 A compound essential for cell growth and the reproduction of red blood cells; also known as folic acid or folacin.
vitamin B_{12} A water-soluble substance that is the common pharmaceutical form of vitamin B; also known as cyanocobalamin. It is involved in the metabolism of protein, fats, and carbohydrates and also in normal blood formation and neural function.
vitamin C A water-soluble vitamin that is essential for the formation of collagen and fibroid tissue for teeth, bones, cartilage, connective tissue, and skin. Vitamin C also aids in fighting bacterial infections, bleeding gums, the tendency to bruise, nosebleeds, and anemia.
vitamin D A fat-soluble vitamin chemically related to the steroids and essential for the normal formation of bones and teeth; also known as calciferol. It is important for the absorption of calcium and phosphorus from the gastrointestinal tract.
vitamin E A fat-soluble vitamin essential for normal reproduction, muscle development, resistance of erythrocytes to hemolysis, and various other biochemical functions; also known as tocopherol.
vitamin K A group of fat-soluble vitamins that are essential for the synthesis of prothrombin in the liver and are involved in the clotting of blood; also known as quinones.
zinc A metallic element that is an essential nutrient in the body and is used in numerous pharmaceuticals such as zinc acetate and zinc oxide.

NUTRITION

Life is nourished by food, and the substances in food on which life depends are the nutrients. These provide the energy and building materials for the countless substances that are essential to the growth and survival of living things. The manner in which nutrients become integral parts of the body and contribute to its function depends on the physiological and biochemical processes that govern their actions. Proteins, fats, and carbohydrates all contribute in varying amounts to the total energy pool, but the energy that they yield is all in the same form. Utilization and conservation of this energy to build and maintain the body require the involvement of vitamins and minerals.

Nutrition is the study of food and drink as related to the growth and maintenance of living organisms. The successive stages include ingestion, digestion, absorption, assimilation, and excretion. Nutrients are essential for growth, reproduction, and maintenance of health (see Figure 31-1).

Protein

Proteins are complex organic nitrogenous compounds composed of large combinations of amino acids. Amino acids are essential constituents of living cells. Twenty-two amino acids have been identified as being vital for proper growth, development, and maintenance of health. The body can synthesize 13 of these, the *nonessential amino acids.* The remaining 9 must be obtained from dietary sources and are termed *essential amino acids.* Protein is the major source of building material for muscles, blood, skin, hair, nails, and the internal organs. It is necessary for the formation of enzymes, antibodies, and hormones. Protein deficiency causes abnormal growth and tissue development in children, leading to kwashiorkor, whereas in adults it results in lack of vigor and stamina, weakness, mental depression, poor resistance to infection, impaired healing of wounds, and slow recovery from disease. Excessive intake of protein may, in some conditions, result in fluid imbalance. Amino acid solutions contain crystalline amino acid (for example Aminosyn®); solutions are also available with electrolytes.

Carbohydrates

Carbohydrates constitute the main source of energy for all body functions, particularly brain functions, and are necessary for the metabolism of other nutrients. Most of the energy needed to move, perform work, and live is consumed in the form of carbohydrates. One gram of carbohydrates yields 4.5 kcal, and one gram of fat yields 9 kcal. Carbohydrates constitute the major source of food for the people of the world. Carbohydrates are either absorbed immediately by the body or stored in the form of glycogen. Current U.S. dietary guidelines recommend that 55% to 60% of total calories should be provided by carbohydrates. Symptoms of deficiency include fatigue, depression, breakdown of essential body protein, and electrolyte imbalance.

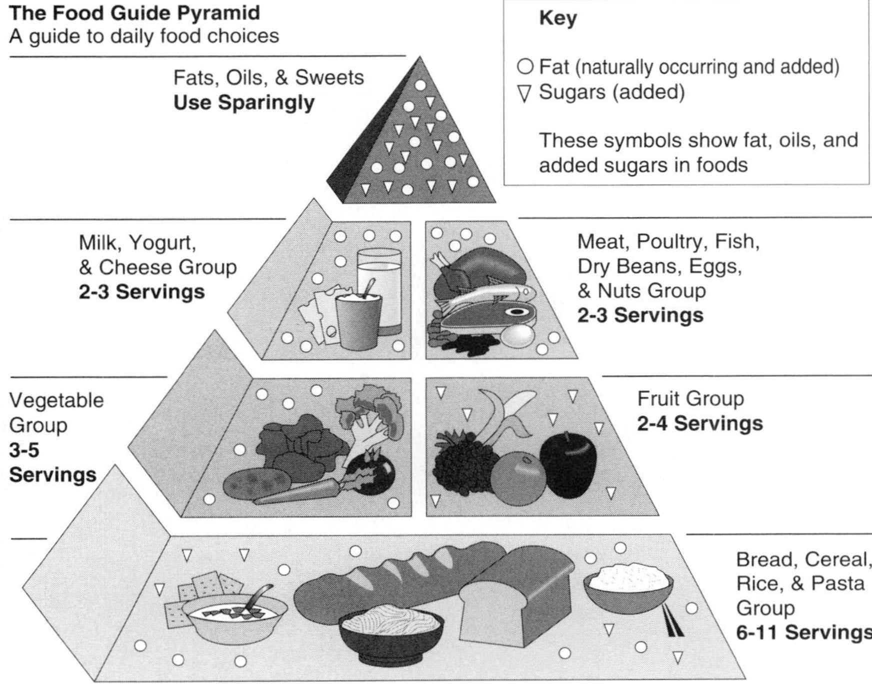

Figure 31-1. The Food Guide Pyramid. (Courtesy of USDA and DHHS, 1992, The food guide pyramid: A guide to daily food choices. Leaflet no. 572, Washington, DC.)

Muscle protein-sparing amounts of food carbohydrates have been estimated to be 50 to 100 g/day for most people. Excessive consumption of carbohydrates may be associated with tooth decay, obesity, and diabetes mellitus.

Lipids (Fats)

Fat constitutes 40% to 50% of the total calories supplied in the average American diet. Lipids are insoluble in water but are soluble in alcohol, chloroform, ether, and other organic solvents. They are stored in the body and serve as an energy reserve but their levels are elevated in various diseases such as atherosclerosis. There are several types of lipids such as **cholesterol**, **fatty acids**, **neutral fat**, **phospholipids**, and **triglycerides**.

Cholesterol

Cholesterol is a sterol found in cell membranes of all animal tissues that is also necessary for production of bile and steroid hormones.

Fatty Acids

Fatty acids are organic acids produced by the hydrolysis of neutral fats. In a living cell a fatty acid usually occurs in combination with another molecule rather than in a free state. Essential fatty acids are polyunsaturated molecules that cannot be produced by the body and must therefore be included in the diet. Some types are linoleic, linolenic, and arachidonic acids. Essential fatty acid deficiency is diagnosed by clinical signs of hair loss, scaly dermatitis, reduced wound healing, decreased platelets, growth retardation, and fatty liver. In this condition the intravenous administration of a fat emulsion is essential to correct the biochemical alteration.

Neutral Fat

Most neutral fats consist of about 95% triglycerides or triacylglycerols. The remaining 5% include traces of monoglycerides, diglycerides, fatty acids, phospholipids, and sterols. Lipids important to nutrition include simple and compound lipids and the fat-soluble vitamins. Table 31-1 shows the classification of lipids.

Phospholipids

Phospholipids are lipids containing fatty acids, an alcohol, and a phosphorus compound. They are widely distributed in cell membranes.

Triglycerides

Triglycerides are lipids consisting of three fatty acid chains esterified to a glycerol molecule.

TABLE 31-1. Classification of Lipids

CATEGORIES	EXAMPLES
Simple lipids	Fatty acids Neutral fats (monoglycerides, diglycerides, triglycerides) Waxes Sterol esters (cholesterol ester) Nonsterol ester (vitamin A ester)
Compound lipids	Phospholipids Glycolipids Lipoproteins
Sterols	Cholesterol Vitamin D Bile salts
Vitamins	Vitamin A, E, and K

VITAMINS

Vitamins are organic compounds that are essential in small quantities for normal physiological and metabolic functioning of the body. With few exceptions, vitamins cannot be synthesized by the body and must be obtained from the diet or dietary supplements. No one food contains all the vitamins. Vitamin deficiency diseases produce specific symptoms usually alleviated by the administration of the appropriate vitamin.

Vitamins are classified according to their fat or water solubility, their physiological effects, or their chemical structures. They are designated by alphabetic letters and chemical or other specific names. The fat-soluble vitamins are A, D, E, and K; the B complex and C vitamins are water soluble.

Hypervitaminosis is an abnormal condition resulting from excessive intake of toxic amounts of one or more vitamins, especially over a long period. Serious effects may result from overdoses of the fat-soluble vitamins A, D, E, or K, but adverse reactions are less likely with the water-soluble B and C vitamins, except when they are taken in megadoses.

Fat-Soluble Vitamins

Each of the fat-soluble vitamins A, D, E, and K has a distinct and separate physiological role. For the most part, they are absorbed with other lipids, and efficient absorption requires the presence of bile and pancreatic juice. They are transported to the liver and stored in various body tissues. They are not normally excreted in the urine.

Vitamin A

Vitamin A (retinol) is one of the fat-soluble vitamins that is essential for skeletal growth, maintenance of normal mucosal epithelium, and visual acuity. Normal stores can last up to 1 year but are rapidly depleted by stress. Vitamin A occupies essential roles in vision growth, bone development, maintenance of epithelial tissue, the immunological process, and normal reproduction. Deficiency leads to atrophy of epithelial tissue, resulting in keratomalacia, xerophthalmia, night blindness, and lessened resistance to infection of mucous membranes. Plasma vitamin A concentrations are reduced in cystic fibrosis, alcohol-related cirrhosis, hepatic disease, and proteinuria. Plasma vitamin A concentrations are elevated in patients with chronic renal disease. The recommended oral intake is 2500 to 5000 IU/day. Contraindications include hypervitaminosis A, oral use in malabsorption syndrome, hypersensitivity, and intravenous use.

Vitamin D

Vitamin D (calciferol) is another fat-soluble vitamin that is chemically related to the steroids and is essential for the normal formation of bones and teeth and for the absorption of calcium and phosphorus from the gastrointestinal tract. Ultraviolet rays activate a form of cholesterol in an oil of the skin and convert it to a form of the vitamin, which is then absorbed. Vitamin D is considered a hormone. Deficiency of the vitamin results in rickets in children, osteomalacia, osteoporosis, and osteodystrophy. Vitamin D hypervitaminosis produces a toxicity syndrome. Vitamin D therapy is contraindicated in hypercalcemia, malabsorption syndrome, and renal dysfunction or if the patient has evidence of vitamin D toxicity or abnormal sensitivity to the effects of vitamin D. The recommended intake is 100 to 400 IU/day. Vitamin D_2 is also called ergocalciferol. A fat-soluble vitamin, it is used for the prophylaxis and treatment of rickets, osteomalacia, and other hypocalcemic disorders (tetany) and hypoparathyroidism. Vitamin D_3 is the predominant form of vitamin D of animal origin. It is found in most fish liver oils, butter, bran, and egg yolk. It is formed in skin exposed to sunlight or ultraviolet rays. It is also called cholecalciferol.

Vitamin E

Vitamin E (tocopherol) is a fat-soluble vitamin that is essential for normal reproduction, muscle, development, and resistance of erythrocytes to hemolysis. It is an intracellular antioxidant and acts to maintain the stability of polyunsaturated fatty acids. Deficiency results in muscle degeneration, vascular system abnormalities, megaloblastic anemia, hemolytic anemia, infertility, and liver and kidney damage. It is stored in the body for long periods of time so that a deficiency is rare. It is considered nontoxic except in hypertensive patients and those with chronic rheumatic heart disease. The recommended oral allowance is 12 to 15 IU/day.

Vitamin K

Vitamin K is essential for the synthesis of prothrombin in the liver. The naturally occurring forms, also called quinone, are vitamin K_1 (phylloquinone), which occurs in green plants and vitamin K_2 (menaquinone), which is formed as the result of bacterial action in the intestinal tract. Water-soluble forms of vitamins K_1 and K_2 are also available. The fat-soluble synthetic compound, **menadione** (vitamin K_3), is about twice as potent biologically as the naturally occurring vitamins K_1 and K_2, on a weight basis. It is another fat-soluble vitamin. It is used for coagulation disorders and vitamin K deficiency. Deficiency results in hypoprothrombinemia and hemorrhage. It is used to increase the clotting time in patients with obstructive jaundice and in hemorrhagic states associated with liver diseases. It is given prophylactically to infants to prevent hemorrhagic disease of the newborn. Natural vitamin K is stored in the body and is not toxic. Excessive doses of synthetic vitamin K can cause anemia in newborns. The suggested oral intake is 0.7 to 2.0 mg/day.

Water-Soluble Vitamins

Most of the water-soluble vitamins are components of essential enzyme systems. Many are involved in the reactions supporting energy metabolism. These vitamins are not normally stored in the body in appreciable amounts and are excreted in small quantities in the urine; thus, a daily supply is desirable to avoid depletion and interruption of normal physiological functions.

Vitamin B Complex

Vitamin B complex is a group of water-soluble vitamins differing from each other structurally and in their biological effects. Heat and prolonged cooking, especially cooking with water, can destroy B vitamins.

Vitamin B_1 (thiamin) is a water-soluble member of the B vitamin complex that is essential for normal metabolism and health of the cardiovascular and nervous systems. Thiamin plays a key role in the metabolic breakdown of carbohydrate. It is not stored in the body and must be supplied daily. Deficiency causes loss of appetite, irritability, sleep disturbance, dyspnea, and arrhythmia. Sever deficiency causes **beriberi**.

Vitamin B_2 (riboflavin) is one of the heat-stable components of the B vitamin complex. It is essential for certain enzyme systems in fat and protein metabolism. It is sensitive to light and plays an important role in preventing some visual disorders, especially cataracts. Deficiency of riboflavin produces cheilosis, local inflammation, glossitis, photophobia, cataracts, and anemia.

Vitamin B_3 (niacin) is made up of parts of two enzymes that regulate energy metabolism. Vitamin B_3 is also called nicotinic acid and nicotinamide. It is essential for healthy skin, tongue, and digestive system. Severe deficiency results in pellagra, mental disturbances, various skin eruptions, and gastrointestinal disturbances.

Vitamin B_6 (pyridoxine) is a coenzyme essential for the synthesis and breakdown of amino acids, the conversion of tryptophan to niacin, the breakdown of glycogen to glucose, and the production of antibodies. Deficiency of pyridoxin may cause anemia, anorexia, neuritis, nausea, dermatitis, and depressed immunity.

Vitamin B_7 (biotin) is a water-soluble vitamin that is synthesized by intestinal flora; therefore, deficiency states are rare. Biotin functions in metabolism via biotin-dependent enzymes.

Vitamin B_9 (folic acid) is essential for cell growth and the reproduction of red blood cells. It functions as a coenzyme with vitamins B_{12} and C in the breakdown of proteins and in the formation of nucleic acid and hemoglobin. It is also essential for fetal development, particularly of the neural tube. Deficiency causes anemia and may cause spina bifida in a fetus. Folic acid is also called folacin.

Vitamin B_{12} (cyanocobalamin) is involved in the metabolism of protein, fats, and carbohydrates. It aids in hemoglobin synthesis, is essential for normal functioning of all cells, and is important in energy metabolism. Deficiency causes pernicious anemia and neurological disorders.

Pantothenic acid is a member of the vitamin B complex. The primary role of pantothenic acid is as a constituent of coenzyme. Thus, it is essential in many areas of cellular metabolism including fatty acid metabolism, the synthesis of sex hormones, and the functioning of the nervous system and the adrenal glands.

Vitamin C

Vitamin C (ascorbic acid) is essential for the formation of collagen tissue and for normal intercellular matrices in teeth, bone, cartilage, connective tissue, and skin. It protects the body against infections and helps heal wounds. Therefore, ascorbic acid has multiple functions as either a coenzyme or cofactor. Its role in enhancing absorption of iron is well recognized. Deficiency causes scurvy, lowered resistance to infections, joint tenderness, dental caries, bleeding gums, delayed wound healing, bruising, hemorrhage, and anemia.

MINERALS AND ELECTROLYTES

Minerals are inorganic substances occurring naturally in the earth's crust that the body needs to help build and maintain body tissues for life functions. They are classified as major and trace elements.

Electrolytes are compounds, particularly salts, that when dissolved in water or another solvent dissociate into ions and are able to conduct an electric current. The concentrations of electrolytes differ in blood plasma and other tissues. Sodium, potassium, and chloride are electrolytes. Minerals help keep the body's water and electrolytes in balance.

Calcium

Calcium (Ca) is the fifth most abundant element in the human body and is mainly present in the bone. The body requires calcium ions for the transmission of nerve impulses, muscle contraction, blood coagulation, and cardiac functions. It is a component of extracellular fluid and of soft tissue cells. The normal daily requirement of calcium is 800 to 1200 mg. The following factors enhance the absorption of calcium: adequate concentrations of vitamin D, calcitonin, parathyroid hormone, large quantities of calcium and phosphorus in the diet, and the presence of lactose. Abnormally high levels of ionized calcium in the extracellular fluid can produce muscle weakness, lethargy, and coma. Hypocalcemia can cause tetanic seizures and hypertension.

Phosphorus

Phosphorus (P) is essential for the metabolism of protein, calcium, and glucose. It aids in building strong bones and teeth and helps in regulation of the body's acid-base balance. Nutritional sources are dairy foods, meat, egg yolk, whole grains, and nuts. A nutritional deficiency of phosphorus can cause weight loss, anemia, and abnormal growth. Anemia, cachexia, bronchitis, and necrosis of the mandible bone characterize chronic poisoning by phosphorus.

Chloride

Chloride (Cl) is involved in the maintenance of fluid and the body's acid-base balance. The most common metal chloride is sodium chloride (table salt).

Sodium

Sodium (Na) is one of the most important elements in the body. Sodium ions are involved in acid-base balance, water balance, transmission of nerve impulses, and contraction of muscles. Major dietary sources of sodium are table salt (sodium chloride), catsup, mustard, cured meats and fish, cheese, and potato chips. Toxic levels may cause hypertension and renal disease. The kidney is the main regulator of sodium levels in body fluids. In high temperatures and high fever, the body loses sodium through sweat.

Potassium

Potassium (K) is the major electrolyte in the intracellular fluids, which helps to regulate neuromuscular excitability and muscle contraction. Sources of potassium in the diet are whole grains, meat, legumes, fruit, and vegetables. Potassium is important in glycogen formation, protein synthesis, and correction of imbalances of acid-base metabolism, especially in association with the action of sodium and hydrogen ions. Potassium salts are very important as therapeutic agents but are extremely dangerous if used improperly. The kidney plays an important role in controlling the secretion and absorption of potassium by the body tissues, especially in the muscles and the liver. Increased renal excretion may be caused by diuretic therapy, large doses of anionic drugs, or renal disorders. Increased gastrointestinal tract excretion of potassium may occur with the loss of gastrointestinal fluid through vomiting, diarrhea, surgical drainage, or chronic use of laxatives. Potassium loss through the skin is rare but can result from perspiration during excessive exercise in a hot environment.

Magnesium

Magnesium (Mg) is an important ion for the function of many enzyme systems. Magnesium is the second most abundant cation of the intracellular fluids in the body. It helps to build strong bones and teeth and aids in regulation of the heartbeat. It is stored in the bone and is excreted mainly by the kidneys. Renal excretion of magnesium increases during diuresis induced by ammonium chloride, glucose, and organic mercurials. Magnesium affects the central nervous, neuromuscular, and cardiovascular systems. Diarrhea, steatorrhea, chronic alcoholism, and diabetes mellitus can produce hypomagnesemia. Hypomagnesemia is often treated with administration of parenteral fluids containing magnesium sulfate or magnesium chloride. Excess magnesium (hypermagnesemia) in the body can slow the heartbeat or cause cardiac arrest. Hypermagnesemia is usually caused by renal insufficiency and is manifested by hypotension, muscle weakness, sedation, and confused mental state.

Iron

Iron (Fe) is a common metallic element essential for the synthesis of hemoglobin and myoglobin. The major role of iron is to transfer oxygen to the body tissues. Inadequate supplies of iron needed to synthesize hemoglobin, poor absorption of iron in the digestive system, or chronic bleeding can cause iron deficiency anemia. Replacement iron may be supplied by ferrous sulfate (Feosol®), preferably the oral form. Iron dextran (Imferon®) is an injectable form of iron supplement.

Iodine

Iodine (I) is an essential micronutrient of the thyroid hormone (thyroxine). Almost 80% of the iodine present in the body is in the thyroid gland. Iodine deficiency can result in goiter or cretinism. Iodine is found in seafood, iodized salt, and some dairy products. Iodine is used as a contrast medium for blood vessels in computed tomography scans. Radioisotopes of iodine are used in radioisotope scanning procedures and in palliative treatment of cancer of the thyroid.

Zinc

Zinc (Zn) is essential for several enzymes, growth, glucose tolerance, wound healing, and taste acuity. It is also used in numerous pharmaceutical agents, such as zinc acetate, zinc oxide, zinc permanganate, and zinc stearate. The best sources are protein foods. Zinc deficiency is characterized by abnormal fatigue, decreased alertness, a decrease in taste and odor sensitivity, poor appetite, retarded growth, delayed sexual maturity, prolonged healing of wounds, and susceptibility to infection and injury.

Fluoride

Compounds of **fluoride** (F) are introduced into drinking water or applied directly to the teeth to prevent tooth decay. It also protects against osteoporosis and periodontal (gum) disease. Excessive amounts of fluoride in drinking water may result in discoloration of the teeth.

Copper

Copper (Cu) is a component of several important enzymes in the body and is essential to good health. Copper is mostly concentrated in the liver, heart, brain, and kidneys. It helps in the formation of hemoglobin and the transportation of iron to bone marrow. Copper accumulates in individuals with Wilson's disease or primary biliary cirrhosis.

Mineral Deficiencies

The diseases and symptoms associated with mineral deficiencies are listed in Table 31-2. The three minerals for

TABLE 31-2. Mineral Deficiency

MINERAL	SYMPTOMS AND DISEASE
Calcium	Rickets (children), osteomalacia (adults), tetany, and osteoporosis
Iron	Iron-deficiency anemia, nutritional anemia
Iodine	Goiter, cretinism (congenital myxedema in children), and acquired myxedema in adults (hypothyroidism)
Phosphorus	Weight loss, anemia, and abnormal growth
Sodium	Water intoxication, confusion and lethargy, leading to muscle excitability, convulsions, and coma
Potassium	Impaired growth, hypertension, bone fragility, renal hypertrophy, bradycardia, death
Magnesium	Nausea, vomiting, muscle weakness, tremors, tetany, lethargy, tachycardia, and arrhythmia
Zinc	Dwarfism, delayed growth, hypogonadism, anemia, and decreased appetite
Fluoride	Tooth decay, osteoporosis, and gum disease
Copper	Anemia, bone disease (copper deficiency is very rare in adults)

which deficiencies are most commonly seen are calcium, iron, and iodine.

HYPERALIMENTATION OR TOTAL PARENTERAL NUTRITION

Nutritional care is the proper intake and assimilation of nutrients, especially for the hospitalized patient. The patient's condition will determine the nutritional requirements that may be provided by regular meals with menus selected from the ordered diet, by tube feeding, or by parenteral hyperalimentation. The treatment of choice for selected patients who are unable to tolerate and maintain adequate enteral intake is hyperalimentation or total parenteral nutrition (TPN). Through TPN all calories, amino acids (proteins), dextrose (carbohydrates), fats, trace elements, vitamins, or other essential nutrients needed for wound healing, immunocompetence, growth, and weight gain are supplied. The basic TPN solution may contain amino acids, carbohydrates, lipids, vitamins, and minerals.

MALNUTRITION

Malnutrition may result from an unbalanced, insufficient, or excessive diet or from impaired absorption, assimilation, or use of foods.

Marasmus

Marasmus is a chronic disease that develops over months or years as a result of a deficiency in total caloric intake. Depletion of fat stores and skeletal protein occurs to meet metabolic needs. In a hypermetabolic state (such as trauma and infection), combined with protein deprivation, this can rapidly develop into severe kwashiorkor malnutrition characterized by hypoalbuminemia, edema, and impaired cellular immune function. In advanced stages, it is characterized by muscular wasting and absence of subcutaneous fat.

Kwashiorkor

Kwashiorkor is an acute process that can develop within weeks and is associated with protein deficiency and impaired immune function. It is due to poor protein intake with adequate to slightly inadequate caloric intake. It is characterized by hypoalbuminemia, edema, and an enlarged, fatty liver.

Obesity

Overweight is a state in which a person's weight exceeds a standard based on height; **obesity** is a condition of excessive fatness, either general or localized. It is possible to be obese at a weight within normal limits according to the standard table, just as it is possible to be overweight without being obese; however, in most people, being overweight and being obese tend to parallel each other.

REVIEW QUESTIONS

1. All of the following are classified as compound lipids, except
A. lipoproteins.
B. triglycerides.
C. glycolipids.
D. phospholipids.

2. Efficient absorption of fat-soluble vitamins requires the presence of
A. pancreatic juice.
B. gastric juice.
C. vitamin B_{12}.
D. thyroid hormone.

3. Which of the following vitamins has a special role in enhancing absorption of iron?
A. Vitamin D
B. Vitamin E
C. Vitamin B_{12}
D. Vitamin C

4. Hypocalcemia can cause titanic seizures and
A. hyperglycemia.
B. hypertension.
C. hyperventilation.
D. hypoglycemia.

5. Which of the following trace elements is an essential for growth, wound healing, and taste acuity?
A. Copper
B. Iodine
C. Zinc
D. Fluoride

6. The proper intake and assimilation of nutrients is called
A. nutrient.
B. excretion.
C. nutritional insufficiency.
D. nutritional care.

Continues

7. Most hormones are made of
   A. lipids.
   B. carbohydrates.
   C. proteins.
   D. trace minerals.

8. Which of the following substances is essential for production of bile?
   A. Cholesterol
   B. Carbohydrate
   C. Vitamins
   D. Proteins

9. Which of the following is the most abundant of neutral fats (about 95%)?
   A. Phospholipids
   B. Triglycerides
   C. Fatty acids
   D. Cholesterol

10. All of the following ions are involved in acid-base balance, transmission of nerve impulses, and contraction of muscles, except
    A. phosphorus.
    B. calcium.
    C. zinc.
    D. sodium.

Special Considerations for the Pediatric and Neonatal Patient

32

OUTLINE

(Courtesy of the Agricultural Research Service, USDA)

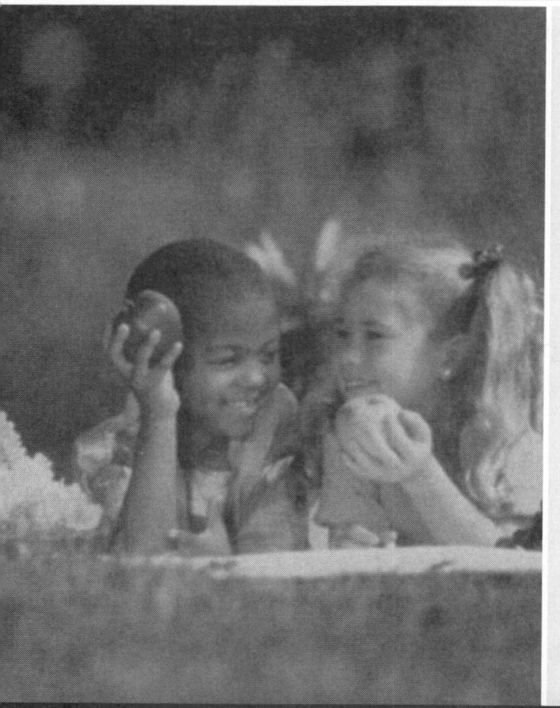

GLOSSARY

asthma A chronic, reversible obstruction of the bronchial airways that is characterized by paroxysmal attacks of dyspnea or difficult respiration on expiration.

bacteremia A condition in which bacteria are recovered from blood cultures of a patient and may or may not be associated with the disease.

patent ductus arteriosus (PDA) A disorder in which the ductus remains patent when pulmonary vascular resistance falls, resulting in aortic blood being shunted into the pulmonary artery.

respiratory distress syndrome (RDS) An acute lung disease of the newborn characterized by airless alveoli, inelastic lung, and an increased respiration rate.

respiratory syncytial virus (RSV) Virus that is the major cause of bronchiolitis and pneumonia in young children.

septicemia A condition in which bacteremia is associated with active disease, localized or systemic.

surfactant A lipoprotein produced by the lungs that keeps the alveoli open.

SPECIAL CONSIDERATIONS FOR THE PEDIATRIC PATIENT

Many medications prescribed for older individuals are also used for neonatal and pediatric patients. However, these patients should not be treated as "smaller adults," which is a common misconception. They are unique, and in many respects, the preparation and administration of their medications requires special attention. Even within a particular age group differing weights, metabolic rates, and organ maturity are found. These factors will affect dosing, therapeutic levels, time of administration, half-life, and excretion of medications. In this chapter selected topics on the use of medications in the pediatric and neonatal patient populations will be presented. To include all medications used would require inclusion of a volume of material that already exists in many texts and is beyond the scope of this text.

DEFINING THE NEONATAL AND PEDIATRIC POPULATION

The neonatal period generally covers the time from birth to approximately 28 days of age. This general category also includes premature infants of varying gestational ages. Gestational age will be a factor in dosing of various medications and may even preclude the use of some. The pediatric period covers a wide range of age, from birth to approximately age 18. To prepare medications for pediatric and neonatal patients accurately requires that the pharmacist or technician know the current weight of the patient because dosages for this population are given per unit of weight. Only during an emergency situation should drugs be given without knowing the actual weight of the child. In these instances, certain devices are used to provide a reasonable estimate of weight. The Broselow tape is one such device. It is placed along the length of the child, and the corresponding color zone on the tape is used to give emergency personnel medication dosages and other pertinent information, such as catheter and endotracheal tube sizes (see Figure 32-1). Patients should be weighed daily, and this information should be sent to the pharmacy so that doses of medications can be adjusted for the rapid weight gains and losses that sometimes occur in children.

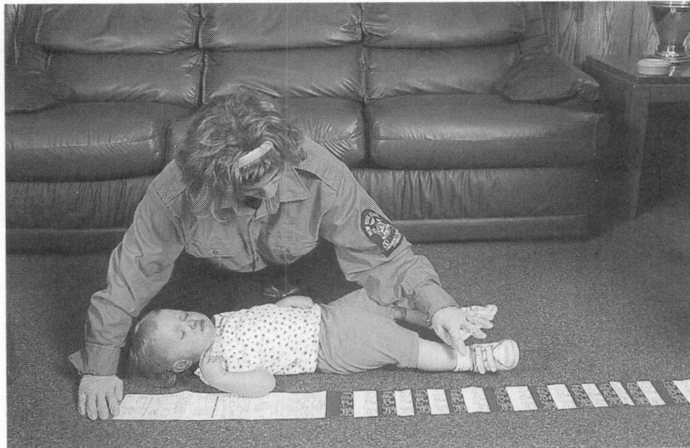

Figure 32-1. The Broselow tape is used to estimate weight in an emergency situation.

CHILDHOOD RESPIRATORY DISORDERS

The patterns of respiratory tract disorders in childhood are affected by age, sex, race, season, geography, and environmental and socioeconomic conditions. Immediately after birth, tuberculosis can be transmitted to the newborn, presenting after several weeks of life as a severe pneumonitis. Lung immaturity and other events related to the perinatal period predispose infants to hyaline membrane disease. The incidence of respiratory tract infections also peaks during the first 2 to 3 school years. Respiratory disorders affect many children each year. Respiratory syncytial virus infection and asthma are two specific problems often treated in the pediatric/neonatal patient population. Apnea is also seen in the neonatal age group, especially in premature infants.

Respiratory Syncytial Virus

Respiratory syncytial virus (RSV) is the major cause of bronchiolitis and pneumonia in infants younger than 1 year of age. It is the most important respiratory tract pathogen of early childhood. It causes mild cold-like symptoms in infants and most children. However, RSV can cause more serious respiratory disease that sometimes requires hospitalization in premature infants. The at-risk group includes infants born at less than 36 weeks of gestation or those with chronic lung disease. The respiratory disease occurs because of the immaturity of the infants' lungs and because these infants have not received sufficient antiviral substances from their mothers. Other high-risk infants include children with certain kinds of congenital heart disease, children with other chronic lung diseases such as cystic fibrosis, children who are immune-deficient, or children who are receiving immune-suppressive medication. In most parts of the United States RSV infection occurs seasonally, generally from fall through spring (October through March). At-risk infants are now being treated before discharge from the hospital to provide some immunoprophylaxis.

Treatments for Respiratory Syncytial Virus

Palivizumab (Synagis) is used for immunoprophylaxis against severe lower respiratory tract RSV infections. In infants with uncomplicated bronchiolitis, treatment is symptomatic.

Humidified oxygen is usually indicated for hospitalized infants because most have hypoxia. Fluids should be carefully administered. Often, intravenous or tube feeding is helpful when sucking is difficult. Bronchodilators should not be routinely used. However, a course of epinephrine should be tried in children with wheezing who are older than 1 year of age. Bronchodilators should be administered if found to be beneficial. The use of corticosteroids is not indicated except as a last resort in children whose condition is critical. Sedatives are rarely necessary. The antiviral drug ribavirin, delivered by small-particle aerosol and breathed along with the required concentration of oxygen for 20 to 24 hours per day for 3 to 5 days, has a beneficial effect on the course of pneumonia caused by RSV.

Asthma

Asthma is a leading cause of chronic illness in childhood and is responsible for a significant proportion of school days missed because of chronic illness. Asthma is a chronic, reversible obstruction of the bronchial airways. The airways become over-reactive because of this inflammation and increased mucus secretion; mucosal swelling and muscle contraction then occur (see Figure 32-2). This leads to airway obstruction, chest tightness, coughing, and wheezing, and, if asthma is severe, to shortness of breath and low blood oxygen levels. Most children experience their first symptoms by 4 to 5 years of age. Allergies, viral respiratory infections, and airborne irritants produce the inflammation that can lead to asthma. Childhood asthma is a disease with a strong allergic component and a genetic predisposition. Approximately 75% to 80% of children with asthma have allergies.

Treatment for Asthma

Treatment generally includes two types of medications: quick-relief medications (also called bronchodilators) and controller medications. Controller medications got their name because they help control inflammation to make breathing easier. These medications must be taken daily to be effective. A list of medications in the bronchodilator and controller groups is provided in Table 32-1.

Respiratory Distress Syndrome

Respiratory distress syndrome (RDS) occurs in preterm newborns and is characterized by impairment of respiratory function due to immaturity affecting the production of enzymes necessary to produce surfactant in the lungs. This is the leading cause of death in premature infants. Symptoms of RSD include a low APGAR score immediately after birth, atelectasis of the lung, impaired blood perfusion of the lung, and reduced pulmonary compliance. Respiratory difficulty will be present and the infant will exhibit signs of cyanosis, tachycardia, and grunting.

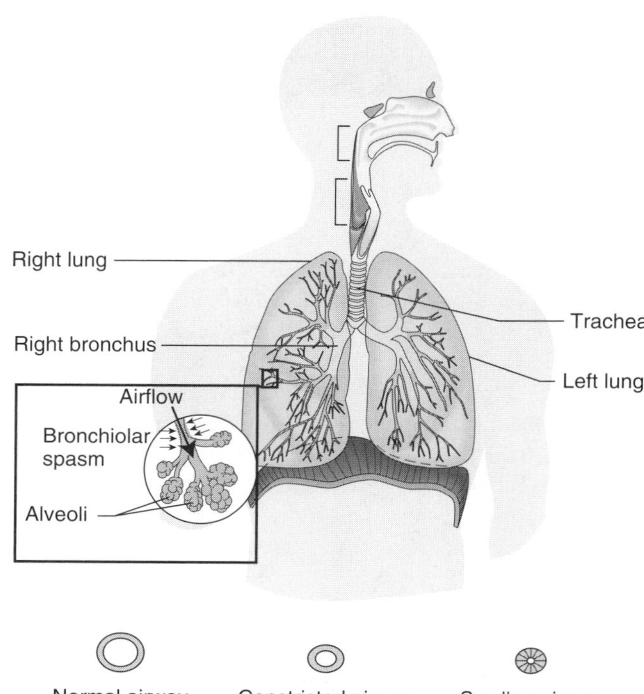

Figure 32-2. Asthma is characterized by bronchoconstriction and swelling of the airways.

Treatment for Respiratory Distress Syndrome

Infants at risk for or those who have RDS as well as infants with respiratory failure due to meconium aspiration syndrome, persistent pulmonary hypertension, or pneumonia, are treated with intratracheal administration of natural, animal-derived, or synthetic surfactant. **Surfactant** is a lipoprotein produced by the lungs that keeps the alveoli open. Its production can be limited in premature infants because of lung immaturity or may be missing or lacking in infants with other disease processes. Continuous positive airway pressure also can be used to prevent alveolar collapse.

FEVER

Fever (pyrexia) has been a sign of disease for a number of years. It is a physiological event that occurs naturally as the core temperature of the body is elevated 1° or more from normal (37°C or 98.6°F). It is the most common complaint voiced by parents when they describe their child as being "sick." Fever is found during both infectious and noninfectious illnesses, but it is highly associated with infections. It is the body's response to pyrogenic substances and helps to stimulate normal defense mechanisms. The higher set point temperature of the body may be detrimental to the bacteria causing the illness. Fever in children younger than 2 months

TABLE 32-1. Medications Used in Asthma

CLASSIFICATION	GENERIC NAME	TRADE NAME	INDICATION
Bronchodilators			
β-adrenergic agonists	albuterol	Proventil®	Used to promote pulmonary smooth muscle relaxation and improve respiratory function
	pirbuterol		
	levalbuterol		
	epinephrine	Sus-phrine®	
	metaproterenol sulfate	Alupent®	
	terbutaline sulfate	Brethaire®	
	theophylline	Bronkodyl®	
Anticholinergic		Atrovent®	
Anti-inflammatory medications			
Antiallergics	cromolyn sodium	Intal®	
	nedocromil sodium	Tilade®	
Corticosteroids	prednisolone	Prelone®	Used to reduce airway reactivity and inflammation
	prednisone	Deltasone®	
Mucolytic agents	acetylcysteine	Mucomyst®	Used to reduce the viscosity of sputum, chiefly in patients with cystic fibrosis
	dornase alfa recombinant human deoxyribonuclease	Pulmozyme®	

of age is uncommon because neonates, infants, and young children are less able to produce a febrile response. Because of this, fever is a significant finding in this age group.

Treatment for Fever

Antipyretic drugs are commonly used to restore the body's normal temperature set point. Aspirin is no longer given to children with fever because of its connection to Reye's syndrome. Acetaminophen (Tylenol) is used instead. However, they should not be routinely administered for fever, unless the temperature is at least 104.9°F (40.5°C). They are usually given if other symptoms associated with fever, such as malaise, headache, and arthralgia, bother the child. Acetaminophen is used at a dose of 10 to 15 mg/kg by mouth or by rectum every 4 to 6 hours, with a maximum dose of 4 g/24 hr or 5 doses in 24 hours. Ibuprofen is used at a dose of 5 to 10 mg/kg/dose by mouth every 6 to 8 hours, with a maximum dose of 40 mg/kg/24 hr.

CARDIOVASCULAR DISORDERS

Medications to support cardiovascular functions in the pediatric/neonatal patient population differ little from those used for adults. Digoxin, diuretics, and, occasionally, antihypertensives are used. Their indications and dosage generally are the same for all groups. Discussion in this section will focus on a topic unique to the neonatal population, patent ductus arteriosus, and the use of inotropic agents to support blood pressure. The pharmacy technician may need to recognize the medications used and to prepare them for proper use.

Patent Ductus Arteriosus

During fetal life most of the pulmonary arterial blood is shunted through the ductus arteriosus into the aorta. Functional closure of the ductus normally occurs soon after birth, but if the ductus remains patent when pulmonary vascular resistance falls, aortic blood is shunted into the pulmonary artery (see Figure 32-3). **Patent ductus arteriosus (PDA)** is one of the most common congenital cardiovascular anomalies associated with maternal rubella (German measles) during early pregnancy. After birth and after a series of physiological changes, the pulmonary and systemic circulations become arranged into two circuits, so that oxygenated blood returns from the lungs and is ejected from the left side of the heart to the systemic circulation. Deoxygenated blood returns from the systemic circulation and is ejected from the right side of the heart to the lungs (the pulmonary circuit). After birth, the onset of breathing causes an increase in pulmonary blood flow and pressure which, among other complex reactions, helps the ductus arteriosus to close. A decrease in the level of one particular chemical, prostaglandin, specifically aids

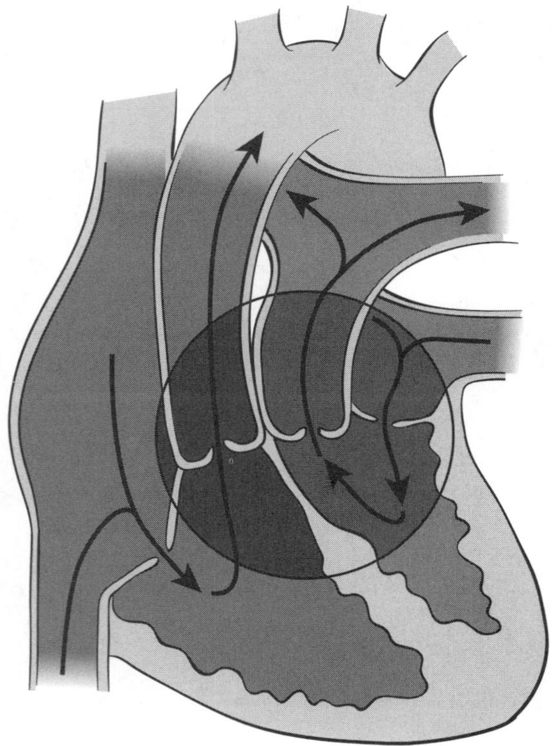

Figure 32-3. Patent ductus arteriosus.

in this closure. The entire phenomenon of transition is not completely understood, and the transition period in infants is a particularly important time. In uncomplicated PDA, the ductus closes spontaneously within the first weeks or months of life.

Treatment for Patent Ductus Arteriosus

When a large symptomatic PDA is present, general treatment may include fluid restriction, correction of anemia, digitalization, and diuretic therapy. Ductus arteriosus patency is mediated through prostaglandins, and the ductus arteriosus in the preterm infant with respiratory distress syndrome can be constricted and closed by administration of inhibitors of prostaglandin synthesis such as indomethacin. Early administration of indomethacin in the course of respiratory distress syndrome associated with large ductal left to right shunts is approximately 80% effective in closing the ductus. Surgical closure is a safe and effective backup technique for management when indomethacin is contraindicated or indomethacin treatment has not been successful. Administration is by intravenous infusion over at least 30 minutes to minimize adverse effects on cerebral, renal, and gastrointestinal blood flow. Usually, three doses per course are given, with a maximum of two courses. Urine output must be closely monitored and if anuria (no urine output) or oliguria occurs, subsequent doses should be delayed.

INFECTIOUS DISEASES

Various types of infectious agents have effects on different body systems in newborns and children and cause infectious diseases. Discussion of the many infectious diseases that exist is beyond the scope of this text, but the following are a few examples that are seen often.

Diarrhea

Diarrhea is one of the most common problems encountered by pediatricians. Diarrhea is defined as an increase in the frequency, fluidity, and volume of feces. During the first 3 years of life it is estimated that a child will experience an acute, severe episode of diarrhea one to three times. It may be caused by a variety of infectious agents, such as bacteria, viruses, protozoans, and parasites. Hospitalization is usually necessary for severe diarrhea because of the possibility of bacterial disease, which should be treated there, and because hydration often requires fluid therapy.

Treatment for Diarrhea

Treatment for diarrhea is symptomatic. Antipyretic drugs are recommended for fever. Codeine, morphine, and the phenothiazine derivatives, often used for pain and vomiting but rarely needed for children, should be avoided because they may induce misleading signs and symptoms.

Bacteremia and Septicemia

The terms bacteremia and septicemia indicate the presence of bacteria in the blood. In **bacteremia**, bacteria are recovered from blood cultures of a patient and may or may not be associated with a disease. **Septicemia** is bacteremia associated with active disease, localized, or systemic. In some patients, bacteremia or septicemia may be associated with focal infection (e.g., pneumonia, osteomyelitis, endocarditis, or meningitis). Primary bacteremia, however, also occurs in normal infants and children.

Treatment for Bacteremia and Septicemia

Treatment may be initiated with ampicillin and a semisynthetic penicillinase-resistant penicillin (methicillin, oxacillin, or nafcillin) administered intravenously. In some patients, the use of chloramphenicol may also be indicated.

Acute Bacterial Meningitis

The incidence of bacterial meningitis (especially that caused by *Haemophilus influenzae* type B or group B β-hemolytic streptococci) is increasing. Mortality and morbidity are significant, but the reported number of deaths has decreased over time. Several types of bacteria may cause acute bacterial

TABLE 32-2. Infective Causes of Meningitis

AGE GROUP	MOST COMMON INFECTIVE CAUSES
Neonates	Group B streptococci, *Escherichia coli*
Infants	*Haemophilus influenzae* type B, *Streptococcus pneumoniae*
Young children	*Streptococcus pneumoniae* or *Neisseriae meningitidis*

meningitis in neonates, infants, and older children. Table 32-2 shows the most common infectious agents that cause meningitis in different age groups.

Treatment for Meningitis

Initial therapy includes immediate administration of multiple antibiotics including a third-generation of cephalosporin (such as ceftriaxone or cefotaxime) after an IV line has been placed and blood has been drawn for cultures. Vancomycin, with or without rifampin, is usually added, as is ampicillin or gentamycin. Heparin therapy should be considered for patients with the syndrome of disseminated intravascular coagulation. The use of corticosteroids has been suggested as a therapeutic adjunct that may reduce cerebral edema and inflammation.

Streptococcal Infections

Streptococci are among the most common causes of bacterial infections in infancy and childhood. Group A streptococci are the most common bacterial cause of acute pharyngitis.

Treatment for Streptococcal Infections

Penicillin is the drug of choice for the treatment of streptococcal infections. The goal of therapy is to maintain, for at least 10 days, blood and tissue levels of penicillin sufficient to kill streptococci.

REVIEW QUESTIONS

1. Two specific and common problems of respiratory diseases that affect many children and neonates are
A. bronchiolitis and cystic fibrosis.
B. asthma and tuberculosis.
C. asthma and respiratory synctival virus infection.
D. asthma and pulmonary edema.

2. The trade name of albuterol is
A. Proventil.
B. Alupent.
C. Brethaire.
D. Intal.

3. Which of the following is a congenital cardiovascular anomaly that is associated with maternal rubella (German measles)?
A. Septicemia
B. Cystic fibrosis
C. Aneurism of aorta
D. Patent ductus arteriosus

4. Initial therapy for bacterial meningitis in neonates includes all of the following, except
A. heparin therapy.
B. corticosteroids.
C. Proventil®.
D. ampicillin.

5. The drug of choice for the treatment of acute pharyngitis in young children, which is caused by a streptococcal microorganism, is
A. penicillin.
B. tetracycline.
C. bacitracin.
D. chloramphenicol.

6. The major cause of bronchiolitis and pneumonia in infants under 1 year of age, is
A. rabies virus.
B. para-influenza virus.
C. respiratory syncytial virus.
D. chickenpox virus.

7. Respiratory distress syndrome in the newborn may be characterized when a respiration rate is greater than _____ per minute.
A. 15
B. 30
C. 40
D. 60

8. Apnea is seen more commonly in which of the following age groups of children?
A. Premature infants
B. Preschool
C. Neonatal
D. A and C

Continues

9. Which of the following is the most common infective cause in neonates?
   A. Haemophilus influenzae Type B
   B. Group B streptococci
   C. Escherichia coli
   D. B and C

10. Treatment for patent ductus arteriosus includes which of the following agents?
    A. Methicillin
    B. Indomethacin
    C. Oxygen
    D. Morphine

11. The goal of therapy for the treatment of acute pharyngitis, which is caused by a streptococcal infection, includes
    A. bacitracin.
    B. chloramphenicol.
    C. penicillin.
    D. tetracycline.

Drug Therapy for Aging Patients

33

OUTLINE

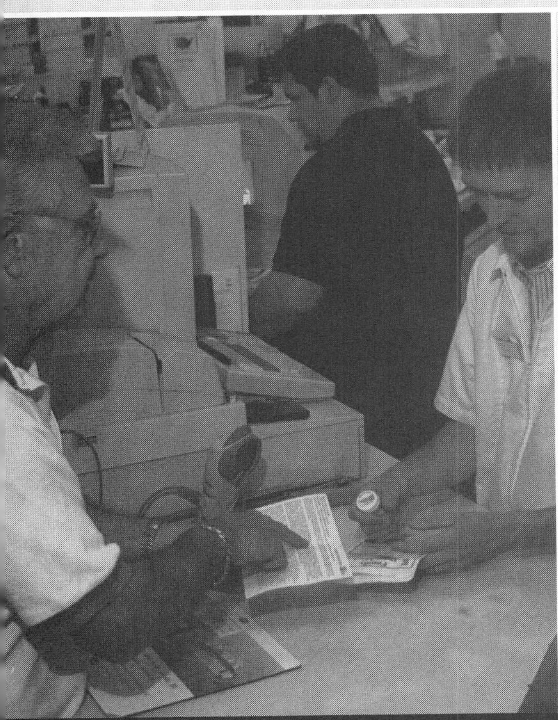

GLOSSARY

pharmacodynamic interaction Differences in effects produced by a given plasma level of a drug.

pharmacokinetic interaction Differences in the plasma levels of a drug achieved with a given dose of that drug.

AGING PATIENTS

The impact of age on medical care is substantial and, thus, a significant alteration in the approach to treatment of the older patient is needed. As individuals age, they are more likely to have a disease or disability or treatment-related side effects. Combined with the decrease in physiological reserve, these added burdens (if present) make the older person more vulnerable to environmental, pathological, or pharmacological illnesses. Understanding these facts is essential for optimal care of older patients. The health problems and medical management of elderly patients differ from those of younger ones in important ways, which explains the development of training in geriatrics as a medical specialty. Prescribing medications for elderly patients is always a challenge for physicians. Body functions decline dramatically in elderly patients. Therefore, the normal aging process can lead to altered drug effects and the need for altered doses.

PRINCIPLES OF DRUG THERAPY IN ELDERLY PATIENTS

There are several reasons for the greater incidence of adverse reactions to drugs in the elderly population. Drug metabolism is often impaired in this group because of a decrease in the glomerular filtration rate and reduced hepatic clearance. The reduction in hepatic clearance is due to decreased activity of microsomal enzymes and reduced hepatic perfusion with aging. The distribution of drugs is also affected. Because elderly persons have a decrease in total body water content and a relative increase in body fat, water-soluble drugs become more concentrated and fat-soluble drugs have longer half-lives. In addition, serum albumin levels decrease, especially in sick patients, so that protein binding of some drugs (e.g., warfarin and phenytoin) is reduced, leaving more free (active) drugs available. In addition, older individuals often have altered responses to a given serum drug level. Thus, they are more sensitive to some drugs (e.g., opioids) and less sensitive to others (e.g., β-blocking agents). Finally, the older patient with multiple chronic conditions is likely to be receiving many drugs, including nonprescribed agents. Thus, adverse drug reactions and dosage errors are more likely to occur, especially if the patient has visual, hearing, or memory deficits.

Drug Interactions

A drug interaction occurs whenever the pharmacologic action of a drug is altered by a second substance. This change may be related to a **pharmacokinetic interaction** (differences in the plasma levels of a drug achieved with a given dose of that drug) and a **pharmacodynamic interaction** (differences in effects produced by a given plasma level of a drug). The duration and intensity of the action of a drug are a function of the plasma level of the drug, which is related directly to the rates of absorption, distribution, metabolism, and excretion of that drug. These rates may be altered by previous drug therapy, dietary factors, and exposure to environmental chemicals (chemicals not used for therapeutic purposes). Physical factors such as ambient temperature and effects of disease (e.g., fever) may also have an effect.

Drug Absorption

Physiological changes with aging such as changes in gastric pH, slowed gastric emptying rate, reduced cardiac output (blood flow), reductions of absorptive surfaces, and slowed gastrointestinal (GI) track motility are factors that affect not only drug absorption but also drug distribution and metabolism. Different diseases and conditions of the GI tract are also obvious factors that affect drug absorption. Examples are peptic ulcer, diarrhea, constipation, and others.

Drug Distribution

Alterations in drug distribution in elderly patients depend upon many factors such as a reduction in total body water content, decreased plasma albumin concentration, reduced lean body mass, and increased body fat. Many drugs, especially acidic ones, bind to plasma proteins. Drugs can compete for plasma protein-binding sites. Plasma protein-binding sites are especially significant when a high percentage of the drug (more than 90%) is normally protein bound, as for coumarin anticoagulants, sulfonamides, salicylates, indomethacin, and most other nonsteroidal anti-inflammatory agents. Lipid-soluble drugs such as lidocaine and diazepam have a large volume of distribution in elderly persons, whereas water-soluble drugs such as ethanol and acetaminophen have a smaller volume of distribution. Digoxin also has a lower volume of distribution in elderly persons, and, therefore, doses of digoxin must be reduced.

Drug Metabolism

The most common and most important cause for differences in plasma levels of a drug is a change in the rate of biotransformation of the drug. Variations in a person's plasma drug levels are more common with drugs that undergo extensive GI metabolism, or first-pass hepatic metabolism. The total liver blood flow declines 40% to 45% with aging because of reduction of cardiac output. Therefore, if severe and progressive liver damage is present in an elderly person, drug metabolism would be affected. Otherwise, the decline in the ability of elderly persons to metabolize most drugs is relatively small and difficult to predict. The effects of cigarette smoking, diet, and alcohol consumption may be more important than physiological changes in the liver.

Drug Elimination

Drugs may be eliminated from the body by many routes, including urine, feces (e.g., unabsorbed drugs or those secreted in bile), saliva, sweat, tears, milk, and lungs (e.g., alcohols and anesthetics). Any route may be important for a given drug, but the kidney is the major and most important route for the elimination of the majority of drugs. Some drugs are excreted unchanged in the urine, whereas other drugs are so extensively metabolized that only a small fraction of the original chemical substance is excreted unchanged. Different responses to drug therapy may be seen in elderly individuals because of a decline in hepatic and renal function, which is often accompanied by a concurrent disease process. The rate of excretion of any drug eliminated by the kidneys is reduced in elderly persons. Examples of these drugs are aminoglycosides, chlorpropamide, digoxin, and lithium carbonate. To prevent drug toxicity, renal function must be estimated, and the dosage of drug should be adjusted. Most elderly patients do not have normal renal function, and the majority require adjustments in the dosages of drugs that are eliminated primarily by the kidneys.

SPECIFIC DRUG CONSIDERATIONS FOR ELDERLY PATIENTS

Several classes of drugs prescribed for elderly patients require specific consideration. These include anticoagulants, glaucoma medications, analgesics, antihypertensives, cold remedies, antiemetics, and benzodiazepines.

Anticoagulants

Many elderly patients with atrial fibrillation are not given anticoagulants because physicians fear injuries and secondary bleeding due to falls. Head injuries are usually of greatest concern. Given that anticoagulation can result in an annual absolute reduction in the risk of stroke, the benefits of anticoagulation outweigh the risks of falling in most instances.

Glaucoma Medications

Topical β-blockers can cause systemic side effects (bradycardia, asthma, or heart failure) as can oral carbonic anhydrase inhibitors. The latter may also produce malaise, anorexia, and weight loss.

Analgesics

Meperidine is associated with an increased risk of delirium and seizures in elderly persons and should be avoided in this population. Of the nonsteroidal anti-inflammatory drugs (NSAIDs), the risk of confusion is highest with indomethacin. For treatment of osteoarthritis, use of acetaminophen on a scheduled basis is safer than use of a NSAID with comparable effectiveness.

Antihypertensives

In most elderly patients, the first choice for treating hypertension is a thiazide at a low dosage. Unfortunately, use of thiazides increases the risk of exacerbation of gout. Use of an NSAID at the same time can worsen hypertension.

Cold Remedies

Over-the-counter cold remedies often cause adverse effects in elderly people. The anticholinergic properties of many of these can create confusion, impair bladder emptying, or cause constipation; decongestants rarely cause urinary hesitancy or retention in men.

Antiemetics

Prochlorperazine and metoclopramide both can cause drug-induced parkinsonism.

Benzodiazepines

Sedative-hypnotics such as benzodiazepines more commonly cause greater central nervous system depression in elderly patients than in other patients. The use of benzodiazepines in elderly patients may cause falling and hip fractures. Smaller doses should be used in elderly patients, and drugs with extremely long half-lives should be avoided in these patients.

REVIEW QUESTIONS

1. Which of the following drugs requires a lower dosage in elderly persons because of reduction of renal function?
   A. Warfarin
   B. Gentamicin
   C. Digoxin
   D. Zantac®

2. Which of the following medications in elderly patients may cause falling and hip fractures?
   A. Thiazides
   B. Diazepam
   C. Vitamin B_{12}
   D. Cimetidine®

3. Physiological changes with aging may alter all of the following, except
   A. reduction of cardiac output.
   B. reduction of absorptive surfaces.
   C. faster gastric emptying rate.
   D. changes of gastric pH.

4. All of the following are reasons for the greater incidence of adverse reaction to drugs in the elderly individual, except
   A. total body fluid increases.
   B. drug metabolism may be impaired.
   C. serum albumin levels decrease.
   D. medication errors are more likely to occur.

5. Which of the following drugs has a large volume of distribution?
   A. Diazepam
   B. Acetaminophen
   C. Digoxin
   D. Ethanol

6. Which of the following body systems is the most important for elimination of the majority of drugs?
   A. Digestive
   B. Respiratory
   C. Reproductive
   D. Urinary

7. Which of the following drugs may cause drug-induced parkinsonism?
   A. Prochlorperazine
   B. Chloramphenicol
   C. Acetaminophen
   D. Thiazide

8. In most elderly patients, the first choice for treating hypertension includes which of the following?
   A. Digitalis
   B. Ethyl alcohol
   C. Thiazide
   D. Aspirin

9. Drug metabolism is often impaired in elderly patients because of which of the following?
   A. Decreased activity of the brain
   B. Increased secretion of stomach acid
   C. Decrease in the glomerular filtration rate
   D. Increased hepatic clearance

10. A difference in the effects produced by a given plasma level of a drug is known as a
    A. pharmacokinetic interaction.
    B. pharmacodynamic interaction.
    C. pharmacognosy.
    D. pharmacology.

11. Anticoagulation can result in an annual absolute reduction in the risk of which of the following diseases?
    A. Stroke
    B. Peptic ulcer
    C. Glaucoma
    D. Gout

12. Which of the following analgesics is associated with an increased risk of delirium and seizures in elderly persons?
    A. Indomethacin
    B. Acetaminophen
    C. Meperidine
    D. Ibuprofen

SECTION

V

Pharmaceutical Calculations

Basic Mathematics 34

OUTLINE

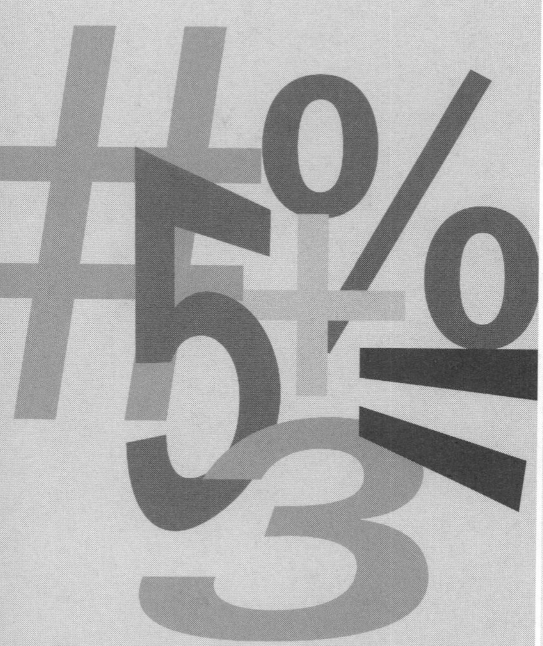

GLOSSARY

Arabic numbers Standard numerical numbers.
denominator The number the whole is divided into.
dividend A quantity to be divided.
divisor The number performing the division.
extremes The two outside terms in a ratio.
fraction An expression of division with a number that is the portion or part of a whole.
means The two inside terms in a ratio.
numerator The portion of the whole being considered.
percent A fraction whose numerator is expressed and whose denominator is understood to be 100.
proportion The relationship between two equal ratios.
quotient The answer to a division problem.
ratio A mathematical expression that compares two numbers by division.

BASIC MATH

The first technical operation that pharmacy technicians must learn is the manipulation of measures of volume, balance, and weights. In this learning process, the various systems of weights and measures, their relationships, and a mastery of basic mathematics is necessary. Pharmacy technicians must learn basic mathematics to be able to calculate the dosage of drugs by weight, measures of volume, and balances. This chapter summarizes the basic mathematics of these operations.

ARABIC NUMBERS AND ROMAN NUMERALS

The system of Roman numerals uses letters to designate numbers. The use of this system is obviously restricted because mathematical procedures would become extremely complicated if the attempt were made to use these numerals in calculations. Most of the medications administered or ordered should be measured by amounts expressed in **Arabic numbers**. The familiar system of whole numbers (0 through 9), fractions (e.g., $\frac{1}{5}$), and decimals (e.g., 0.7) is used widely in the United States and internationally. Table 34-1 shows some examples of Arabic numbers and Roman numerals.

FRACTIONS

Pharmacy technicians need to understand fractions to be able to interpret and act on practitioners' orders, read prescriptions, and understand patient records and information in the pharmacy literature. Fractions are used in apothecary and household measures for dosage calculations. A **fraction** is an expression of division with a number that is the portion or part of a whole. Fractions can stand alone or can be part of a mixed number, which is a whole number and a fraction. A fraction has two parts. The bottom is referred to as the **denominator** and is the number the whole is divided into. The **numerator** is the portion of the whole being considered. See Figure 34-1, which is a diagram representing fractions of a whole.
Four parts shaded out of six parts represents:

$$\frac{4}{6} = \frac{\text{Numerator}}{\text{Denominator}}$$

TABLE 34-1. Examples of Arabic Numbers and Roman Numerals

ARABIC NUMBER	ROMAN NUMERAL
1	I
2	II
3	III
4	IV
5	V
6	VI
7	VII
8	VIII
9	IX
10	X
20	XX
30	XXX
50	L
100	C
500	D
1000	M

Classification of Fractions

There are two types of fractions: common fractions and decimal fractions. Common fractions usually are referred to simply as fractions (e.g., $\frac{1}{4}$). Decimal fractions are commonly referred to simply as decimals (e.g., 0.5). There are four types of common fractions: proper, improper, mixed, and complex fractions.

Proper Fractions

A proper fraction has a numerator that is smaller than the denominator and designates less than one whole unit. Whenever the numerator is less than the denominator, the value of the fraction must be less than 1.

Example

$$\frac{3}{5} = \frac{\text{Numerator}}{\text{Denominator}} = <1$$

Improper Fractions

Improper fractions have a numerator that is greater than or equal to the denominator. The value of the improper fraction is greater than or equal to 1.

Example

$$\frac{6}{4} = >1$$

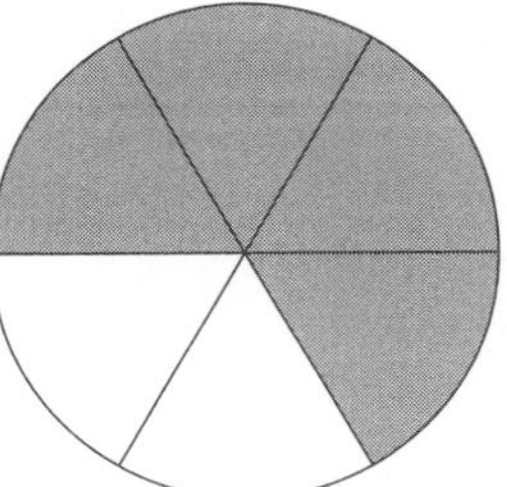

Figure 34-1. Four parts shaded out of six parts represents:
$\frac{4}{6}$ = Numerator/Denominator

Whenever the numerator and denominator are equal, the value of the improper fraction is always equal to 1.

Example

$$\frac{6}{6} = 1$$

Mixed Fractions

Mixed fractions have a whole number and a proper fraction that are combined. The value of the mixed number is always greater than 1.

Example

$$1\frac{3}{5} = 1 + \frac{3}{5} = >1$$

Complex Fractions

Complex fractions have a numerator or denominator or both as a whole number, proper fraction, or mixed number. The value may be less than, greater than, or equal to 1.

Examples

$$\frac{3/5}{1/2} = >1 \qquad \frac{3/5}{1/2} = <1$$

$$\frac{1\,3/5}{1/5} = >1 \qquad \frac{1/2}{2/4} = 1$$

Comparing Fractions

When calculating some drug dosages, it is helpful for the technician to know whether the value of one fraction is greater than or less than the value of another fraction. The size of a fraction can be determined by comparing the numerators when the denominators are the same or comparing the denominators if the numerators are the same. If the numerators are the same, the fraction with the smaller denominator has the greater value.

Example

Compare $\frac{1}{2}$ and $\frac{1}{3}$
Numerators are both 1
Denominator 2 is less than 3

Therefore, $1/2$ has the greater value.

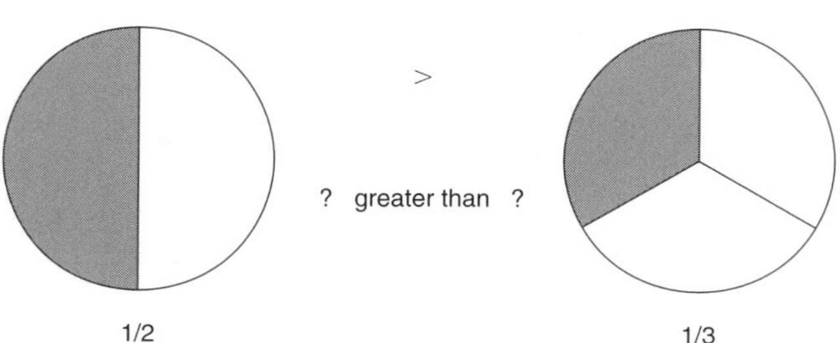

On the contrary, if the denominators are both the same, the fraction with the smaller numerator has the lesser value.

Example

Compare $\frac{2}{5}$ and $\frac{4}{5}$
Denominators are both 5
Numerators: 2 is less than 4

Therefore, $2/5$ has a lesser value.

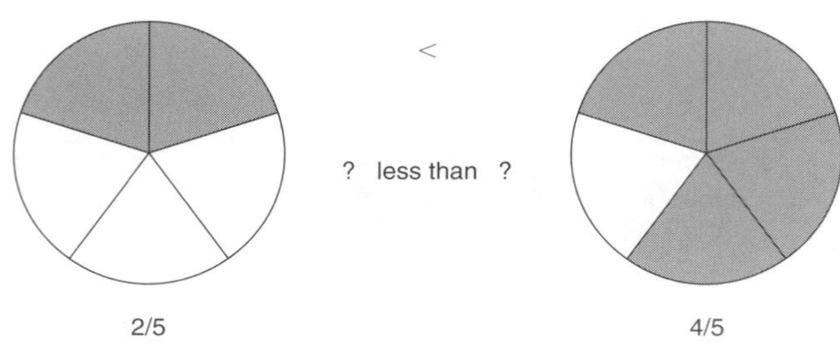

Adding Fractions

To add two fractions, it is necessary to find a common denominator first. Next, the numerators are added together and the value of the common denominator is kept the same. Finally, the resulting value is reduced to its lowest terms.

Examples

Add $1/6$ and $4/12$. To obtain a common denominator of 12, it is necessary to multiply the numerator and denominator of $1/6$ by 2:

$$1 \times \frac{2}{6} \times 2 = \frac{2}{12}$$

Now we have a common denominator and are able to simply add the numerators. Be sure to reduce the final answer:

$$\frac{2}{12} + \frac{4}{12} = \frac{6}{12} = \frac{1}{2}$$

$6/12$ is reduced to lowest terms, which is $1/2$.

Subtracting Fractions

The first step in subtracting fractions is to find a common denominator. Then the numerator is subtracted, and, finally, the result is obtained by keeping the denominator the same and taking the difference of the numerator. The resulting value is reduced to its lowest terms to obtain the final answer.

Example

Subtract $1/2$ from $8/10$. To obtain a common denominator, multiply the numerator and denominator by 5 to produce 10 as the common denominator:

$$\frac{1}{2} \times \frac{5}{5} = \frac{5}{10}$$

Subtract the numerator:

$$\frac{8}{10} - \frac{5}{10} = \frac{3}{10}$$

The answer cannot be reduced further. The final answer is $\frac{3}{10}$.

Multiplying Fractions

To multiply fractions, first, the numerators are multiplied. Second, the denominators are multiplied, the product of the numerators is placed over the product of the denominators, and finally, the resulting value is reduced to its lowest terms.

Example 1

$$\frac{3}{4} \times \frac{2}{5} = \frac{6}{20} = \frac{3}{10}$$

Example 2

$$\frac{2}{4} \times \frac{3}{4}$$

Reduce $\frac{2}{4}$ to $\frac{1}{2}$, then multiply:

$$\frac{1}{2} \times \frac{3}{4} = \frac{3}{8}$$

Dividing Fractions

To divide fractions, first, the divisor is inverted (or turned upside down). Second, the two fractions are multiplied, and the resulting value is reduced to its lowest terms.

Example 1

$$\frac{3}{4} + \frac{2}{3} =$$

$$\frac{3}{4} \times \frac{3}{2} =$$

$$3 \times \frac{3}{4} \times 2 = \frac{9}{8}$$

Example 2

$$\frac{3}{4} + \frac{8}{9} =$$

$$\frac{3}{4} \times \frac{9}{8} =$$

$$3 \times \frac{9}{4} \times 8 = \frac{27}{32}$$

DECIMALS

Decimal fractions or decimals are used with the metric system, which is the system most often used in the calculation of drug dosages. It is very important for the pharmacy technician to be able to manipulate decimals easily and accurately. Each decimal fraction consists of a numerator that is expressed in numerals, a decimal point placed so that it designates the value of the denominator, and the denominator that is understood to be 10 or some power of 10. In writing a decimal fraction, always place a zero to the left of the decimal point so that the decimal point can readily be seen. This also ensures that the decimal will not be mistaken for the whole number 1. Table 34-2 shows some examples.

For reading and writing decimals, observe Figure 34-2, which shows that all whole numbers are to the left of the decimal point and all fractions are to the right.

TABLE 34-2. Fractions and Their Related Decimal Fractions

FRACTION	DECIMAL FRACTION	DESCRIPTION
$\frac{4}{10}$	0.4	Because 10 has **1** zero, the decimal point of 4 is moved to the left **once**.
$\frac{17}{100}$	0.17	Because 100 has **2** zeros, the decimal point of 17 is moved to the left **twice**.
$\frac{334}{1000}$	0.334	Because 1000 has **3** zeros, the decimal point of 334 is moved to the left **three** places.

Multiplying Decimals

To multiply decimals, first, the product is found as usual. Second, the number of decimal places in both the multiplicand and the multiplier are counted. Finally, the total number of decimal places in the product is marked and a decimal point is inserted.

Example

Multiply 2.05 × 0.3.

Step 1

2.05 (multiplicand)
× 0.2 (multiplier)
0410 (product)

Step 2

Count the number of decimal places in the multiplicand and the multiplier:

2.05
× 0.2 = Total of three decimal places

Step 3

Mark off three decimal places in product.

New decimal = 0.410

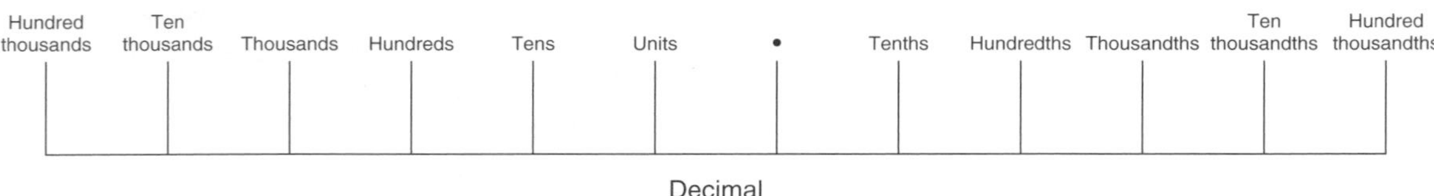

Figure 34-2. Decimals.

Dividing Decimals

To divide a decimal by a whole number, first, the problem is written as usual. Second, a decimal point is placed in the quotient line directly above the decimal in the dividend, and then the quotient is found. Division is written using several symbols, such as 1 ÷ 2 or $\frac{1}{2}$. The **divisor** (the number performing the division) is on the right of the first symbol, and the bottom of the second symbol. The answer to a division problem is called the **quotient**. The divisor must be a whole number (a number with no decimal point), and the decimal point must be correctly placed in the answer. When a decimal number is being divided by a whole number, the decimal point is placed directly above the decimal point in the **dividend** (number being divided). When a number is being divided by a decimal number, the decimal point in the divisor must be moved to the right as many places as needed to make the divisor a whole number. The decimal point in the dividend must be moved the same number of places to the right. The decimal point in the quotient is placed directly above the new position of the decimal point in the dividend.

Example

$$1{:}3.25 \div 0.5$$

To divide decimal numbers, convert the divisor to a whole number. Move the decimal point in the dividend the same number of places to the right:

$$3.25 \div 0.5$$

Place the decimal point in the quotient directly above its new position in the dividend:

$$32.5 \div 0.5$$

Perform the calculation:

$$\frac{32.5}{5} = 6.5$$

Adding Decimals

To add decimals, the decimals are written in a column, with the decimal points placed directly under each other. Then, the numbers are added as in the addition of whole numbers, and the decimal point is placed in the sum directly under the decimal points in the addends.

Example 1

$$0.8 + 0.0 = \begin{array}{r} 0.8 \\ \underline{0.9} \\ 1.7 \end{array}$$

Example 2

$$0.9 + 0.03 + 2 = \begin{array}{r} 0.90 \\ 0.03 \\ \underline{2.00} \\ 2.93. \end{array}$$

Subtracting Decimals

To subtract decimals, the decimals are written in columns, keeping the decimal points under each other. Then, they are subtracted as with whole numbers (zeros may be added after the decimal without changing the value), and the decimal point is placed in the remainder, directly under the decimal point in the subtrahend and minuend.

Example 1

$$0.10 - 0.423 = \begin{array}{r} 0.800 \\ \underline{-\ 0.423} \\ 0.377 \end{array}$$

Example 2

$$0.7 - 0.239 = \begin{array}{r} 0.700 \\ \underline{-\ 0.239} \\ 0.461 \end{array}$$

RATIOS

A **ratio** is a mathematical expression that compares two numbers by division. It is used to indicate the relationship of one part of a quantity to the whole. When written, the two quantities are separated by a colon (:). The use of the colon is a traditional way to write the division sign within a ratio and is expressed as "3 is to 7."

Example 1

$\frac{3}{7}$ may be expressed as a ratio: 3:7

Example 2

1:150 may be expressed as a fraction: $\frac{1}{150}$

PROPORTIONS

A **proportion** shows the relationship between two equal ratios. A proportion may be expressed as

$$4:8 :: 1:2$$

or

$$4:8 = 1:2$$

where, in the first case, (::) is read as "so as." Thus, 4 is to 8 so as 1 is to 2. These are equal because multiplying 1 and 2 by 4 will result in 4 and 8, respectively. In a proportion, the terms have names. The **extremes** are the two outside terms, and the **means** are the two inside terms. This relationship is shown in Figure 34-3. In a proportion, the product of means is equal to the product of extremes.

Most of the time we know only three terms of a proportion. The term we do not know is the *unknown*, and in this book it is labeled *X*. To solve unknown proportion terms, first, the extremes and the means are multiplied. Their products are set as equal. Then, both sides of the equation are divided by the number to the left of *X*.

Example 1

$$2:4 = X:10$$
$$4X = 2 \times 10$$
$$4X = 20$$
$$X = \frac{20}{4} = 5$$

Example 2

$$\frac{1}{2}:X = 1:8$$

$$1X = 4(8 \times \frac{1}{2})$$

$$X = \frac{4}{1} = 4$$

Terms
Means ? ? 2 : 4 : : 8 : 16 ? Proportion ? ? Extremes

Figure 34-3. Expression of proportions.

PERCENTAGES

The term **percent** and its symbol % mean hundredths. A percent number is a fraction whose numerator is expressed and whose denominator is understood to be 100. It can be changed to a decimal by moving the decimal point two places to the left to signify hundredths or to a fraction by expressing the denominator as 100.

Example 1

7% means 7/100 or 0.07

Example 2

$$\frac{1}{5}\% \text{ means } \frac{1/5}{100} \text{ or } 0.0025$$

When the percentage is unknown, you can use the formula of X.

Example 3

What percent of 10 ounces is 3 ounces? You are looking for a percentage in this case:

$$3 = X \times 10$$
$$3 = 10X \text{ or } 10X = 3$$
$$X \text{ divided by } 10 = 3 \text{ divided by } 10$$
$$X = \frac{3}{10} \text{ or } X = 30\%$$

REVIEW QUESTIONS

1. Which of the following defines how to multiply fractions?
A. Find the least common denominator and then add
B. Multiply numerators by numerators and denominators by denominators
C. Multiply numerators by denominators and denominators by numerators
D. Do not worry about how; just use a calculator

2. Rate per hundred means
A. variation.
B. decimal.
C. density.
D. percentage.

3. Which of the following Arabic numerals is expressed by the letter "C" in the Roman system?
A. 100
B. 1000
C. 10
D. 5

4. When dividing two fractions, it is necessary to
A. divide the numerators first and then divide the denominators.
B. invert the divisor and then multiply.
C. divide the denominators and then divide the numerators.
D. None of the above

Continues

5. In order to add or subtract two fractions, one must
A. add/subtract the numerator and denominator.
B. keep the numerator the same and add/subtract the denominators.
C. invert one fraction and then add/subtract.
D. find a common denominator first.

6. The Roman numeral that stands for 29 is which of the following?
A. XXIX
B. IIIX
C. XXVIIII
D. IXXX

7. The mixed fraction for 6 and $^{2}/_{3}$ is which of the following?
A. $^{11}/_{3}$
B. $^{20}/_{6}$
C. $^{20}/_{3}$
D. $^{55}/_{3}$

8. If you were to multiply the fractions $^{6}/_{7}$ and $^{3}/_{5}$, which of the following would be the answer?
A. $^{30}/_{21}$ (or 1 and $^{3}/_{7}$)
B. $^{18}/_{35}$
C. $^{42}/_{15}$ (or 2 and $^{4}/_{5}$)
D. $^{21}/_{30}$

9. If you divided $^{1}/_{4}$ by $^{2}/_{16}$, what would the answer be?
A. 2
B. 4
C. $^{2}/_{64}$ (or $^{1}/_{32}$)
D. 3 and $^{1}/_{4}$

10. 5:12 = X:8. What does X stand for?
A. 1.33
B. 3.00
C. 2.65
D. 3.33

Measurement Systems

35

OUTLINE

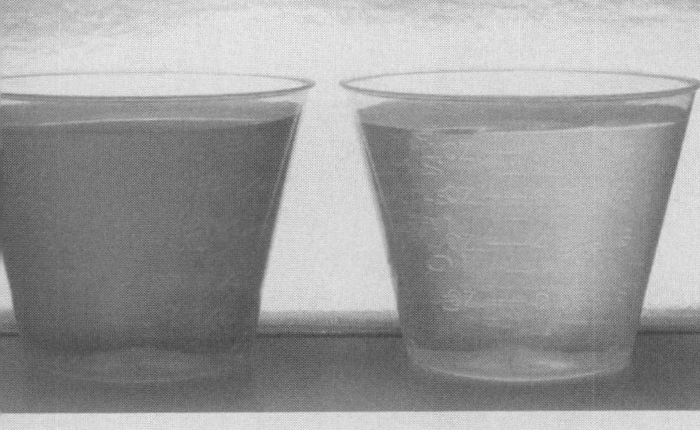

GLOSSARY

dram A unit of weight in the apothecary system; 1 dram equals 60 grains.
grain The basic unit of weight in the apothecary system.
gram The basic unit of weight in the metric system.
liter The basic unit of volume in the metric system.
meter The basic unit of length in the metric system.
minim The basic unit of volume in the apothecary system.
ounce A unit of weight in the apothecary system; 1 ounce equals 8 drams.

MEASUREMENT SYSTEMS

Most medications and measurements used in the health care field are calibrated and calculated using the metric system. Whereas some medications are still prescribed in apothecary and household terms, health care workers will find that the majority of medication calculation and administration skills involve *accurate* use of the metric system. Pharmacy technicians must have a complete knowledge of the weights and measures used in the prescription and administration of medications. Three systems are used by health professionals: metric, household, and apothecary. It is essential for pharmacists and technicians to be familiar with each system and to be able to convert from one system to another.

THE METRIC SYSTEM

This system of measure was introduced in France in the late eighteenth century. Its use in the United States was legalized in 1866. By an Act of Congress in 1893, it became our legal standard of measure, and all other systems refer to it for official comparison. It is now the standard for scientific and industrial use and measurements. The metric system is used in approximately 90% of the world's developed countries. Today, the metric system is the system of choice when one deals with the weights and measures involved in the calculation of drug dosages. Its accuracy and simplicity is based on the decimal system. The use of decimals can eliminate errors in measuring medications. The three basic units of the metric system are the following:

1. **Gram**: the basic unit for weight
2. **Liter**: the basic unit for volume
3. **Meter**: the basic unit for length

Parts of these basic units are named by adding a prefix. Each prefix has a numerical value, which is shown in Table 35-1. It is also important that pharmacy technicians be familiar with common metric abbreviations, which are shown in Table 35-2.

TABLE 35-1. Metric Prefixes

PREFIX		VALUE
nano (n)	=	$^1/_{1,000,000,000}$ (one-billionth of basic unit)
micro (mc)	=	$^1/_{1,000,000}$ (one-millionth of basic unit)
milli (m)	=	$^1/_{1000}$ (one-thousandth of basic unit)
centi (c)	=	$^1/_{100}$ (one-hundredth of basic unit)
deci (d)	=	$^1/_{10}$ (one-tenth of basic unit)
kilo (k)	=	1000 (one thousand times basic unit)

Gram

The gram is the basic unit of weight in the metric system. Some medications are ordered as fractions of grams. The milligram is 1000 times smaller than a gram; medications may be ordered in milligrams. Table 35-3 shows values of the gram.

Liter

The liter (L) is the basic unit of volume used to measure liquids in the metric system. It is equal to 1000 cubic centimeters (cc) of water. One cubic centimeter is equivalent to 1 milliliter (mL); thus, 1 L = 1000 mL.

Meter

The meter is used for linear (length) measurements. Linear measurements (meter and centimeter) are commonly used to measure the height of an individual and to determine growth patterns and is not used in the calculation of doses. Therefore, only the units of weight and volume are discussed in this chapter.

HOUSEHOLD MEASUREMENTS

Household measurements are not accurate enough for health care professionals to use in the calculation of drug dosages in the hospital or pharmacy. This system, however, is still in use for doses given primarily at home, as indicated by the name. The household system is the least accurate of the three systems of measure. Capacities of utensils such as teaspoons, tablespoons, and cups vary from one house to

TABLE 35-2. Common Metric Abbreviations

nanogram	ng	liter	L
microgram	mcg	millimeter	mm
milligram	mg	centimeter	cm
kilogram	kg	meter	m
milliliter	mL	kilometer	km
deciliter	dL		

TABLE 35-3. Gram Values

GRAM		VALUE
1000 grams (g)	=	1 kilogram (kg)
1000 milligrams (mg)	=	1 gram
1000 nanograms (ng)	=	1 microgram (mcg)
1000 microgram	=	1 milligram

another. Table 35-4 shows a list of approximate equivalents between the metric and household measurement systems.

THE APOTHECARY SYSTEM

The apothecary system is also called the wine measure or United States liquid measure system. This system is a very old English system. It has slowly been replaced by the metric system. There are few units of measure in this system that are used for medication administration. In the following paragraphs, some basic units for weight and volume in the apothecary system are discussed.

Weight

The basic unit for weight is the **grain**. The abbreviation for grain is gr. **Dram** is also a unit of weight; 1 dram is equal to 60 grains. The dram is usually abbreviated as dr. **Ounces** are larger than drams; 1 ounce is equal to 8 drams. The ounce is usually abbreviated as oz.

Volume

The basic unit for volume is the **minim**. The abbreviation for minim is a lower case letter "m." A minim is extremely small, perhaps the size of 1 drop. Volume can also be measured by drams and ounces. In summary, the units of the apothecary system are as follows:

Weight:	grain (gr)
	dram (dr)
	ounce (oz)
Volume:	minim (m)

CONVERTING WITHIN AND BETWEEN SYSTEMS

In pharmacy and medicine, use of the metric system currently predominates over that of the other commonly used systems. Most prescriptions and medication orders are written in the metric system, and labeling on most prepackaged pharmaceutical products shows drug strengths and dosages described in metric units, replacing to a great extent the use of the other systems of measurement. Medications are usually ordered in a unit of weight measurement such as grams or grains. Pharmacy technicians must be able to convert and calculate the correct dosage of drugs. The technician can convert between units of measurement within the same system or convert units of measurement from one system to another. He or she must also interpret the order and administer the correct number of tablets, capsules, tablespoons, milligrams, or milliliters.

TABLE 35-4. Metric and Household Measurement Equivalents

METRIC MEASURE		HOUSEHOLD MEASURE
1 milliliter (mL)	=	15 drops (gtt)
5 milliliters	=	1 teaspoon (tsp)
15 milliliters	=	1 tablespoon (tbsp)
180 milliliters	=	1 cup (c)
240 milliliters	=	1 glass
1 kilogram (kg) or 1000 grams (g)	=	2.2 pounds (lb)
2.5 centimeters (cm)	=	1 inch

Conversion of Weights

To convert units of weight, one must remember that 1000 mg = 1 g and that 1000 micrograms (mcg) = 1 mg. To convert grams to milligrams, always multiply by 1000 or move the decimal point 3 places to the right.

Example

2 g = 2000. mg
0.2 g = 200. mg
0.02 g = 020. mg

Alternatively, to convert milligrams to grams, divide by 1000 or move the decimal point 3 places to the left.

Example

250 mg = 0.250 g
50 mg = 0.050 g
5 mg = 0.005 g

To convert milligrams to micrograms, multiply by 1000 or move the decimal point 3 places to the right.

Example

3 mg = 3000. mcg
0.5 mg = 500. Mcg
0.08 mg = 080. mcg

To convert micrograms to milligrams, divide by 1000 or move the decimal point 3 places to the left.

Example

1,500 mcg = 1.500 mg
600 mcg = 0.600 mg
20 mcg = 0.020 mg

The microgram, milligram, and gram are the most commonly used measurements in medication administration. Tablets and capsules are most often supplied in milligrams. Antibiotics can be provided in grams, milligrams, or units. For small dosages or for very powerful drugs in pediatric and critical care patients, micrograms are used.

Conversion of Liquids

To convert and calculate the correct dosage of liquid medications, remember the units of the metric system for volume.

Example

Convert 0.02 L to mL:

Equivalent: 1 L = 1000 mL
Conversion factor is 1000

Multiply by 1000: 0.02 L = 0.02 × 1000 = 20 mL, or move decimal point 3 places to the right: 0.02 L = 0.020. = 20 mL.

To convert milliliters to liters, one must divide. Remember that the equivalent of 1 L = 1000 mL and then divide the number of milliliters by 1000.

Example

Convert 3000 mL to L:

Equivalent: 1 L = 1000 mL
Conversion factor is 1000.

Divide by 1000: 3000 mL = 3000 ÷ 1000 = 3 L, or move decimal point 3 places to the left: 3000 mL = 3.000 = 3 L.

REVIEW QUESTIONS

1. Which of the following measurement systems was introduced in France first?
A. Household
B. Metric
C. Apothecary
D. Household and metric

2. The prefix *milli* (m) has a value of
A. $\frac{1}{1,000,000}$.
B. $\frac{1}{1000}$.
C. $\frac{1}{100}$.
D. 1000.

3. Which of the following is the basic unit of weight in the metric system?
A. Nanogram
B. Milligram
C. Kilogram
D. Gram

4. One milliliter is equivalent to how many drops?
A. 5
B. 15
C. 25
D. 50

5. Which of the following measurement systems is an Old English system?
A. Metric
B. Household
C. Apothecary
D. None of the above

6. All of the following are units of the apothecary system for weight and volume, except
A. minim.
B. dram.
C. gram.
D. grain.

7. When you convert 0.3 g to milligrams, which of the following is the correct answer?
A. 300
B. 0.003
C. 0.030
D. 0.300

8. All of the following weight values are commonly used measurements in medication administration, except
A. grain.
B. milligram.
C. microgram.
D. gram.

9. If the equivalent of 1 L is 1000 mL and the conversion factor is 1000, which of the following conversions of 0.02 L is the correct answer?
A. 2 mL
B. 0.2 mL
C. 20 mL
D. 200 mL

10. A patient should drink 48 oz of fluid every day. How many cups should the patient be advised to drink each day?
A. 2
B. 4
C. 6
D. 8

11. A pharmacy technician tells a patient to drink a pint of juice. How many ounces will the patient need to drink to equal a pint?
A. 6
B. 12
C. 16
D. 24

Continues

12. Approximately how many pounds is 79 kg equivalent to?
A. 198.8 lb
B. 173.8 lb
C. 163.8 lb
D. 143.8 lb

13. How many glasses is 360 mL of fluid equivalent to?
A. ½ glass
B. 1 glass
C. 1½ glasses
D. 2 glasses

14. How many milligrams is 400 grams equivalent to?
A. 40
B. 4,000
C. 40,000
D. 400,000

15. How many drops is 12 mL equivalent to?
A. 192 gtt
B. 180 gtt
C. 142 gtt
D. 135 gtt

16. How many mL is equivalent to four glasses of water?
A. 860 mL
B. 898 mL
C. 960 mL
D. 998 mL

17. How many teaspoons is equivalent to 45 mL?
A. 9
B. 7
C. 3
D. 2

18. How many milliliters is 16 tablespoons equivalent to?
A. 276
B. 256
C. 240
D. 126

19. How many grams is 529 mg equivalent to?
A. 5.29 g
B. 0.529 g
C. 0.029 g
D. 52.9 g

20. How many milligrams is 8.92 kg equivalent to?
A. 8,920 mg
B. 80,920 mg
C. 800,920 mg
D. 8,920,000 mg

21. How many qt are in 4 gal?
A. 4 qt
B. 8 qt
C. 12 qt
D. 16 qt

22. How many mL are equivalent to two glasses?
A. 240
B. 280
C. 380
D. 480

23. How many pounds is equivalent to 100kg?
A. 120 lb
B. 160 lb
C. 220 lb
D. 260 lb

24. How many milliliters is equivalent to five cups?
A. 500 mL
B. 600 mL
C. 700 mL
D. 900 mL

25. How many milliliters is equivalent to one quart?
A. 250 mL
B. 500 mL
C. 800 mL
D. 1000 mL

26. How many gallons is equivalent to four qt?
A. 1 gal
B. 2 gal
C. 3 gal
D. 4 gal

27. How many milligrams is equivalent to one grain?
A. 20
B. 30
C. 50
D. 60

28. How many centimeters is equal to one inch?
A. 1.54
B. 2.54
C. 2.84
D. 3.84

29. How many cubic centimeters (cc) is equivalent to one mL?
A. 1
B. 2
C. 3
D. 4

30. How many qt is equivalent to 750 mL?
A. ½ qt
B. ¾ qt
C. 1½ qt
D. 1¾ qt

Calculation of Dosages 36

OUTLINE

Calculation of Dosages
Calculation of Oral Drugs
- Dosing of Tablets and Capsules
- Dosing of Oral Liquids

Calculation of Parenteral Drugs
- Drug Dosage in Standardized Units
- Dosing of Intravenous Medications
- Dosing of Total Parenteral Nutrition

Pediatric Dosage Calculations
- Clark's Rule
- Young's Rule
- Fried's Rule

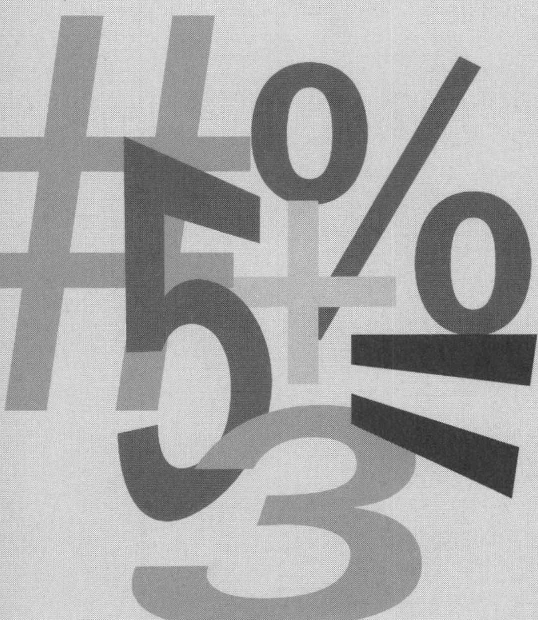

GLOSSARY

drop rate The number of drops at which an intravenous infusion is administered over a specified period of time.

meniscus The dip in fluid level when an oral liquid medication is dispensed.

CALCULATION OF DOSAGES

The common practice in hospitals today is for the pharmacist to calculate and prepare the drug dosage form for administration to the patient. Most of the time, the drug is provided in a unit-dose package. However, pharmacy technicians must understand the concept of calculating medication dosages that patients receive. Learning to correctly calculate drug dosages is an extremely important skill, because it can often be the difference between life and death for the patient. Calculating incorrect dosages could result in undertreatment with the patient's condition not improving or even worsening or an overdose that causes the patient harm. The ability to calculate drug dosages is a skill that should not be taken lightly. In fact, all health care professionals who deal with the preparation and/or administration of medications should aim for 100% success in performing this task. Recall the seven rights of drug administration discussed in Chapter 5: right patient, right drug, right dose, right time, right route, right technique, and right documentation.

The use of calculators is recommended for complex calculations of dosages to ensure accuracy and save time. These types of calculations require basic math skills to use calculators properly.

CALCULATION OF ORAL DRUGS

There are a variety of forms of drugs that are commonly administered orally. Medications administered by mouth may be solid or liquid. Solid-form drugs are generally intended to be given as a whole to achieve a specific effect in the body.

Dosing of Tablets and Capsules

Tablets and capsules are solid medications that are supplied in different strengths or dosages. Their dosages can be expressed in apothecary or metric measures, for example, grains or milligrams.

Converting drug measures from one system to another and from one unit to another to determine the dosage to be administered can result in discrepancies, depending on the conversion factor used. For example, one must remember the following:

- The label for Tylenol® may indicate 325 mg (5 grains). This is based on the equivalent 65 mg = 1 gr. On the other hand, the label for aspirin may indicate 300 mg (5 grains). Here the equivalent 60 mg = 1 gr was used. Both of the equivalents are correct. *Remember that equivalents are not exact.* Use the common equivalents when making conversions, for example, 60 mg = 1 gr.
- If the precise number of tablets or capsules is determined and administering the amount calculated is unrealistic or impossible, always use the following rule to avoid an error in administration: *No more than 10% variation should exist between the dose ordered and the dose administered.* For example, one may determine that a patient should receive 0.9 tablet or 0.9 capsule. Administration of such an amount accurately would be impossible. In this case, 1 tablet or 1 capsule could be safely administered.
- Capsules are not scored and cannot be divided. They are administered in whole amounts only. Never crush or open a timed-release capsule or empty its contents into a liquid or food.
- In the calculation of oral doses, measures other than apothecary or metric may be encountered. For example, with electrolytes such as potassium the number of milliequivalents (mEq) per tablet will be indicated. Another measure that may be seen for oral antibiotics or vitamins is units. For example, the label for vitamin E capsules will indicate 400 U per capsule. Units and milliequivalent measurements are specific to the drugs they are being used for. There is no conversion between these and apothecary or metric measures.

Dosing of Oral Liquids

Liquid medications include elixirs, syrups, tinctures, and suspensions. Certain liquid drugs are irritating to the stomach mucosa and must be well diluted before administration. An example is potassium chloride (KCl). Tincture medications are always diluted. Any liquid medication that may cause discoloration of the teeth should be diluted and taken through a drinking straw. In general, liquid cough medicines are not diluted. Liquid medications contain a specific amount of drug in a given amount of solution. Figure 36-1A and B show the labels of solutions.

When a liquid medication is measured, hold the transparent measuring device at eye level. The liquid curve in the center is called the **meniscus**. All liquid medication is measured at the meniscus level (see Figure 36-2).

For medications in liquid form, calculate the volume of the liquid that contains the ordered dosage of the medication. The label of drugs bottled may indicate the amount of drug per 1 mL or per multiple milliliters of solution, for example, 20 mg/5 mL, 250 mg/5 mL, or 1.4 g/30 mL. Liquid drugs must be calculated with the formula:

$$\frac{D}{H} \times V = X$$

In this formula, *D* represents the desired dosage or the dosage ordered. *H* represents the dosage you have on hand per a quantity. *V* represents the volume of the drug.

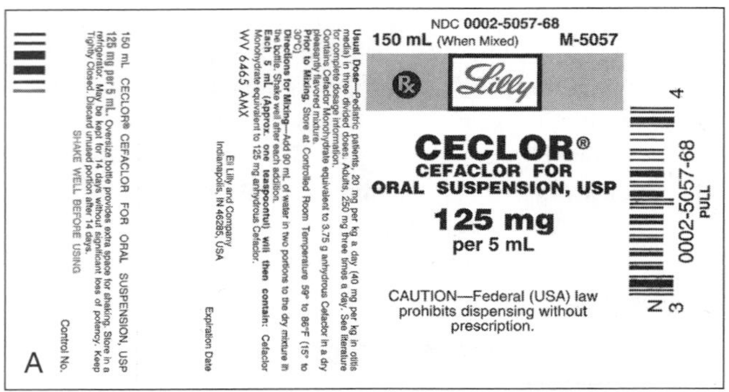

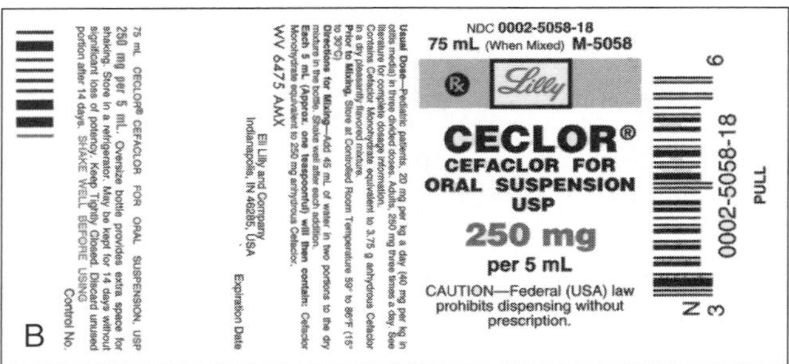

Figure 36-1. Labels typically found on an oral liquid. (Courtesy of Eli Lilly and Company.)

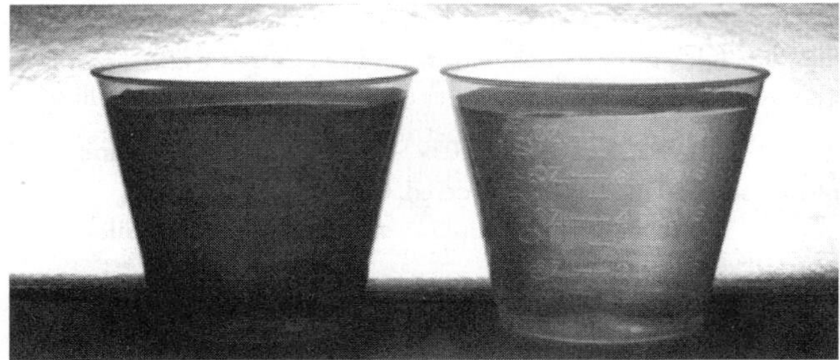

Figure 36-2. Measure oral liquids by the level of the meniscus.

Example 1

A prescription is written to give 4 mL of ampicillin with a dosage strength of 125 mg/5 mL. The following formula is used:

$$\frac{D}{H} \times V = \frac{100 \text{ mg}}{125 \text{ mg}} \times 5 \text{ mL} = X$$

$$\frac{4}{5} \times 5 \text{ mL} = \frac{20}{5} \text{ mL} = 4 \text{ mL}$$

Example 2

A prescription is written to give 100 mg of ampicillin. The medication is available with a dosage strength of 250 mg/5 mL. The following formula is used:

$$\frac{D}{H} \times V = \frac{100 \text{ mg}}{250 \text{ mg}} \times 5 \text{ mL} = X$$

$$\frac{2}{5} \times 5 \text{ mL} = \frac{10}{5} = 2 \text{ mL}$$

CALCULATION OF PARENTERAL DRUGS

Medications administered by injection can be given intradermally (within the skin), subcutaneously (SC, into fatty tissue or under the skin), intramuscularly (IM, into the muscle), and intravenously (IV, into the vein). Injectable drugs are ordered in grams, milligrams, micrograms, grains, or units. The preparations of injectable drugs may be packaged in a solvent (diluent or solution) or in a powdered form. Intramuscular injection is a common method of administering injectable drugs. The volume of solution for an intramuscular injection is 0.5 to 3.0 mL, with the average being 1 to 2 mL. A volume of drug solution greater than 3 mL causes increased muscle tissue displacement and possible tissue damage. Occasionally, 5 mL of certain drugs, such as magnesium sulfate or immunoglobulin (given after exposure to rabies), may be injected in a large muscle, such as the dorsogluteal. Dosages greater than 3 mL are usually divided and given at two different sites. Drug solutions for injection are commercially premixed and stored in vials and ampules for immediate use. At times there may be enough drug solution left in a vial for another dose, and the vial may be saved. The balance of a drug solution in an ampule is always discarded after the ampule has been opened and used. For calculating intramuscular dosage, the following example can be used.

Example 1

An order is given for gentamicin 60 mg IM. The available dosage strength of gentamicin is 80 mg/2 mL in a vial. The following formula is used:

$$\frac{D}{H} \times V = \frac{60}{80} \times 2 = \frac{120}{80} = 1.5 \text{ mL}$$

or

$$
\begin{aligned}
&H{:}V{::}D{:}X \\
&= 80 \text{ mg}{:}2 \text{ mL}{::}60 \text{ mg}{:}X \text{ mL} \\
&= 80X = 120 \\
X &= \frac{120}{80} = 1.5 \text{ mL}
\end{aligned}
$$

Example 2

The physician's order is for atropine 0.2 mg SC stat. The drug is available at a dosage of 400 mcg/mL (0.4 mg/mL). The following formula is used:

$$\frac{H}{D} \times V = \frac{0.2 \text{ mg}}{0.4 \text{ mg}} \times 1 \text{ mL} = \frac{0.2}{0.4} \times 1 = 0.5 \text{ mL}$$

Drug Dosage in Standardized Units

Several drugs that are obtained from animal sources can be standardized in units according to their strengths rather than on weight measures such as milligrams and grams. Some hormones such as insulin are too complex to be completely purified to obtain the exact weight of the drug per unit of volume. Therefore, insulin and many other drugs are measured in units for parenteral administration. The labels of such medications indicate how many units are needed per milliliter.

Insulin Dosage

Insulin orders must be written clearly and contain specific information to prevent errors. The order for insulin should include the brand name, supply dosage, number of units to be given, and the route and time or frequency of administration.

Example

An order is given for Humulin R Regular U-100®, 14 U SC stat or for Iletin 11 NPH U-100® 24 U SC ½ hour after breakfast.

Insulin is supplied in 10-mL vials labeled with the number of units per milliliter; thus, 100-U insulin means there are 100 U/cc. In the past, insulin was administered in 40- and 80-U dosage forms. Today, however, the 100-U form has almost totally replaced the weaker strength forms. The smaller volume required per dose decreases local reactions at the injection site, as well as simplifying mathematical calculations. The simplest and most accurate method to measure insulin is within an insulin syringe. The syringe is calibrated in units, and the desired dose may be read directly on the syringe. Figure 36-3A and B shows both sides of a standard U-100 syringe with Novalin®.

If an insulin syringe is not available, a tuberculin syringe may be used, and the unit dosage may be converted to the equivalent number of cubic centimeters, using the proportion method.

Example

Give 40 units of insulin, using 100-U insulin and a tuberculin syringe. The amount administered is calculated as follows:

$$\frac{40}{100} \times 1 \text{ mL} = 0.4 \text{ mL}$$

Heparin Dosage

Heparin is also derived from animal sources and is standardized for its activity as an anticoagulant. It is obtained in unit-dose or multiple-dose vials and in strengths ranging from 10 to 20,000 U/mL. There is often no set dose for the use of heparin; the patient's requirements are obtained from blood clotting studies done initially every 4 hours. Heparin is often given intravenously to produce a rapid effect and then is given in deep subcutaneous injections in larger and more infrequent doses. The normal adult heparin dosage is 20,000 to 40,000 U every 24 hours. When given IV, heparin is ordered in units per hour. Heparin is available in different strengths; therefore, it is important to read labels carefully when it must be administered.

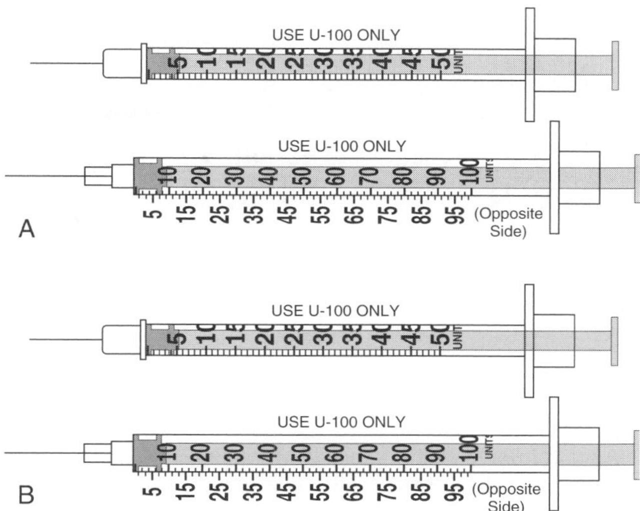

Figure 36-3. Units found on insulin syringes.

Example 1

A physician's order is for heparin 7,500 U SC. Heparin is available in a dosage of 10,000 U/mL (see Figure 36-4). The amount administered is calculated as follows:

$$10{,}000 \text{ U} = 1 \text{ mL} = 7{,}500 \text{ U}:X \text{ mL}$$
$$10{,}000X = 7{,}500$$
$$X = \frac{7{,}500}{10{,}000}$$
$$X = 0.75 \text{ mL}$$

Example 2

A physician's order is for D5W (5% dextrose in water) 1000 mL containing 20,000 U of heparin, which is to be infused at 30 mL/hr. The dose of heparin the patient is to receive per hour is

$$20{,}000 \text{ U}:1{,}000 \text{ mL} = X \text{ U}:30 \text{ mL}$$
$$1{,}000X = 20{,}000 \times 30$$
$$\frac{1{,}000X}{1{,}000} = \frac{60{,}000}{1{,}000} = 600 \text{ U/hr}$$

Antibiotic Dosage

The dosages of many antibiotics are still standardized in units. These may be prepared for injection in the form of a liquid containing a specified number of units per cubic centimeter. Antibiotics are also available in the form of a dry powder in a vial that must first be diluted with water or another diluent. The powder should be diluted so that the desired dose is in 1- or 2-cc (mL) amounts if the dose is to be given IM. If it is to be given IV, a larger amount of diluent may be used.

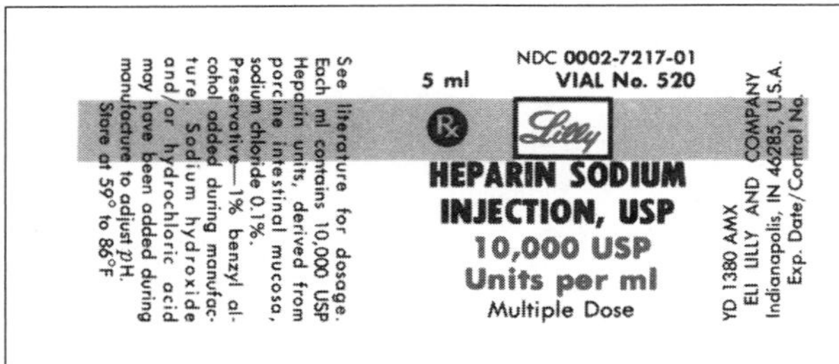

Figure 36-4. Heparin label. (Courtesy of Eli Lilly and Company.)

Example

A vial of powdered penicillin G contains 1,000,000 units. The amount of diluent to be added to obtain a solution containing 100,000 U/mL is

$$100{,}000{:}1\text{ mL} = 1{,}000{,}000{:}X\text{ mL}$$

$$100{,}000X = 1{,}000{,}000 \times 1$$

$$X = \frac{1{,}000{,}000}{100{,}000}$$

$$X = 10\text{ mL}$$

Dosing of Intravenous Medications

The term *intravenous* literally means "within a vein." Intravenous infusion is the slow introduction of a substance such as a solution, whole blood, plasma, or antibiotics into a vein. Intravenous solutions fall into four functional categories: replacement fluids, maintenance fluids, therapeutic fluids, and agents to keep the vein open. If the patient is dehydrated and unable to eat or drink or if he or she has lost blood, replacement fluids are ordered. Maintenance fluids help patients maintain normal electrolyte and fluid balances. Therapeutic fluids deliver medication to the patient. Some intravenous lines provide access to the vein for emergency situations. Fluids prescribed to keep the vein open include 5% dextrose in water. Thus, the pharmacy technician must learn how to effectively calculate infusion rates and the administration of these agents.

Intravenous Solution Concentrations

Solutions may have different concentrations of dextrose (glucose) or saline (sodium chloride). For example, 5% dextrose contains 5 g of dextrose per 100 mL. Figure 36-5 shows a label for a 5% dextrose solution.

Normal saline is 0.9% saline; it contains 900 mg, or 0.9 g, of sodium chloride per 100 mL (see Figure 36-6).

Equipment for Intravenous Infusion

Equipment used to administer intravenous medications is available in several forms. They are either completely manual or electronic.

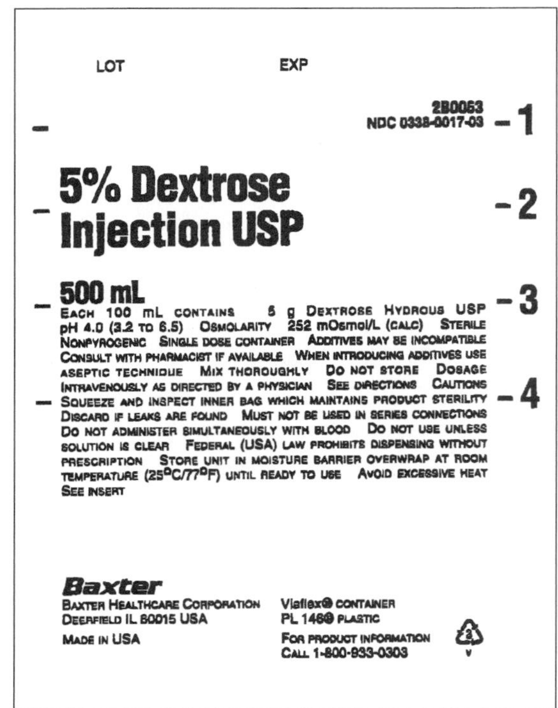

Figure 36-5. Label for 5% dextrose. (Courtesy of Baxter.)

The primary intravenous line may consist of a bag or bottle of solution and tubing. Bags for intravenous infusion come in different sizes. The solution of fluid to be infused is often 500 or 1000 cc (mL). The tubing, which is the primary line, usually includes a drip chamber, roller clamp, and injection ports (see Figure 36-7).

To measure the flow rate, the drip chamber must be squeezed until it is half full, making it easier to appropriately count the number of drops falling into the chamber. The roller clamp is used to adjust the speed of the infusion either up or down, as needed. The injection port is available to inject medications into the primary line or to attach a second intravenous line. There are two sizes of tubing available: macrodrop and microdrop. Macrodrop tubing is used for fluids infused at a higher rate, for example, infusions that are set at 80 mL/hr or higher. Microdrop tubing is used for slower infusions for which accuracy of dosage delivery is essential, such as in the critical care or pediatric settings.

Monitoring the Intravenous Infusion

The infusion of intravenous fluids is monitored in many different ways. Most times, for manual monitoring the bag containing the intravenous solution is hung 36 inches above the patient's heart so that gravity will draw the fluid into the patient. When the infusion is monitored, the roller clamp is used to adjust the rate of delivery. Another method of monitoring is the use of an electronic infusion pump, which applies a set amount of pressure so that a set volume is infused over a set time period (see Figure 36-8). The flow rate is generally programmed

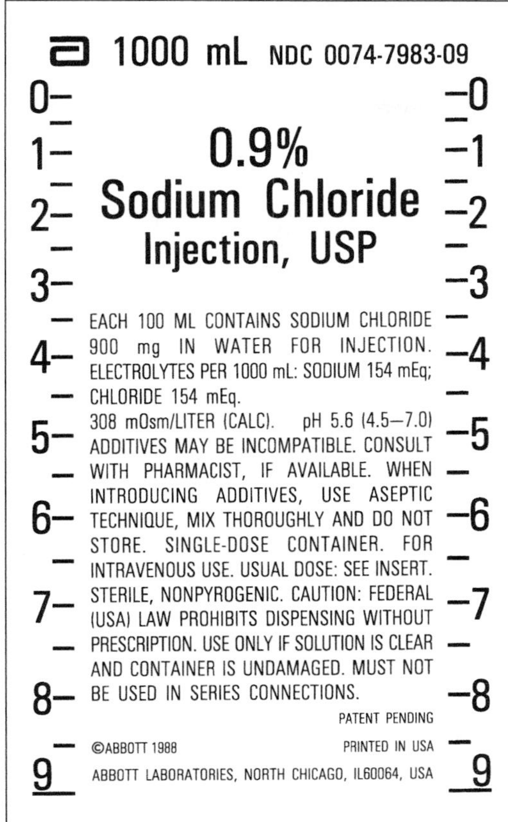

Figure 36-6. Label for 0.9% sodium chloride. (Courtesy of Abbott Laboratories.)

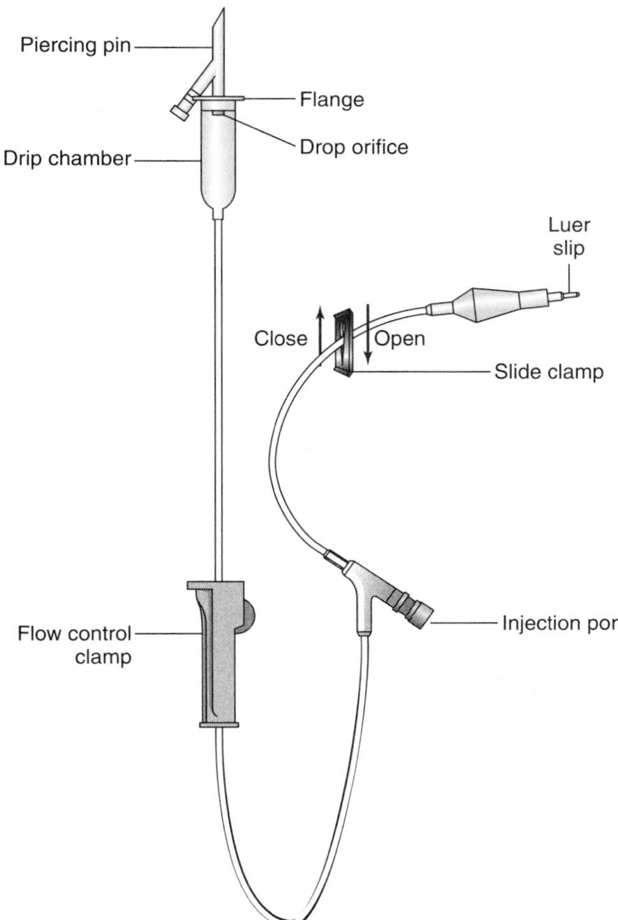

Figure 36-7. Primary administration set.

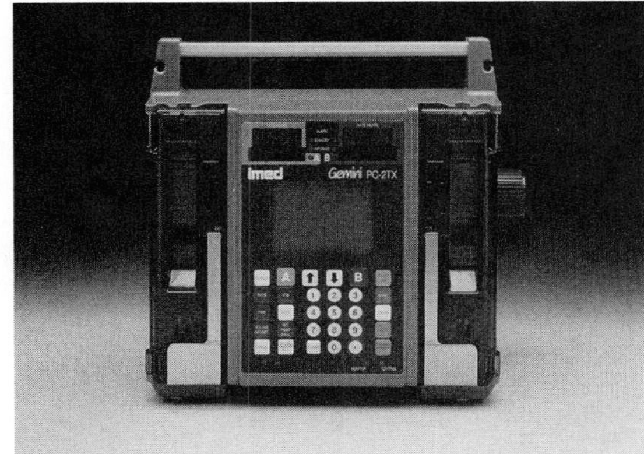

Figure 36-8. Electric infusion pump. (Courtesy of Alaris Medical System.)

into the device in milliliters per hour. The pumps do not rely on gravity but rather on pressure that the pump creates to force the solution through the tubing and into the patient's vascular system. Most electronic pumps are armed with sensors that sound when the bag of solution is empty or if the rate cannot be properly maintained. Despite advances in technology, there is no substitute for a vigilant health care provider to ensure that the right patient is receiving the right medication, at the right time, and at the right infusion rate.

Calculation of Intravenous Flow Rates

A flow rate is the speed at which intravenous fluids are infused into a patient. Allowing the patient to receive a prescribed fluid too fast or too slow can result in adverse reactions. The ability of the pharmacy technician to correctly and efficiently calculate flow rates of intravenous fluids is critical to the well-being of the patient. Flow rates are generally prescribed or written as 125 mL/hr or 500 mL/2 hr, meaning that the fluids should be infused into the patient at a rate of 125 mL over a period of 1 hour or at a rate of 500 mL over a period of 2 hours, respectively. Flow rates can be regulated either by the use of an electronic pump or by manually adjusting the intravenous equipment to achieve the prescribed flow rate. When an electronic pump is used, the flow rate is calculated in milliliters per hour and can be arrived at by using the following formula:

$$\frac{\text{Total amount ordered (mL)}}{\text{Total number of hours}} = (\text{hr}) = \frac{\text{mL}}{\text{hr}}$$

After the flow rate is successfully calculated, the rate is then programmed into an electronic infusion device. For example: Jane Doe is a patient for whom a **500-mL** bag of intravenous fluids to be infused over **2 hours** has been prescribed. To calculate the flow rate, use the preceding formula:

$$\frac{\text{Total amount ordered (mL)}}{\text{Total number of hours (hr)}} = \frac{500\text{ mL}}{2\text{ hr}} = \frac{250\text{ mL}}{\text{hr}}$$

Therefore, the infusion device is programmed for 250 mL/hr. Another formula is especially helpful when flow rates that have a prescribed infusion time of ½ hour or less are calculated. For example, J.P. Ellen is a patient for whom 500 mg of an IV antibiotic in a **100-mL** bag of fluid to be infused over **30 minutes** has been prescribed. To calculate the flow rate for this patient, use the following formula (remember that 60 minutes = 1 hr):

$$\frac{\text{Total milliliters ordered}}{\text{Total hours ordered}} = \frac{X\text{(mL)}}{1\text{ hr}} \rightarrow \frac{100\text{ mL}}{30\text{ min}} = \frac{X\text{ mL}}{60\text{ min}}$$

Cross-multiply to get

$$30X = 6000$$

and then divide both sides by 30 to get

$$X = 200\ \frac{\text{mL}}{\text{hr}}$$

Thus, the electronic infusion pump should be set at 200 mL/hr for the 100-mL bag of fluid to be infused over 30 minutes.

Manually Calculating Drop Rates

The pharmacy technician may, depending on the setting, have to calculate a **drop rate** of an intravenous fluid and then manually regulate the equipment to control the speed at which the fluid is being infused. To calculate the drop rate the technician must determine how many drops (abbreviated as gtt) per minute should be infused over a prescribed time period. The number of drops per minute depends on the type of intravenous tubing used. Two types of tubing are available: standard or macrodrop and microdrop. Standard tubing has a drop factor of 10, 15, or 20 gtts/mL, whereas microdrop tubing has a drop factor of 60 gtt/mL. The drop factor is generally found on the outside packaging of the tubing. The following formula is used to calculate flow rates in drops per minute:

$$\frac{V\text{(total volume to be infused in mL)}}{T\text{(total time in minutes)}} \times C\text{(drop factor in gtt/mL)} = R\text{(rate of flow in gtt/min)}$$

or the formula can also be written as

$$\frac{V}{T} \times C = R$$

For example, John Brown is to receive **200 cc** of intravenous fluids over **2 hours**. Macrodrop tubing has been selected, which has a drop factor of **20 gtt/min**. The job of the technician is to calculate how many drops per minute are needed so that all 200 cc is infused over 30 minutes. The first step is to convert 2 hours into minutes (reminder: 1 hour = 60 minutes): 2 × 60 = 120 min. The second step is to set up the problem using the formula $V/T \times C = R$:

$$\frac{200}{120} \times 20 = 33.3\text{ gtt/min}$$

Note that the number of drops per minute needs to be rounded to the nearest whole number. In this example, round down to get 33 gtt/min. The third step is to set the drop rate by adjusting the roller clamp and counting the amount of drops per minute that fall into the drip chamber.

Many people may see the ability to adequately calculate and manually adjust drop rates to be outdated because of the improved technology available with electronic infusion pumps, which can be easily programmed. However, the opposite is true. It is important for pharmacy technicians to know the math behind what electronic pumps do because an electronic pump may not be available. In addition, emergency situations require immediate attention, and the ability to correctly determine intravenous infusion drop rates without the aid of an infusion pump is an invaluable skill.

Dosing of Total Parenteral Nutrition

Total parenteral nutrition (TPN), also called hyperalimentation, is an intravenous infusion that provides a patient with all of his or her daily nutritional requirements in the form of a liquid infusion. TPN is generally prescribed for patients who, because of their disease process or surgical intervention, are unable to eat. It includes fluids such as dextrose, electrolytes, amino acids, trace elements, and vitamins. In some cases, other substances such as fat, insulin, or other drugs can be added to the infusion. The contents of TPN are determined by the patient's individual nutritional requirements. TPN is not infused through a peripheral vein (veins in the hands and arms) but rather through a central vein such as the subclavian vein or internal jugular vein. Figure 36-9 shows veins commonly used to place central lines.

Central lines are used to deliver TPN because its higher concentration of agents, such as concentrated dextrose solutions, could potentially damage peripheral veins. In addition, central lines, once established, can be left in place long-term, whereas peripheral lines are inserted for short-term use. The contents of TPN can be changed on a daily basis as the physical and caloric needs of the patient change.

PEDIATRIC DOSAGE CALCULATIONS

Children are not able to tolerate adult doses of drugs. Dosage must be measured accurately according to the age

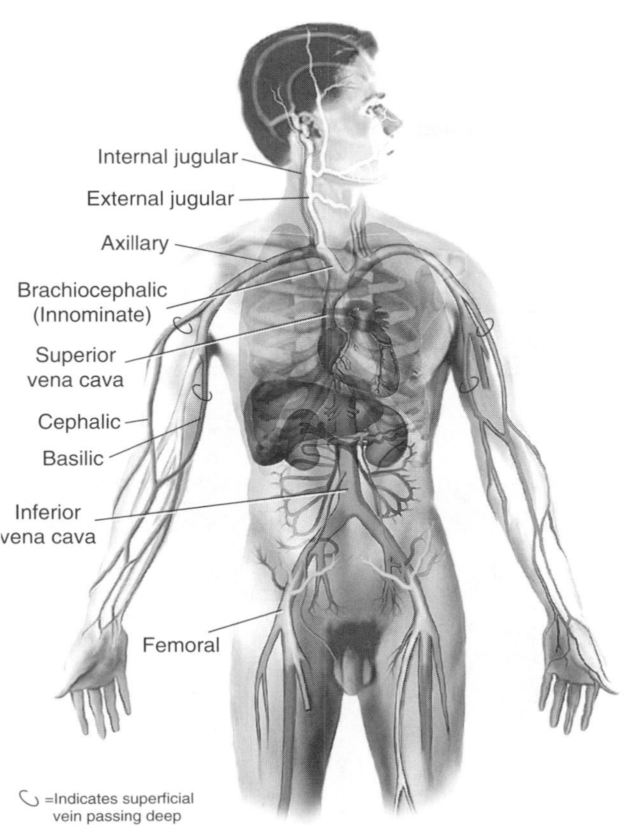

Figure 36-9. Sites for insertion of central lines.

and weight of infants and children. Several methods are used for calculating dosage for this group of patients. The dosage form per kilogram or pound of body weight is more accurate than dosage calculated by age. The body surface area method is another way to measure the dosage for children. Charts are available to determine the body surface area in square meters, according to height and weight. Many drugs are not advised for administration to children because of their potential for harmful side effects in the growing child or because they have not been sufficiently tested in children to give a recommended dosage range. Three formulas are used to calculate dosage for infants and children: Clark's rule, Young's rule, and Fried's rule.

Clark's Rule

Clark's rule is calculated as follows:

$$\frac{\text{Weight of child}}{150} \times \text{average adult dose} = \text{child's dose}$$

Example

Find the dose of cortisone for a 30-lb infant (adult dose = 100 mg). The calculation is

$$\frac{30}{150} \times 100 \text{ mg} = 20 \text{ mg}$$

Young's Rule

Young's rule is calculated as follows:

$$\frac{\text{Age of child}}{\text{Age of child} + 12} \times \text{average adult dose} = \text{child's dose}$$

Example

Find the dose of acetaminophen for a 4-year-old child (adult dose = 1000 mg). The calculation is as follows:

$$\frac{4}{4 + 12} \times 1000 \text{ mg} = \frac{4000}{16} = 250 \text{ mg}$$

Note that Young's rule is not valid after 12 years of age. If the child is small enough to warrant a reduced dose after 12 years of age, the reduction should be calculated on the basis of Clark's rule.

Fried's Rule

Fried's rule is sometimes used for calculating dosages for infants younger than 2 years of age. The formula is as follows:

$$\frac{\text{Age in months}}{150} \times \text{average adult dose} = \text{child's dose}$$

Example

Find the dose of phenobarbital for a 15-month-old infant (adult dose = 400 mg). The calculation is as follows:

$$\frac{15}{150} \times 400 \text{ mg} = 40 \text{ mg}$$

Pediatric drug dosages are calculated in three steps. For example, Amoxil® 25 mg/kg/day given every 12 hours is being ordered for a 24-lb baby. The first step in calculating the correct dosage for this baby is to convert pounds to kilograms. The conversion rule is

$$1 \text{ kg} = 2.2 \text{ lb}$$

$$1 \text{ kg}/2.2 \text{ lb} = \frac{X \text{ kg}}{24 \text{ lb}}$$

Cross-multiply this ratio:

$$2.2X = 24$$

$$X = 10.9 \text{ kg (round up to 11.0 kg)}$$

The next step is to calculate the drug dosage based on 25 mg/kg of body weight:

$$\frac{25 \text{ mg}}{1 \text{ kg}} = \frac{X \text{ mg}}{11 \text{ kg}}$$

Cross-multiply this ratio:

$$X \text{ mg} = 275$$

$$X = \frac{275 \text{ mg}}{24 \text{ hr}}$$

The third and final step is to calculate out how much Amoxil this patient receives per dose. Remember, the patient is to receive a dose once every 12 hours or 2 divided doses in one 24-hour period. The calculation is as follows:

$$\frac{275 \text{ mg}}{2} = 137.5 \text{ mg per dose}$$

Amoxil is available in 250 mg/5 mL dosages so the exact number of milliliters to give the patient per dose needs to be calculated:

$$\frac{250 \text{ mg}}{5 \text{ mL}} = \frac{137.5 \text{ mg}}{X \text{ mL}}$$

Cross-multiply this ratio:

$$250X = 687.5$$

$$\frac{687.5}{250X}$$

$$X = 2.75 \text{ mL}$$

Therefore, the patient would receive 2.75 mL of Amoxil every 12 hours.

Calculating drug dosages for the pediatric patient is not as time-consuming as it initially appears. After a technician has practiced doing several dosage calculations, he or she will soon become proficient.

REVIEW QUESTIONS

1. Learning to correctly calculate ______ ______ is extremely important because it can often be the difference between life and death.
A. unit doses
B. common practices
C. digital timings
D. drug dosages

2. Oral medications may be solid or
A. liquid.
B. ointment.
C. IM.
D. SC.

3. All of the following are formulas used to calculate drug dosage for infants and children except
A. Clark's rule.
B. Fried's rule.
C. Franklin's rule.
D. Young's rule.

4. Oral liquid drugs and medications include
A. suspensions, tinctures, intravenous infusions, and elixirs.
B. elixirs, stirrups, tinctures, and sublinguals.
C. elixirs, syrups, tinctures, and suspensions.
D. none of the above.

5. The liquid curve in the center of a transparent device (used for measuring liquid medications) is called the
A. meniscus.
B. menstruiscus.
C. liquiscus.
D. curve.

6. In the formula $\frac{D}{H} \times V = X$, what does the D stand for?
A. Diuretic
B. Drug
C. Desired dosage
D. Drop

7. Parenteral medications can be given in all of the following ways, except
A. intradermally.
B. intravenously.
C. subcutaneously.
D. interocularly.

8. The balance of a drug solution in an ampule is always ______ after the ampule has been opened and used.
A. poured into another ampule for reuse later
B. discarded
C. tested
D. reordered

9. Insulin and many other drugs are measured in ______ for parenteral administration.
A. units
B. ampules
C. milliliters
D. cubic centimeters

10. The most popular syringe for insulin administration holds which amount?
A. 10 U
B. 100 U
C. 40 U
D. 80 U

11. To determine how much heparin a patient needs, blood clotting studies are initially done every
A. 14 hours.
B. 4 days.
C. 4 hours.
D. 40 minutes.

12. Antibiotics are available in the form of a liquid and a/an ______ that must be diluted.
A. elixir
B. suspension
C. grain
D. powder

Continues

13. Normal saline is ______% saline. It contains 900 mg of sodium.
A. 0.9
B. 90
C. 9.09
D. 10

14. Two sizes of intravenous tubing are available, which are called
A. minidrop and maxidrop.
B. monodrip and multidrip.
C. macrodrop and microdrop.
D. medidrop and minidrop.

15. A flow rate is the speed at which
A. sodium is infused into the patient.
B. intravenous fluids are infused into the patient.
C. blood is drawn from the patient.
D. sodium is drawn from the patient's blood.

16. To calculate flow rate, one formula requires dividing the total amount ordered (in milliliters) by
A. total number of drops.
B. total number of minutes.
C. total number of hours.
D. total number of days.

17. A drop is abbreviated as
A. gdd.
B. ged.
C. gtt.
D. drp.

18. Total parenteral nutrition (TPN) is generally prescribed for patients who
A. are unable to see.
B. are unable to drink.
C. are able to drink but not able to taste or smell.
D. are unable to eat.

19. A physician orders heparin 3500 U SC q12h. Heparin 5000 U/mL is available. The nurse must give which of the following amounts?
A. 0.1 mL
B. 0.3 mL
C. 0.7 mL
D. 1.0 mL

20. A prescription is written for Lasix 60 mg IV stat. In your hands you have Lasix 20 mg per 2 mL ampule. How many mL will you administer to the patient?
A. 1 mL
B. 3 mL
C. 5 mL
D. 6 mL

21. A nurse received an order from a physician for heparin 8000 U SC stat. The technician brought heparin 10,000 U/1 mL to the floor. Which of the following is the correct calculation of heparin for the patient?
A. 0.2 mL
B. 0.4 mL
C. 0.6 mL
D. 0.8 mL

22. A pediatrician ordered ampicillin 50 mg/kg/day IV in equally divided doses every 6 hours for an infant who weighs 26 lbs. Ampicillin 125 mg/5 mL is available. How many mL of this medication should the baby receive?
A. 0.5 mL
B. 1.25 mL
C. 1.5 mL
D. 2.0 mL

23. A prescription is written for 1500 mL D5W for 12 h. The drop factor is 15 gtt/mL. Which of the following flow rates (in gtt/min) is correct?
A. 11
B. 21
C. 31
D. 41

24. Ceclor suspension 225 mg p.o., b.i.d. is prescribed. There is only Ceclor suspension, 375 mg per 5 mL available. Which of the following is the right dose?
A. 1.5 mL
B. 3.0 mL
C. 4.5 mL
D. 6.0 mL

25. A patient needs Pepcid 20 mg p.o., q.i.d., but it is only available as 80 mg/10 mL. Which of the following is the right dose?
A. 1.5 mL
B. 2.5 mL
C. 3.5 mL
D. 5.0 mL

26. A tablet contains 0.125 milligrams of medication. A patient receives three tablets a day for five days. How many milligrams of medication does the patient receive over the five days?
A. 0.625
B. 0.925
C. 1.375
D. 1.875

27. If you want to give a patient 1 1/2 teaspoons of cough syrup four times a day, how many teaspoons of cough syrup will you give each day?
A. 2.5
B. 4.0
C. 6.0
D. 7.5

Continues

28. Determine the amount to administer.
Ordered: Depakene syrup 125 mg p.o. q12h
On hand: Depakene syrup 250 mg/5 mL
Which of the following is the correct amount?
A. 1.25
B. 2.00
C. 2.50
D. 3.00

29. Determine the amount to administer.
Ordered: ranitidine HCL (Zantac) 35 mg, IM, q8h
On hand: ranitidine HCL (Zantac) 25 mg/mL
How many milliliters (mL) of Zantac should the patient receive every day?
A. 1.5
B. 4.2
C. 5.5
D. 6.2

30. Determine the amount to administer. Ordered: Cedax susp 300 mg p.o. qd 2h after breakfast
On hand: Cedax oral suspension 90 mg/5 mL
Which of the following is the correct amount?
A. 1.7 mL
B. 5.7 mL
C. 13 mL
D. 17 mL

APPENDIX

A Additional Questions

1. Which of the following medications should be prepared under a vertical laminar airflow hood?
   A. Trimethoprim/sulfamethoxazole
   B. Methotrexate
   C. Magnesium
   D. TPN

2. According to federal law, which of the following medications must be distributed along with patient package inserts?
   A. Minocin®
   B. Premarin®
   C. Dilantin®
   D. Prilosec®

3. How much 1:1000 stock solution is required to prepare 1000 mL of a 1:4000 solution?
   A. 4000 mL
   B. 1000 mL
   C. 460 mL
   D. 250 mL

4. Regarding the proper operation of horizontal laminar airflow hoods, which of the following statements is most accurate?
   A. The hood and HEPA filter should be cleaned often throughout the compounding period.
   B. All aseptic manipulations should be performed at least 3 inches within the hood.
   C. Interior working surfaces should be cleaned from back to front.
   D. Laminar airflow hoods should be tested and certified by qualified personnel every 2 years.

5. A pharmacy receives an order for acetaminophen with codeine elixir (120 mg and 12 mg/5 mL) that reads "Sig: 1 tablespoon PO q6h p.r.n. Disp: 4 oz." Each prescribed dose will contain
   A. 360 mg of acetaminophen and 36 mg of codeine.
   B. 300 mg of acetaminophen and 30 mg of codeine.
   C. 240 mg of acetaminophen and 24 mg of codeine.
   D. 120 mg of acetaminophen and 12 mg of codeine.

6. What is the chemical formula for sodium bicarbonate?
   A. $NaCl$
   B. $NaCO_3$
   C. $NaHCO_3$
   D. $NaOH$

7. The desired result is a 1000 mL solution of 3.5% amino acid in 15% dextrose. Which of the following formulas will provide the desired result?
   A. Amino acid 7% 400 mL + dextrose 30% 600 mL
   B. Amino acid 7% 500 mL + dextrose 30% 500 mL
   C. Amino acid 10% 300 mL + dextrose 30% 700 mL
   D. Amino acid 10% 500 mL + dextrose 30% 500 mL

8. If you calculate a result by dividing the total dollars spent on purchasing drugs for 1 year by the actual value of the pharmacy inventory at any point in time, what is the result called?
   A. Median drug cost
   B. Average monthly inventory
   C. Inventory turnover rate
   D. Wholesale markup factor

9. To dispense 20 doses of 75 mg, the amount of 125 mg/5 mL solution required would be
   A. 50 mL.
   B. 60 mL.
   C. 80 mL.
   D. 100 mL.

10. If running at an hourly dose of 15 mL/hr, a solution of heparin 25,000 U in D5W 500 mL is delivered at a rate of
    A. 750 U/hr.
    B. 250 U/hr.
    C. 50 U/hr.
    D. 15 U/hr.

11. When a recall notice is received, a pharmacy technician should first do which of the following?
    A. Remove the product from the shelf, regardless of lot number.
    B. Notify patients of the recall.
    C. Order replacement stock.
    D. Check to see whether the product is in stock.

12. Which of the following tasks is a pharmacy technician allowed to do?
    A. Recommend a medication to a patient or someone representing the patient.
    B. Discuss a potential drug interaction.
    C. Counsel a patient on the use of an OTC product.
    D. Enter a written order into a computer.

13. To administer a dose of 8 mg of a solution, what volume of the solution (labeled "0.05 g = 1 mL") would be required?
   A. 0.60 mL
   B. 0.45 mL
   C. 0.16 mL
   D. 0.08 mL

14. 48 Fleet® enema kits cost a pharmacy $56.70. The pharmacy sells them at a markup of 50%. What is the retail price for one kit?
   A. $2.36
   B. $2.09
   C. $1.77
   D. $1.19

15. What volume will deliver a dose of 6 mg, if the label on a multidose vial reads 25 mg/mL?
   A. 4.1 mL
   B. 2.5 mL
   C. 0.48 mL
   D. 0.24 mL

16. A pharmacy technician has been given 100 mL of a 10% acetic acid solution. The pharmacist asks the technician to dilute the solution to 500 mL with sterile water and to label the solution. What percentage should appear on the label?
   A. 3.0%
   B. 2.5%
   C. 2.0%
   D. 1.5%

17. DEA Form 222 is used to order controlled substances listed in which of the following schedules?
   A. Schedule V
   B. Schedule IV
   C. Schedule III
   D. Schedule II

18. To make a 120 mL bottle of 0.8 mg/mL solution, what amount of a 16 mg/mL solution is needed?
   A. 2400 mL
   B. 96 mL
   C. 6 mL
   D. 3 mL

19. What is a pharmacist trying to determine if he asks a pharmacy technician to collect data for a creatinine clearance monitoring program?
   A. What a patient's liver function is, and, therefore, the need to adjust medication doses
   B. What the patient's renal function is, and, therefore, the need to adjust medication doses
   C. Whether any of a patient's current medications are altering blood-clotting properties
   D. Whether any of a patient's current medications are causing neurotoxicity

20. To compound a formula reading "camphor 0.3%, menthol 0.25%, hydrocortisone 1%, Aquaphor qs ad 600 g," how much camphor is required?
   A. 3.8 g
   B. 3200 mg
   C. 1800 mg
   D. 180 mg

21. To dispense a 0.030 g dose using stock 5 mg tablets, the pharmacist would give the patient
   A. 6 tablets.
   B. 4 tablets.
   C. $\frac{1}{4}$ tablet.
   D. $\frac{1}{6}$ tablet.

22. How should NSAIDs such as ibuprofen be taken?
   A. At bedtime
   B. With food or milk
   C. With a sip of water
   D. On an empty stomach

23. If a pharmacy technician learns that the patient is allergic to the drug prescribed, what should he or she do?
   A. Tell the patient to see a different physician.
   B. Notify the pharmacist.
   C. Process the prescription.
   D. Refuse to process the prescription.

24. Which of the following is a Schedule I drug?
   A. Heroin
   B. Phenobarbital
   C. Morphine
   D. Tylenol® with codeine

25. A DEA Form 222 is required for the purchase of which medication?
   A. Methylphenidate
   B. Methotrexate
   C. Methyltestosterone
   D. Methylphenobarbital

26. Bisacodyl is
   A. an anticholinergic.
   B. an antidiarrheal.
   C. a sedative.
   D. a laxative.

27. Find the final fee for a prescription with an average wholesale price (AWP) of $25.00. The selling price of the prescription medication is the AWP less 12% plus a dispensing fee of $3.00.
   A. $31.00
   B. $25.50
   C. $25.00
   D. $24.64

28. To deliver a dose of 1.5 mg, what volume of haloperidol injection supplied in 5 mg/mL ampules is required?
A. 3.00 mL
B. 1.50 mL
C. 0.30 mL
D. 0.03 mL

29. A pharmacy technician questions the pharmacist about the following prescription: "Fosamax® 10 mg #30 Sig: 1 qd w/food, 2 refills." Why is the pharmacy technician questioning it?
A. Prescriptions for this medication are not renewable.
B. This product is not available in the strength specified.
C. This medication is usually prescribed qid.
D. This medication is not supposed to be administered with food.

30. You must determine an exact count of which of the following medicines when conducting a DEA-required Schedule drug inventory?
A. Demerol®, Ritalin®, Vicodin®, Darvocet-N®, and Phenergan® with codeine
B. Demerol® and Ritalin®
C. Demerol®, Ritalin®, Vicodin®, and Darvocet-N®
D. Ritalin® and Vicodin®

31. To prepare six 2-oz bottles of 10% trichloroacetic acid, what volume of 36% trichloroacetic acid solution is needed?
A. 136 mL
B. 100 mL
C. 36 mL
D. 17 mL

32. According to federal law, to secure a supply of __________, a registrant must complete a DEA Form 222.
A. triazolam
B. lorazepam
C. pentazocine
D. oxycodone

33. Hypodermic syringes are commonly used to administer medication by which of the following routes?
A. Subcutaneous
B. Intravenous
C. Intramuscular
D. Intradermal

34. __________ is what online processing of a third-party claim to determine payment is called.
A. Restriction
B. Adjudication
C. Processing degree
D. Reconciliation

35. In a crash cart awaiting patient use, how should nitroglycerin SL tablets be stored?
A. The manufacturer requires that the tablets be placed in a plastic bag before dispensing.
B. The unopened bottle of tablets should be stored in the original container.
C. The bottle should be opened and the tablets should be placed in a pharmacy vial for dispensing.
D. The manufacturer requires that the container be broken and put in unit-dose packaging for dispensing.

36. Automated medication dispensing systems offer the primary benefit of
A. replenishment by nurses.
B. prevention of narcotic diversion.
C. better tracking and control of drug inventory.
D. tracking of adverse drug reactions.

37. When pharmacy staff are handling hazardous chemicals, which of the following is the most important item to have readily available?
A. An approved first-aid kit
B. A "code" box
C. A spill kit
D. Dilute isopropyl alcohol

38. For mixing intravenous solutions with automated compounders, which of the following statements is most accurate about?
A. Operator error should be the main focus of a quality assurance program, because it is the primary reason for compounding errors.
B. Compounding errors associated with these machines are often associated with mechanical failure.
C. These machines should be used rarely, because in most instances, pharmacy technicians can prepare the solutions faster and more accurately.
D. The manufacturers of these machines have installed highly sophisticated monitoring devices, such as audio and visual alarms, so that additional monitoring of pump malfunction is not warranted.

39. Which of the following is likely to aggravate peptic ulcer disease?
A. Guaifenesin
B. Ibuprofen
C. Omeprazole
D. Acetaminophen

40. For storing etoposide (VP-16) capsules, which of the following is the recommended temperature storage range?
A. 30°C to 40°C (86°F to 104°F)
B. 15°C to 30°C (59°F to 86°F)
C. 8°C to 15°C (46°F to 59°F)
D. 2°C to 8°C (36°F to 46°F)

41. To prepare 1 L of 0.1% sodium hypochlorite disinfecting solution, what volume of 5% sodium hypochlorite is required?
A. 25 mL
B. 20 mL
C. 2.5 mL
D. 2.0 mL

42. The following radiation therapy mixture is written by a physician:
"Mix: Mylanta® 88 mL Lidocaine viscous 2% 20 mL, Diphenhydramine elixir 12 mL. Sig: i or ii tbsp ac & hs." What size bottle is most appropriate for dispensing the final mixture?
A. 1 liter
B. 1 pint
C. 4 ounce
D. 2 ounce

43. What are universal claim forms used for?
A. Insurance billing
B. HMO group purchasing credits
C. FICA submissions
D. Public aid prescription payments

44. Via which of the following routes are dosage forms such as sequels and spansules normally administered?
A. Oral
B. Intramuscular
C. Topical
D. Transdermal

45. The extent to which a dosage form retains its properties and characteristics between the current time and the time of its preparation is known as
A. expiration.
B. pH.
C. concentration.
D. stability.

46. For increased clotting, which of the following vitamins is involved?
A. Vitamin A
B. Vitamin E
C. Vitamin K
D. Vitamin B_3

47. To prepare an IV bag containing 2 g of $MgSO_4$, what amount of 50% magnesium sulfate solution should be injected?
A. 8 mL
B. 6 mL
C. 4 mL
D. 2 mL

48. Which of the following resources contains broad general statements of philosophy and detailed guidelines for implementing them in hospital pharmacies?
A. U.S. Pharmacopeia
B. Human resources manual
C. Policy and procedure manual
D. Material safety data sheet (MSDS)

49. On an IV administration set, the purpose of the filter is to prevent the
A. entry of air into the administration set.
B. entry of particulate matter into the vascular system.
C. separation of an emulsion.
D. contamination of blood products.

50. On an insurance claim form, the required ICD-9 code refers to the
A. geographical location.
B. national drug code.
C. average wholesale price.
D. diagnosis.

51. The trade name for lidocaine is
A. Pontocaine®.
B. Cocaine®.
C. Novocaine®.
D. Xylocaine®.

52. Bentyl® is the trade name for
A. diazepam.
B. dicyclomine.
C. dimenhydrinate.
D. diphenhydramine.

53. On IV tubing, a Y-site refers to the
A. drip chamber of the tubing.
B. roller clamp located at the end of the tubing.
C. medication port in the tubing.
D. primary set of tubing.

54. To ensure the safety of employees, hazardous drugs must be
A. stored in a biological safety cabinet.
B. listed on a quarterly report filed with the EPA.
C. labeled to indicate that special handling is required.
D. unpacked and inventoried by the pharmacist only.

55. Of the following drugs, which one is an H_2 receptor antagonist medication?
A. Clemastine
B. Loratadine
C. Ranitidine
D. Clonidine

56. Which of the following approves changes in the drug formulary?
A. FDA
B. Pharmacy and therapeutics (P&T) committee
C. Drug use review committee
D. DEA

57. Which of the following drugs reduces viscosity of tenacious secretions and increases respiratory tract fluids?
A. Expectorant
B. Antihistamine
C. Antitussive
D. Emollient

58. In the event of a recall of medications, the most important pieces of information to have on record are the
A. lot number and expiration date.
B. drug name and controlled substance status.
C. drug manufacturer and drug distributor.
D. National Drug Code (NDC) number and package size.

59. Over 24 hours, a patient is to receive 1 L of D5/0.45 NS with 20 mEq of KCl IV solution. The flow rate is
A. 84 mL/hr.
B. 42 mL/hr.
C. 24 mL/hr.
D. 21 mL/hr.

60. Assume that 1 lb = 454 g. An order for 1 lb of 4% zinc oxide paste is prepared using the pharmacy's stock 10% paste and 1% paste. How much of each stock paste must be mixed to obtain the desired concentration?
A. 115 g of 10%, 330 g of 1%
B. 330 g of 10%, 115 g of 1%
C. 151 g of 10%, 303 g of 1%
D. 303 g of 10%, 151 g of 1%

61. Using the following manufacturer's invoice figures, what amount should be remitted if it is paid within 30 days? The total is $520.00 with the terms 2% net.
A. $530.40
B. $520.00
C. $509.60
D. $490.00

62. Find the final percentage concentration using the following figures: an IV solution contains 25 g of a medication in 1000 mL of stock solution.
A. 0.25%
B. 1.25%
C. 2.5%
D. 12.5%

63. For influenza A and B, which of the following drugs is used as an inhaled neuraminidase inhibitor?
A. Tamiflu®
B. Relenza®
C. Xenical®
D. Vioxx®

64. In which classifications do federal regulations require that a "C" designation be placed on the drug manufacturer's label?
A. Schedules I and IV
B. Schedules I, II, III, IV, and V
C. Schedules III, IV, and V
D. Schedules I and II

65. Which of the following is an insurance or entitlement program that reimburses for products of services?
A. Universal claim plan
B. Home health care plan
C. Third-party plan
D. Cash payment

66. What is the trade name for glyburide?
A. Glucotrol®
B. Glucophage®
C. Micronase®
D. Diabinese®

67. Which 1970 federal legislation established drug schedules and registration requirements pertaining to potentially addictive medications?
A. Kefauver-Harris Amendments
B. Drug Abuse Control Amendments
C. Controlled Substance Act
D. Harrison Narcotic Act

68. The generic equivalent of Percodan® consists of
A. acetaminophen and hydrocodone.
B. acetaminophen and oxycodone.
C. aspirin and codeine.
D. aspirin and oxycodone.

69. What would the total daily dose be of the following if 100 mg is administered qid? The drug concentration is 100 mg/2.5 mL.
A. 10 mL containing 40 g
B. 10 mL containing 0.4 g
C. 5 mL containing 0.4 g
D. 2.5 mL containing 400 g

70. Which of the following should be stored in a refrigerator?
A. Procaine penicillin
B. Tetracycline
C. Cimetidine
D. Fluoxetine

71. Investigational drugs must initially be ordered by the
A. pharmacy technician.
B. oncology nurse.
C. physician.
D. pharmacy director.

72. What is the maximum number of refills within 6 months permitted for a prescription for a Schedule III drug, according to federal law?
A. Five
B. Two
C. One
D. None

73. The most widely used agent for the treatment of acute gouty arthritis is
A. indomethacin.
B. phenylbutazone.
C. colchicine.
D. probenecid.

74. What should the pharmacy technician do when a nurse calls for missing drugs?
A. Dispense the missing pills at once.
B. Tell the nurse to use the patient's own medication.
C. Tell the nurse that the physician has to write orders for them again.
D. Check the patient's profile to verify the physician's order.

75. What volume of injection will be used to prepare a 2500 mL TPN bag for the following order? The order includes folic acid 2 mg/L filled using a stock vial that delivers 5 mg/mL.
A. 2.5 mL
B. 1 mL
C. 0.5 mL
D. 0.1 mL

76. "Extemporaneous compounding" means
A. making stock solutions.
B. using mortar and pestle only.
C. preparing medication for a specific patient.
D. compounding with a controlled substance.

77. Which of the following is most often used in combination with KCl supplements?
A. Ibuprofen
B. Lisinopril
C. Phenytoin
D. Hydrochlorothiazide

78. The following prescription, in a 2 oz increment, is frequently ordered by a dermatologist: "LCD 2% Salicylic acid 5% QSAD yellow petrolatum." The pharmacy technician wants to prepare a 500 g bulk amount and then prepackage it in 2 oz containers. How much salicylic acid will be needed to compound the 500 g?
A. 25 g
B. 5 g
C. 2.5 g
D. 0.5 g

79. To deliver a dose of 0.125 mg, which of the following volumes of a 0.5 mg/2 mL digoxin injection is correct?
A. 2.0 mL
B. 1.5 mL
C. 0.75 mL
D. 0.5 mL

80. For a 6-year-old patient, the following prescription is ordered: "Cipro 500 mg tablets; take 1 tablet bid for 10 days; disp 20." In assessing this prescription, the pharmacy technician recognizes that the
A. medication is inappropriate for the patient's age.
B. prescription is acceptable as written.
C. dosage form is not available.
D. duration of therapy will be 14 days.

81. "Sig," a prescription term, refers to
A. directions to the patient.
B. physician's name and address.
C. medication dose and strength.
D. directions to the pharmacist.

82. An inventory control system principle is which of the following?
A. Fast movers first
B. Manufacturer rebate
C. First out, last in
D. First in, first out

83. Basically a collection of drug product package inserts, which of the following is a commonly used reference?
A. *Handbook of Nonprescription Drugs*
B. *Remington's Pharmaceutical Sciences*
C. *Physicians' Desk Reference* (PDR)
D. *American Hospital Formulary Service* (AHFS)

84. The prefix "neur(o)" represents which of the following?
A. Kidney
B. Lung
C. Heart
D. Nerve

85. What is the name of the agreement involved when an institution agrees to purchase 80% to 90% of its pharmaceuticals from a single vendor?
A. Prime vendor agreement
B. Borrow and loan agreement
C. Manufacturer agreement
D. Direct purchasing agreement

86. For a patient requesting "nerve pills," which of the following medications on the profile would the pharmacy technician refill?
A. Chlorpropamide
B. Chlorpheniramine
C. Chlorothiazide
D. Chlordiazepoxide

87. A class III prescription balance has been moved onto a secure level surface by a pharmacy technician. Before weighing any substance, the technician should
A. lock the balance and level it to "1."
B. place the desired weight on the left-hand pan.
C. unlock the balance and level it to zero.
D. place the substance on the right-hand pan.

88. Determine which of the following answers would not be an appropriate dosage regimen, using the information provided. A drug is available in the following strengths and dosage forms: 125 mg tablets, 250 mg capsules, and 125 mg/5 mL liquid. A child weighs 55 lb and the recommended dose is 10 mg/kg/24 hr (to be given in 6- or 12-hour intervals).
A. ½ of a 125 mg tablet every 6 hours
B. 5 mL of 125 mg/5 mL liquid every 12 hours
C. One 250 mg capsule every 12 hours
D. One 125 mg tablet every 12 hours

89. The following prescription has been given to a patient: "Captopril 12.5 mg. Sig: ss tab bid." How much of the drug will the patient take in 1 week?
A. 262.5 mg
B. 175 mg
C. 87.5 mg
D. 43.8 mg

90. Which of the following product elements do the middle four characters of an NDC number represent?
A. Package size and product strength
B. Manufacturer and dosage form
C. Product, strength, and dosage form
D. Package size, manufacturer, and strength

91. A sensitivity to which of the following will most likely be exhibited if the patient has a penicillin allergy?
A. Tetracycline
B. Erythromycin
C. Gentamicin
D. Cephalexin

92. Once it has been refilled and dated, the crash cart should be
A. sealed and stored.
B. sent to central sterile supply.
C. checked and sealed.
D. sent to the nursing unit.

93. What would the technician dispense if he or she received a prescription for "tetracycline 250 mg capsules, #C"?
A. 1000 capsules
B. 100 capsules
C. 50 capsules
D. 10 capsules

94. What does the abbreviation "Na" stand for?
A. Zinc
B. Iron
C. Sodium
D. Potassium

95. What do the last two digits of the NDC indicate?
A. Unit package size
B. Dosage strength
C. Product manufacturer location
D. Number of units per case

96. The first dose of cefazolin 1 g IV q8h was administered to the patient at 1:00 PM. When should the next two doses be given?
A. 1.00 AM and 12:00 noon
B. 9:00 PM and 5:00 AM
C. 6:00 PM and 4:00 AM
D. 8:00 PM and 8:00 AM

97. How much codeine is contained in a tablet composed of acetaminophen with ½ grain of codeine?
A. 60 mg
B. 50 mg
C. 30 mg
D. 15 mg

98. A pharmacy technician learns that because of failure to release a drug within the specified period, an estradiol patch has been recalled. How should this recall be classified?
A. Class IV: Use of the product caused no harm to patients, and the FDA handled the problem in its own office without pharmacists' intervention.
B. Class III: Use of this product is not likely to have caused adverse health consequences.
C. Class II: Use of this product may have caused temporary or medically reversible adverse health consequences, with little probability of serious adverse health consequences.
D. Class I: Use of or exposure to this product may have caused serious adverse health consequences or death.

99. For DUE criteria, which of the following drug categories may be selected?
A. Drugs that are classified as controlled substances
B. Drugs frequently backordered by the manufacturer
C. Drugs in Phase III of a clinical trial
D. Drugs known to cause adverse reactions or drug interactions

100. Of the following parenteral medications, one must be prepared inside a biological safety cabinet. Select the correct choice.
A. Dactinomycin
B. Erythromycin
C. Streptomycin
D. Vancomycin

101. To increase the folic acid content by 0.5 mg/5 mL, how many 1 mg tablets of folic acid would be added to 360 mL of vitamin preparation?
A. 72 tablets
B. 36 tablets
C. 18 tablets
D. 6 tablets

102. In the *Orange Book*, generic drugs are required to be identical to the innovator or brand-name product listed, in terms of active ingredient and dosage form, as well as
A. route of administration and color.
B. color and strength.
C. size and identification markings.
D. route of administration and strength.

103. A prescription order for amoxicillin 500 mg PO q8h is received by the pharmacy technician. The current pharmacy profile shows an active order for cephalexin 250 mg tid. The pharmacy technician should
A. not prepare the amoxicillin for dispensing, because the patient is taking cephalexin.
B. discontinue the cephalexin, because the amoxicillin is the most recent antibiotic order.
C. prepare the amoxicillin for dispensing.
D. notify the pharmacist of a potential therapeutic duplication.

104. "Protection of the identity and health information of patients" is most specifically referred to by which of the following professional concepts?
A. Compatibility
B. Mortality
C. Confidentiality
D. Motility

105. The pharmacy and therapeutics (P&T) committee's primary function is to
A. create credentialing requirements for pharmacy employees.
B. fund independent research to verify therapeutic claims by manufacturers of pharmaceutical products and medical devices.
C. enforce state pharmacy laws and FDA regulations.
D. formulate policies governing selection and therapeutic use of pharmaceutical products and medical devices.

106. Automated dispensing systems include all of the following, except
A. Kirby-Lester KL 25.
B. McKesson's Baker APS.
C. Sure-Med.
D. Pyxis.

107. On a graduated cylinder, where is the volume of aqueous liquid read?
A. Top of the meniscus
B. Volume when drawn up into a syringe
C. Top surface of the liquid
D. Bottom of the meniscus

108. __________ is classified as a Schedule II controlled substance.
A. Restoril®
B. Halcion®
C. Persantine®
D. Ritalin®

109. In a 1:10,000 solution, how much gentian violet is in 500 mL?
A. 50 g
B. 5 g
C. 50 mg
D. 5 mg

110. Dextrose solution of 12.5% has been ordered via prescription. The pharmacy technician would mix the stock solutions of 20% dextrose and 5% dextrose solutions in which ratio?
A. 2:1
B. 1:3
C. 1:2
D. 1:1

111. A physician may prescribe a listing of the medications within a given setting, such as a third-party plan. This listing is called a
A. closed panel.
B. pharmacy benefit manager.
C. formulary.
D. risk contract.

112. What are the directions for a dispensed prescription that reads "ii gtt OU bid prn pain"?
A. Instill 2 drops in each eye twice a day as needed for pain.
B. Instill 2 drops in each eye three times a day as needed for pain.
C. Instill 2 drops in the right eye twice a day as needed for pain.
D. Instill 2 drops in the left eye twice a day as needed for pain.

113. The recommended storage temperature for a phenobarbital injection is
A. 15°C to 30°C (59°F to 86°F).
B. 2°C to 8°C (36°F to 46°F).
C. −20°C to −10°C (−4°F to 14°F).
D. 30°C to 40°C (86°F to 104°F).

114. Which medications from the patient's profile should be refilled for an order prescribing refills of metoprolol and lovastatin?
A. Tenormin® and Mevacor®
B. Lopressor® and Zocor®
C. Tenormin® and Zocor®
D. Lopressor® and Mevacor®

115. To prepare 4 oz of 2% hydrocortisone cream, the quantity of hydrocortisone powder needed is
A. 2.40 g.
B. 1.20 g.
C. 0.240 g.
D. 0.120 g.

116. When an investigational drug expires, the pharmacy technician should do which of the following?
A. Remove the expired drug from inventory and return it to the FDA.
B. Record the quantity on the inventory record and return the product to the wholesaler for credit.
C. Record the quantity of each lot number on the perpetual inventory record and return the product to the sponsor.
D. Remove the expired drug from inventory and destroy it according to EPA guidelines.

117. For repackaging of injectable medications, containers must be sterile and
A. clear and colorless.
B. made of glass.
C. pyrogen-free.
D. made of low-density plastic.

118. Prices in a pharmacy are based on average wholesale price (AWP) plus a professional fee, as follows:

Fee	AWP
$2.00	$25.00 and under
$5.00	$25.01–$50.00
$10.00	$50.01–$75.00
$20.00	$75.01 and over

A prescription is received that reads "Sig: 2 tabs bid × 25 days." If the AWP of this drug is $321.66 for 500 tablets, what will be the retail price of the prescription?
A. $85.25
B. $74.33
C. $70.20
D. $66.53

119. From a 10 g vial of cefazolin, how many 500 mg doses can be prepared?
A. 50 doses
B. 25 doses
C. 20 doses
D. 15 doses

120. Photosensitivity is caused by which of the following drugs?
A. Fluoxetine
B. Estradiol
C. Ketorolac
D. Sulfamethoxazole

121. A particular drug costs $1.50 for 100 tablets. What would the dispensing charge have to be to yield a 40% gross profit?
A. $5.00
B. $2.50
C. $2.10
D. $2.00

122. To deliver 8 g of zinc oxide, how many grams of 20% zinc oxide ointment would be required?
A. 160 g
B. 80 g
C. 40 g
D. 20 g

123. A prescription reads: "clindamycin 1%, propylene glycol 5%, isopropyl alcohol qs ad 480 mL." How many 150 mg clindamycin capsules are required to compound this prescription?
A. 56 capsules
B. 48 capsules
C. 32 capsules
D. 5 capsules

124. Which of the following medications should be protected from exposure to light?
A. Nitroprusside
B. Ampicillin
C. Diphenhydramine
D. Ondansetron

125. What is the charge to the customer for a prescription for 30 tablets, using the following information? The pharmacy pricing formula is the average wholesale price (AWP) plus $4.50 and the AWP is $90 for 100 tablets.
A. $94.50
B. $31.50
C. $30.50
D. $27.50

126. Insulin is classified as which of the following types of drugs?
A. Prophylactic
B. Palliative
C. Replacement
D. Diagnostic

127. When one reads a prescription, which of the following abbreviations means "four times a day"?
A. qd
B. qh
C. qid
D. qod

128. Which of the following is equivalent to 500 mg?
A. 0.5 g
B. 1.0 g
C. 2.5 g
D. 5.0 g

129. Ibuprofen (Motrin®) is classified as which of the following types of drugs?
A. Anticoagulant
B. Antiemetic
C. Anti-inflammatory
D. Antitussive

130. Which of the following elements of a prescription provides directions for the patient?
A. Subscription
B. Signa
C. Inscription
D. Repetatur

131. Which of the following terms refers to decreased susceptibility to the effects of a drug after continued use?
A. Cumulative action
B. Idiosyncrasy
C. Immunity
D. Tolerance

132. Ciprofloxacin (Cipro®) 500 mg bid × 7 days is prescribed for a patient. The pharmacy technician has only the 250 mg dose in stock. How many 250 mg caplets will the pharmacist dispense to the patient?
A. 7
B. 14
C. 21
D. 28

133. A physician will most likely prescribe which of the following drugs for hormone replacement therapy?
A. Zolpidem (Ambien®)
B. Levothyroxine (Levoxyl®)
C. Lisinopril (Zestril®)
D. Alendronate (Fosamax®)

134. When a patient with hypertension is given a prescription for a diuretic, he or she should be advised that which of the following is an excellent source of potassium?
A. Bananas
B. Cheese
C. Milk
D. Rice

135. A physician prescribes 0.15 mcg of levothyroxine (Synthroid®) for a patient. Levothyroxine is available in 0.075 mcg tablets. How many tablets should the patient receive?
A. 0.5
B. 1.0
C. 1.5
D. 2.0

136. Each of the following is classified as one of the "seven rights" of proper drug administration EXCEPT
A. right patient.
B. right physician.
C. right route.
D. right dose.

137. Which of the following terms means "the life of the drug"?
A. Bioequivalence
B. Bioavailability
C. Pharmacokinetics
D. Pharmacodynamics

138. To keep privileged information about a customer from being disclosed without his or her consent is called
A. confidentiality.
B. professionalism.
C. protocol.
D. morals.

139. Which of the following abbreviations means "legend drug"?
A. Dx
B. Vx
C. Tx
D. Rx

140. Which of the following is called a biological catalyst?
A. Cofactor
B. Enzyme
C. Vitamin
D. Intrinsic factor

141. Indications for metformin (Glucophage®) include which of the following diseases or conditions?
A. Insomnia
B. Panic disorder
C. Diabetes
D. Migraines

142. The trade name of cetirizine is
A. Zyrtec®.
B. Fosamax®.
C. Allegra®.
D. Flagyl®.

143. The best treatment for tuberculosis is the combination regimen of
A. isoniazid, gentamicin, and rifampin.
B. kanamycin, penicillin G, and amikacin.
C. erythromycin, ethambutol, and cycloserine.
D. rifampin, isoniazid, and ethambutol.

144. If a heparin order is 4,000 U SC and the drug in stock is available as 10,000 U/1 mL, how many milliliters of the drug should the nurse administer?
A. 0.25 mL
B. 0.2 mL
C. 0.4 mL
D. 0.5 mL

145. Which of the following muscles is the best choice for injecting an infant who is only 4 months old?
A. Deltoid
B. Vastus lateralis
C. Gluteus maximus
D. Pectoralis major

146. A physician orders NPH insulin 35 U SC. The drug is available in U100 insulin syringe. How much insulin should be withdrawn, as indicated on the insulin syringe?
A. 35 U
B. 50 U
C. 70 U
D. 100 U

147. The trade name of doxycycline is
A. Tobramycin®.
B. Lincomycin®.
C. Vancomycin®.
D. Vibramycin®.

148. Which of the following vitamin deficiencies may cause pernicious anemia?
A. Vitamin D
B. Vitamin C
C. Vitamin B_1
D. Vitamin B_{12}

149. Vertical flow hoods use air that originates from which of the following parts of the hood?
A. Roof
B. Floor
C. Back
D. Side

150. Which of the following abbreviations means "immediately"?
A. Sat
B. NPO
C. Stat
D. USP

Answer Key

1. B
2. B
3. A
4. C
5. A
6. C
7. B
8. C
9. B
10. A
11. D
12. D
13. C
14. C
15. D
16. C
17. D
18. C
19. B
20. C
21. A
22. B
23. B
24. A
25. A
26. D
27. C
28. C
29. D
30. B
31. B
32. D
33. D
34. B
35. B
36. C
37. C
38. A
39. B
40. D
41. B
42. C
43. A
44. A
45. D
46. C
47. C
48. C
49. B
50. D
51. D
52. B
53. C
54. C
55. C
56. B
57. A
58. A
59. B
60. C
61. C
62. C
63. B
64. B
65. C
66. C
67. C
68. D
69. B
70. A
71. C
72. A
73. C
74. D
75. B
76. C
77. D
78. A
79. D
80. A
81. A
82. D
83. C
84. D
85. A
86. D
87. C
88. D
89. C
90. C
91. D
92. C
93. B
94. C
95. A
96. B
97. C
98. B
99. D
100. A
101. B
102. D
103. D
104. C
105. D
106. A
107. D
108. D
109. C
110. D
111. C
112. A
113. A
114. D
115. A
116. C
117. C
118. B
119. C
120. D
121. C
122. C
123. C
124. A
125. B
126. C
127. C
128. A
129. C
130. C
131. D
132. D
133. B
134. A
135. D
136. B
137. B
138. A
139. D
140. B
141. C
142. A
143. D
144. C
145. B
146. A
147. D
148. D
149. A
150. C

APPENDIX

B

Case Studies

1. A patient with chronic glaucoma is also receiving treatment for chronic obstructive pulmonary disease. He is referred for evaluation of a sudden increase in intraocular pressure. Which drug used in pulmonary disease is most likely to be responsible?
   A. Epinephrine
   B. Pilocarpine
   C. Atropine
   D. Timolol

2. A 27-year-old woman in the 32nd week of pregnancy with her first child is seen with a blood pressure of 160/110, 3+ proteinuria, confusion, and retinal hemorrhages. Which medication would be indicated in the treatment of this patient?
   A. Magnesium sulfate
   B. Progesterone
   C. Indomethacin
   D. Terbutaline

3. Andrew is a pharmacy technician. He receives a prescription that orders 12.5% dextrose solution. There are 20% dextrose and 5% dextrose solutions available in stock. If the technician wants to mix these stock solutions, which of the following ratios will be correct?
   A. 2:1
   B. 1:1
   C. 1:2
   D. 1:3

4. A patient brings a prescription to your pharmacy. The order is "tetracycline 250 mg #30 Sig: 1. q.i.d. w/food or milk, no refills." You, as a pharmacy technician, question the pharmacist about this prescription because
   A. this medication is not available in the strength specified.
   B. this product is off the market.
   C. this medication is usually prescribed only once a day.
   D. this product is not supposed to be administered with milk or dairy products.

5. A pharmacy technician was asked to compound a formula reading "camphor 0.3%, menthol 0.25%, hydrocortisone 1%, and Aquaphor qs ad 600 g." How much camphor is required for this composition?
   A. 3.8 mg
   B. 2500 mg
   C. 1800 mg
   D. 0.25 mg

6. A child is brought to the emergency department with an asthma attack. His weight is 64 lb, and he requires aminophylline IV at 1 mg/kg/hr. The solution is prepared using premixed aminophylline 400 mg in 500 cc D5W. Which of the following will be the correct rate?
   A. 18.18 cc/hr
   B. 32.32 cc/hr
   C. 64.64 cc/hr
   D. 128.128 cc/hr

7. The prescriber orders 20 mg IM of a drug for his patient. The drug is available in a 10-mL vial that contains 50 mg of the drug. How many milliliters will be needed to supply the dose of 20 mg?
   A. 1 mL
   B. 4 mL
   C. 6 mL
   D. 7 mL

8. The recommended dose of meperidine (Demerol®) is 6 mg/kg/24 hr for pain. It is given in divided doses every 4 to 6 hours. How many milliliters of Demerol injection (50 mg/mL) should be administered to a 33-lb child as a single dose every 6 hours?
   A. 0.45 mL
   B. 0.75 mL
   C. 1.25 mL
   D. 1.50 mL

9. A pharmacy technician student needs 233 hours of practical work experience to complete a college course. If the student has completed 175 hours, how many hours remain to fulfill the requirement?
   A. 37
   B. 42
   C. 58
   D. 63

10. Barbara Forrest, a technician working in the unit-dose cart fill area, notices that the 25 mg and 50 mg strengths of Benadryl® are mixed together in the same storage bin. What can Barbara do to correct this error?
A. Modify the stock shelf so that each strength has its own section or bin.
B. Change the label to indicate that both strengths are in the bin.
C. Make no changes, because technicians are responsible to read labels carefully.
D. Store the 25 mg strength under Benadryl® and the 50 mg strength under diphenhydramine.

11. In the typical IV setup, a large-volume parenteral (LVP) port is attached to a primary set that is then attached to the catheter and inserted into the patient. Drugs given intermittently are usually given
A. by adding them to the LVP solution.
B. through another IV line (not through the one used for the LVP).
C. through a Y-site injection port or flashbulb on the primary set.
D. by none of the methods that are mentioned above.

12. A nurse is giving potent drugs that are adjusted for their effect on the patient and their amounts must be controlled carefully. Which of the following devices allows this type of control?
A. A wrist watch
B. A roller clamp
C. A spirometer
D. An electronic infusion

13. The recommended dose of ampicillin to treat an ear infection is 50 mg/kg/day, given q6h. If a child weighs 20 kg, how much ampicillin should she receive per day?
A. 250 mg
B. 500 mg
C. 750 mg
D. 1000 mg

14. How much drug will she receive per dose?
A. 100 mg
B. 150 mg
C. 250 mg
D. 500 mg

15. A pharmacy technician is looking for information about a new drug and cannot find information in the many references available in his pharmacy. He should
A. make up information.
B. assume that the information does not exist.
C. call a physician to get help.
D. consult a pharmacist to help him redefine his search strategy.

16. Kimberly Ross, a pharmacy technician at Wuesthoff Pharmacy, has the flu and has been taking antihistamines to dry her runny nose. She decides to work her scheduled shift because she knows how busy the pharmacy has been this week. However, she feels terrible, and the antihistamine is making her sleepy and dizzy. Kimberly is trying to fill prescriptions accurately, but her eyes are watering and she is having trouble reading. What should Kimberly do to prevent medication errors from occurring?
A. Drink lots of water, and have chicken soup for lunch.
B. Drink a few cups of tea or coffee to help avoid being sleepy.
C. Ask the pharmacist if she can go home because she is ill.
D. Ask the patients to read their prescriptions to her.

17. A pharmacy technician is documenting the receipt of pharmaceuticals for which the purchase order or manufacturer's invoice cannot be located. Which of the following information should be recorded?
A. Date of receipt, product name, and amount
B. Date of receipt, name of receiver, product name, strength, dosage form, and amount
C. Product name, strength, and amount
D. Product name and amount only

18. Sharon is a nurse who received an order to administer 5 mEq of potassium acetate per hour. The bag of IV fluid contains 30 mEq/L. How many drops per minute would be needed to provide the prescribed dose using a set that delivers 15 gtts/mL?
A. 5
B. 18
C. 42
D. 57

19. A mother comes to the prescription counter and asks the pharmacy technician to recommend an OTC product for her 2-year-old child who has an earache. The technician should
A. take the mother to the ear drop section and select a product.
B. refer the mother to a physician.
C. refer the mother to the pharmacist.
D. tell the mother to go to the emergency department of the hospital.

20. A pharmacy technician is mixing an IV admixture containing calcium gluconate and potassium phosphate in D5W. After the product is prepared, the technician notices a cloudy precipitate forming. The technician should do all of the following except
A. check the IV reference for calcium gluconate and potassium phosphate incompatibility.
B. not dispense the product.
C. consult with the IV room pharmacist.
D. filter the solution with an in-line filter.

21. A pharmacy technician is filling a prescription for an adult for Compazine® syrup 5 mg/5 mL. The physician's directions are to take 10 mg three times daily. How many teaspoonfuls should the technician indicate on the prescription label?
A. One teaspoonful
B. Two teaspoonfuls
C. Three teaspoonfuls
D. None of the above

22. An inpatient order is received from the pediatrician for ampicillin 75 mg/kg/24 hr to be given in divided doses every 8 hours for 10 days. The child weighs 44 lb. The pharmacy has a 150 mL bottle that contains 250 mg/5 mL. What is the patient's weight in kg?
A. 40 kg
B. 30 kg
C. 20 kg
D. 10 kg

23. What is the single dose in milligrams of ampicillin?
A. 500 mg
B. 250 mg
C. 125 mg
D. 75 mg

24. What is the dose in milliliters that the nurse must administer?
A. 2.5 mL
B. 5 mL
C. 7.5 mL
D. 10 mL

25. What is the dose in teaspoonfuls that the mother must administer?
A. 1 teaspoonful
B. 2 teaspoonfuls
C. 3 teaspoonfuls
D. 4 teaspoonfuls

26. The pharmacy technician notices that the inventory on Demerol® tablets is low and must be reordered. The technician should
A. call in an order for the Demerol® to the supplier.
B. ignore the situation.
C. alert the pharmacist.
D. call around to find the Demerol®.

27. A pharmacy technician is checking in an order of prescription drugs and receives an unfamiliar drug. The technician desires to determine the storage conditions for this drug. The best way to determine the storage conditions for the drug is to
A. refer to the manufacturer's label.
B. refer to the U.S. Pharmacopeia.
C. guess and store at room temperature.
D. ask the pharmacist.

28. A patient's goal is to lose 36 lb. The physician wants the patient to lose these pounds slowly, over a 24-month period. How many pounds should the patient attempt to lose each month?
A. 0.75 lb
B. 1.50 lb
C. 1.75 lb
D. 2.50 lb

29. Laura, a pharmacy technician, receives a prescription which reads as follows: "Fosamax® 10 mg #30 Sig: 1 qd w/food, 3 refills." Laura questions the pharmacist about this prescription because
A. the product is not available in the strength specified.
B. the medication is not refillable.
C. the medication is not supposed to be administered with food.
D. the medication is usually prescribed qid.

30. A pharmacist dispensed a Schedule II drug. He is asking you to fill out a special form to order controlled substances listed in this schedule. Which of the following forms is the most appropriate form to use?
A. DEA Form 224
B. DEA Form 363
C. DEA Form 222
D. DEA Form 510

31. Mrs. Johnson tells the pharmacist that her son became deaf from a medication he was taking in the neonatal intensive care unit when he was a newborn. Which of the following agents may cause deafness?
A. Lasix®
B. Detrol®
C. Winstrol®
D. Simron®

32. A teenager calls your pharmacy to tell you that she is experiencing a racing heartbeat, nervousness, and feels "hyped-up." She says she takes asthma medication. You refer her to the pharmacist and hear the pharmacist telling the patient that she is probably having an adverse reaction to which of the following?
A. Singulair®
B. Intal®
C. Albuterol®
D. Primatene Mist®

33. A child's mother describes the fact that her child's gums seem bigger and are more prone to bleeding. The child has been receiving a medication for 6 months. Which of the following is it likely to be?
A. Dilantin®
B. Intal®
C. Prevacid®
D. Bactrim®

34. Sometimes the available dosage of medication on hand is not the same as that which the physician has ordered. The pharmacy technician must determine how much of the medication should be used. In the equation used for the calculation of how much is needed, the needed dosage is indicated by
A. the numerator.
B. the denominator.
C. a whole number.
D. both the numerator and denominator.

35. The cost of 250 tablets of Zocor® 20 mg is $246.84. If your pharmacy marks up the cost by 13% and adds a $2.35 dispensing fee, what would be the retail charge for 60 tablets?
A. $23.57
B. $27.54
C. $54.51
D. $69.29

ANSWERS TO CASE STUDY QUESTIONS

1. C
2. A
3. B
4. D
5. C
6. C
7. B
8. A
9. C
10. A
11. C
12. D
13. D
14. C
15. D
16. C
17. B
18. C
19. C
20. D
21. B
22. C
23. A
24. D
25. B
26. C
27. A
28. B
29. C
30. C
31. A
32. C
33. A
34. A
35. D

APPENDIX C

Answers to Review Questions

CHAPTER 1

1. C
2. C
3. A
4. B
5. D
6. D
7. B
8. D
9. C
10. A

CHAPTER 2

1. B
2. D
3. B
4. B
5. B
6. D
7. D
8. D
9. C
10. D
11. B
12. A
13. D
14. D
15. B
16. D
17. B
18. C
19. D
20. B
21. C

CHAPTER 3

1. D
2. C
3. D
4. B
5. B
6. C
7. B
8. A
9. C
10. D
11. C
12. D
13. C
14. C
15. D
16. A
17. D
18. C
19. D
20. C
21. C
22. A
23. D
24. A

CHAPTER 4

1. B
2. D
3. B
4. B
5. C
6. C
7. D
8. B
9. D
10. C
11. D
12. D
13. D
14. A
15. A

CHAPTER 5

1. B
2. C
3. D
4. C
5. C
6. A
7. A
8. D
9. B
10. B
11. C
12. D
13. C
14. C
15. A
16. C
17. D
18. A

CHAPTER 6

1. D
2. A
3. B
4. C
5. B
6. C
7. D
8. B
9. A
10. D

CHAPTER 7

1. C
2. B
3. C
4. A
5. B
6. A
7. D
8. C
9. B
10. D
11. C
12. B
13. A
14. D
15. D

CHAPTER 8

1. D
2. B
3. C
4. D
5. A
6. B
7. A
8. C
9. B
10. D
11. D

CHAPTER 9

1. B
2. A
3. D
4. A
5. D
6. B
7. D
8. C
9. B
10. C
11. B
12. B
13. B
14. D
15. B

CHAPTER 10

1. C
2. A
3. D
4. C
5. B
6. C
7. B
8. D
9. A
10. C
11. D
12. C
13. A
14. D
15. B
16. B
17. D
18. C
19. B
20. A

CHAPTER 11

1. C
2. B
3. D
4. C
5. C
6. A
7. D
8. B
9. B
10. C
11. D
12. A
13. B
14. D
15. C

CHAPTER 12

1. B
2. C
3. B
4. A
5. B
6. C
7. A
8. C
9. C
10. C
11. A
12. C
13. B
14. C
15. A

CHAPTER 13

1. B
2. C
3. D
4. D
5. D
6. D
7. D
8. C
9. A
10. C
11. B
12. C
13. D
14. B
15. A

CHAPTER 14

1. C
2. A
3. B
4. B
5. C
6. D
7. A
8. C
9. C
10. D
11. C
12. B
13. B
14. D
15. A
16. C
17. C
18. D
19. C
20. B
21. B

CHAPTER 15

1. C
2. A
3. D
4. A
5. B
6. C
7. A
8. D
9. C
10. A

CHAPTER 16

1. C
2. A
3. D
4. A
5. B
6. D
7. C
8. B
9. A
10. B
11. B
12. D
13. C
14. D
15. A
16. B

CHAPTER 17

1. D
2. C
3. B
4. B
5. C
6. A
7. C
8. A
9. D
10. B

CHAPTER 18

1. D
2. C
3. C
4. A
5. C
6. D
7. B
8. C
9. D
10. A
11. C
12. D
13. A
14. D
15. B

CHAPTER 19

1. C
2. C
3. B
4. A
5. B
6. D
7. D
8. B
9. D
10. C
11. B
12. A
13. B
14. C
15. B
16. C
17. A
18. C
19. A

CHAPTER 20

1. B
2. A
3. D
4. A
5. C
6. A
7. D
8. C
9. B
10. C
11. A
12. D
13. D
14. C

CHAPTER 21

1. A
2. B
3. D
4. D
5. C
6. A
7. D
8. B
9. D
10. A
11. C
12. B

CHAPTER 22

1. C
2. A
3. A
4. D
5. B
6. B
7. D
8. C
9. D
10. C
11. A
12. D
13. A
14. B
15. D
16. B
17. C
18. C
19. D
20. C

CHAPTER 23

1. B
2. B
3. C
4. A
5. D
6. B
7. C
8. D
9. A
10. C
11. D
12. B
13. A
14. C
15. B

CHAPTER 24

1. B
2. D
3. D
4. B
5. D
6. B
7. C
8. C
9. B
10. A
11. B
12. A
13. B
14. D
15. D
16. C
17. D
18. C
19. D
20. B

CHAPTER 25

1. D
2. C
3. C
4. A
5. D
6. B
7. D
8. B
9. C
10. C
11. C
12. C
13. A
14. D
15. D

CHAPTER 26

1. C
2. D
3. B
4. C
5. A
6. C
7. A
8. B
9. A
10. B
11. B
12. B
13. B
14. A
15. D
16. B
17. C
18. B
19. A
20. B

CHAPTER 27

1. D
2. C
3. A
4. B
5. C
6. A
7. D
8. D
9. A
10. B
11. C
12. A
13. D
14. C
15. C

CHAPTER 28

1. C
2. D
3. A
4. C
5. B
6. B
7. D
8. A
9. D
10. C
11. B
12. D
13. B
14. D
15. B

CHAPTER 29

1. B
2. D
3. C
4. B
5. A
6. C
7. D
8. B
9. A
10. C
11. B
12. C
13. D
14. D
15. A

CHAPTER 30

1. D
2. B
3. B
4. A
5. D
6. A
7. C
8. B
9. D
10. B
11. C
12. C
13. C
14. D
15. C

CHAPTER 31

1. B
2. A
3. D
4. B
5. C
6. D
7. C
8. A
9. B
10. C

CHAPTER 32

1. C
2. A
3. D
4. C
5. A
6. C
7. D
8. D
9. D
10. B
11. C

CHAPTER 33

1. C
2. B
3. C
4. A
5. A
6. D
7. A
8. C
9. C
10. B
11. A
12. C

CHAPTER 34

1. B
2. D
3. A
4. B
5. D
6. A
7. C
8. B
9. A
10. D

CHAPTER 35

1. B
2. B
3. D
4. B
5. C
6. C
7. A
8. A
9. C
10. D
11. C
12. B
13. C
14. D
15. B
16. C
17. A
18. C
19. B
20. D
21. D
22. D
23. C
24. D
25. D
26. A
27. D
28. B
29. A
30. B

CHAPTER 36

1. D
2. A
3. C
4. C
5. A
6. C
7. D
8. B
9. A
10. B
11. C
12. D
13. A
14. A
15. B
16. C
17. C
18. D
19. C
20. D
21. D
22. A
23. C
24. B
25. B
26. D
27. C
28. C
29. B
30. D

Glossary

abbreviations Shortened forms of words.

abciximab A platelet aggregation inhibitor.

absorption The movement of a drug from its site of administration into the bloodstream.

accounting A system of recording, classifying, and summarizing financial transactions for preparing a pharmacy budget.

acetaminophen An analgesic and antipyretic commonly used instead of aspirin, particularly for patients who are allergic to aspirin, are taking anticoagulants, or have a peptic ulcer.

acetylcholine (ACh) A neurotransmitter that stimulates nerve endings of parasympathetic and sympathetic nervous systems.

acid Any substance with a hydrogen ion that is released in a solution and reacts with metals to form salts; pH less than 7.

active immunity Immunity resulting from the development of antibodies within a person's body that renders the person immune; it may occur from exposure through a disease process or from immunizations.

addition The combined effect of two agents, which is equal to the sum of the effects of each drug taken alone.

administrative law Regulations set forth by governmental agencies, such as the Internal Revenue Service (IRS) and the Social Security Administration (SSA).

adrenal glands Glands that synthesize glucocorticoids, mineralocorticoids, and androgens.

agonist The drug that produces a functional change in a cell.

alkali Any of a class of compounds such as sodium hydroxide that form salts with acids and soaps with fats.

alkyalting agents Antineoplastic drugs the affect cell growth.

allergic rhinitis Inflammation of the nasal mucosa that is due to the sensitivity of the nasal tissue to an allergen.

allergy A state of hypersensitivity induced by exposure to a particular antigen.

Alzheimer's disease An illness characterized by progressive memory failure, impaired thinking, confusion, disorientation, personality changes, restlessness, speech disturbances, and inability to perform routine tasks.

ambulatory care Medical care that is given on an outpatient basis. Patients are able to come and go to an office or clinic for diagnostic tests or treatments.

amebicides Drugs used to treat a protozoal infection.

aminoglycosides A group of potent bactericidal agents that are usually reserved for serious or life-threatening infections.

amortize To spread the cost of services out over the period of several years.

ampule A sealed glass container that usually contains a single dose of medicine. The top of the ampule must be broken off to open the container.

anabolic steroids Synthetically produced androgens.

anabolism The metabolic process by which substances are converted into other chemical components of an organism's structure.

analgesics Pain-relieving drugs.

anaphylactic reaction A life-threatening allergic reaction that is characterized by a drop in blood pressure with difficulty breathing.

anesthetics Agents that act on nervous tissue to produce a loss of sensation or unconsciousness.

angina pectoris An episodic, reversible insufficiency of oxygen to the heart muscle.

antacids Alkaline compounds used to neutralize hydrochloric acid in the stomach.

antagonism The combined effect of two drugs that is less than the effect of either drug taken alone.

anthrax A zoonotic disease caused by the anthrax bacillus that can infect humans in a number of ways and can be fatal.

antibiotics Substances that have the ability to destroy or interfere with the development of a living organism.

antibody Protein that develops in response to the presence of an antigen in the body and reacts with the antigen on the next exposure. Antibodies may be formed from infections, immunization, transfer from mother to child, or unknown antigen stimulation.

anticholinergics Medications that block acetylcholine.

anticoagulants Chemical substances that inhibit blood coagulation.

antiemetics Drugs used to prevent or relieve nausea and vomiting that may be associated with many different disorders.

antigen A substance that is either introduced into the body or formed by the body to induce the formation of antibodies specific to that antigen.

antihistamine A drug that counteracts the action of histamine.

antimetabolites Substances that prevent cancer growth by affecting DNA production.

antineoplastic agents Drugs used to treat cancers and malignant neoplasms.

antiparasitics Agents that are used to treat worms.

antiplatelet agent Any agent that destroys platelets or inhibits their function.

antipyretics Fever-relieving drugs.

antithyroid agent A chemical agent that lowers the basal metabolic rate by interfering with the formation, release, or action of thyroid hormones.

antitubercular Drugs that are used to treat tuberculosis.

antitussives Agents that relieve or prevent coughing.

antiviral agents Substances used to treat viral infections by influencing viral replication.

Arabic numbers Standard numerical numbers.

arrhythmia Loss of rhythm.

arteriosclerosis Hardening and narrowing of the arteries resulting from age.

Arthus reaction A severe local inflammatory reaction that occurs at the site of injection of an antigen in a previously sensitized individual.

aspirin (acetylsalicylic acid) An analgesic, antipyretic, antiheumatic, and anti-inflammatory agent.

assignment of benefits An authorization to an insurance company to make payment directly to the pharmacy or physician.

asthma A chronic, reversible, obstruction of the bronchial airways that is characterized by paroxysmal attacks of dyspnea or difficult respiration on expiration.

atherosclerosis Narrowing of the arteries due to build up of plaque and fatty deposits on the walls of the arteries.

atropine An anticholinergic alkaloid found in belladonna; it acts as a competitive antagonist of acetylcholine at muscarinic receptors.

autoclave A sterilizing machine. An autoclave uses a combination of heat, steam, and pressure to sterilize equipment.

autonomy The right of an individual to make informed decisions for his or her own good.

auxillary labeling Supplementary or secondary labeling.

Bacillus anthracis Bacteria causing anthrax with a cell shape that is cylindrical (longer than it is wide).

bacteremia A condition in which bacteria are recovered from blood cultures of a patient and may or may not be associated with the disease.

bactericidal agents Antibiotic drugs that kill bacteria.

bacteriostatic agents Drugs that tend to restrain the development of the reproduction of bacteria.

barbiturates Chemical derivatives of barbituric acid that have a depressant effect on the central nervous system.

batch repackaging The reassembling of a specific dosage and dosage form of medication at a given time.

benign Nonprogressive.

benzene A liquid hydrocarbon obtained mainly as a by-product of the destructive distillation of coal. It is used as a solvent. Benzene is an irritant and is toxic and carcinogenic.

benzodiazepines Drugs used to treat anxiety that has a depressive action on the central nervous system.

beriberi A disease of the peripheral nerves caused by a deficiency of or an inability to assimilate thiamine.

β-adrenergic agents Drugs that work as both a cardiac and respiratory agonist.

β-adrenergic blockers Drug that reduce oxygen demand by decreasing heart rate and contraction of the myocardium while also decreasing arterial blood pressure.

bile acid sequestrants Drugs that are nonabsorbable and used for lowering cholesterol.

bioavailability Measurement of the rate of absorption and total amount of drug that reaches systemic circulation.

bioethics A discipline dealing with the ethical and moral implications of biological research and applications.

biohazard symbol An image or object that serves as an alert that there is a risk to organisms, such as ionizing radiation or harmful bacteria or viruses.

biotransformation The conversion of a drug within the body; also known as metabolism.

black box warning A warning located in the *Physician's Desk Reference* to alert physicians to high risks involved in administration of a particular drug.

body language The use of gestures, movements, and mannerisms to communicate something.

broad spectrum antibiotics A type of antibiotic that is used in the treatment of multiple organisms.

bronchodilators Agents that relax the smooth muscle of the bronchial tubes.

buccal Pertaining to the inside of the cheek.

calcium An alkaline earth metal element. The body requires calcium ions for the transmission of nerve impulses, muscle contraction, blood coagulation, cardiac functions, and other processes.

calcium channel blockers Drug that prevent and reverse coronary spasm and decrease oxygen requirements, causing vasodilation.

caplet A tablet shaped like a capsule.

capsule A solid dosage form in which the drug is enclosed in either a hard or soft shell of soluble material.

carbohydrate The major source of energy for all body functions.

carbon monoxide (CO) A colorless, odorless, tasteless gas, formed by burning carbon or organic fuels with a scant supply of oxygen. It is the number one cause of unintentional poisoning around the world.

cardiac glycosides Drugs derived from digitalis that increase cardiac output and renal blood flow.

cardiac toxicity Adverse effects on the cardiovascular or hematopoietic systems that result from exposure to chemical substances.

case law Law established by judicial decision in legal cases and used as legal precedent.

cell-mediated immunity The type of immune responses brought about by T cells (T lymphocytes).

cellular hypersensitivity reaction The result of the activity of many leukocyte actions. The T^1 lymphocytes become sensitized by their first contact with a specific antigen. Subsequent exposure to an antigen stimulates multiple reactions aimed at destroying or inactivating the offending antigen.

Centers for Medicare & Medicaid Services (CMS) The federal organization that administers Medicare and Medicaid. Its official Web site offers information about programs, statistical highlights, and the full text of laws and regulations affecting the agency. Formerly known as the Health Care Financing Administration (HCFA).

cephalosporins Semisynthetic antibiotics structurally and pharmacologically related to penicillins.

CHAMPVA Civilian Health and Medical Program of the Veterans Administration; a program to cover medical expenses of dependent spouse and children of veterans with total, permanent service-connected disabilities.

chemical sterilization A method of cleaning equipment used for instruments that cannot be exposed to the high temperatures of steam sterilization.

chloride An anion of chlorine. The most common form is sodium chloride (table salt).

cholesterol A waxy lipid found only in animal tissues. A member of a group of lipids called sterols, it is widely distributed in the body.

cilostazol A drug that inhibits platelet aggregation.

clopidogrel A drug that inhibits platelet aggregation.

coagulation The complex process that leads to the conversion of fibrinogen to fibrin to form a blood clot; also referred to as hemostasis.

coagulation factor One of 12 factors in the blood, the interactions of which are responsible for the process of blood clotting.

common law Derives authority from ancient usages and customs affirmed by court judgments and decrees.

compensation An unconscious mechanism by which one tries to make up for fancied or real deficiencies.

computerized physician order entry system (CPOE) A process in which the physician enters medication orders directly into a computerized system to eliminate the need for interpretation and thus reduce the risk for medication error.

congestive heart failure A condition in which the output of the heart is insufficient to supply adequate levels of oxygen for the body.

constitutional law Deals with interpretation and implementation of the United States Constitution.

contraindication A condition that increases the chance of a serious adverse reaction.

convulsion Abnormal motor movements.

coordination of benefits The prevention of duplicate payment for the same service.

co-payment Most policies have a coinsurance, or cost-sharing requirement, that is the responsibility of the insured.

copper A metallic element that is a component of several important enzymes in the body and is essential to good health.

corticosteroids The most potent and consistently effective anti-inflammatory agents that are currently available for relief in respiratory conditions.

cost control The implementation of managerial efforts to achieve cost objectives.

cream A semisolid emulsion of either the oil-in-water or the water-in-oil type, ordinarily intended for topical use.

cross-dependence The ability of one drug to substitute for another drug in the same drug class to maintain a dependent state or prevent withdrawal.

cross-tolerance Tolerance to one drug conferring tolerance to other drugs in the same drug class.

cyanide A binary compound that prevents tissue use of oxygen; most of its compounds are deadly poisons.

cytotoxic reaction Severe damage to or destruction of cells by a substance.

data The raw facts the computer can manipulate.

decongestants Drugs that cause vasoconstriction of nasal mucosa and reduce congestion or swelling.

deductible A specific amount of money that must be paid each year before the policy benefits begin (e.g., $50, $100, $300, or $500).

denominator The number the whole is divided into.

Department of Public Health (DPH) An organization in which sciences, skills, and beliefs that are directed to the maintenance and improvement of the health of all the people are combined.

dependence The total psychophysical state of one addicted to drugs or alcohol who must receive an increasing amount of the substance to prevent the onset of withdrawal symptoms.

dependents The insured's spouse and children under the terms of the policy.

detergent An agent that purifies or cleanses.

diabetes mellitus A disorder of carbohydrate metabolism that involves either an insulin deficiency, insulin resistance, or both.

dicoumarol A synthetic anti-coagulant used for the prophylaxis and treatment of thrombosis and embolism.

dipyridamole A coronary vasodilator used for the long-term treatment of angina.

disease-modifying antirheumatic drugs (DMARDs) Immunosuppressive drugs useful in the treatment of lupus nephritis, seropositive progressive rheumatoid arthritis, and vasculitis syndromes.

disinfection Destruction of pathogens by physical or chemical means.

dispensing fee A pricing mechanism calculated by adding the operating expenses and profit margin and dividing by the total work units, either unit doses or inpatient prescriptions.

displacement The transfer of impulses from one expression to another, as from fighting to talking.

distribution The process by which blood leaves the bloodstream and enters the tissues of the body.

diuretics Drugs that reduce left ventricular pressure, decrease left ventricular volume, and lower oxygen demand.

divisor The number performing the division.

dopamine antagonists A major category of antiemetics.

dram A unit of weight in the apothecary system; 1 dram equals 60 grains.

drive through An external site at a pharmacy that can be accessed by driving up in the car.

drop rate The number of drops at which an intravenous infusion is administered over a specified period of time.

drug abuse Nonmedical use of a drug that is deemed unacceptable by society.

dry heat sterilization A method of sterilization that uses heated dry air at a temperature of 320 to 356°F (160 to 180°C) for 90 minutes to 3 hours.

dry powder inhaler (DPI) A device used to deliver medication in the form of micronized powder into the lungs.

electrolyte A compound that dissociates into ions when dissolved in water.

eligibility The specific terms of coverage under a policy.

elixir A clear, sweetened, hydroalcoholic liquid intended for oral use.

emetics Agents used to promote vomiting.

emulsion A system containing two liquids that cannot be mixed together in which one is dispersed, in the form of very small globules, throughout the other.

endogenous depression Feelings of intense sadness, helplessness, and worthlessness that have no external cause and may be the result of genetic factors or biochemical changes in the brain.

enteral nutrition Feedings given into the gastrointestinal system. Although normal eating qualifies as enteral nutrition, the term is usually applied to specially prepared liquid feedings.

enunciation Clearing speaking and forming words.

epilepsy A group of disorders that are characterized by hyperexcitability within the central nervous system.

essential (primary) hypertension A chronic cardiovascular disease with no known origins.

estradiol A chemical derivative of natural estrogen.

estrogen A female sex hormone produced by the ovaries and the placenta.

ethics The branch of philosophy that deals with the distinction between right and wrong with the moral consequences of human actions.

ethinyl A chemical derivative of natural estrogen.

ethylene glycol A chemical used in automobile antifreeze.

exogenous depression Feelings of intense sadness, helplessness, and worthlessness in response to a loss, disappointment, or illness.

expectorants Agents that promote the removal of mucous secretions from the lung, bronchi, and trachea, usually by coughing.

exposure control plan A written procedure for the treatment of persons exposed to biohazardous or similar chemically harmful materials.

extemporaneous A medication that is made based upon a particular set of circumstances or criteria.

extravasation Leakage of fluid from vessels into surrounding tissues.

extremes The two outside terms in a ratio.

fat A substance composed of lipids or fatty acids and occurring in various forms.

fatty acid Any of several organic acids produced by the hydrolysis of neutral fats.

file A set of data or a program that has been given a name.

fire safety plan A written procedure that includes fire extinguisher locations, fire alarm pull-box locations, sprinkler system location, exit signs, and clear directions to the quickest and safest exit of a building during an emergency.

first-pass metabolism The degree to which a drug is chemically altered as it circulates through the liver for the first time.

floor stock system A system of drug distribution in which the pharmacy buys medications in bulk and distributes bulk orders to patient care units, where they are stored in medication rooms. Nurses are then responsible for preparing individual doses of medications.

fluidextract A pharmacopeial liquid preparation of vegetable drugs, made by filtration, containing alcohol as a solvent or as a preservative or both.

fluoride Any binary compound of fluorine.

formaldehyde A gaseous compound with strong disinfectant properties. It is used in a 37% solution (formol or formalin) as a disinfectant and as a preservative and fixactive for pathological specimens. The gas is toxic and carcinogenic.

fraction An expression of division with a number that is the portion or part of a whole.

gas sterilization The use of a gas such as ethylene oxide to sterilize medical equipment.

gel A jelly or the solid or semisolid phase of a colloidal solution.

gelcap An oil-based medication that is enclosed in a soft gelatin capsule.

glucocorticoids A hormone that increases the formation of glycogen from fatty acids and proteins rather than from carbohydrates, exerts an anti-inflammatory effect, and influences many body functions.

grain The basic unit of weight in the apothecary system.

gram The basic unit for weight in the metric system.

granule A very small pill, usually gelatin- or sugar-coated, containing a drug to be given in a small dose.

gray baby syndrome A disorder caused by administration of chloramphenicol to pregnant women or to neonates. The newborn baby exhibits an ashen-gray color within 24 hours after administration of the drug. The newborn may also have other signs and symptoms such as vomiting, irregular respiration, and cyanosis.

group purchasing Procurement contracts are negotiated on behalf of the members of a group (e.g., hospitals, nursing home pharmacies, and home infusion pharmacies). The group purchasing organization uses the collective buying power of its members to negotiate discounts from manufacturers, wholesalers, and other suppliers.

half-life The time it takes for the plasma concentration to be reduced by 50%.

hardware The parts of the computer that you can touch.

hazard communication plan Use of warning labels for all hazardous chemicals.

health insurance A contract between a policy-holder and an insurance carrier or government program to reimburse the policyholder for all or a portion of the cost of medical care rendered by health care professionals.

heparin sodium A mucopolysaccharide that enhances the effects of antithrombin III. It is used as an anti-coagulant for laboratory testing and as a therapeutic agent.

hepatitis Inflammation of the liver caused by microorganisms, especially viruses, or drugs such as alcohol and other poisons.

highly active antiretroviral therapy (HAART) A substance that combines two reverse transcriptase inhibitors and one protease inhibitor in a cocktail that interrupts the human immunodeficiency virus in two different phases of its life cycle.

histamine A chemical substance found in all the body tissues, that protects the body from factors in the environment that produce allergic and inflammatory reactions.

histamine H_2 receptor antagonists Drugs that inhibit the interaction of histamine (H_2) at the H_2 receptors, which predominate in gastric parietal cells.

hormonal agents Substances consisting of a heterogenous compound that either blocks hormone production or blocks hormone action.

hormone A natural chemical secreted into the bloodstream from the endocrine glands to regulate and control the activity of an organ or tissues in another part of the body.

hospice Originally a facility, usually within a hospital, intended to care for the terminally ill, in particular, by providing physical comfort to the patient and emotional support and counseling to the patient and the family.

human immunodeficiency virus (HIV) The virus that causes acquired immunodeficiency syndrome.

human rabies immune globulin A sterile solution of antirabies immune globulin for intramuscular administration. It is prepared from the plasma of human donors hyperimmunized with the rabies vaccine. It should be administered to patients as soon as possible after exposure to the disease.

humeral immunity Protective molecules (mostly B lymphocytes) carried in the fluids of the body.

hydrophobia A fear of water; a symptom caused by rabies as the disease progresses.

hypersensitivity An unpredictable reaction to a drug due to the development of antibodies against it; also known as an allergy.

hypervitaminosis An abnormal condition resulting from excessive intake of toxic amounts of one or more vitamins, especially over a long period.

hypnosis An increased tendency to sleep.

idiosyncratic reaction Experience of a unique, strange, or unpredicted reaction to a drug.

immunity An immunological reaction that destroys or resists antigens.

immunoglobulin A blood product that contains disease-specific antibodies for passive immunity.

implant An insert or a graft.

inactivated vaccines Vaccines in which the infectious components have been destroyed by chemical or physical treatments.

independent practice association (IPA) A type of health maintenance organization (HMO) in which the HMO contracts directly with physicians, who continue in their existing practices.

independent purchasing The pharmacist or technician works alone and deals directly with pharmaceutical companies or wholesalers to negotiate price, quantity, and delivery.

informed consent A consent in which there is understanding of what treatment is to be undertaken and of the risks involved, why it should be done, and what alternative methods of treatment are available.

insulin A hormone synthesized and secreted by the pancreas.

international law Law based on treaties and other agreements between two or more countries.

intradermal injection Between the layers of the skin. A dose of an agent administered between the layers of the skin.

intramuscular injection Inside a muscle. Normally used in the context of an injection given into a muscle.

intravenous injection Into a vein. Most commonly used in the context of an injection given directly into a vein.

inventory The stock of medications a pharmacy keeps immediately on hand.

invoice A form describing a purchase and the amount due.

iodine A nonmetallic trace element that is an essential micronutrient of thyroid hormone.

iron A common metallic element essential for the synthesis of hemoglobin.

ischemic heart disease A condition in which there is insufficient blood supply to the myocardium.

isopropyl alcohol A transparent, volatile, colorless liquid used as a solvent and disinfectant and applied topically as an antiseptic. It is also called isopropanol.

Joint Commission on Accreditation of Healthcare Organizations (JCAHO) Not-for-profit organization that sets standards to ensure effective quality services (e.g., optimal standards for the operation of hospitals).

kwashiorkor An acute process associated with protein deficiency and impaired immune function.

laminar airflow hood A system of circulating filtered air in parallel-flowing planes in hospitals or other health care facilities. The system reduces the risk of airborne contamination and exposure to chemical pollutants in surgical theaters, food preparation areas, hospital pharmacies, and laboratories.

law A principle or rule that is advisable or obligatory to observe.

lead A chemical element; excessive ingestion or absorption causes lead poisoning.

legend drug A medication that may be dispensed only with a prescription; also known as a prescription drug.

lentiviruses A group of retroviruses that cause slow-developing diseases.

leukotrienes Substances that contribute to the inflammation associated with asthma.

liniment A liquid preparation for external use, usually applied by friction to the skin.

liter The basic unit of volume in the metric system.

live attenuated vaccines Vaccines containing living organisms or intact viruses that have undergone radiation or temperature conditioning to produce safe vaccinations which will help the patient become immune to a specific disease.

long-term care A wide range of health and health-related support services.

long-term care pharmacy organization An organization involving a licensed professional pharmacy or practice that provides medications and clinical services to long-term care facilities and their residents.

lozenge A small, disk-shaped tablet composed of solidifying paste containing an astringent, an antiseptic, or an oil-based drug used for local treatment of the mouth or throat. It is held in the mouth until dissolved. Also known as a troche.

lymphocytes The second most common form of white blood cells.

macrolides Broad-spectrum antimicrobials, which include erythromycins and erythromycin derivatives.

magnesium A silver-white mineral element. It is the second most abundant cation of the intracellular fluids in the body. It is essential for many enzyme activities.

magnesium sulfate An anticonvulsant and electrolyte replenisher. It is also used as a laxative and local anti-inflammatory agent.

mail order pharmacy A licensed pharmacy that uses the mail or other carriers (e.g., overnight carriers or parcel services) to deliver prescriptions to patients.

malignant Spreading.

malnutrition A disease resulting from unbalanced, insufficient, or excessive diet.

Mantoux test An intradermal screening for tuberculin hypersensitivity. A red, firm patch of skin at the injection site greater than 10 mm in diameter, after 48 hours, is a positive result that indicates current or prior exposure to tubercle bacilli.

marasmus A chronic disease that develops as a result of a deficiency in caloric intake.

markup fee system A pricing mechanism in which the price charged to the patient is calculated by adding a percentage markup, in addition to a dispensing fee, to the acquisition cost of the drug.

means The two inside terms in a ratio.

Medicaid A federal/state medical assistance program to provide health insurance for specific populations.

medical asepsis The destruction of organisms after they leave the body.

Medicare A federal health insurance program created as part of the social security act.

medication A substance used in the treatment or maintenance of an illness.

medroxyprogesterone acetate A long-acting injectable drug that is a highly affective contraceptive.

menadione A water-soluble injectable form of the product of vitamin K_3.

meningitis An inflammation of the meninges (membranes) that surround and protect the brain. It is often caused by bacteria.

meningococcal vaccine Vaccine aiding antibodies in the attacking of the gram-negative coccus bacteria that are responsible for meningitis.

meniscus The dip in fluid level when an oral liquid medication is dispensed.

mercury A chemical element that can be absorbed by the skin and mucous membranes, causing chronic poisoning.

mestranol A chemical derivative of natural estrogen.

metabolism The conversion of a drug within the body; also known as biotransformation.

metastasize Uncontrollable growth characteristic of cancer cells.

meter The basic unit of length in the metric system.

metered dose inhaler (MDI) A hand-held pressurized device used to deliver medications for inhalation.

methyl alcohol A poisonous, colorless liquid used as a solvent and fuel; ingestion may cause blindness or death. It is also called methanol.

mineral An inorganic substance occurring naturally in the earth's crust, having a characteristic chemical composition.

mineralocorticoid A hormone that regulates sodium and potassium balance in the blood.

minim The basic unit of volume in the apothecary system.

mixture A mutual incorporation of two or more substances, without chemical union, in which the physical characteristics of each of the components are retained.

modem A device used to transfer information from one computer to another.

monamine oxidase inhibitors (MAOIs) Drugs that reduce the activity of the enzyme monoamine oxidase and act to increase central nervous system activity.

motor nerve A nerve that originates in the spinal cord and stimulates several muscle fibers; also called somatic nerve.

mucolytic Destroying or dissolving the active agents that constitute mucus.

myocardial infarction (MI) A condition in which a portion of the cardiac muscle suffers a severe and prolonged restriction of oxygenated coronary blood.

narrow-spectrum antibiotics A type of antibiotic that is effective against only a few organisms.

National Drug Code (NDC) A unique and permanent product code assigned to each new drug as it becomes available in the marketplace; identifies the manufacturer or distributor, the drug formulation, and the size and type of its packaging.

National Formulary (NF) A database of officially recognized drug names.

natural fat Consists of about 95% triglycerides or triacylglycerols.

negative feedback A decrease in function in response to a stimulus.

neoplasm A tumor.

neurohormones Neurotransmitters.

neuromuscular junction The area where the motor nerve meets the muscle.

neuron The basic structure of a nerve consisting of dendrites, cell body, and axon.

nicotine A constituent of tobacco, along with various gases and particulate matter.

nitrates Antianginal drugs that relax vascular smooth muscles, dilating the vessels and lowering oxygen demand to decrease the work of the heart.

nitrosoureas Newer forms of alkylating agents that are lipid soluble.

non-nucleoside reverse transcriptase inhibitors (NNRTIs) A substance that inhibits the action of the reverse transcriptase neuraminidase by preventing the formation of proviral DNA.

nonsteroidal anti-inflammatory drugs (NSAIDs) Drugs that inhibit the synthesis of the prostaglandin responsible for causing pain and inflammation.

nuclear pharmacy A pharmacy that is specially licensed to work with radioactive materials. Previously called radiopharmacy.

nucleoside reverse transcriptase inhibitors (NRTIs) Competitive inhibitors of the HIV enzyme that convert viral RNA into DNA and act as DNA chain terminators.

numerator The portion of the whole being considered.

nutrition The sum of the processes involved in the taking in of nutrients and their assimilation and use for proper body functioning and maintenance of health.

obesity A condition of excess fatness.

ointment A semisolid preparation that usually contains medicinal substances and is intended for external application.

opioid Any synthetic narcotic that has opiate-like activities, but is not derived from opium.

oral Pertaining to the mouth. Medication given by mouth.

ounce A unit of weight in the apothecary system; 1 ounce equals 8 drams.

over-the-counter (OTC) A medication that may be purchased without a prescription directly from the pharmacy.

overpayment Payment by the insurer or by the patient of more than the amount due.

pancreas An organ of digestion that lies behind the stomach and produces digestive juices, insulin, and glucagons.

pantothenic acid A member of the vitamin B complex. It is widely distributed in plant and animal tissues and may be an important element in human nutrition.

parenteral Administered by some means other than through the gastrointestinal tract; referring particularly to introduction of substances into an organism by intravenous, subcutaneous, intramuscular, or intramedullary injection.

parenteral nutrition A combination of amino acids, dextrose, fats, vitamins, minerals, electrolytes, and water administered intravenously. Parenteral nutrition is capable of providing all the nutrients needed to sustain life.

Parkinson's disease A disorder characterized by resting tremor, rigidity or resistance to passive movement, akinesia, and loss of postural reflexes.

passive immunity Immunity acquired from the injection or passage of antibodies from an immune person or animal to another for short-term immunity, or immunity passed from mother to child.

patent ductus arterious A disorder in which the ductus remains patent when pulmonary vascular resistance falls resulting in aortic blood being shunted into the pulmonary artery.

patient prescription system A system of drug distribution in which the nurse transcribes a physician's medication order on an order form for the pharmacy and the pharmacy provides a 3-day supply of the medication for the nurse to prepare upon use.

penicillins Natural or semisynthetic antibiotics produced by or derived from certain species of the fungus *Penicillium.*

percent A fraction whose numerator is expressed and whose denominator is understood to be 100.

percentage markup system A system of establishing price that assumes that total operating expenses are directly related to the acquisition cost.

petroleum distillates Made from the vaporization of natural oil.

pharmaceutical care The role of the pharmacist in ensuring "the responsible provision of drug therapy for the purpose of achieving definite outcomes that improve a patient's quality of life."

pharmacist An individual who is educated and licensed to dispense drugs and to provide drug information.

pharmacodynamic interaction Differences in effects produced by a given plasma level of a drug.

pharmacodynamics The study of the biochemical and physiological effects of drugs.

pharmacokinetic interaction Differences in the plasma levels of a drug achieved with a given dose of that drug.

pharmacokinetics The study of the absorption, distribution, metabolism, and excretion of drugs.

pharmacy The art and science of dispensing and preparing medication and providing drug-related information to the public.

pharmacy compounding The preparation, mixing, assembling, packaging, or labeling of a drug or device.

pharmacy technician An individual who helps licensed pharmacists provide medication and other health care products to patients.

Pharmacy Technician Certification Board A national organization that provides certification to pharmacy technicians based on a national examination and continuing education.

phenol An extremely poisonous compound, used in dilute solution as an antimicrobial, anesthetic, and antipruritic.

phospholipid A phosphorus-containing lipid.

phosphorus A nonmetallic chemical element occurring extensively in nature as a component of phosphate rock. Phosphorus is essential for the metabolism of protein, calcium, and glucose.

physical dependence The necessity to continue drug use to avoid a withdrawal syndrome.

pill A small, globular mass of soluble material containing a medicinal substance to be swallowed.

pitch The tone and level of one's voice.

pituitary gland A small gland situated at the base of the brain that secretes hormones that regulate other endocrine glands.

placebo An inert substance given to a patient instead of an active medicine. Placebos are often given to people who participate in studies intended to evaluate the effectiveness of a medicine.

placebo effect A decreased drug effect when the feeling of the patient toward the medication is negative.

plaster A solid preparation that can be spread when heated and that becomes adhesive at the temperature of the body.

point of service Payment of services outside of an insurance plan at the time the service is rendered.

policy and procedure manual A set of standard procedural statements or documents that aid an organization in operating effectively and efficiently and support the goals of the overall organization.

policy limitation Policies that exclude certain types of coverage.

policy terms and financial obligations Policy that becomes effective only after the company offers the policy and the person accepts it and pays the initial premium.

potassium An alkali metal element. Potassium salts are necessary to the life of all plants and animals. Potassium in the body helps to regulate neuromuscular excitability and muscle contraction.
potentiation An effect that occurs when a drug increases or prolongs the action of another drug, the total effect being greater than the sum of the effects of each used alone.
powder A dry mass of minute separate particles of any substance.
preauthorization The requirement of notification and permission to receive additional types of services before one obtains those services.
precaution Specific warning to consider when medications are prescribed or administered.
preferred provider organization (PPO) A managed care organization that contracts with a group of providers, who are called *preferred providers,* to offer services to the managed care organization's members.
prefix A part of a word structure that occurs before or in front of the word and modifies the meaning of the root.
premium The cost of the coverage that the insurance policy contains; this may vary greatly, depending on the age and health of the individual and the type of insurance protection.
prn As needed.
professionalism The conduct or qualities characterized by or conforming to the technical or ethical standards of a profession; exhibiting a courteous, conscientious, and generally businesslike manner in the workplace.
progesterone A hormone secreted by the corpus luteum at the time of ovulation.
programs A set of electronic instructions that tell the computer what to do.
projection A defense mechanism by which a repressed complex in the individual is denied and conceived as belonging to another person, such as when faults that the person tends to commit are perceived in or attributed to others.
proportion The relationship between two equal ratios.
protamine sulfate A heparin antagonist derived from fish sperm.
protease inhibitors A substance used to block the action of enzymes.
protein A complex organic nitrogenous compound composed of large combinations of amino acids.
psychological dependence The overwhelming need to take a drug to maintain a sense of well-being.
psychosis A mental illness accompanied by bizarre behavior and altered personality with failure to perceive reality.
pulmonary toxicity Adverse effects on the functioning and structure of the pulmonary system that result from exposure to chemical toxins.
purchase order The document created when an order is placed.
quinolones Bactericidal agents that are effective against most gram-negative and many gram-positive bacteria.
quotient The answer to a division problem.
rabies The only rhabdovirus that infects humans; it is a zoonotic disease characterized by fatal meningoencephalitis.
radiopharmaceutical A drug that is or has been made to be radioactive. Although a few radiopharmaceuticals are used to treat diseases (e.g., radioactive iodine), most are used as diagnostic agents.
ratio A mathematical expression that compares two numbers by division.
rationalization A psychoanalytic defense mechanism through which irrational behavior, motives, or feelings are made to appear reasonable.
receptor The cell that a drug has an affinity to.
regression An unconscious defense mechanism involving a return to earlier patterns of adaptation.
regulatory law Regulations set forth by governmental agencies. It is also called administrative law.
repression A defense mechanism of removing from consciousness an unacceptable idea or impulse.
respiratory distress syndrome (RDS) An acute lung disease of the newborn characterized by airless alveoli, inelastic lung, and an increased respiration rate.
respiratory syncytial virus (RSV) Virus that is the major cause of bronchiolitis and pneumonia in young children.
reteplase A human tissue enzyme produced by recombinant DNA techniques.
root The main part of a word that gives the word its central meaning.
salicylates Nonopoid analgesic and anti-inflammatory medications.
salicylism Toxic effects of overdosage with salicylic acid or salicylates, usually marked by tinnitus, nausea, and vomiting.
secondary hypertension A chronic cardiovascular disease related to an underlying abnormal condition.
sedation A state of consciousness characterized by decreased anxiety, motor activity, and mental acuity.
seizure An epileptic event.
selective serotonin reuptake inhibitor (SSRI) A type of antidepressant that blocks the reuptake and inactivation of serotonin in the brain.
septicemia A condition in which bacteremia is associated with active disease, localized or systemic.
serotonin antagonists The most effective drugs for suppressing nausea and vomiting caused by antineoplastic drugs.
side effect An outcome other than that intended. Most commonly used in the context of drug therapy in which a side effect is an unwanted consequence of the drug in use.
smallpox Acute viral disease that was essentially eradicated in 1979. It causes a disfiguring rash, headache, vomiting, and fever.
soap A kind of detergent used as a cleanser.
sodium One of the most important elements in the body. Sodium ions are involved in acid-base balance, water balance, transmission of nerve impulses, and contraction of muscles.
software A set of electronic instructions that tell the computer what to do.
solution The incorporation of a solid, a liquid, or a gas into a liquid.
somatic nerve A nerve that originates in the spinal cord and stimulates several muscle fibers; also called motor nerve.
specific affinity The attraction a drug has for particular cells.
spirits An alcoholic or hydroalcoholic solution of volatile substances.
standard precautions A set of guidelines for infection control.
standards Established by authority, custom, or general consent as a model or example; something set up and established by authority as a rule for the measure of quantity, weight, extent, value, or quality.
starter kit A group of medications provided to a hospice patient to treat urgent problems that develop in the last days of life.
statin drugs Drugs used to lower high blood cholesterol concentrations.
statutory law The body of laws enacted by a legislative body with the power to make law.
sterile product One that contains no living organisms.
sterilization Complete destruction of all forms of microbial life.
streptokinase A fibrinolytic activator that enhances the conversion of plasminogen to the fibrinolytic enzyme plasmin. It is produced by strains of streptococci and is used in the treatment of certain instances of pulmonary and coronary embolism.
subcutaneous injection The administration of medication by means of a needle and syringe into the layer of fat and blood vessels beneath the skin.

sublimation An unconscious defense mechanism in which unacceptable instinctual drives and wishes are modified into more personally and socially acceptable channels.

sublingual Pertaining to the area under the tongue.

subscriber The individual or organization protected in case of loss under the terms of an insurance policy.

suffix A word ending that modifies the meaning of the root.

sulfonamides Synthetic derivatives of sulfanilamide; these agents were the first drugs to prevent and cure human bacterial infections successfully.

suppository A small, solid body shaped for ready introduction into one of the orifices of the body other than the oral cavity (e.g., rectum, urethra, or vagina), made of a substance, usually medicated, that is solid at ordinary temperature but melts at body temperature.

surfactant A lipoprotein produced by the lungs which keeps the alveoli open.

surgical asepsis The complete destruction of organisms before they enter the body.

suspension A class of pharmacopeial preparations of finely divided, undissolved drugs dispersed in liquid vehicles for oral or parenteral use.

synergism A combined action of two or more agents that produces an effect greater than would have been expected from the two agents acting separately.

syrup A liquid preparation in a concentrated aqueous solution of a sugar used for medicinal purposes or to add flavor to a substance.

tablet A solid dosage form containing medicinal substances with or without suitable diluents.

tetracyclines Antibiotics and semisynthetic antibiotic derivatives obtained from cultures of *Streptomyces*.

tetraiodothyronine (T_4) A hormone produced by the thyroid that increases the rate of metabolism for most cells; also called thyroxine.

The State Board of Pharmacy The organization responsible for the registration of pharmacists, pharmacy interns, and pharmacy technicians.

Third-party payers The fee for services provided is paid by the insurance company and not by the patient.

thromboembolism A condition in which a blood vessel is blocked by an embolus carried in the bloodstream from the site of formation of the clot.

thrombolytic agents The agents that dissolve thrombi.

thrombus An aggregation of platelets, fibrin, clotting factors, and the cellular elements of the blood attached to the interior wall of a vein or artery, sometimes occluding the lumen of a vessel.

thyroxine A hormone produced by the thyroid that increases the rate of metabolism for most cells; also called tetraiodothyronine.

ticlopidine A platelet aggregation inhibitor, used to reduce the risk of stroke. It works by preventing excessive blood clotting. Its trade name is Ticlid.

time limit The amount of time from the date of service to the date (deadline) the claim can be filed with the insurance company.

time purchase The time that the purchase order was made.

tincture An alcoholic solution prepared from vegetable materials or from chemical substances.

tine test In this test, the tuberculin antigen is injected just under the skin with a multi-pronged instrument. The antigen is located on the spikes (tines) that penetrate the skin. If positive, the skin around the injection site will be red and swollen like a mosquito bite, 48 to 72 hours after the injection. It is not as accurate as the Mantoux test.

tissue plasminogen activator (TPA) A clot-dissolving substance produced naturally by cells in the walls of blood vessels. It is also manufactured synthetically by genetic engineering techniques. TPA activates plasminogen to dissolve clots and has been used therapeutically to dissolve blood clots blocking coronary arteries.

tolerance Increasing resistance to the usual effects of an established dosage of a drug as a result of continued use.

toluene An aromatic solvent similar to xylene. It is found in many paints and removers and is considered to be a neurotoxin.

topical Pertaining to a drug that is applied to the surface of the body.

total parenteral nutrition (TPN) An intravenous feeding that supplies all of the nutrients necessary for life.

transdermal drug delivery (TDD) Pertaining to a passage through the skin. Dosage forms that release minute amounts of drug at a consistent rate.

TRICARE A federally funded comprehensive health benefits program for dependents of personnel serving in the uniformed services.

tricyclic antidepressant (TCA) A drug that inhibits the uptake of norepinephrine and serotonin in the central nervous system.

triglycerides A simple fat compound consisting of three molecules of fatty acid and glycerol. Triglycerides make up most animal and vegetable fats, and are the principal lipids in the blood, where they circulate within lipoproteins.

triiodothyronine (T_3) A hormone produced by the thyroid that increases the rate of metabolism for most cells.

troche A small, disk-shaped tablet composed of solidifying paste containing an astringent, antiseptic, or oil-based drug used for local treatment of the mouth or throat. It is held in the mouth until dissolved. Also known as a lozenge.

tuberculin A glycerinated broth culture of *Mycobacterium tuberculosis* that is evaporated and filtered. Formerly used to treat tuberculosis, tuberculin is now used chiefly for diagnostic tests.

tuberculosis A chronic granulomatous infection caused by *Mycobacterium tuberculosis*. It is generally transmitted by the inhalation or ingestion of infected droplets and usually affects the lungs.

unit-dose drug distribution system A system of drug distributions in which a copy of the physician's order is sent to the pharmacy, the pharmacist prepares individual doses of medication, and a 24-hour supply of medication is delivered to the patient care floor.

unit-of-use packaging The packaging from bulk containers into patient-specific containers.

urokinase An enzyme produced in the kidney and found in urine that is a potent plasminogen activator of the fibrinolytic system.

U.S. Pharmacopeia (USP) A database of drugs and their preparation that serves as the standard for drugs used in the United States.

uterine relaxants Drugs that inhibit the contractility of uterine smooth muscle and stop labor.

vaccination The process of immunization for prevention of diseases.

vial A small glass or plastic bottle intended to hold medicine.

vitamin An organic compound essential in small quantities for normal body functioning.

vitamin A A fat-soluble vitamin essential for skeletal growth, maintenance of normal mucosal epithelium, reproduction, and visual acuity; also known as retinol.

vitamin B complex A group of water-soluble compound vitamins.

vitamin B_1 A water-soluble, crystalline compound of the B complex; also known as thiamin. It is essential for normal metabolism and health of the cardiovascular and nervous systems.

vitamin B_2 One of the heat-stable components of the B complex; also known as riboflavin. It is involved as a coenzyme in the oxidative processes of carbohydrates, fats, and proteins.

vitamin B_3 A compound made up of two enzymes that regulate energy metabolism; also known as niacin.

vitamin B_6 A water-soluble vitamin that is part of the B complex; also known as pyridoxine. It acts as a coenzyme essential for the synthesis and breakdown of amino acids.

vitamin B_7 A water-soluble B complex vitamin that acts as a coenzyme in fatty acid production and in the oxidation of fatty acids and carbohydrates; also known as biotin.

vitamin B_9 A compound essential for cell growth and the reproduction of red blood cells; also known as folic acid or folacin.

vitamin B_{12} A water-soluble substance that is the common pharmaceutical form of vitamin B; also known as cyanocobalamin. It is involved in the metabolism of protein, fats, and carbohydrates. Vitamin B_{12} is also involved in normal blood formation and neural function.

vitamin C A water-soluble vitamin that is essential for the formation of collagen and fibroid tissue for teeth, bones, cartilage, connective tissue, and skin. Vitamin C also aids in fighting bacterial infections, bleeding gums, the tendency to bruise, nosebleeds, and anemia.

vitamin D A fat-soluble vitamin chemically related to the steroids and essential for the normal formation of bones and teeth; also known as calciferol. It is important for the absorption of calcium and phosphorus from the gastrointestinal tract.

vitamin E A fat-soluble vitamin essential for normal reproduction, muscle development, resistance of erythrocytes to hemolysis, and various other biochemical functions; also known as tocopherol.

vitamin K A group of fat-soluble vitamins known as quinones that are essential for the synthesis of prothrombin in the liver and are involved in the clotting of blood.

waiting period The period of time that an individual must wait to become eligible for insurance coverage (e.g., 30 days) before coverage commences or for a specific benefit.

want book A list of drugs and devices that routinely need to be reordered.

warfarin An oral anticoagulant agent used for the prophylaxis and treatment of thrombosis and embolism.

water A mixture of distilled water with an aromatic volatile water.

wheal An intensely itchy skin eruption larger than a hive.

xanthine derivatives A substance that is effective for relief of bronchospasm in asthma, chronic bronchitis, and emphysema.

zinc A metallic element that is an essential nutrient in the body and is used in numerous pharmaceuticals such as zinc acetate and zinc oxide.

Z-track method A method of intramuscular injection of medication in which the skin must be pulled to one side before the tissue is grasped for the injection of such medication. It is used when a drug is highly irritating to subcutaneous tissues or has the ability to permanently stain the skin.

References

American Pharmacists Association. (1999). *The pharmacy technician.* Morton/Perspective Press.

American Society of Health-System Pharmacists (1998). *Manual for pharmacy technicians* (2nd ed.). Washington, DC: Author.

Anthony, P. K. (2000). *Pharmacy technician certification—Exam review.* Albany, NY: Thomson Delmar Learning.

Ballington, D. A. (2003). *Pharmacy practice for technicians* (2nd ed.). St. Paul, MN: EMC-Paradigm.

Briggs, G. G., Freeman, R. K., & Yaffe, S. J. (2002). *Drugs in pregnancy and lactation* (6th ed.). Baltimore: Lippincott Williams & Wilkins.

Brody, T. M., Larner, J. & Minneman, K. P. (1998). *Human pharmacology—Molecular to clinical* (3rd ed.). St. Louis, MO: Mosby.

Brooks, M. L. (2002). *Exploring medical language—A student-directed approach* (5th ed.). St. Louis, MO: Mosby.

Drug facts and comparisons (58th ed.). (2004). St. Louis, MO: Facts & Comparisons.

Durgin J., & Hanan, Z. (1999). *Pharmacy practice for technicians* (2nd ed.). Albany, NY: Thomson Delmar Learning.

Fremgen, B. F. (2002). *Medical law & ethics.* Upper Saddle River, NJ: Prentice Hall.

Grajeda-Higley, L. (2000). *Understanding pharmacology—A physiologic approach.* New York: Appleton & Lange.

Grogan, J. (2001). *Pharmacy simplified—A glossary of terms.* Albany, NY: Thomson Delmar Learning.

Hitner, H., & Nagle, B. T. (2005). *Pharmacology—An introduction* (5th ed.). New York: McGraw Hill.

Holland, N., & Patrick, M. (2003). *Core concepts in pharmacology.* Upper Saddle River, NJ: Prentice Hall/PharMedia.

Issel, L. M. (2004). *Health program planning and evaluation—A practical, systematic approach for community health.* Sudbury, MA: Jones and Bartlett.

Karch, A. M. (2004). *2004 Lippincott's Nursing Drug Guide* Baltimore: Lippincott Williams & Wilkins.

Kongstvedt, P. R. (2002). *Managed care—What it is and how it works* (2nd ed.). Rockville, MD: Aspen.

McCarthy, R. L., & Schafermeyer, K. W. (2001). *Introduction to health care delivery—A primer for pharmacists* (2nd ed.). Rockville, MD: Aspen.

Moisio, M. A., & Moisio, E. W. (2002). *Medical terminology—A student-centered approach.* Albany, NY: Thomson Delmar Learning.

Newby, C. (2004). *Hospital billing using Just Claims software.* New York: McGraw Hill.

Olsen, J. L., & Patrick, A. (2000). *Medical dosage calculations* (7th ed.). Upper Saddle River, NJ: Prentice Hall Health.

Pickar, G. D. (1999). *Dosage calculations* (6th ed.). Albany, NY: Thomson Delmar Learning.

Reiss, B. S., & Evans, M. E. (2002). *Pharmacological aspects of nursing care* (6th ed.). Albany, NY: Thomson Delmar Learning.

Ross, A., Williams, S. J., & Pavlock, E. J. (1998). *Ambulatory care management* (3rd ed.). Albany, NY: Delmar/Medical Group Management Association.

Salerno, E. (1999). *Pharmacology for health professionals.* St. Louis, MO: Mosby.

Sanderson, S. M. (2001). *Computers in the medical office* (3rd ed.). New York: Glencoe/McGraw-Hill.

Saxton, D., O'Neill, N. E., & Glavinspiehs, C. (1998). *Math & meds for nurses.* Albany, NY: Thomson Delmar Learning.

Shier, D., Butler, J., & Lewis, J. (2003). *Hole's essentials of human anatomy and physiology* (8th ed.). New York: McGraw-Hill.

Smith, C. M., & Reynard, A. M. (1992). *Textbook of Pharmacology.* Philadelphia: Saunders.

Stoogenke, M. M. (2002). *The pharmacy technician* (3rd ed.). Upper Saddle River, NJ: Prentice Hall.

Thompson, J. E., & Davidow, L. (1998). *A practical guide to contemporary pharmacy practice* (2nd ed.). Baltimore: Lippincott Williams & Wilkins.

Warn, B. A., & Woodcock, E. W. (2001). *Operating policies and procedures manual for medical practices* (2nd ed.). Washington, DC: Medical Group Management Association.

Wolper, L. F. (2004). *Health care administration—Planning, implementing, and managing organized delivery systems* (4th ed.). Sudbury, MA: Jones and Bartlett.

Wong, D. L., Hockenberry-Eaton, M., Wilson, D., Winkelstein, M. L., & Schwartz, P. (2001). *Wong's Essentials of pediatric nursing* (6th ed.). St. Louis, MO: Mosby.

Woodrow, R. (2002). *Essentials of pharmacology for health occupations* (4th ed.). Albany, NY: Thomson Delmar Learning.

INDEX

A

B

I

Q

R

S

T

Practice Exams for the Pharmacy Technician

SETUP INSTRUCTIONS:

1. Insert disc into CD-ROM player. The program should start up automatically. If it does not, go to step 2.
2. From My Computer, double click the icon for the CD drive.
3. Double click the *start.exe* file to start the program.

SYSTEM REQUIREMENTS:

- Operating system: Microsoft® Windows™ 98, Me, NT 4.0, 2000, XP, or newer
- Processor: Pentium (120 MHz) processor or faster
- Memory: 24 MB
- Hard disk space: 16 MB
- Monitor: VGA-compatible color
- CD-ROM drive: 4x

Microsoft® is a registered trademark and Windows® and Windows NT® are trademarks of Microsoft Corporation.